Always Stay Young!

"*Prolonging Health* by James Williams is an excellent review of the aging processes and the various theories of aging. Most importantly, it offers practical advice on how to take care of yourself so that you may live as long and healthy a life as possible. Dr. Williams offers sensible advise regarding hormone replacement as well as sensible advise on those vitamins, minerals, herbs and metabolites that may have a positive impact on health. He also reviews those laboratory tests that will tell you how well you are doing. Well referenced and a good resource section. I really enjoyed reading it."

–Sheldon S. Hendler, Ph.D., M.D., FAIC

Also by J. E. Williams, O.M.D.

Viral Immunity

Prolonging Health

Mastering the 10 Factors of Longevity

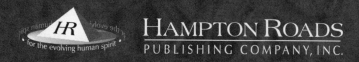

HAMPTON ROADS
PUBLISHING COMPANY, INC.

for the evolving human spirit

J. E. Williams, O.M.D.

Cover design by Steve Amarillo
Cover art © 2003 Nova Development Corporation
Medical/Scientific Illustrations by Anne L. Louque

Hampton Roads Publishing Company, Inc.
1125 Stoney Ridge Road
Charlottesville, VA 22902

434-296-2772
fax: 434-296-5096
e-mail: hrpc@hrpub.com
www.hrpub.com

If you are unable to order this book from your local
bookseller, you may order directly from the publisher.
Call 1-800-766-8009, toll-free.

Library of Congress Cataloging-in-Publication Data

Williams, J. E. (James Eugene), 1949-
Prolonging health : mastering the 10 factors of
longevity / J.E. Williams.
    p. cm.
Includes bibliographical references and index.
ISBN 1-57174-338-3 (7 x 9 TP : alk. paper)
1. Longevity. 2. Aging--Prevention. 3. Health. I.
Title.
RA776.75.W536 2003
612.6'8--dc22

2003016266

ISBN 1-57174-338-3
10 9 8 7 6 5 4 3 2 1
    •   Printed on acid-free paper in the United States

Disclaimer

This book is written as a source of information to educate the reader. It is not intended to replace medical advice or care, whether provided for by a primary care physician, a specialist, or a licensed alternative medicine medical professional. The author took a great deal of time and energy to support the information contained in this book with published documentation from scientific and clinical research; however, this research is not meant to be used as justification for any of the recommendations contained in the book. When medications are recommended, dosages are given in ranges for the average adult and are to be used as generalized guidelines only. Effects from any medication can vary a great deal from person to person and applications must be adjusted to meet individual requirements.

The author has no financial ties to any of the products, clinics, services, or medications cited in the text. Specific products and medications are recommended solely to help the reader get better results. These recommendations are not endorsements, but are given because, based on long clinical experience, they are those that the author uses for his patients. This is not to say that other products may not be equally effective. The author is not responsible if the reader does not obtain health benefits from these medications.

Neither the author nor the publisher shall be liable or responsible for any adverse effects arising from the use or application of any of the information contained herein, nor do they guarantee that everyone will benefit or be healed by these techniques and are not responsible if they are not. Please consult your doctor before beginning any new medications, diet, nutrients, or any form of health program.

Table of Contents

Dedication

To my friend and mentor, Taoist master Share K. Lew, a living example of health and happiness, and to my mother, Bernice Barbara Beauks, R.N. (retired), still strong and enthusiastic at 89.

Preface

It seems to me that we humans have strange notions of how our life should unfold. During the first half of it, we live as if we were immortal; then our own mortality overshadows all of the second half when the permanence of death, the finality of closing one's eyes forever, can be incomprehensible and frightening. Two emotions, wonder and fear, appear to control our desire to live forever—the one, to experience life at its best and to its fullest; the other, to avoid death at all cost. Both are archetypal driving forces in the search for longevity and immortality—an endeavor in which humans have engaged since time immemorial.

However, the nature of this perennial quest has changed in recent times. Modern longevity practices have taken on new meaning for Baby Boomers and the affluent aging population. An intensity of purpose to forestall what once was considered inevitable has fostered an explosion of life-extension regimens, anti-aging medical clinics, magazines and scientific journals on aging, and longevity centers.

Currently, we are in the mid-stage of an anti-aging and longevity revolution that started several decades ago with the natural health and fitness movement. It gained momentum after the introduction of human growth hormone injections as a rejuvenation medication in the late 1980s, and will likely not only continue well into the twenty-first century, but will undoubtedly accelerate as new biomedical technologies are discovered and made available to the public and doctors.

Postmodern anti-aging practices will be driven by genomics (the science of genetics and its practical application in medicine) and targeted pharmaceutical therapies, as well as by still undreamed of bioelectric devices that will promote the body's ability to repair and heal itself. In addition, specialized nutraceuticals (medicinal substances derived from natural sources but prepared by pharmaceutical standards into concentrated extracts, making them more therapeutically active), botanical medicines, and advanced forms of vitamins, minerals, amino acids, enzymes, and other natural products will be available. New advances in hormone therapies will greatly enhance the outcome of anti-aging programs and make people look and feel younger.

The future of anti-aging technologies could be startling.

To illustrate one such futuristic scenario, imagine a boy who looks 13 years old, sitting in front of you. His body is perfectly symmetrical and he has the smooth facial skin of an adolescent before beginning to shave. When he stands to greet you, you notice that he is tall for his age and slightly more muscular than the average teenager. You shake hands, and upon starting up a conversation, immediately recognize that he is unusually bright, in fact, much smarter than anyone you've ever met.

In the course of talking, you find out that what at first sounded like historical references to places and times were actual events he experienced over 150 years ago. During that time span, he earned three doctoral degrees, each in a different field, wrote 80 books, learned seven languages, outlived all of his doctors, and witnessed unparalleled changes in political systems, cultures, and the environment. Stunned, you step back and observe thin tubes and wires under his shirt connected to a small device on his belt.

You've just had an encounter with one of the first postmodern immortals. Impossible? Not according to Stanley Shostak, Ph.D., associate professor of biological sciences at the University of Pittsburgh and the author of *Becoming Immortal* (Shostak 2002).

To construct such a creature, according to Shostak, requires that molecular engineers start with a cloned individual genetically selected for perfect physical traits and the absence of genes for hereditary diseases and that he undergo a medical procedure that makes him permanently a juvenile. This guarantees that he'll stay young, provided that he has a continual supply of new stem cells (like those in your skin that divide without limit). Artificially renewing tissues may perpetuate youth, but along with a stem cell generator, our postmodern man requires a pump. This is necessary to release hormones, and it serves as an extra endocrine organ. In addition, this youth would need antibiotics and other drugs to prevent infections and maintain physiological function.

Theoretically, biotechnological advances in the near future will be capable of creating such an individual—the first postmodern human. The appearance of such an individual would signal the "posthuman stage of history" as Francis Fukuyama, Ph.D., a member of the President's Council on Bioethics, describes it in his book *Our Posthuman Future: Consequences of the Biotechnology Revolution* (Fukuyama 2002).

However, the use of this Pandora's box of possibility, though technologically feasible, raises numerous biological and ethical questions. Once we head down the road of humans by human design, will we gradually cease to be who we are? In a world of ever-decreasing natural resources and declining biodiversity, will we become cloned versions bearing less of what we once were—wild, free, unpredictable, and creative individuals—and being instead cybergenetic beings without emotional unpredictability and therefore spiritually sterile? Questions such as these make us think about our very essence as humans and the elusive truths philosophers have struggled with for centuries.

We are closer today to a genetically modified human than you might think. Human enhancement already occurs in plastic surgery, pharmacological manipulation of mood and certain physical functions such as heart rate and rhythm. Human cloning, though banned in many countries, will undoubtedly take place experimentally in others. Will we wake up in time and choose the high road, content with the natural course of life, extended to perhaps age 95 but lived out in good health? So if we could live longer in optimal health with the help of natural medicines, would we choose to?

This book is not about cloning, nor an artificially induced extension of life. It is about *natural longevity*—how to remain in good health with a sound mind for a long time. I leave the pursuit of technologically enhanced immortality for other, hopefully wiser generations. Technology should be the servant of humanity, not the other way around as it unfortunately is now.

Though decoding the human genome, accomplished in 2000, may be the scientific high point of our times, in the twenty-first century the quest for a long and healthy life is rapidly becoming the most important pursuit of an expanding and aging population. As more people live longer, they want to stay healthy and active into their later years. Many are rejecting the former myths of aging where to be elderly meant frailty and mental feebleness, or worse, to have age-related diseases and their complications, such as Alzheimer's, cancer, stroke, congestive heart failure, and diabetes. The senior citizens of tomorrow will be healthier, use more natural medicines, and lead productive and creative lives well into their eighties and nineties. This is not surprising given the statistics.

Americans are aging at an astonishing rate, and so are people in the rest of the world. In the industrialized countries, life expectancy has increased by 31 years in the last century—from 46 in 1900 to 77 in 1998—and the average age of the world's population is continuing to increase each year. At the time of America's declaration of independence in 1776, the average life expectancy was 35 years. By 2020, one in six Americans will be over 65, and by 2050 one of every three people on Earth will be over 60. Women will continue to outlive men; in fact, half of all girls born in 2000 are predicted to live to see the twenty-second century. If you are now between 45 and 75, are reasonably healthy, free of a major disease, and have no major accidents, you have a high probability of living to between 85 and 100, and some to 110 or even older. It is likely that if you are now younger than 45, you will live to 100, and perhaps to 120, or older.

So what if we are living longer? Current reports show that older people have more disease, spend more time at the doctor's, and that as they become increasingly feeble many require full-time nursing care. However, the idea presented in this book is not just to live longer, but to have *good health* for the *longest* amount of time. The goal is prolonging health.

So what does the natural postmodern healthy individual look like?

In his book *Spontaneous Healing*, Andrew Weil puts it nicely, "You would not contract heart disease or cancer in middle age, be crippled by arthritis in later life, or lose your mind to premature senility" (Weil 1995).

For those who choose not to use technological enhancement for pseudo-immortality, for which the cost would be out of reach except for the richest, what is the best way to achieve a healthy older age? In essence, the best way is to *prolong* your health as long as possible. People have done this, and it can be accomplished in a natural manner without drugs or technology. However, on the matter of *how* to optimize one's vitality and energy, and retain mental ability, is where the current debate begins. Can antioxidants, hormones, herbal medications, and other substances increase vigor and extend life? An ever-increasing volume of aging and longevity research data suggests that they can, and in this book I discuss the most important of these substances and what they can do to prolong your health and extend your life span.

In researching this book, I found that no gerontologist or doctor of anti-aging medicine had all of the answers, though many proclaim they have. In its best form, I call this the "rule of 100/10," when someone is 100 percent right about only 10 percent of the issue. At its worst, it is simply misleading and in some cases dangerous because you could be basing your program on only a small part of the solution. I also found several interesting things.

First, many people have lived to be over 100 without the assistance of science or medicine. Second, though there is a significant amount of research on the subject of longevity, there is no consensus among the experts on why we age, why some people live longer than others, and what is the best way to extend life. Third, there is no integrated theory of aging, and no comprehensive manner in which to approach anti-aging and longevity therapies, making it a complicated and difficult endeavor to follow.

To help people understand the overwhelming amount of information on aging, I took on the challenge of distilling the most significant information in this field into a coherent and comprehensive manual and organizing this knowledge into ten longevity factors and four strategies for prolonging health and extending the natural life span.

My own interest in longevity started 35 years ago, well before my 20-year career began as a doctor of Oriental medicine and naturopathic physician. One brilliant late winter day in the Siberian Eskimo village of Savoong, on St. Lawrence Island in the Bering Sea just below the Arctic Circle, where I lived with a traditional Eskimo family in 1967–1968, I went to visit Koviq, one of the village elders. Koviq was 82 years old and a quiet man about five feet tall, with a thin white beard, broad shoulders, erect posture, and powerful legs. He had a wealth of knowledge of traditional customs and a vivid memory of details from Eskimo life before the Cold War between the Soviet Union and the United States separated his people from relatives on the Siberian mainland. I frequently visited him to listen to his stories. However, on that day, he was not home.

Even though the island was still snow-covered, the days were beginning to lengthen and the way the sunlight reflected off the snow provided ten hours of daylight. Koviq's great-grandnephew informed me that his uncle was out for a walk. Raising his hand he pointed to where Koviq was. Following his fingertip beyond the village boundaries, across the shore ice, and along a series of high cliffs to the southeast was a small dark spot moving slowly across the snowfield. Koviq, still vigorous in his eighties, was out for an eight-mile walk on snowshoes. His routine, a feat beyond my New England capabilities, inspired me from that day forward to emulate him, and I promised myself that I would be as healthy and strong as he when I reached his age.

By 1972, I was intensively engaged in esoteric Taoist and yogic longevity methods. Though that was more than 30 years ago, I recall the glacial streams on Mount Rainier, a silent volcano south of Seattle, Washington, the penetrating cold, and the piercing air scented with the smell of pine from giant Douglas fir trees. Practicing meditation and breathing techniques in nature far from urban areas produced strength and health, but I needed more training, so I returned to college to study biology and continued independently to study herbology and Eastern methods of healing.

Then in 1978, while I was studying under the world-renowned natural healer Bernard Jensen, D.C., N.D. (1908–2001), my interest in longevity was kindled further. In his book *World Keys to Health and Long Life*, Dr. Jensen described the attributes that he believed contribute to longevity. He detailed his travels to Hunza and other areas of the world in search of the secrets of health and longevity, and summarized his research into easily practiced keys. This work convinced me that the pursuit of rejuvenation and longevity practices was worthy of all of my professional intent. Dr. Jensen himself was an example of health in older age. A short man with the intensity of an army of men, even in his seventies and eighties his skin was smooth and radiant, and he often worked 12 to 14 hours a day with his office and editorial assistants, writing and publishing books on natural health.

Another turning point occurred for me in my quest for longevity when in 1981 I was introduced to the Taoist Sifu Share K. Lew by my Chinese medicine teacher, Dr. York Why Loo. After Dr. Loo passed away in 1989, Sifu Lew guided me deeper in the principles of Taoism. *Sifu* is the Chinese term for "teacher."

Now in his eighties, Sifu Lew is a great example of radiating physical and mental health, and I often asked him about the essential teachings of Taoism. Repeatedly, he reminded me, "Follow the way of nature; don't force anything."

A picture of Sifu Lew at age 80 hangs in my office. His hair is full and black, there are no wrinkles on his face, and he has a thin dark mustache and long beard. One day, a patient of mine, an athletic Scotsman, age 56, commented, "What I want to know is how come at age 80 he looks younger than me?"

"You are looking at the secrets of longevity in action," I replied.

Since then, I have pursued with great passion the science of life extension as well as the natural health practices that foster longevity. I have practiced them on myself and on my patients, many of whom you'll meet in this book. The benefits of a natural longevity program to prolong your health speak for themselves: freedom from degenerative disease, increased energy, youthful appearance, sexual vigor, and good memory.

Based upon my experiences and education in natural medicine, my patients' successes in overcoming illness, achieving optimal health, and extending their life span, and the ever-growing body of scientific evidence, one thing is certain: the better your health, the longer you will live, and live well. A Baby Boomer myself, I want to remain professionally, physically, and intellectually active for as long as possible, and I've met many others who have the same wish. I wrote this book for those of us hitting our fifties who don't want to end up like most of our parents—undergoing coronary bypass surgery, suffering strokes, dealing with the consequences of obesity and Type II diabetes, getting Alzheimer's—and who prefer a natural approach to managing the consequences of aging.

To learn more about the science of aging and longevity, I've attended several international scientific symposiums on aging, including the Sixth International Symposium on the Neurobiology and Neuroendocrinology of

> *Based upon my experiences and education in natural medicine, my patients' successes in overcoming illness, achieving optimal health, and extending their life span, and the ever-growing body of scientific evidence, one thing is certain: the better your health, the longer you will live, and live well.*

Aging in Bregenz, Austria, and the Buck Institute Symposium 2002 on Neuroendocrine Systems and Life Span Determination at America's premier private institute on aging in Novato, California. I have had valuable interactions with several international research groups on the prevention of aging, notably the St. Petersburg Institute of Bioregulation and Gerontology in St. Petersburg, Russia.

This book constitutes the results of a lifetime of personal and clinical practice, as well as extensive investigation and inquiry. It also introduces, summarizes, and draws upon the achievements of many others in the field of human aging. These include Linus Pauling, Bernard Strehler, Nathan Shock, and George C. Williams, among many others. Thanks in particular go to the following physicians for elucidating the clinical application of hormone therapy and laboratory evaluation: Thierry Hertoghe, M.D., of Brussels, Belgium; James Webber, M.D., of San Diego, California; and Brett Jacques, N.D., associated with AAL Laboratories in Irvine, California. A number of scientists provided inspiration and generously provided information during the writing of this book. These comprise a very long list that most notably includes Andrzej Bartke, Ph.D., of Southern Illinois Carbondale; William E. Sonntag, Ph.D., at Wake Forest University School of Medicine, Winston-Salem, North Carolina; Steve N. Austad, Ph.D., from the University of Idaho; Bret S. Weinstein, Ph.D., of the University of Michigan; and Michael R. Rose, Ph.D., of the University of California at Irvine. Most of us in the functional and integrative medical field owe a great deal to Jeffrey Bland, Ph.D., who illuminated the path of nutritional neuroendocrinology and positive genetic expression well before it was recognized as a valid clinical endeavor.

Others I wish to thank include Chef Everett Williams of Lifetime Health and Nutrition; Tony Montagne of Advanced Training in San Diego, California; Michael Garrett of Bikram's College of India; Tim Miller of the Ashtanga Yoga Center in Encinitas, California, for keeping me fit and flexible; and Nandu Menon, M.S., R.P.T. (the tantric priest Amarananda Bhairavan), for his advice on the physiology of yoga.

The manuscript has been reviewed by a number of people, who've all offered solutions to its many deficiencies. In particular, I'd like to thank Leon Seltzer, Ph.D., for his generous assistance in fine-tuning it, and my editor, Richard Leviton, for his confidence in the book and for turning it into a polished work. Aging and longevity is an extensive subject to tackle in a single book. Any deficiencies that remain are solely due to my own limitations, and the immensity of the subject.

Introduction

Prolonging Health is a strategic guide to help you design a comprehensive, safe, and effective program to prevent disease, preserve and extend your health, and live longer. It combines well-documented, scientific, and proven natural health methods into a new approach to aging, which I call the clinical science of integrative longevity medicine. Though many anti-aging therapies require medical assistance, with the guidance found in this book you can use most of them safely and effectively without a doctor.

I call this book *Prolonging Health* because the longer we remain healthy, the better our chances are of living longer. By "prolonging health," I mean the extension of the natural vibrant state of the body, which is one of mental, emotional, and physical wellness, and this allows you to fulfill your purpose in life and to live happily and healthily to an advanced age.

The life-transforming program described in this book will improve the way you live and greatly enhance the quality of your health during the second half of your life. It will help prevent and reverse age-related degenerative diseases, prevent cancer, increase your vitality and sexuality, elevate your mood, and make you look and feel younger. The secret to living long is to live well, and to live well you have to prevent disease, maintain an attitude that fosters contentment

and happiness, and prolong your health. Prolonging health is the key to successful aging.

Prolonging health is a serious and complex matter. In an article printed in *Time* magazine in January of 2002 (Kluger 2002), senior staff writer Jeffrey Kluger wrote, "For scientists and physicians, there has been no goal more seductive than extending human life, and none that has been harder to achieve." Not only is it a complicated clinical field, but as more people take the practice of prolonging health into their own hands, the greater the necessity for accurate information becomes. I've attempted to provide the keys to help you achieve your goal of living a long and healthy life.

Let's clarify some more of the commonly used terms in the book including anti-aging, longevity, life extension, prolongevity.

Anti-aging: This term was first coined by Sheldon Hendler, Ph.D., M.D., in his book *The Complete Guide to Anti-Aging Nutrients* (Hendler 1985). Later it was popularized by Ronald Klatz, D.O., the cofounder of the American Academy of Anti-Aging Medicine, and it caught the public imagination in the late 1990s. However, the word "anti-aging" implies methods that actually reverse or prevent aging. This is misleading, as there is no proven way to effectively and permanently reverse or stop aging. Therefore the term itself is scientifically incorrect. Instead of anti-aging, the term preferred by scientists who study aging is anti-senescence, which is the specific process by which biological age, the physical characteristics and laboratory biomarkers that define aging, is lowered. The net effect, of course, is that you look and feel younger.

Longevity: Anti-aging and longevity are often used as synonyms, but they are not the same. Longevity is the attainment of a long life, the process of achieving a long, healthy, normal life span. It suggests achieving your maximum life span in good health. Longevity is the term preferred by Asian and most European researchers, whereas anti-aging is mainly used in America, specifically by doctors practicing anti-aging medicine. In this book, I use the terms anti-senescence and longevity.

Anti-aging Medicine: This refers to the medical practice of preventing the degenerative diseases of aging and the promotion of longevity. However, since the term anti-aging itself is scientifically inaccurate, I prefer to call the medical approaches described in this book integrative longevity medicine. This is a completely new frontier in health care, where advanced scientific discoveries meet clinical medicine in an integrated fashion to emphasize natural medications over drugs, and where an informed patient with a cooperative physician co-creates a program that fosters a long life free from disease, enabling one to express one's full potential.

Complementary Medicine: Susan Aldridge, Ph.D., a British science writer says "Complementary medicine could help older people function at a higher cognitive, physical, psychosocial, and spiritual level"(Aldridge 2001). In England, combining the best of alternative and traditional medical therapies is called complementary medicine, or sometimes complementary and alternative medicine (CAM).

Life Extension and Prolongevity: These terms were popularized by Durk Pearson and Sandy Shaw, the authors of *Life Extension: A Practical Scientific Approach* (Pearson 1982). They suggest the proactive involvement of an individual in promoting longevity through the practice of methods such as taking vitamins and minerals, and using hormones to extend life span. Those who follow such practices are called life extensionists.

How to Use This Book

A considerable number of natural medicines that help prevent and reverse the common diseases and degenerative changes that occur during aging are discussed in this book. Using them wisely may not only create a healthier life for you, but may also promote disease-free longevity. To avoid the frailty associated with typical aging and to lead an active, healthy life, read the information in this book carefully and study it well. It may save your life and add healthy years to it.

This book provides instructions on how to navigate the changes that accompany aging and provides a profile of healthy aging based on three fundamental premises:

1. A disease-free long life is possible, with a healthy life span of at least 95, and possibly 120 to 150 years.

2. Long-life genes are important, but healthy aging depends mostly on a lifestyle and environment that promote longevity.

3. Prolonging health throughout life minimizes the effects of aging.

In order to prolong your health and achieve longevity, specific physiologic directives need to be followed:

- Prolong health by preventing degenerative and genetically caused disease.

- Improve quality of life by relieving depression, improving strength, increasing energy, instilling enthusiasm, and maintaining independence in later life.

- Reverse premature aging and lower your biological age.

- Achieve maximum life span.

The book is divided into two parts, and each covers several aspects of a complete plan for prolonging health and extending your life span. I call this mastering the factors of longevity. So that you can manage your program safely, I also inform you about the risks involved in longevity practices and any possible adverse reactions from medications.

Part 1 lays the foundation for understanding the aging process. I discuss the aging process in detail and explain how to evaluate the influences of aging on your body. I also explain the main theories of aging and the perspective of evolutionary biology, which helps in understanding the bigger picture about human aging. I guide you through common tests you can do on your own to determine the impact age has on your body. Obtaining biochemical information on how well you are aging, what your hormone levels are, and what your risks are for degenerative diseases is an important aspect of a comprehensive longevity program. So I outline a number of specialized laboratory tests that provide information used to determine your health and aging status.

Aging is a fascinating study, and learning more about how we age and how age-related changes are measured makes the aging process less mysterious. This understanding helps us formulate a plan to prevent many of the unpleasant changes that occur with aging and to promote longevity.

Part 2 gives advice about how to prolong your health. I discuss ten important factors that influence aging, cause the degenerative diseases associated with aging, shorten our life span, and rob us of our health. All of these aging factors are *modifiable* with proper diet, healthy lifestyle, nutritional supplementation, natural hormones, adaptogenic herbs, and other specialized prolongevity medications—natural substances that promote health and longevity. By *modifiable* I mean two things.

First, our environment (diet, lifestyle, medications, stressors, where we live, and other factors) exerts a positive or negative influence on our health. To prevent disease and achieve health, it's necessary to emphasize positive environmental influences and minimize negative ones like stress. By emphasizing positive influences, we prolong our health as we age, and therefore live longer and healthier.

Second, through positive environmental factors we not only prevent disease, but we influence our genes. For example, if you are genetically prone to heart disease and you reduce your stress, lower your cholesterol by eating a healthy diet rich in green leafy vegetables and low in saturated fats, as found in processed spreads, and take extra vitamin E—all positive environmental factors—you lower your risk for a heart attack or stroke because all of these improve how your genes work. In addition, if you take specific natural medications such as coenzyme Q10, you can even reverse the underlying causes of cardiovascular disease.

In this case, then, you prevent cardiovascular disease by controlling what is known as gene expression—the hereditary potential carried inside your genetic material. I also explain how you take this concept a step further by using hormones and natural medicines to enhance longevity genetic potential.

The ten modifiable aging factors presented in *Prolonging Health* are:

Modifiable Aging Factor 1: Oxidative Damage. I discuss the cellular effects of aging caused by the utilization of oxygen in our body, and how to use antioxidants to prevent the major degenerative diseases of aging.

Modifiable Aging Factor 2: Genetic Damage. I explain how to guard your genome (your total gene package) with DNA repair medications.

Modifiable Aging Factor 3: Impaired Detoxification. I outline a plan to renew your cells and tissues with detoxification therapies.

Modifiable Aging Factor 4: Insulin Resistance. I discuss why our ability to utilize glucose (blood sugar) falters as we age and how it controls the rate at which we age, and I show how to improve glucose tolerance and insulin sensitivity.

Modifiable Aging Factor 5: Impaired Protein Synthesis and Glycation. I discuss the importance of proteins in building our body and their roles in preventing aging, and I show how to reverse the end products of protein glycation. Protein glycation is the result of a chemical reaction between proteins and sugar that forms abnormal (damaged) proteins.

Modifiable Aging Factor 6: Chronic Inflammation. I explain the reason chronic inflammation contributes to the degenerative diseases of aging and provide advice on how to reduce accelerated inflammation.

Modifiable Aging Factor 7: Impaired Cardiovascular Function and Sticky Blood. I discuss the importance of a strong heart and healthy blood circulation, and explain how to strengthen your heart and improve your blood flow.

Modifiable Aging Factor 8: Declining Hormone Function. Improving your hormone levels offers some of the greatest health benefits during aging. I explain how maintaining high levels of key hormones helps to prolong health and discuss how to restore optimal hormone levels.

Modifiable Aging Factor 9: Immune System Decline. I discuss how to prevent immunosenescence, the progressive age-related weakening of your immune system. I also describe numerous natural medicines to enhance your immune system and tell you how to prevent the common viral and bacterial infections that occur during aging.

Modifiable Aging Factor 10: Neurodegeneration. I explain how to revitalize your aging brain. I discuss neuroregeneration and explain how to use natural medications to improve memory and cognition.

Until now, most anti-aging books were too general and simplistic or too narrowly focused, such as those on only human growth hormone. These books suggest that taking one substance alone will provide the answer to reversing aging. This, of course, is not how the body or any biological system works. I contend that a comprehensive plan that follows a deeper understanding of biological principles plus the use of medications that work synergistically is a better, more effective approach.

In *Prolonging Health,* I discuss the ten modifiable factors of longevity and provide five comprehensive strategies for mastering each of these factors to prolong your health and promote a maximum life span.

The five longevity strategies are:

Longevity Strategy I—Restore Homeostasis: I explain how to restore your body's physiological balance (called homeostasis) by resetting your body's biological clock; rehydrating your body's fluids and replacing mineral stores called electrolytes; reenergizing your metabolism; rebuilding the functional reserves of your organs; and neutralizing stress. All of these are based on lifestyle and are thus environmental factors that influence aging.

Longevity Strategy II—Eat for Longevity: I present the most important dietary principles for the prevention of disease and the promotion of healthy aging. I list special longevity foods and give sample recipes.

Longevity Strategy III—Practice Periodic Calorie Restriction: I discuss the research on calorie restriction and how it promotes health and longevity. I outline how to practice periodic calorie restriction.

Longevity Strategy IV—Exercise for Maximum Longevity: I introduce five key aspects of exercise. These are balance, flexibility, core strength, muscle mass and strength, and cardiovascular fitness.

Longevity Strategy V—Use Life-Extending Nutritional Supplements: I out-line a comprehensive nutraceutical plan to prevent and reverse the degenerative diseases of aging, prevent cancer, and achieve maximum life span. These substances have specific purposes in the body and are necessary for longevity. They include a multivitamin and mineral, antioxidants, calcium, essential fatty acids, digestive enzymes, and longevity nutraceuticals.

In an epilogue, I discuss the importance of spirituality in later life and touch upon the quest for immortality. In the appendices, I provide resource lists and other useful information to help you to prolong your health and slow the aging process.

PART I

The Process of Aging and How to Determine Your Aging Status

"The first quarter century of your life is spent under the cloud of being too young for things, while the last quarter century would normally be shadowed by the still darker cloud of being too old for things."

—James Hilton, in *Lost Horizons*

"Ageing seems to be the only available way to live a long time."

—Daniel-François-Esprit Auber (1782–1871), French composer

Introduction to Part I: Aging and Anti-Aging

Aging has been defined as "an irreversible, time-dependent, functional decline that converts healthy adults into frail ones, with reduced capacity to adjust to everyday stresses, and increasing vulnerability to most diseases, and to death" (Kamel 2000). This definition coincides with the accepted medical belief that aging itself displays symptoms of disease and that as people live longer they experience more of the so-called "age-related" diseases such as heart disease, stroke, arthritis, Alzheimer's disease, Parkinson's disease, osteoporosis, and cancer, all which require increasing degrees of medical and pharmaceutical intervention.

But is aging really a disease or is it a natural process experienced by all living organisms, and do these diseases *inevitably* accompany aging or are they better viewed as late-onset conditions caused by other reasons and not induced by aging?

Three different camps have set up to answer these questions: scientists who study aging, conventional medical doctors, and doctors who practice anti-aging medicine. Scientists inform us that aging is a biological process, not a disease, and is controlled by basic biochemical and genetic mechanisms that can be studied and eventually understood. Conventional medical doctors also tell us that

aging is not a disease, but are entrenched in the belief that degenerative diseases are inevitable during aging and require drugs and surgery. Anti-aging doctors would have us believe that aging is a disease that is treatable with hormones and drugs. Which camp is correct?

Most of the diseases associated with aging develop gradually over a long period of time, and often do not show symptoms until the condition is well established in the body. They start as functional disorders and only in their end-stages become organic diseases. Functional diseases are those that affect physiological activity, as when your blood pressure becomes unstable or rises inappropriately, while organic diseases are those with cellular and tissues changes, such as when high blood pressure leads to a stroke where brain cells are destroyed.

Also, all of these diseases can occur even in middle-aged or younger individuals, and though more frequent in later life they are not exclusively confined to people above the age of 65. Therefore, though aging involves both functional and organic changes, it cannot be medically defined as a disease, and there is no official diagnostic code for it. In light of that, it is more accurate, though less descriptive, to call the degenerative diseases associated with aging delayed-onset diseases rather than age-related. This is because they have a slow fuse and develop gradually over a long period of time, often several decades, only appearing when we are older. They are not associated exclusively with aging nor do they occur in everybody when they age.

Some medical doctors would disagree. Many of the doctors who practice anti-aging medicine, a style of medical practice that emphasizes using hormone therapies to treat the symptoms of aging, deem aging itself a curable disease. This, of course, is not the case. No

Whether aging is a disease or not doesn't change our goals, which are healthy disease-free aging, the prevention of unhealthy disease-ridden aging, prolonging health, and achieving our maximum life span potential. Essentially, that is what this book is about—successful aging through prolonging health—and that is why prevention is the best medicine for most of the diseases associated with aging.

medical doctor has ever stopped aging or prevented it from occurring with the use of drugs.

Though the aging *process* itself is unavoidable, the *combination* of the delayed-onset degenerative diseases and aging is not only unnatural and unnecessary, but deadly. It robs us of vitality, causes considerable pain and dysfunction, costs much time and money for treatment, and shortens our life span. For the most part, these degenerative delayed-onset diseases are *indicators* of unhealthy aging—*effects*, not causes. In fact, they are mostly caused by unhealthy lifestyle choices, improper nutrition, chronic exposure to toxic

environmental chemicals in our food, water, and air, and the unnecessary overuse of pharmaceutical drugs. The stress of modern life also contributes considerably to the development of many of these diseases. In other words, they are largely environmentally induced rather than spontaneously arising during aging.

That is not to say that genetics don't play a critical role, because heredity is a significant factor in what type of disease we might develop. There is the exception of rare genetic diseases such as Hutchinson-Gilford Progeria Syndrome, a condition that accelerates the aging process to about seven times the normal rate, creating symptoms in children associated only with advanced aging. However, heredity comprises your genetic tendencies or predisposition, but it does not predetermine or doom you to unavoidable events that automatically end in disease and decrepitude.

In fact, there is no consensus among researchers as to how much of aging is genetic and how much is environmentally induced. Remember as you read this book that these are genetic *tendencies*, not fixed rules. By implementing the information in this book, you can start to prevent their negative expression and see how to manifest your optimal genetic patterns to prolong health and foster longevity.

Whether aging is a disease or not doesn't change our goals, which are healthy disease-free aging, the prevention of unhealthy disease-ridden aging, prolonging health, and achieving our maximum life span potential. Essentially, that is what this book is about—successful aging through prolonging health—and that is why prevention is the best medicine for most of the diseases associated with aging. It is also why natural medicine is better for their treatment than pharmaceutical drugs. Of course, modern medicine is great at lifesaving intervention, but to actually reverse the disease process, natural therapies hold the most promise.

As we begin the first part of the book, I'd like to introduce you to two of my patients who are examples of healthy natural aging. These two individuals demonstrate just how far a healthy lifestyle and good genes can take us.

When Maurine, an 82-year-old retired dance teacher, first came to see me, she was dressed in an elegant gray outfit. Her long silver hair, tied behind her head, was full and thick. I immediately recognized that this woman was someone to pay attention to. Sitting erect in her chair opposite me, my small writing table between us, she described her complaints, which were numbness in her feet and legs, lack of balance, and fatigue. She told me that all of these had been slowly progressing for about five years, and that before that she had had no health complaints. On the contrary, she was very active with dancing and yoga classes several times weekly, and she walked daily.

"My doctors say there is nothing wrong with me," she told me. Upon reviewing her blood chemistry tests and the other laboratory work she brought with her, I saw that she did indeed look good on paper.

After I conducted a physical examination, we discussed her case, and then I asked her, "What do you want to get out of this visit and working with me?"

Maurine said, "Doctor Williams, if I can have another five to eight years of healthy and active living, I'll be happy."

I told her that, based upon my examination and her medical history, there was nothing about her condition that should prevent her from reaching her goal. However, something was causing her symptoms and further tests were necessary to find exactly what that might be. I referred her to several specialists, ordered additional blood testing including hormone levels, obtained a magnetic resonance imaging (MRI) of her spinal column and a computerized tomography (CT) of her heart and cardiac blood vessels, and did a bone density study. After all of these tests, I reviewed my clinical impressions with her, describing how arthritis had affected the bones in her spine, how low hormone levels cause fatigue and reduce the body's ability to regenerate itself, and why it was important to effectively manage her blood sugar levels.

In cooperation with her internist, Maurine started a regimen of low-dose human growth hormone therapy, weekly vitamin B_{12} injections, and a nutritional supplement plan. She also began receiving weekly chiropractic adjustments and acupuncture treatments for her back and neck pain. In only a few weeks she felt remarkably better, without fatigue, and the lack of balance cleared up.

My second patient, Ted, didn't like to be referred to as "retired," though when I first met him he had sold his successful chain of restaurants and was working part-time as a consultant to businesses in locations as far away as Shanghai, China, and Michoacan, Mexico. At 68, he devoted his life to international peace causes and the promotion of organic farming. When he was 70, he met with Fidel Castro in Havana to discuss ways to market organic food products, and when he was 72, he returned to Cuba as a keynote speaker at an international symposium on sustainable economies.

Just after that, Ted came in for an office visit to discuss how I might optimize his already good health. Like Maurine, he wanted to extend his healthy and active years as much as possible. Also like Maurine, he preferred the natural healing approach and was suspicious of the allopathic model that used several pharmaceutical drugs at a time to treat conditions that commonly occur during aging. After laboratory tests on Ted, I found that his DHEA and growth hormone levels were low, and started him on a program to enhance his hormone function. This included DHEA, herbal rejuvenation medications such as ginseng, low-dose growth hormone injections, and a complete nutritional supplementation plan. The results were beyond what I expected. In a matter of weeks, he was feeling better than he had in 20 years, and was so active that his office staff, family, and friends, most of whom were half his age, could not keep up with him.

Granted, both of these people are not your average overweight, junk-food-eating elderly American. However, they demonstrate that people can live long, active, disease-free lives well into their seventies and beyond, and they show how with the addition of a well-designed longevity plan, each person improved their health and vitality to levels they hadn't experienced in 15 or more years. Maurine and Ted are still active, vigorous, older people with new interests and projects. In fact, Ted recently finished building a custom home in one of the world's most beautiful locations near the southern tip of Baja California in Mexico.

Models of healthy aging not only exist among individuals, but are also present in groups of people such as the Okinawans, the world's longest-lived and healthiest people. Okinawans have 80 percent fewer heart attacks than Americans, 80 percent less breast and prostate cancer, and 8 percent higher bone density at the hip and 13 percent higher in the lumbar spine. Twice as many Americans as Okinawans suffer from Alzheimer's dementia (Willcox 2001).

What is their secret? They have learned to live in harmony with their environment and to maximize their genetic potential through a healthy lifestyle and diet. In this book, you will learn how the Okinawans preserve their health

and attain longevity, as well as other longevity secrets from many parts of the world.

We begin our exploration of how to prolong health by discussing why we age and what changes occur during the aging process. In chapters 1–3, I present concepts to help you understand the complex changes that occur with aging. These concepts are based upon current scientific theories of aging; the evolutionary view of aging and why it will change the way we look at aging in the future; the concept of "aging zones" and an "aging axis point" and why it is crucial for you to know this in order to be successful in your *Prolonging Health* program; and the different effective methods used to extend life. In chapters 4 and 5, I discuss how you can assess the effects of aging on you, including detailed descriptions of laboratory tests that are used to evaluate diseases associated with aging and the effects of aging on your body.

Specificity of medical knowledge about the *individual* is a key component of anti-aging medicine and the *Prolonging Health* program. Not all of the tests covered in these chapters are necessary. However, the ones I recommend are valuable and important in assessing your aging status, defining early stages of degenerative diseases, and evaluating progress of your program. They can be expensive and your medical insurance may not cover the costs for these tests. But how much is your health and the chance to prolong your health to the age of 100 or more worth to you?

In chapter 6, I summarize the material discussed in part 1 and explain how to determine how well you are aging by determining your age-point. This is the guiding point of your entire program. If you are aging rapidly, you must reverse the aging trend and return to you individual age-point. If you are at your age-point, you must practice the *Prolonging Health* recommendations to remain there.

1 Why We Age

Though there are many different theories on aging, the experts agree that maintaining wellness into advanced age prevents disease and promotes longevity. Successful natural aging is defined by the ability to live a healthy, happy, and productive life into the eighth or even tenth decade. But effectively increasing longevity requires several components. Of course, there's no underestimating the importance of genetics, though experts disagree on how much one's health depends on having good genes—ranging from 10 to 90 percent (hardly a precise science). Still, following a healthy lifestyle is critical.

L. Stephen Coles, M.D., Ph.D., director of the Los Angeles Gerontology Research Group at the University of California, Los Angeles, splits the difference at 50 percent for genetics and 50 percent for environmental influences (Coles 2001). Diana Schwarzbein, M.D., an endocrinologist practicing in Santa Barbara, California, and the author of *The Schwarzbein Principle*, an excellent book on diet and hormone health, suggests that 90 percent of the causes of aging are environmental (Schwarzbein 2002).

There are many reasons for this lack of consensus. One of them is called *pleiotrophy*, a term introduced by the American evolutionary biologist George C. Williams (Williams 1957), that describes the characteristic of genes to change function, in the process altering the messages they send to cells—thus changing cellular structure and function according to different environmental pressures. This ability of genes to alter cell function suggests just one of the difficulties in calculating the effects of genes on cells. Therefore, the debate among scientists goes on: Do genes program aging, or is aging caused by environmental pressures?

Actually, aging cannot be reduced to any specific percentage of genetic influence, as each part of the body has its own genetic predisposition; and though it appears that we age overall at the same rate, different parts of our body age differently and at different times during our life. Also, genetic and environmental influences—as we will see throughout this book—interact with one another. However, for the purposes of this book, I think we can safely compromise with Drs. Coles and Schwarzbein and say that conservatively at least 70 percent of the aging factors are environmentally induced, and only 30 percent genetic.

Since environmental causes play a crucial role, and you can control many of them, such as diet, nutritional supplements, and exercise, this requires you to have the most up-to-date

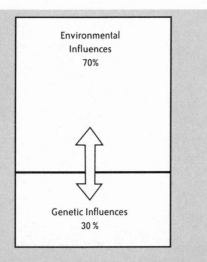

Genetic and Environmental Influences on Aging
Though environment appears to play the more significant role in influencing the rate of aging and the degenerative diseases associated with aging, genes also have an important function. Environmental and genetic factors also interact and influence each other.

knowledge on how to incorporate longevity techniques into your life. It requires you to have practical and accurate information on how to prolong your health and age well. In this book you will find precisely that information presented as a comprehensive approach to modifying these environmental influences as well as promoting positive gene expression and minimizing negative genetic tendencies.

In addition, to exert a positive influence over the environmental causes of aging, you need the endurance to practice a prolonging health lifestyle year in and year out. You also need a philosophy of life and an attitude that keeps the daily stresses—and even the larger losses that accompany living—in perspective. Perhaps a dose of lucky genes is needed as well.

As you read this book, you will come to understand that successful aging is associated with lifelong good health, and that though you

can start your *Prolonging Health* program at any age, it is best to start as young as possible. Indeed, one of the main premises of this book is that a lifestyle that promotes optimal health supported by natural medicines practiced over a lifetime can foster longevity. However, good genes and a healthy lifestyle are only the beginning. To truly prolong health and live long, you need an effective strategy. But before I discuss what the most effective strategies are, which I explain in detail in part 2, let's find out how scientists study aging, what evolutionary biologists are saying about aging, and how aging occurs—the main topics of this chapter—and why it is important that we change the way we look at aging and how we live as we age in order to achieve these health goals. This information will help you better understand the strategies in part 2.

The Study of Aging

The field of gerontology, the scientific study of human aging, is relatively new in the West. The late Nathan W. Shock, Ph.D., known as the "father of gerontology," began his career at the National Institutes of Health in 1941, where he initiated the first long-term study of aging in the United States, called the Baltimore Longitudinal Study of Aging. Dr. Shock took up the debate of whether aging was a disease or not and declared, "aging is not a disease."

Presently, the study of aging is not only the realm of gerontologists, scientists who study human aging, but has been taken up by microbiologists, geneticists, endocrinologists, neurobiologists, evolutionary biologists, medical doctors, and scientists in other disciples including physics. Doctors of Oriental and naturopathic medicine, like me, also work in the aging field. But despite recent advances in the study of aging, many of which I discuss in this chapter, a firm conceptual and scientific foundation by which to understand aging in a comprehensive manner is still missing. The lack of a clear guiding principle makes it monumentally difficult for anyone to develop a specific therapy for aging. This is because aging is such a complex process, and scientific research, until now, has followed a linear model, looking for one gene or one process that explained all of aging.

In order for modern Westerners to understand aging fully, inclusive of its biological, chemical, psychological, social, and spiritual aspects, a completely new paradigm is required. It should include science and medicine, but would do well to also include Eastern methods. That is because for over two thousand years Chinese, Tibetan, and Indian scholars and physicians, Buddhist monks, yogis, and Taoists have not only studied the effects of aging on living things, but also successfully practiced longevity techniques on themselves and established a conceptual basis and pragmatic foundation for these practices. Also, sociology, psychology, and anthropology can contribute their methodologies and insights.

This consilience[1] of East and West, of the social sciences with biology and genetics, will provide not only broader but deeper insights into the phenomena of aging. In the process of changing how we look at aging scientifically, our attitudes towards aging require transformation to allow us to look upon aging as a gift rather than a disgrace, as the natural extension of a full life, not its ultimate failure requiring costly medical intervention.

There are many reasons why aging is difficult to study. One is that it occurs so slowly. Another is that there have been so few people who have lived long enough and healthy enough lives to serve as study models. However, this is changing as greater numbers of people live longer; not only is this of scien-

tific interest, but it has political and economic interest as well because in no other time in recorded history will as many older people be alive as will be the case later in this century. But more on demographics later; for now, let's continue with how scientists study aging.

Scientists approach the study of aging in several different ways, including basic molecular research on cell cultures; study of mammalian and non-mammalian animals; the study of disease processes associated with aging—the delayed-onset disease discussed earlier; diseases of accelerated aging; and the sociological, psychological, physiological, and biochemical changes that occur in older people. Of the latter, one of these models is to investigate those who have aged well.

One such study is the MacArthur Foundation Study on Successful Aging. This was founded in 1984 by John D. and Catherine T. MacArthur, who gathered leading scholars and scientists to develop the conceptual foundation for a "new gerontology" based upon how people age successfully rather than on the disease model of aging. The disease model of aging parallels the current view taken by Western allopathic medicine, in which the clinical focus is on pathology and the symptoms of disease along with objective laboratory studies that lead to the naming of the disease (the diagnosis), rather than on prevention and the improvement of physiologic function to rid the body of disease.

The findings of this study, summarized and published in *Successful Aging*, hold that we can attain "high-quality, vital, disease-free late years" (Rowe 1998). The MacArthur Study has made an excellent contribution to dispelling the former medical myths of aging.

The study of individual centenarians, those who have navigated the long journey of living successfully to 100 years and older, is another way that we gain clues about successful aging. The New England Centenarian Study, begun in 1994 at Beth Israel Deaconess Medical Center, a teaching hospital of Harvard Medical School in Cambridge, Massachusetts, was the first North American investigation of the world's oldest people. Thomas T. Perls, M.D., M.P.H., the director of this study, wrote in *Living to 100* that successful aging "takes effort," and emphasized good health practices, effective stress management, maximizing your genetic potential, getting exercise, and eating lots of fruits and vegetables (Perls 1999). Like the MacArthur Study, the work of Dr. Perls and his colleagues has contributed to a more sensible approach to healthier aging, based on practical lifestyle changes that prevent age-related diseases and improve quality of life for older people.

European centenarian studies have a longer history than those in the United States, and include the Swedish Centenarian Study, as well as ongoing studies in Germany, Italy, Russia, Austria, Denmark, Japan, and China.

A method similar to the study of long-lived individuals is to study groups of people in cultures or societies that have a high percentage of healthy elderly people. From this we obtain clues about lifestyle, diet, and cultural attitudes that foster longevity. The most well known of these groups are the Hunzas of Northern Pakistan, the residents of the village of Vilcabamba in the Ecuadorian Andes, and people in the Caucasus Mountains of Georgia, Armenia, and Azerbaijan. All three regions claim to have a high percentage of supercentenarians, those over 110. However, researchers have found that the ages were exaggerated and there were far fewer centenarians than first reported; even though true ages had to be shifted downwards, we still learned valuable clues about longevity from these mountain

people, such as the benefits of eating yogurt and the value of exercise in maintaining health during advanced age.

The most well-documented study of this kind is the Okinawa Centenarian Study. In this study, 25 years of irrefutable scientific documentation attest to the remarkable health of the people of the island of Okinawa, including detailed birth records (the three areas mentioned above were unable to produce this), medical analyses, and meticulous notes taken by the research group. We can gather many more clues to healthy aging from *The Okinawa Program,* by Bradley Willcox, M.D., Craig Willcox, Ph.D., and Makoto Suzuki, M.D., the principal researchers of the study; the authors describe in detail the lifestyle, diet, and attitudes toward life of the Okinawan people (Willcox 2001).

According to the authors, the main lifestyle determinants to successful aging among the Okinawans are diet, regular exercise, moderate use of alcohol, non-smoking, blood pressure control, and a psycho-spiritual outlook on life that minimizes stress. In addition, the researchers found that these determinants enabled the Okinawans to maintain healthy arteries and heart function, reduce cancer risk, and keep the bones of Okinawa's elderly stronger than those of their American counterparts.

The longest ongoing study of this type in America is the Baltimore Longitudinal Study on Aging, sponsored by the National Institute on Aging. Begun in 1958 and still going, the study has scientists working with more than 1,200 volunteers to learn what happens as people age. Studies like these provide a great deal of observational data on the effects of aging, and in the next chapter, I discuss these data in detail.

From the results of studies such as these and others, we can conclude that prolonging health not only prevents disease, but also promotes longevity. We can also guess that, since the people in the study have similar cultural and genetic heritages, genetic and environmental factors play important and perhaps equal roles.

Scientists also garner information on human aging by studying rare diseases that mimic aging such as Werner syndrome, Seip-Berandinelli syndrome, and Hutchinson-Gilford syndrome, or progeria (Martin 2000). These conditions are characterized by tissue changes that are similar, but not identical to, those that occur during aging. Another way to study aging is to evaluate the changes that occur in hormone deficiency diseases such as insulin-dependent diabetes or Addison's disease, a condition characterized by the lack of adrenal hormones, and compare them to the effects of the hormone decline that occurs during aging. Unfortunately, none of these diseases accurately conveys the complexity of age-related decline in healthy older people.

In the early 1980s, observational and longitudinal studies, at the time the only way to study aging, gave way to molecular and genetic studies, which today remain the main arena for basic aging research. Through these methods, a considerable amount of information has been accumulated, much of it on how individual genes influence aging and longevity, but valuable information has also been uncovered on the various diseases associated with aging as well as the fundamental biology of aging.

Much of the basic research in aging uses small animals as models to determine the influence of genetics on life span. Called by researchers the "four bestiary" models of aging—yeast, worms, flies, and mice—these four constitute the main models for research on aging in living organisms. Because of its anatomical and biological simplicity, the lowly

nematode worm *(Caenorhabditis elegans)* is the current focus of genetic research, but the animal model that contributed the most in the early stages of genetic research was the fruit fly *(Drosophila melanogaster)*.

Surprisingly, though it has a more complex body and is considerably larger in size (the nematode requires a microscope to see it), the fruit fly has fewer genes than the nematode (14,000 genes compared to 19,000), and due to its rapid reproduction rate it has enthralled scientist for decades. From the third bestiary, the yeast *Saccharomyces cerevisiae*, scientists have identified 30 genes that are thought to be involved in the aging process.

Only a few mammalian models have been routinely used to study aging, mainly genetically altered mice, though in some studies primates have been used. Studies using these animals are in progress at the University of California, in Los Angeles and Berkeley, at the University of Arizona in Tucson, and at many other leading universities and private research institutes in North America, such as the Orentreich Foundation for the Advancement of Science in Cold Springs-on-Hudson, New York,[2] as well as in Europe. The life span of laboratory mice and rats is about six years, which allows for experiments to be completed in five to ten years. Although mice are mammals and may be more useful than worms or flies in studying effects of environmental and other factors on aging, they are biologically very different from humans. Genetically similar to people, monkeys are commonly used as research models, but their disadvantage is that they live longer and the studies take longer.

Because they breed readily in captivity, the monkey most commonly used for aging research is the rhesus macaque, though squirrel monkeys are also used. The rhesus monkey's maximum life span is about 40 years, making for lengthy research in life extension using these animals in whom 95 percent of their DNA is identical to those of humans. However, results take much longer than with rodents, requiring a minimum of ten years to evaluate, and longer studies in aging require 20 or more years to complete.

Among the few researchers using nonhuman primates is George S, Roth, Ph.D., a senior guest scientist at the National Institute on Aging (NIA). He leads a team of scientists in the primate diet restriction project based in Baltimore, Maryland. Since primates are the closest animal research model to humans, attention to detail is necessary in order to form as complete a picture as possible of how aging takes place.

This complete picture includes measuring hormone levels and blood glucose levels; following reproductive cycles and capacity; measuring bone growth, mineral content, and the composition of muscles; following activity and rest cycles; and evaluating cognitive function, body temperature, calorie expenditure, and other physiological parameters that are used to measure age-related changes in the body (Mattison 2003). Information gathered from primate studies may one day find use in human aging research or in the development of medicines that treat the degenerative diseases associated with aging.

Obviously it is unethical to study humans in the same way as laboratory animals, but we can examine and measure the physiological changes that happen as we age, such as changes in body temperature, blood pressure, skin and hair, blood sugar levels, and hormones, as in the Baltimore Longitudinal Study.

Another basic research method is based on laboratory culture of specific cell lines. This model dates back to 1961 when Leonard Hayflick, Ph.D., a professor of anatomy at the University of California at San Francisco, and Paul Moorhead, Ph.D., used human diploid cells taken from lung and skin samples to study aging. Diploid cells contain two sets of genetic information, one copy from each parent; all cells in your body, with the exception of sperm and egg cells, are diploid.

Dr. Hayflick, credited as the father of cellular gerontology, discovered that cultured normal cells undergo a limited number of cell divisions, after which they become senescent, undergoing less efficient replication, and finally die. This phenomenon is known as the "Hayflick limit," or the finite capacity of cells to duplicate. Since then, cell model studies have been expanded to include other types of cells such as arterial smooth muscle cells, and scientists are beginning to look at cells from long-lived animals, such as whales, and those that show little signs of aging, such as birds.

One such researcher is João Pedro de Magalhães, Ph.D., a young gerontologist from Portugal working in the Department of Biology, Unit of Cellular Biochemistry and Biology at the University of Namur in Belgium. Namur is a small town of old gray stone buildings set among wooded hills about an hour by local train west of Brussels. I was impressed with the depth of information on Dr. Magalhães's website[3] and contacted him for an interview while I was in Europe on the way to the Sixth International Symposium on the Neurobiology and Neuroendocrinology of Aging in Austria.

Over lunch in a local tavern, Dr. Magalhães, his dark hair long enough to brush his shoulders and dressed in a loose white T-shirt, energetically described to me his interest in studying cells from long-lived animals, especially tortoises, such as the Marion's tortoise capable of living over a century, or humpbacked whales that might live even longer, though no one really knows exactly what a whale's life expectancy is. Expressing his dismay and concern at the difficulty of obtaining cells from large animals, especially endangered ones, he suggested that aging research was limited by the current models and that we needed new ones to progress (Magalhães 2002). Without new models, it is unlikely that new findings will occur.

However, most aging researchers contend that there is still more to learn from our existing models even though they are decades old. One researcher in the field of molecular biology of aging is Peter Schmeissner, Ph.D., of the Department of Molecular Biology and Biochemistry at Rutgers University in Piscataway, New Jersey. A thoughtful young scientist who works with nematode worms *(Caenorhabditis elegans)* and who carefully phrases his answers, Dr. Schmeissner explained to me why nematodes were still an important model for aging research.

First, the nematode genome is now completely sequenced, making its biological architecture more available to scientists. When scientists sequence an organism's genome, they tabulate a list of all the genetic material found in that organism, such as was done with the human genome project completed in 2000. Second, its life span is short, only two to three weeks, which allows scientists to follow several generations in a relatively short period of time. Third, nematodes are large enough that their life cycles can be observed without much difficulty. Compared to bacteria, nematodes are giants.

Dr. Schmeissner's view, shared by many researchers, is that since all living organisms have a similar if not common biological base, if we solve the riddle of aging in any one organism, even the lowly nematode worm, we may discover the key to unlocking the door to aging in other organisms, including humans (Schmeissner 2002).

But why study worms and flies or microscopic cells of other animals for that matter, when what we ultimately want to know is why humans age? The answer, though perhaps simplistic because we are in the infancy of our understanding of the cellular biology of living things, is that by studying aging "under glass" in simpler life forms we can learn a great deal about the fundamental biological mechanism of aging (Shay 2000).

Though we have gathered a great amount of information on cellular aging from this type of basic research and though it is accepted that the biochemistry of aging is similar among different life forms, these studies are obviously not easily translated to human aging since they are based on animal models and isolated cells in the laboratory. Such investigation may never directly help us learn how to practice anti-aging techniques; however, researchers mine the biological field in this manner and over the last few decades have extracted much valuable information on the molecular mechanisms of aging, which perhaps may one day provide a window on why living things age, including us.

Among the most fascinating of these studies is research on the so-called longevity genes sir2 and daf16. The discovery of these genes led scientists to the next stage of aging research—insulin/IGF signaling pathways. Insulin and insulin-like growth factor (IGF) are hormones produced by the body to regulate glucose (blood sugar). By manipulating these genes in nematodes, along with making environmental changes, such as caloric restriction, that influence metabolism, scientists have doubled the life span of nematodes. Sir2, primarily researched by Leonard Guarente, Ph.D., of the Massachusetts Institute of Technology in Cambridge, Massachusetts, and daf16, intensively investigated by Cynthia Kenyon, Ph.D., of the University of California in San Francisco, are just two of several gene complexes that appear to promote longevity.

Though important for fundamental knowledge of how aging takes place on the subcellular level, such information does not help us as individuals to live longer. In order to extract practical knowledge on aging and longevity, we need new ways. One gaining more attention (because of the number of people involved) is

Over the course of my own 25-year career in natural medicine, I have made a habit of asking those among my patients and even chance acquaintances who have lived long and aged successfully for their longevity secrets. From such people I gleaned valuable clues, confirming much of what the researchers are suggesting, that a long life depends on wellness and that wellness is reflected in an optimistic attitude towards living and a healthy lifestyle.

to evaluate individuals who have practiced anti-aging and life extension methods. Granted, this method is not pure science, being more sociological and anthropological in nature, but it can undoubtedly produce valuable insights into how humans modify the affects of aging on themselves, which may provide leads for scientists to follow.

There are three branches to this method of investigation. The first is to look at non-Western models, primarily those found in Taoism from China, and Ayurvedic and yogic practices from India. These civilizations have a

history of several thousand years reaching to the present, and from them we can gain a considerable amount of practical information on natural longevity methods. Unfortunately, few Western researchers are pursuing this direction, partly because of the difficulty in working in a country as foreign to Westerners as China and partly because of the prejudice against anything but laboratory science. The second way is to observe those individuals who have reviewed the scientific studies on anti-aging, such as caloric restriction using lab animals, and tried the results on themselves. These are often the same scientists working with laboratory animal models.

The third way is to interview living practitioners of longevity practices. Called life-extensionists, these people use nutrients and drugs to prevent aging. They can be interviewed and laboratory tests taken to see how successful they have been in preventing aging and to what they attribute their success. The foremost organization for this type of information is the Life Extension Foundation in Fort Lauderdale, Florida.[4]

Over the course of my own 25-year career in natural medicine, I have made a habit of asking those among my patients and even chance acquaintances who have lived long and aged successfully for their longevity secrets. One such individual, a Cuban merchant marine, who at 85 looked like a healthy 60-year-old, attributed his good health to long sea voyages away from pollution and stress, abstinence from sex during these trips, and one fine Cuban cigar daily. From such people I gleaned valuable clues, confirming much of what the researchers are suggesting, that a long life depends on wellness and that wellness is reflected in an optimistic attitude towards living and a healthy lifestyle.

Interestingly, for the most part none of these long-lived individuals were experts in gerontology, knew anything about the science of longevity, or used anti-aging medicines. Most did not even use health foods, hormones, or vitamin supplements. This tells us that people can live a long and healthy life without assistance from technological medicine or nutritional supplements. Imagine what we could achieve if we knew more about the aging process *and* used advanced methods for prolonging health. This book will sketch out some of the possibilities along these lines.

Life Expectancy

Life expectancy, also called the mean life span, is defined as the average maximum age a person might expect to reach. Gerontologists arrive at this mean by calculating the average maximum life span of all individuals alive in a population with the age of death from all causes. When early deaths from childhood infections are factored in, the average life expectancy of previous centuries is amazingly low, often only 35 to 40 years.

Conversely, in modern times in the industrialized countries, life expectancy is greater for the average person because there are considerably fewer deaths from infection or accidents. This method of arriving at an average age for

Table 1: Selected Life Expectancies

Country	Average Life Expectancy
Okinawa	81.2
Japan	79.9
Sweden	79.0
France	79.0
Italy	78.3
Greece	78.1
United States	76.8
France	75.2
Cuba	74.8
Australia	73.2
Chile	73.0
United Kingdom	71.7
Mexico	65.0
China	62.3
Brazil	59.1
India	53.2

Sources: World Health Organization's Healthy Life Expectancy Ratings based on the Disability Adjusted Life Expectancy (DALE); United Nations Statistics Division, Trends and Statistics 200—Life Expectancy and Infant Mortality; National Center for Health Statistics, 1998

life expectancy may be a useful way of attributing statistical measurements to aging, but it is highly misleading because it does not accurately reflect the rate of aging or the potential maximum life span of an individual.

Another term used by gerontologists is maximum life span, which is the age reached by the oldest member of a species. For example, some trees like the giant sequoias *(Sequoiadendron giganteum)*, an evergreen tree found in California along the western slopes of the southern Sierra Nevada mountain range, have circumferences up to 100 feet in diameter and live over 5,000 years. On the other end of the spectrum, *Drosophila*, the fruit fly used in aging research, lives less than 70 days. Tortoises can live upwards of 250 years, bowhead whales live 210 years and perhaps considerably longer, and some cranes live over 80 years. Interestingly, the tortoise, crane, and the pine tree are symbols of longevity in Chinese culture, confirming the correct observation in Eastern cultures of long-lived animals and plants.

Humans fall roughly in the middle on the life span scale. The average life expectancy in the United States is now 76.8 years, ranked eighteenth compared to other countries; the longest average life span is 81.2 years, found among the Okinawans. In contrast, developing nations in the third world have a life expectancy 15–20 years lower than that in the developed nations of North America, Europe, and Japan.

Although life expectancy is increasing in all countries, especially in Europe and North America, the maximum life span does not appear to have changed over time. Indeed, according to S. Jay Olshansky, Ph.D., who researches the upper limits of human longevity at the University of Chicago, this trend is expected to peak and begin to level off before mid-century. Dr. Olshansky believes that an average life expectancy of 100 may be unrealistic (Olshansky, Carnes, and Desesquelles 2001). Other experts think this is too pessimistic and believe that humans not only are living longer, but will continue to achieve longer life spans with an upper limit that has not yet been defined.

What Is the Maximum Human Life Span?

Though the life expectancy of a greater number of people in the developed countries has nearly doubled in the last 100 years, experts are in disagreement over the limits of life expectancy for the next 50 years. However, in general they agree that more people will live to over 100 than have in the past. Marie-Françoise Schulz-Aellen, Ph.D., of the Institutions Universitaires de Geriatrie et de Psychiatrie in Geneva, Switzerland, says: "If slow deterioration of all physiological functions associated with aging proceeds normally, the human body has the potential to live significantly longer than one hundred years. In fact, the human life span is shorter mainly because of infections or noninfectious age-associated diseases" (Schulz-Aellen 1997).

How long can we expect to live? Genetic science has extended the life span of fruit flies, the soil nematode, mice, and even monkeys under controlled laboratory situations. And though none of this research has yet been proven on humans, from these and other studies, some researchers speculate that humans might also be able to extend their life span upward to between 150 and 200 years. Among the more optimistic is Steven Austad, Ph.D., of the University of Idaho department of biological sciences and the author of several books on aging. He thinks that 150 or older is possible (McCann 2002).

Dr. Austad's research suggests that such a possibility is on the horizon. I met Dr. Austad during a conference at the Buck Institute in Novato, California, a small town tucked into the hills about 20 minutes north of San Francisco. Friendly, with a casual manner but full of profound insights, he proposed that long-ignored environmental influences on aging will combine with advanced molecular techniques to help us understand the interaction of environment and genes. The results of this integrated way of studying aging will open the gates to a new paradigm in aging research where "environment, gender differences, multiple interactivity of genes, and pleiotrophy all count" (Austad 2002).

Realistically, looking at the limits of aging and the maximum range of the human life span from what we know about aging, the upper limit appears to be 120–125 years. The oldest (documented) person of modern times was Madam Jeanne Louise Calment of France, who died on August 4, 1997, at the age of 122. But, if some people can reach this age, why can't more? Why do they fall short by 45 years?

The simple answer is that it is possible and more people are beginning to live longer, though we haven't yet seen what that upper limit is and won't for at least another 40 to 50 years when the effects of life extension practices and modern medicine come to fruition. By making the right choices *now*, such as utilizing an effective longevity strategy as presented in part 2, we should be able to prolong our health and live to between 85 and 100, and perhaps even longer.

Who Are Those Who Have Aged Successfully?

There are many examples of people who have aged successfully. In fact, as I mentioned earlier, average life expectancy is only a measure of the mean life span and does not reflect the quality of life during aging or individual differences in health or variations in the aging process. The healthy elderly include people from all walks of life and different nationalities and races. The commonality among them is that they are people who remain free from major diseases and who stay physically active and mentally astute into their seventies, eighties, and some even into their nineties and longer.

Historically, plenty of people lived beyond 80 years old, including the Greek philosopher Plato, who lived to at least 80, and the dramatist Sophocles, who was 90, when he died. Undocumented reports of humans having lived this long or longer are found in China and India, countries where longevity techniques have been practiced for centuries. Hua Tuo, a famous physician during the Han dynasty, was close to 100 when he died, and there are numerous reports of others living even longer. Wang Lie from Handan, China, reportedly lived to 238, and Gan Shi from Taiyuan was said to be 300 years old when he died (Campany 2002). One can only imagine if science were to join forces with Eastern longevity practices just how long we might live.

Contemporary examples of such people include Jack La Lanne, the "godfather of physical fitness," who at 86 is still active and in good health; Paul Bragg, the "father of the American health movement" who died at 96 while swimming in rough seas in Hawaii; Bill Haast of the Miami Serpentarium, who, attributing his vigor to daily injections of snake venom, at 90 was still handling poisonous snakes; and Frank Lloyd Wright, who at 92 designed and began construction of the Guggenheim Museum in New York.

Another example is Scott Nearing (1883–1983), who inspired several generations of contemporary homesteaders through his book *Living the Good Life*, coauthored with his wife, Helen (Nearing 1970). Actively working on his farm in Maine, Nearing, called one of the truly great vegetarians of the twentieth century and an American radical, died at the age of 100 by simply ceasing to eat. His wife, Helen, writing and lecturing at 90 years old, died in a car accident.

Though they aged, these individuals are examples of what we can accomplish with a healthy lifestyle that includes physical fitness, a positive mental attitude, and a healthy diet. Even more fascinating are those that lived beyond age 100.

The Centenarians and Supercentenarians: According to *Centenarians in the United States*, there were 37, 306 people over 100 years old living in the United States in 1999. With people living longer and the population increasing, the expected number of centenarians in the United States may reach over 265,000 by the year 2050 (Kruch and Velkoff 1999).

Supercentenarians, those over 110 years of age, are found throughout the world, though there are very few of them. At the time of this writing, there are 32 known supercentenarians in the world, the oldest being Kamato Hongo, a Japanese woman who in January 2002 was 114 and still alive (Coles 2002). By another calculation, by the Los Angeles Gerontology Research Group, the number of known supercentenarians in 2001 was 28, and 20 of them were women (Coles 2001). Of the 28, 8 are Japanese; 4 are from the United States, and the remaining 12 are from different European countries and Australia.

All of these countries are places where accurate birth and medical records are kept, making documentation easier than in third-world countries such as Pakistan or Ecuador, countries who claim to have long-lived people. However, people of very advanced age are also found in other countries as well. In Dominica, an island in the Caribbean, Elizabeth "Ma Pampo" Israel is reported to be 127 years old, but documentation of her exact age is lacking; thus she is not included in the official list of supercentenarians.

Now let's turn our attention to the results of these investigations and what scientists consider the causes of aging.

Theories of Aging

Theories on aging attempt to make sense of the complexity of human aging by looking for specific causes such as a gene that turns on the aging process. These are different from theories about how to extend life, explained in a following section and which this book is about: practical solutions that will help you prolong health and extend life. However, in order to appreciate those solutions, it is first necessary to review a few of the most important theories on aging, giving credit along the way to those individuals who have made significant contributions to the field.

The Main Theories of Aging

- Free Radical Theory: Your cells burn out from oxygen utilization.

- DNA Damage-Repair Theory: Your DNA looses its ability to repair itself.

- Telomere Theory: Your chromosomes can't make copies of themselves anymore.

- Neuroendocrine Theory: Your body runs out of hormones and growth factors.

- Immunological Theory: Your immune system runs down.

- Thermodynamic Theory: Your metabolism stops working.

The Free Radical Theory: Since first proposed in 1956 by Denham Harmon, M.D., Ph.D., an emeritus professor at the University of Nebraska Medical Center in Omaha, the free radical theory has proven to be one of the classic models of aging. Though many researchers once believed the free radical theory was the fundamental cause of aging, after significant study, most agree that the oxidative process influences the pathology of many diseases *associated* with aging, but is not the single determinant of the aging process or life span. Still, cumulative oxidative processes influence health, disease, and aging, and because of this and in light of how these diseases are treated with natural therapies, it's worth taking a closer look at the free radical theory.

Essentially this theory states that aging is the result of the process by which oxygen from the air is used to make energy, a process termed oxidation. Over time, free radical damage accumulates because repair processes cannot keep up with the damage caused by oxygen, and our cells and tissues gradually become useless. Free radicals, also called reactive oxygen species (ROS), are unstable toxic molecules with a missing electron, which are formed during all metabolic activity in the body.

To compensate for the effects of oxidation, nature designed sophisticated methods to manage free radical activity by providing naturally occurring *anti*oxidants, substances that work against oxidants and neutralize reactive oxygen species. Free radical activity is normalized by naturally occurring antioxidants such as glutathione, and the enzymes catalase and superoxide dismutase (SOD), as well as dietary antioxidants such as vitamins C and E, and the minerals zinc and selenium.

A Quick Explanation of Genetics

Genes are found in the nucleus of cells. They store hereditary information, the instructions for an organism's life. Genes are made of deoxyribonucleic acid (DNA) and ribonucleic acid (RNA). DNA is the molecule that stores genetic information. An organism's total DNA content, transmitted from generation to generation, is known as its genome. The human genome contains 30,000 known genes, and scientists suggest that we may have up to 75,000. Genes encode information to make specific proteins, which are the building blocks of the body. DNA and protein combine together to form chromosomes. Humans have 23 pairs of chromosomes. RNA is made from DNA to synthesize proteins.

Other naturally occurring substances in our body also have antioxidant activity, including uric acid, a substance produced as the end product of purine metabolism. Purine is a protein used by the body as the building block for the manufacture of RNA and DNA, our genetic material. Most uric acid in the body is filtered out of the blood by the kidneys and excreted in the urine. However, when uric acid levels are too high, crystals may be deposited in the joints, mostly the large toe joint or the ankle, causing the painful condition called gout. Excess uric acid levels are also thought to contribute to cardiovascular disease (Fang 1992).

Interestingly, because of its antioxidant effect higher levels (but not too high) of uric acid may guard against aging and have been shown to protect against central nervous system damage as occurs in multiple sclerosis (Hooper 1998). The paradoxical utilization of uric acid in the body is another example of how nature provides effective solutions to the evolutionary challenges of life.

The greatest degree of the free radical damage in the body occurs in the mitochondria, the organelles within the cells where most cellular metabolism occurs and where energy is manufactured in the form of adenosine triphosphate (ATP), the energy currency of the cell. The mitochondria utilize nearly 90 percent of the body's oxygen sources and consequently form many of the free radicals found in cells, particularly in brain and muscle tissue.

In addition, mitochondria have their own genetic material called mitochondrial DNA (mtDNA), and researchers have shown mtDNA to be more susceptible to free radical damage than the DNA in the cell nucleus. Also, it appears that mtDNA has fewer repair mechanisms than nuclear DNA, contributing to cumulative damage because it cannot repair itself as readily as other parts of the cell.

However, supplying extra antioxidants in the diet or from supplements hasn't seemed to greatly influence maximum life span, though it has been shown that antioxidants can prevent and may even reverse many degenerative diseases associated with aging.

The DNA Damage-Repair Theory: The individual cell is the basic unit of life for all multicellular higher organisms from insects to humans, and all cells store hereditary information in the same chemical code in specialized structures within the cell. This code, which provides biochemical messages informing the cell what to do, is stored inside the cell's nucleus in a group of sugars called nucleotides, specifically DNA. The collective content of all DNA in your body is known as the genome. Think of the genome as the archives of all the hereditary and evolutionary information necessary for *you* to survive and of DNA as the books or computer discs where the information is stored, copied, and passed on to each new generation of cells. However, for it to be useful your cells must convert this information into proteins, the basic building blocks of all life processes.

From the moment of your conception, these processes are repeated millions upon millions of times with a variety of biochemical consequences along the way. At any part or stage in the process of replication or protein building, damage to the DNA may occur. This may be due to ultraviolet radiation from the sun or man-made sources such as x-rays, or to toxic chemicals in the environment, including cigarette smoke. Genetic damage is also caused by free radicals, which are unstable and highly reactive molecules associated with aging, heart disease, cancer, and the chronic inflammation that often accompanies aging, and from chronic viral, bacterial, or parasitic infections.

However, when you are young, under normal circumstances your cells have highly effective mechanisms to prevent this damage or to repair it when it occurs. But as you age, your body's ability to repair damaged genetic material is reduced. Due to the cumulative effects of radiation and the other causes of genetic damage, mutations occur in the DNA, causing alteration in the normal genetic expression of your cells. Abnormal genetic expression may lead to cancer, cardiovascular disease, and other illnesses, as well as accelerated aging and death.

Over a lifetime, it appears that deterioration of a person's genome takes place and that the structure of the genetic material becomes changed through mutation. Therefore, according to this theory, these mutations combined with failure of repair mechanisms lead to age-related tissue changes. Researchers have found that without damage, the function of DNA itself does not change with age, suggestive of a still undiscovered mechanism for longevity.

The Telomere Theory: The telomere theory of aging attempts to explain Dr. Hayflick's limit of cellular senescence. That limit states that the gradual degradation of cellular function and reduced ability to repair genetic damage are due to the cells' limited capacity to replicate. Normal cells reach this capacity after 60–80 replications. Cells grow when the chromosomes divide (replicate) into two identical offspring, each with all the same genetic material as the parent cell.

During replication, telomeres are repeatedly shortened. Telomeres are specialized proteins at the tips of the chromosomes thought to be essential in their maintenance and to prevent abnormal cell division. Once shortened beyond a certain limit, a mechanism that prevents further replication is turned on and cell division slows or is halted. According to the telomere theory, when the chromosome cannot replicate any longer, aging and eventual cellular death occur.

However, nature provides a mechanism that prevents excessive shortening of the telomeres in the form of telomerase, an enzyme that protects telomeres by helping to reconstruct the broken tips, thereby preserving the integrity of the chromosomes. Scientists have discovered that an interesting twist of events takes place with telomerase. In certain cell lines and in most human cancer cells, telomerase creates an *immortality effect*—by lengthening telomeres, it causes cells to live longer.

Ironically, though gradual shortening of telomeres appears to play a role in aging and telomerase prevents shortening and thus cellular aging, this same mechanism also seems to work *for* cancer cells. Cancer cells are immortal and apparently use telomerase to keep them alive. Cancer researchers are investigating ways to turn off telomerase, thought to be responsible for the proliferation of tumor cells, but when telomerase is inhibited, life span is greatly shortened. In the aging field, telomere researchers are looking for ways to maintain telomere length and not trigger cancer; if successful, this research could help us live longer.

Besides the telomere-cancer paradox, there are other contradictions in telomere research. For example, Elizabeth Blackburn, Ph.D., of the University of California at San Francisco, found that the most significant telomere shortening takes place between birth and the age of four, with a gradual shortening of telomere length as one approaches old age (Blackburn 2000). Since we aren't aged at four years old and cancer is rare in young children, the general telomere theory of aging is questioned by this data. Though there are still many unanswered questions in telomere biology, as the data accumulates, it appears that the telomere theory as an age determinant has potential for explaining at least part of the aging process from the molecular level, and much like counting the rings on a tree trunk, only in reverse, it is part of the puzzle of the complete picture of aging.

The Neuroendocrine Theory: The simple version of this theory proposes that failure in the production of hormones is the cause of aging. It is well known by doctors that reduced hormone levels have profound effects on all systems of the body. For example, when thyroid hormone is low, this causes hypothyroidism. Medical experts agree that if the neuroendocrine theory is not central to aging, age-related hormonal decline certainly speeds up the process. These changes are most apparent during menopause when the production of estrogen and progesterone by the ovaries declines considerably. Estrogen deficiency is

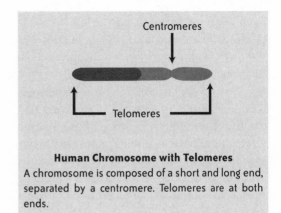

Human Chromosome with Telomeres
A chromosome is composed of a short and long end, separated by a centromere. Telomeres are at both ends.

associated with fatigue, frailty, memory loss, insomnia, depression, dry skin, reduced bone density, all of which are conditions associated with aging.

When a woman is given estrogen to replace her own production of this important hormone, she generally feels more alive and happier, her memory improves, she sleeps better, and she has fewer wrinkles. These results have led many physicians to believe that hormonal replacement therapy is the fountain of youth. However, though hormones do help to reduce many of the symptoms of the aging process, they do not reverse aging itself as some proponents of the basic neuroendocrine theory suggest.

To anti-aging physicians, the star of hormone replacement is human growth hormone. Originally researched for its relevance in aging by the late Daniel Rudman, M.D. (Rudman 1990), whose work brought growth hormone to the forefront of the anti-aging field, it has since been promoted as the antidote to aging. Unfortunately, answers to aging are not that easy to come by, and I will discuss both the positive and negative sides of growth hormone replacement in considerable detail in later chapters. Though estrogen, growth hormone, and the adrenal hormone DHEA have received most of the attention during the last decade, it is actually insulin that may be more critical to the process of aging; I discuss insulin's role in hormone balancing in detail in part 2.

A more sophisticated version of the neuroendocrine theory emerged in the early part of the twenty-first century. Based upon research evidence, scientists found that signaling mechanisms operate in the body to instruct hormones to work better. Mainly involving insulin, the hormone that regulates blood sugar and therefore metabolism, and a related molecule, insulin-like growth factor (IGF), these signaling molecules communicate messages to specific genes, such as sir2, that have active roles in promoting cellular life and death.

Several mechanisms have been proposed for the insulin/IGF signaling and neuroendocrine process of aging. One of them suggests that aging actually starts in the brain. Marc Tatar, Ph.D., an assistant professor in evolutionary and ecological genetics at Brown University in Providence, Rhode Island, may have discovered the first evidence of a hormone-based aging mechanism in a gene called insulin-like receptor (InR), found in fruit flies.

It appears that InR regulates hormonal secretion, and thereby aging, through the interaction of another substance called juvenile hormone, or neotenin, a hormone secreted by glands near the brain of insects, which affects molting, the process of shedding the outer skeleton (Tatar 2001). Though a similar mechanism in humans has yet to be found, lower levels than normal of insulin in the blood are associated with longevity, and researchers are actively investigating how diet, metabolism, hormones, and genetics influence aging.

The pineal hormone melatonin is also a candidate for a neuroendocrine aging-triggering substance. Walter Pierpaoli, M.D., Ph.D., director of the Jean Choay Institute for Biomedical Research in Riva San Vitale, Switzerland, believes that the pineal gland, situated in the brain, controls aging by regulating neuroendocrine and immune system modulation through a genetically determined program (Pierpaoli 1998). Other researchers are equally passionate in favor of the hypothalamus, another gland in the brain, as being the regulating center for aging.

The Immunological Theory: The capacity of the immune system to protect us against infection from microbial organisms declines significantly with age. Proponents of this theory suggest that the immune system is worn down by repeated exposure to infectious and noninfectious antigens, substances that trigger an immune response. These include viruses, bacteria, parasites, protozoa, pollutants, pollens and other allergenic substances, and even food. It is well known that older people are more easily infected by microorganisms such as *Streptococcus pneumoniae* and *Klebsiella pneumoniae*, bacteria that cause common pneumonia, or influenza A virus, which causes the flu.

An autoimmune condition develops when the body's immune function turns on itself, as in rheumatoid arthritis. Cancer, particularly of the epidermal tissue (skin), as in basal and squamous cell cancers, is more common in older people. Declining hormone function, particularly of the thymus gland where the T-lymphocytes (cells that form part of the main architecture of the immune system) mature, further weakens the immune system. At the same time, the ongoing activity of the immune system to defend the body against tumor formation and infectious disease may contribute to many of the cellular changes described above, thus causing aging.

The Thermodynamic Theory: The term thermodynamics is used in physics and refers to the exchange of energy in closed systems.

The thermodynamic theory of aging explains biological aging in chemical and mathematical terms. The first and second laws of thermodynamics state that there is a tendency for energy to be conserved and that while energy is used some must be lost or transformed into something else. In the body and other biological systems, this mechanical view doesn't describe all of the complex biological processes that make up a living organism.

However, it does serve to explain some of the occurrences that happen during the aging process. Extrapolating from physics, it says that the general tendency during metabolism is to conserve energy, mostly manifested in the form of body heat; as a person ages, these continuous metabolic processes gradually use up energy. As a consequence, the loss of metabolic control that follows initiates the onset of the irreversible aging process.

Citing that many, but not all, of the world's oldest and healthiest people live in mountainous regions, Professor Georgi P. Gladyshev of the International Academy of Creative Endeavors in Moscow believes that though heredity is the first factor that influences aging, the second factor is the body's thermodynamic mechanisms, which are influenced by climate, physical conditioning, and diet (Gladyshev 1999). From a similar perspective, Karlis Ullis, M.D., a professor at the University of California at Los Angeles and the author of *Age Right*, suggests that the way energy is metabolized in the body plays a key role in managing aging, and that metabolism can be controlled through diet, hormones, exercise, and nutrients (Ullis 1999). I discuss this concept in more detail in the next chapter.

The thermodynamic model forms a continuity between physics and biology. The possibilities that it suggests deepen our perception of how the aging process might work as seen from a broader, less molecular view, and it is a view based more on systems than single mechanisms. In this model, the laws of thermodynamics do not contradict life processes and may eventually show that our body's biochemistry works on chemical gradients. These are fluid patterns of ever-changing pleiotrophic cellular function. It may also show that energy patterns are as important as laboratory statistics, that we're dealing with mosaics of living cells. We are still in the very early stages of the development of this theory of aging, but it may prove to be one of the more interesting of all the models.

Evolution and Aging

The Darwinian idea of evolution, proposed by the British naturalist Charles Darwin (1809–1882) in the mid-1800s, theorized that all things worked toward greater perfection based on *natural selection*. From this point of view, all biological processes, including aging, work towards survival of the individual and therefore the species. From the standpoint of this view, reproductive capability, the rearing of offspring, and the biological contributions one makes to society—all of which decline and eventually become absent as one ages—are the determining factors in why species and individuals age. This theory makes intuitive sense, but scientists have found it difficult to prove, and not all evolutionary biologists agree with each other, or even with Darwin.

Alfred Russell Wallace (1823–1913) was a contemporary of Darwin and credited with formulating the first evolutionary theory of aging published in 1858, a year before Darwin's *On the Origin of Species*. Wallace suggested that natural selection favored reproduction at the expense of longevity, that aging and death were required to winnow the population; otherwise overpopulation and starvation would result.

Quixotic and energetic, Wallace, who lived to 90 despite bouts of malaria he contracted in New Guinea, possessed a spiritual side and suggested that evolution advanced guided by unseen forces. Wallace's ideas were not accepted at the time, while scholars and clergy debated the Darwinian notion of evolution ver-

This concept is important because it informs us that our cells, and therefore our body, are capable of evolutionary activity and hereditary genetic expression, while simultaneously having the ability to express an entirely different nature based on their environment. Therefore, by providing an optimal environment, your cells will work towards prolonging health rather than manifesting disease.

sus creationism. Such ideas, though radical during Victorian times, now seem naïve and overly simplistic, and it was not until the mid-twentieth century that newer ideas of evolution emerged.

In 1957, George C. Williams, Ph.D., America's preeminent evolutionary biologist, proposed that natural selection could both favor the reproductive potential of youth and oppose senescence through a property of cellular function he termed "pleiotropy," the state in which a cell can have more than one function (Williams 1957). In other words, under one set of environmental circumstances, a cell may express its potential to resist environmental stress, for example, while in an entirely different circumstance the same cell may display a completely different trait.

Pleiotropic consequences have confounded scientists because one cell can express multiple traits, and it is not easy to tell under which circumstances it will express which trait, or if it is only one cell causing different genetic expressions or many different cells causing multiple effects. You might think of it in terms of how a chameleon changes colors to match its surroundings: it is the same animal each time, only appearing different.

As regards aging, scientists find that during our youth a particular gene can express a specific function, but later in life the same gene may alter its expression and convey messages to the cell communicating that it is time to age. How or why this happens is still unknown.

You might also look at this pleiotropic trait as the "quantum cell." Johnjoe McFadden, Ph.D., a professor of molecular biology at the University of Surrey in England, in his book *Quantum Evolution* explains it this way: the cell should no longer be thought of as a particle pursuing an "independent trajectory through intercellular space," but be seen as a "dynamic mosaic" (McFadden 2000). The idea of a *mosaic cellular effect*, the quantum or pleiotropic cell, recurs repeatedly in this book, and for our purposes the idea suggests that the cells of your body, though not having volitional action independent of the entire living organism (in other words, they do not operate on their own, with the exception perhaps of cancer cells), have multiple and complex functions based upon millions of years of evolution.

This concept is important because it informs us that our cells, and therefore our body, are capable of evolutionary activity and hereditary genetic expression, while simultaneously having the ability to express an entirely different nature based on their environment.

Therefore, by providing an optimal environment, your cells will work towards prolonging health rather than manifesting disease.

Returning to the evolutionary theory of aging, in this case, we are speaking less of the origin and evolution of species, but of molecular evolution of the genome and the traits that influence aging, which have been conserved over our history. I have already described how within our bodies there exists a mosaic of cellular patterns and functions, more like clouds building in a weather system than mechanical objects such as trains or clocks. In this scenario, it is possible that within our genetic heritage encoded in DNA may be the key to understanding aging and the possibility of altering evolution through the extension of life beyond the known maximum life span. But it is highly unlikely that a simplistic solution will emerge to such a complex question as why we age.

In Dr. Williams's *Why We Get Sick: The New Science of Darwinian Medicine,* he suggests that if aging were as devastating a process as humans think, natural evolution would have eliminated it eons ago (Nesse 1994). But it hasn't, and aging remains. Therefore, by understanding molecular and cellular evolution, we may gather insights into the mechanisms of aging, but since evolutionary processes actually select for genes that cause senescence, a more complete understanding of aging may only come through broader knowledge hidden in the genome and in life itself. In any case, we are still "doomed" to age, but as you will find by reading further, we are not destined to become feeble and disease-ridden. We may prolong our health even as we age.

The New Paradigm of Aging

Based upon advances in evolutionary biology and ecology, the confluence of physics and biology, along with the newest research on cellular aging, and spurred on by a growing interest by the public, a new paradigm of aging, anti-aging practices, and life extension methods is unfolding. This paradigm underscores all the information you will learn in this book, so before we go on to the next chapters, let's explore the main ideas of the new paradigm of aging. Let's also look at one of the main questions poised by evolutionary biologists: why does senescence occur at all?

Senescence is not synonymous with aging, which is our experience as biological organisms over the course of our life span as marked by the arrow of time. Senescence is the measurable decline in cellular function and the observable changes in bodily processes that accompany aging. It is also referred to as the aging phenotype. A phenotype is the composite of characteristics expressed by genes through our cells and which ultimately creates how we look, function, and what types of diseases we're subject to. Molecular biologists and geneticists look at very minute pieces of the puzzle of life, health and disease, and aging. Evolutionary biologists look at the bigger picture. However, previous evolutionary concepts, until the time of George Williams's theories on pleiotropy, were linear. To understand life, and aging, a more comprehensive, less linear view is needed.

Another way of viewing evolution, and perhaps one more consistent with the ecological and spiritual needs of our times, is to consider that nature and the phenomena of life, as well as living and nonliving things themselves, are constantly changing. According to Eric J. Chaisson, Ph.D., a research professor in astrophysics at Tufts University near Boston, Massachusetts, biological evolution is only part of a much broader evolutionary scheme.

Dr. Chiasson suggests that "cosmic evolution is the study of change" (Chaisson 2001).

The word "cosmic" implies the immensity of the universe and the forces that work to shape all things in the universe, including our planet and the countless organisms that inhabit it.

Nature is not only in constant flux, but it works towards greater complexity. In order to survive, the complexity in nature evolves towards the perfection of each organism, enriching and becoming more specialized in the process. For example, can you imagine a more perfect tiger? It is true that we may be able to clone a tiger, but only over extended periods of time would tigers evolve different, more perfect traits, characteristics, and abilities. In fact, cloning may actually cause de-evolution, the regression of traits that enhance survival. This was seen in the sheep Dolly, the first cloned animal, in 1997; it developed severe arthritis and had a shortened life span.

Natural selection, considered by traditional evolutionary biologists to act for the benefit of the individual, also works for the good of the group. Bret Weinstein, Ph.D., a doctoral candidate in tropical ecology at the University of Michigan in Ann Arbor, says that science cannot expect to simply discover one gene that effects a single disease and then find a way to switch it on and off at will without consequences. He suggests: "If it were so simple, then natural selection would have done it long before we ever became aware that we had a problem" (Royte 2001).

In *The Hidden Connections*, Fritjof Capra, Ph.D., the world-renowned physicist who wrote *The Tao of Physics*, proposes an even more radical departure than Dr. Weinstein (Capra 2002). The central dogma of molecular biology, in vogue for more than four decades, is flawed, says Dr. Capra. In this model, genes are the hereditary units of the cell and therefore the main determinant of the lives of individual organisms, including how they age and what their maximum life span potential might be. Dr. Capra says this line of reasoning will have to be abandoned in favor of a more complex genetic landscape involving the entire genome rather than isolating single genes. Such a landscape is composed of nonlinear networks, multiple interactive pathways, and multiple effects of pleiotropy—much like the mosaic effect discussed in this chapter.

Besides the theories of aging that I have introduced here, there are hundreds of other ideas and concepts as to why we age. None have proven conclusive or to explain all the phenomena associated with aging. A unified theory of aging is still undeveloped. Researchers looking for a specific cause for aging have yet to find one gene, type of cell, or site in the body that controls aging. Perhaps they are looking too closely. Perhaps aging, like all life processes, is not narrowly designed but composed of broad interrelated mechanisms that often occur simultaneously, such that even individual components have multiple functions.

In this scenario, aging appears to occur from a random accumulation of repetitive damage to cells and programmed processes that are genetically controlled, as well as from biological and biochemical events occurring in our bodies that reduce the fine-tuning function of homeostasis. In addition, all of these processes are influenced by biological evolution, as well as by cosmic forces that are part of a universal scheme. Though it is not the purpose of this book to propose a unified theory of aging, by approaching aging from a *multifactorial perspective* we can better design a prolongevity program that is comprehensive and prolongs health and extends life. In fact, more of the scientific experts on aging agree that our primary goal should not be extension of life, but as Dr. Olshansky said, to "prolong the duration of healthy life" (Olshansky 2002).

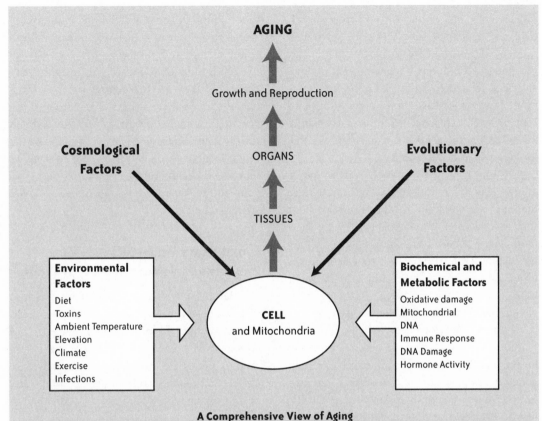

A Comprehensive View of Aging
Cells, the basic functional units of life, are influenced by a variety of factors and conditions resulting in growth, reproduction, and finally aging.

Since there is no single theory that explains the entire process of aging, and since aging may be a broad phenomenon involving numerous, if not all, systems of the body, it is useful to place the many theories into a more manageable perspective. Let's organize these concepts into a coherent scheme in order to better understand the aging process in preparation for learning how we can influence it to prolong our health.

First, we know that individual cells constitute the basic structure of biological life and that they organize themselves in a manner to create different tissues and organs built from proteins according to the genetic information stored in their DNA. In turn, the organs carry on countless physiological processes including reproduction, metabolism, and immune function. However, the biological mosaic that makes up life is vastly more complex than a simple linear model suggests. It also involves highly organized networks, biochemical and neuroendocrine chemical communication systems, the pleiotropy of individual genes, the interplay of longevity genes, and other factors.

Second, cells are influenced not only by genetics, but by external and internal environmental factors such as diet, pollutants, infectious microorganisms, and radiation, as well as by chemicals within the body such as free radical molecules, hormones, and other subcellular and molecular substances. They are also influenced by cosmic forces such as the Earth's gravitational field, our body's internal biological clock related to lunar phase changes, and other factors that have more to do with quantum physics than most gerontologists, mainly schooled in the central dogma of molecular biology, would like to admit.

Third, physical and nonphysical forms of energy play an important role in maintaining life and are involved in the aging process through metabolism, as explained in the thermodynamic theory of aging. Bodily processes are also influenced by laws of physics, and in order for a person to be healthy and live long, these processes must be in harmony with genetic, cellular, and cosmological factors.

Fourth, nature has been at work at this for countless millennia in the process we term evolution, and this plays a substantial role in how genes develop, what their functions are, and how our body responds to environmental factors and stresses such as oxidative damage.

Four Key Concepts of Aging

1. Genetic influences on aging are complex.

2. Environmental factors, including cosmological influences, significantly influence aging and age-related diseases.

3. Physical laws, such as thermodynamics, influence our rate of aging.

4. Evolutionary factors influence why and how we age.

So, welcome to the new paradigm of aging, which I suggest is based upon a comprehensive view and includes all of the theories discussed in this chapter along with the four general concepts of why we age. However, this paradigm goes a step further than integrating individual

theories and is one in which both evolutionary and cosmological processes interplay and where biology and physics intertwine. Cells are the basic functional unit of life in the human body, and they are the central point of influence for all of these factors. They are also the key to prolonging health. When you exert a positive influence on a cell, you improve its function, ability to repair itself, and capacity to reproduce healthy new cells, and by doing so, your body's health is prolonged and your life span extended.

Evolutionary Trade-Offs—Cell Proliferation Versus Cancer Prevention

Before we finish this chapter, let's look at one more critical aspect of aging: cancer. Nature manipulates evolutionary trade-offs and biological balance in ways science is just beginning to appreciate. According to researchers, if evolutionary forces work through natural selection involving reproduction of the individual to maintain the survival of the species, senescence may be the late-life trade-off for a cancer-free youth.

This provocative idea was published in the journal *Nature* in 2002. Scientists working with the p53 gene, a protein that suppresses the development of tumors, found that laboratory mice that lack p53 grow normally but have more cancer, and therefore die young; those bioengineered to have high levels of p53 are resistant to tumors (Tyner 2002). Paradoxically, though these mice don't develop cancer, they age more quickly. The rampant cell proliferation that characterizes cancer and the cellular processes that control it may be linked to normal aging.

Judith Campisi, Ph.D., one of the world's authorities on aging and cancer and a senior scientist at the Life Sciences Division of the

Lawrence Livermore National Laboratory at the University of California, Berkeley, explores how nature solves the cancer problem. According to her studies, this is accomplished in two ways: apoptosis, or programmed cell death, and senescence—tumor cells either die on their own, or we get old and die along with the cancer. Dr. Campisi's evidence suggests that cancer and senescence are related and that tumor suppression evolved at the expense of cellular senescence in the body.

This doesn't mean that if we were to solve the cancer problem an individual wouldn't age, because many supercentenarians are tumor free but still age and die. But perhaps if we were to eliminate cancer, evolutionary processes over several generations would select for longevity genes instead of senescent ones. Biological immortality might then be within reach.

The evolutionary processes of nature are far wiser than modern humans imagine. Instead of trying to find a genetic fix for aging, as if it were a disease, a better solution is to achieve a balance between anticancer activity and the pro-aging effects that the body already naturally possesses. This would thereby reduce the incidence of cancer and slow aging at the same time. In part 2 of this book, you will learn several strategies to effectively bring these two forces, cancer and senescence, into balance.

We will age, but we have considerably more control over how we age than once thought. Gerontologists and other scientists investigating aging have found many significant clues, yet they remain daunted by the mystery of aging. The next step in aging research is the combining of advanced genomic techniques with environmental factors, but to truly advance in our understanding of aging, the new paradigm needs to be accepted first. In this paradigm, the linear view of aging gives way to a comprehensive view in which the genetic mosaic communicates with a variety of environmental factors.

Science is important, but it is not the whole story. The changes that occur during aging are observable and therefore easy to define, but they are difficult to measure. We can learn more about aging by observing long-lived people and those who practice life extension methods. Those who live beyond the average life expectancy do so because they are generally healthier. They also stay more active and curious, have less depression, and maintain their independence well into their ninth decade or longer. They not only live longer, they age more slowly and more evenly than others.

In this chapter we learned several important clues to healthy natural aging:

- Lifelong health contributes to longevity.

- Degenerative diseases shorten life span.

- Environment influences your genes.

- Getting exercise, eating plenty of fresh fruits and vegetables, and drinking sufficient amounts of pure water help you live longer.

- Handling stress effectively and practicing stress-reducing techniques prevent degenerative diseases and improve our chances for longevity.

- Cultural attitudes influence how we think about aging.

- Not smoking and drinking alcohol in moderation help prevent diseases associated with aging.

- Antioxidants help limit the effects of aging and prevent degenerative diseases.

- Natural medicines help prolong health.

• If you don't get cancer, you have a better chance of living to 100 or older.

From the information discussed in this chapter, several basic points surfaced that will influence our discussion on prolonging health and aging throughout the book:

• Successful aging requires good health.

• Successful aging does not require technological medicine, though it may be supported or helped through good medical practices.

• Successful aging largely depends on a healthy environment and lifestyle to support good genes and promote positive genetic expression.

• Successful aging depends on preventing cancer.

In addition, a new paradigm of how we think about aging is emerging. Here is a summary of its key points:

• Aging does not have to be associated with disease.

• We will still age, but we can age more slowly.

• We can age more evenly, and more gracefully.

• We can remain productive and active well into our eighties and nineties, and even longer.

• We may not live forever, but we will live well.

• Prolonging health means we prolong the duration of a healthy life.

2 The Way We Age

In the previous chapter we considered several of the most important theories of aging and organized these many different ideas into an integrated model in order to better understand the variety of influences on aging. We saw that though aging may be inevitable, we have considerable control over its effects; that some people age better and live considerably longer than others; and that our body's biological mechanisms, when in balance, support health and longevity. We also examined the research evidence to prove these assertions, and I stated that my personal and clinical experience indicates that an extended, disease-free life is possible.

Fundamentally, a healthy lifestyle—preferably one that begins early, rather than only when one has gotten older—promotes healthy aging. By promoting lifelong health, the effects of aging may be minimized. However, it is never too late to start improving your health, and you can start increasing your longevity at any age. Prolonging health is a matter of finding ways to cooperate with biological and evolutionary processes that guide our cells, energize our system, and regulate the quality of our aging.

Not only do evolutionary processes promote wellness, they may also select for senescent genes, or the expression of senescence. This suggests we age because we are programmed to do so by evolutionary forces beyond the ability of the current scientific paradigm to understand. Therefore, because we inevitably will age, it is important to know how our body systems age. In this chapter, I discuss the different ways in which we age and the effects of aging on our body and mind.

What Happens Biologically As We Age?

The many causes of aging are at work concurrently, though not simultaneously, over time. Therefore, the physical changes that accompany aging affect every system of the body but appear only gradually. This is because aging occurs first at the cellular level and only later do tissue changes become apparent. Underlying the cellular mechanisms of aging are genetic, molecular, and bioenergetic changes, factors we've called thermodynamic. Eventually the accumulation of molecular, cellular, and tissue changes leads to alterations in organ function. This causes disruptions in your body's systems such as the immune and cardiovascular systems, and that in turn causes senescence, or what scientists call the aging phenotype. These are the biological changes that generate the outward physical expression of an old person.

Additionally, as changes that promote aging occur within the cells, our cells begin to function abnormally. Then not only is organ function reduced, but systemic abnormalities appear and, if environmental influences are out of balance, disease processes associated with aging develop, such as cardiovascular disease, diabetes, and arthritis. Keep in mind that though these diseases are more common in older people, normal aging can and does take place without disease.

In addition to system-wide age-related changes, during the process of normal metabolism (how the body produces and uses energy) we accumulate toxic waste substances that cause direct tissue damage and further alter organ function. For example, a fatty material called lipofuscin, an age-related pigment, collects in the tissues, resulting in disruption of normal cell function. Cell membrane changes occur, causing a reduction in the ability to transfer nutrients and oxygen into the vital components within the cells, and cellular waste products, like carbon dioxide, cannot move as readily out of the cells. Some of our cells become larger (hypertrophy), while others shrink (atrophy); some increase in number (hyperplasia), while others lose their normal organization and change shape (dysplasia).

These cellular changes are effects of aging and the body's attempt to compensate for loss of organ function by altering cellular dynamics. The cells falter because they are unable to keep up with the repair of worn-out parts, and eventually die. However, as you know, the aging process is not as simple as this wear-and-tear concept, but it illustrates the point that cells change over time.

So far, we have been discussing processes that happen within our body, but the external environment also takes its toll. Lifelong sun exposure causes visible wrinkling and damages our skin, and predisposes us to cellular changes; precancerous lesions can appear. The ultraviolet radiation from sunlight also damages our immune function, leaving us more vulnerable to viral infections such as herpes simplex virus. Repetitive use of specific muscles and joints causes the wearing out of cartilage leading to the inflammation and chronic pain of arthritis. Exposure to toxic chemicals and hormone-disrupting substances in the environment (polychlorinated biphenyls [PCBs], 1,1-dichloro-2,2-bis ethylene [DDE], and dichloro-diphenyl trichloro-ethane [DDT]) taxes the functional ability of our liver to detoxify, imbalances our hormone secretion and function, leading to neuroendocrine disorders such as thyroid disease, and weakens our immunity, predisposing us to an ever-increasing risk of cancer.

As these changes take place, our appearance is gradually altered from smooth skin to wrinkles; erect posture to a stooped stance; our natural hair color to gray; from clearly defined gender differences to the androgyny of older people. Connective tissue, such as muscle and tendons, becomes stiff and rigid. Our bones become more porous and brittle. We become frail and feeble—aged.

One of the goals of *Prolonging Health* is to show you how to reverse premature aging and lower your biological age, so it is important that we have an idea of the many changes our body endures as we age in order to create a comprehensive strategy to prevent and reverse these effects. So, let's begin by discussing the main systems that contribute to physiological function and see what happens to them as we age.

How Aging Affects the Body's Main Functional Systems

The body's main functional systems are the cardiovascular (heart and blood vessels);

Physical Changes During Aging

Body System	Changes
Cardiovascular	Your heart gets bigger, the valves thicker, blood stickier, and the vessels rigid. Blood pressure rises, hardening of the arteries appears, and we are more prone to heart disease, heart attacks, and strokes.
Respiratory	Your lungs become less elastic, less air gets into the body, and your breathing becomes more difficult.
Neurological	Your brain shrinks, brain cell function is reduced, and neurotransmitter levels drop. You can't think as well, can't remember things, and may even develop Alzheimer's disease or dementia.
Urinary	Your kidneys shrink and their filtering capacity is reduced. Bladder and prostate gland problems appear, and you have difficulty urinating; incontinence may develop.
Liver	Your liver shrinks and its ability to detoxify drugs and chemicals is reduced.
Pancreas	Your pancreas loses its ability to secrete insulin and you are more prone to Type II diabetes.
Gastrointestinal	Your mouth is drier, you produce less stomach acid, and food is harder to digest. Peristalsis is reduced and nutrients are absorbed from the small intestine. You have more gas and bloating, constipation, and inflammatory bowel disease.
Sensory	Your eyesight diminishes, cataracts form, and macular degeneration is more common. Your hearing is reduced and you can't smell as well.
Connective Tissue, Muscle, and Bone	Your skin becomes thinner, wrinkles appear, and age spots show up. Your bones become weaker. You lose muscle and become weaker.
Neuroendocrine	Your hormone levels drop, causing many of the changes in all of the other systems. You become infertile, have less sex drive, and have difficulty handling stress.
Immune	Your immune function falters. You are at increased risk for cancer, and autoimmune and infectious diseases.

respiratory (air passages and lungs); neurological (brain, central and peripheral nervous system); renal (kidneys and urinary tract); and metabolic, which manages glucose (blood sugar), including the liver and pancreas, and along with the stomach and large and small intestines, make up the gastrointestinal system.

These body systems function in coordination with other systems and biochemical substances to maintain homeostasis, the state of equilibrium between the internal and external environment. This is especially so with the neuroendocrine system, which due to its importance in aging, I discuss separately later. This physiological balance maintains our health, provides restorative capacity to repair and regenerate tissue, and contributes to defending our body from infection and cancer.

Cardiovascular Changes in Aging: A number of changes happen to our heart and vascular system during the aging process. Most are preventable by exercising, eating a healthy diet, and taking nutritional supplements such as coenzyme Q10. As we age, our heart cannot keep up under the strain of physical exercise, which causes lack of aerobic fitness and reduced oxygen supply to the tissues due to the reduced capacity of the heart to pump blood. In addition, the arteries become less elastic (Bortolotto 1999). This stiffening and hardening of the arteries (atherosclerosis) are due to calcium deposits, increased collagen, and fatty deposits (lipid plaques) that tend to accumulate along the inner arterial walls and in the heart tissue itself.

As we age, blood pressure levels tend to go up, especially the systolic pressure (the upper number of your blood pressure reading) (Franklin et al. 2002). High blood pressure is clinically defined as a systolic reading of 140 millimeters of mercury (mmHg) or higher over a diastolic (the lower number) of 90 mmHg or higher. Older people are at risk for stroke and heart disease when the systolic reading is above 140 mmHg, even if the diastolic reading is normal. The optimal blood pressure reading for older people is 120/80 mmHg. Clinically speaking, though I am usually satisfied with this pressure, I counsel my patients to try for 110/70 mmHg.

The heart itself may enlarge, the aorta (the main artery that emerges from the heart) may increase in diameter, and the heart valves can thicken (Kitaman 2000). Doctors call this enlargement of the heart muscle congestive heart failure (CHF), which is a form of progressive heart disease common in elderly people, but one that can be improved with natural therapies.

Relationships between the cardiovascular system and other body systems, such as hormonal imbalances that can affect cardiac function, also occur with aging. For example, abnormalities in the production of aldosterone, an adrenal hormone that promotes sodium retention in order to regulate body fluids, may cause hypertension; low levels of human growth hormone and testosterone may contribute to congestive heart failure; and low estrogen and progesterone levels can increase blood pressure.

Age-related cardiovascular changes can affect the autonomic nervous system, causing sleep disruption, and influence other neurocardiovascular relationships such as the ability of the blood pressure to normalize during rest or after exercise. Though frequently associated with aging, these conditions can be prevented and even reversed through proper diet, exercise, and nutritional supplements.

Respiratory Changes in Aging: During the aging process, the lungs lose their capacity to take in oxygen and distribute it throughout the lobes of both lungs. This happens because the lungs, like the blood vessels, become less elastic, with the result that less air gets into the lower part of the lungs, the area where most of the blood goes, thereby further reducing the oxygen-carrying capacity of the blood. By age 50, breathing capacity can be reduced by 20 percent. In addition, due to this reduced respiratory function, old air cannot get out of the lungs and stays trapped in the lower lobes where toxins and waste chemicals accumulate, causing poor health and difficulty in breathing.

Like cardiovascular disease, this process is preventable. You can improve your respiratory function with physical exercise, breathing techniques, a healthy diet, nutritional supplements, and herbal medicines.

Neurological Changes in Aging: Aging causes extensive changes in the brain and nervous system. In fact, the brain actually shrinks by about ten percent of its youthful size by the age of 80; the prefrontal cortex can lose eight percent of its volume in five years. Though it was previously thought that our brain cells (neurons) were reduced in number by as much as 50 percent, it is now known that we actually retain most, if not all, of our neurons. However, their function declines significantly with age. These losses, in both tissue volume and neuron function, contribute to the lapses in memory, reduced cognitive ability, depression, and even dementia seen in aging individuals.

Brain chemistry is also considerably altered during aging, including loss of the neurotransmitter dopamine, which is associated with pleasure and reward; loss of approximately six percent of dopamine receptors in the brain; and disruption of glucose metabolism and utilization. Other neurotransmitters such as serotonin, a substance associated with mood changes and energy, are affected. Estrogen and thyroid hormone play a particularly important role in brain function; deficiencies of these and other hormones, common during aging, contribute to memory loss, depression, and disrupted sleep.

Changes in brain function can be improved with exercise, specialized brain-enhancing medications called nootrophics, nutritional supplements, and diet.

Kidney Changes in Aging: Among other functions, the kidneys filter the blood and help to manage body fluids and electrolytes (sodium, potassium, calcium, magnesium, and chloride) in the blood. As the kidneys age, the number of filtering cells (nephrons) are reduced, and the kidneys can shrink (atrophy), causing a reduction in the rate of blood filtration. The kidneys may also lose their ability to filter out creatinine, a protein produced by the muscles and contained in the blood. Laboratory tests, such as creatinine clearance, used by doctors to evaluate renal function, measure the ability of kidneys to remove creatinine from the body.

Bladder problems are also common in older people, and vary from increased frequency of urination and frequent urination at night (nocturia) to prolapsed bladder, incontinence, and chronic inflammation of the tissues that line the urinary tract. Enlargement of the prostate gland is a common cause of urinary problems in men as they age, and this affects urinary flow, resulting in difficulty in starting and stopping urination, along with a weakened stream.

Proper kidney, bladder, and prostate function can be maintained during aging through improving hormonal activity, managing chronic inflammation, a healthy diet, adequate fluid intake, herbal supplements, and exercise.

Changes in Liver Function and Metabolism During Aging: Though the liver's cellular function and architecture change with age, the overall function of the liver can continue to work well even into advanced age. However, due to overuse of pharmaceutical drugs including over-the-counter medications (such as acetaminophen), chronic alcohol abuse, viral infections such as hepatitis C, and overeating of high-fat foods, considerable loss of liver function can occur. If the liver is overloaded with chemical toxins from drugs and environmental pollutants, its function is considerably diminished. These conditions can lead to a variety of problems, including cirrhosis, and contribute to accelerated aging.

The liver is the principal organ involved in metabolism of the food we eat, as well as in the detoxification of harmful substances in the blood, including pharmaceutical drugs. That is why maintaining good liver function is so critical to prolonging health. So it is worthwhile discussing the liver's role in aging in more detail.

Based on autopsy studies, males over 65 years have a 24 percent reduction in liver weight and females 18 percent, with a total loss of size for both genders between 25 and 35 percent (Couteur 1998). Even with reduced size and weight, the liver can continue to function normally well into advanced age, and studies, as well as my own clinical experience, show that patients in their eighties and nineties can have normal liver function tests. (For more information on these tests, see part 3.) However, blood flow in the liver can be reduced by 35–45 percent, and bile flow by up to 50 percent. Both of these can adversely influence liver function and therefore digestion, assimilation of nutrients, and metabolism.

Perhaps more important, the liver's ability to detoxify chemical substances, including its ability to clear drugs from our system, may be reduced during aging. Older people tend to use more pharmaceutical drugs, and in combination with decreased liver function, the potential for adverse drug interactions and even lethal side effects from drugs is increased with age. Such increased vulnerability to doctor-prescribed or over-the-counter drugs results from an as yet not understood reduction in the critical detoxification enzyme cytochrome P450 (Zeeh 2002). Not only does this enzyme assist in the removal of drugs from the body, it also plays a significant role in the detoxification of environmental toxic substances. Therefore, avoiding the routine use of drugs is an important consideration for those attempting anti-aging or life extension practices.

Like the liver, the pancreas holds up reasonably well during aging, as long as it is not bombarded with a diet high in refined carbohydrates such as white bread or white sugar. The pancreas secretes insulin, the hormone that regulates blood sugar, and is directly influenced by the amount of sugar in the diet. Age-related changes, complicated by a diet high in simple sugars and refined carbohydrates, cause a significant reduction in glucose tolerance, the abil-

ity of the hormone insulin to keep the blood sugar (glucose) within normal limits after eating. This results in increased incidence of low blood sugar (hypoglycemia), Type II diabetes, and metabolic illnesses such as Syndrome X, a condition characterized by insulin resistance, elevated triglyceride levels, abdominal obesity, and hypertension (high blood pressure).

When people eat too much sugar and refined carbohydrate, their glucose levels increase. Since it is necessary to keep glucose levels in check in order to prevent diabetes, more insulin, the hormone that lowers glucose, is released by the pancreas. When too much insulin is present, cells resist the uptake of insulin because it disrupts their normal function. Too much insulin also accelerates aging, as does too much sugar. That's because triglycerides are blood fats (lipid molecules related to cholesterol) manufactured directly from sugars.

Liver function and glucose tolerance can be improved with diet, exercise, nutritional supplementation, and herbal medications.

Changes in the Gastrointestinal System: Our gastrointestinal system begins in the mouth and ends at the anus, and as we age it changes. Our salivary glands make less saliva and we tend to have a drier mouth and the enzymes contained in the saliva that assist with digestion are reduced. Hydrochloric acid production in the stomach to help break down food and assist in protein digestion is often considerably deficient in elderly people; this is one of the reasons why many naturopathic physicians prescribe extra hydrochloric acid to be taken with meals. The secretion of pancreatic enzymes is also less such that fat and carbohydrate digestion are less effective, and as mentioned above, the liver's secretion of bile is reduced, which impairs fat digestion.

The rhythmical contraction and expansion (peristalsis) of the small and large intestines is weaker during aging; absorptive capacity through the small intestine is lessened; and chronic inflammation of the lining of this organ is more common. The large intestine, whose job is to solidify and compact waste material from the digestive process and remove it from the body as fecal matter during a bowel movement, can become sluggish, resulting in constipation and bloating. Like the small intestine, it is prone to chronic inflammation. However, the large intestine, if taken care of through a good diet, sufficient fiber intake, and exercise, can maintain normal function throughout life.

Gastrointestinal health can be maintained even into advanced age through a healthy lifestyle, a good diet with plenty of fiber, exercise, supplementing with digestive enzymes, prevention of chronic inflammation, the use of probiotic substances such as acidophilus, nutritional supplements, and herbal medicines.

Age-Related Changes to Other Systems

Now that we have discussed the main functional systems that cause some of the most pronounced changes during aging, let's look at some other body systems and see how aging affects them.

The Sensory System: One of the first signs of aging is the need for reading glasses, which usually occurs before age 50. Eyesight gradually diminishes, cataracts form, and in some cases macular degeneration (an age-related eye condition associated with gradual deterioration of central vision) and glaucoma (a condition characterized by increased intraocular pressure, nerve damage, and loss of the

Summary of Selected Characteristics of Senescence	
Increased	**Decreased**
Susceptibility to disease	Ability to repair
Cortisol	Androgenic hormones
Insulin	Glucose tolerance
Parathyroid function	Thyroid function
Cancerous lesions	Skin and tissue tone
Dryness	Moisture
Fatigability	Energy
Stiffness	Muscle tone and strength
Bone brittleness	Bone density and mass
Irritability	Emotional stability
Sexual dysfunction	Sexual interest

visual field) occur. Our ability to perceive color diminishes, and the muscles of the eyes and pupils become less flexible, making it difficult to focus, and we require more light to read by.

Hearing is also impaired in aging, which researchers think is mostly due to the decrease of outer hair cells in the ear that transmit sound waves. Older people have a loss of hearing in the high frequency ranges, difficulty in speech recognition when there is background noise, and may have trouble differentiating tones of complex sounds as in classical music. High blood pressure and atherosclerosis of the arteries in the inner ear and the blood vessels in the neck cause a reduction in the blood flow that supplies the ears and also contribute to hearing loss. Cumulative noise damage over a lifetime of exposure to loud noises, as well as from infection, also causes hearing loss. Tinnitus, the annoying condition of ear ringing that is still poorly understood by medicine, is also more common in older people.

Our sense of smell becomes diminished and though we lose very few taste buds as we age, our experience of taste is reduced. Older people are less tolerant to changes in heat and cold, and their sense of touch becomes more acute.

Since many of these age-related sensory changes are influenced by higher neurological functions in the brain, and since many of these changes actually occur early in life between ages 30 and 50, there is little to do to reverse them once they are established. However, by following the *Prolonging Health* strategies outlined in part 2, you can prevent serious decline in sensory ability and in some cases even improve it.

The Connective Tissue and Muscles: Though the outer layer of skin does not change much with aging, except due to cumulative damage from sunlight and toxic chemical exposure, the underlying layers (dermis) become looser and are affected by reduced blood supply as well as loss of collagen and elastin (protein fibers that give skin and muscle elasticity and fullness). Wrinkling occurs, and the aging pigments lipofuscin and melanin accumulate in the skin, causing the familiar brown spots on the back of the hands and across the face characteristic of elderly people. A lifetime of sun damage predisposes older people to precancerous skin changes, which are often seen as raised dry lesions or moles, and epithelial cancers are also more common among the elderly.

Total bone mass gradually declines from about age 30, but after sex hormone levels fall during menopause and andropause (the male menopause) along with falling levels of growth hormone, DHEA, and other hormones, bone density may decline precipitously, leading to osteoporosis, a condition characterized by the loss of bone density primarily in the spine and hip joint. However, except in rare cases, the end stage effects, spontaneous fracture, don't show up until age 80 or older when the incidence of hip fracture rises steeply. Cartilage is lost around the joints and osteoarthritis can develop with the characteristic stiffness, joint pain, and enlarged joints of older people.

Muscle mass is gradually lost during aging, and this loss is accelerated by inactivity due to arthritic joint pain, lack of energy, and a sedentary lifestyle. Muscle strength can remain fairly stable until after age 50, with a 20 percent reduction occurring during the following two decades; by the eighties we can have lost 40 percent of our original strength with the greatest loss in the arms and hands. Loss of muscle mass and strength change our appearance, gait, posture, and balance. We look spindly in the legs, and lack the muscle tone to hold them up; our remaining muscle and skin seem to hang down. This condition is called sarcopenia, and is considered one of the causes of accelerated aging. Loss of muscle strength also contributes to reduced bone mass (Blain 2001). Weakened back musculature contributes to poor posture, and we stoop (Sorkin 1999).

As muscle mass declines, fat increases, causing an apple-shaped body to appear, with more fat around the waist, hips, and thighs, and less muscle in the arms and legs. This is called lipodystrophy, and is a sign of metabolic disease and unhealthy aging. The cartilaginous discs between our vertebrae deteriorate and we can lose several inches in height; older people frequently suffer from chronic low back pain as a result of this.

Regular exercise, sufficient dietary protein, nutritional supplements, and proper hormonal balance prevent, and in many cases, effectively reverse much of the age-related decline in our muscles, bones, and connective tissue.

Changes in the Neuroendocrine System: As we age, a significant decline in hormone production takes place. Indeed, low hormone levels are one of the most significant factors in age-related changes, affecting all other systems of the body. Because hormonal changes have global effects on all systems and tissues of the body (the basis for the neuroendocrine theory of aging introduced in chapter 1 and discussed in detail in parts 2 and 4), it is worth discussing age-related changes in the neuroendocrine system at this point.

From studying body changes that occur during menopause, researchers have gained considerable information on the aging effects of hormone deficiency. Estrogen drops steeply and ovulation ends in women at about 48–50 years of age, often triggering menopausal symptoms, including hot flashes, night sweats, fatigue, depression, memory loss, and vaginal dryness. In addition, bladder changes occur and there is a tendency to have more frequent urination, bladder infections (cystitis), and even incontinence.

In men, testosterone gradually drops as they approach 50, and this decline (andropause) is involved in tissue changes in the prostate gland, leading to enlargement and difficulty urinating, as well as declining sex drive, reduced interest in activities, and loss of muscle strength resulting in reduced fitness.

However, age-related hormonal changes begin in the brain well before menopause or andropause. The hypothalamus, a gland located in the central portion of the brain that secretes hormones and controls the endocrine system (made up of glands that produce hormones, such as the thyroid gland and adrenal glands), is largely responsible for these changes. Changes in hormonal activity first occur in the hypothalamus, followed by changes in hormonal secretion by the pituitary gland situated in the front part of the brain, and these changes cause modifications in how hormones are synthesized in the target glands such as the thyroid and ovary.

During aging, cells become more resistant to hormones, causing reduced utilization of them by the tissues, as in insulin resistance, where the body fails to respond to insulin. The variety of hormone and hormone-related activity in the body causes global changes in every other system, including the cardiovascular, immune, nervous, and urogenital, and it influences mood, energy, and metabolism.

Let's look at some of the individual hor-

As we age, a significant decline in hormone production takes place. Indeed, low hormone levels are one of the most significant factors in age-related changes, affecting all other systems of the body.

mones that decline during aging. Thyroid function (the endocrine glands in the neck) gradually declines as we age, causing dry skin, fatigue, anemia, thinning hair, and depression. Some anti-aging experts believe that declining thyroid hormone secretion and reduced hormonal activity actually drive senescence. Because low thyroid (hypothyroidism) sharply reduces metabolism, it can cause a number of conditions associated with aging, such as increased cholesterol levels, constipation, dry skin, hair loss, memory loss, depression, intolerance to heat or cold, increased susceptibility to infections, and fatigue. However, in my clinical opinion, though thyroid hormone is important to maintain quality of life for older people, it does not directly trigger senescence.

Levels of anabolic hormones (growth-promoting and muscle-building hormones such as testosterone and DHEA) drop sharply, causing reduced muscle mass, fatigue, and weakness. DHEA levels plummet with aging beginning relatively early in adult life, and this clearly defined drop is considered a reliable biomarker of biological age.

Another hormone with considerable anabolic activity and also considered a biomarker of aging is human growth hormone. It too declines sharply in older people, contributing to sagging skin, poor muscle tone, and many of the other structural changes that occur during aging. Growth hormone has received considerable attention as a possible candidate as a fountain of youth drug, and I discuss it in considerable detail in part 2.

Not only do levels of the female hormones estrogen and progesterone drop, but imbalances between them and the different types of estrogens can cause considerable age-related dysfunction in women, as well as precipitate the cellular changes that lead to a variety of cancers, predominantly breast cancer.

The pineal hormones melatonin and thalamine also decrease during aging, causing dysregulation in the body's natural circadian rhythms, mostly noticed in sleep disruption but with wider-ranging consequences such as reduced immune function and changes in body temperature.

Though declining hormone levels are generally characteristic of aging, the levels of some hormones, such as parathyroid hormone and insulin, can increase. Increased insulin levels cause insulin resistance and can lead to Type II diabetes. Excess parathyroid hormone can lead to osteoporosis. Levels of cortisol, a hormone produced in the adrenal gland, can fall or rise. If it falls, you are more tired, have a tendency to hypoglycemia, and have difficulty handling stress. If it rises, which can also be induced by stress, there is a tendency towards insulin resistance, loss of muscle, and increased fat deposits, especially around the waist, face, and upper back. Levels of leptin, a hormone also associated with metabolism and weight gain, may rise.

The reproductive system is profoundly influenced by hormones, and during aging reproductive function declines and eventually ceases to function. Interest in sex declines with age, and for women with menopausal-related vaginal dryness, intercourse can be painful. Sperm count decreases in men over 50. The incidence of impotence increases with age and even if able to have an erection, many older men find it difficult to maintain it.

The hippocampus is a horseshoe-shaped region in the brain with roles in emotion, sexuality, memory, and cognition; it constructs mental positioning "maps" that help us navigate through our environment. Its function also declines with age. Hippocampal function is highly dependent on hormones such as estrogen (a steroid), melatonin, and a variety of neurotransmitter substances.

Restoration of the normal neuroendocrine balance is critical in order to prolong health, and you do this by supplementing hormonal deficiencies with bio-identical hormones, vitamins and minerals, herbal medicines, diet, and exercise.

Immunosenescence—The Aging Immune System: Our immune system protects us from invading pathogenic microorganisms such as bacteria and viruses, neutralizes allergens such as pollens, and prevents the runaway cell proliferation associated with cancer. During aging, our immune function is considerably reduced and we become increasingly more vulnerable to infections such as pneumonia, are at greater risk for developing cancer, and experience more autoimmune diseases such as rheumatoid arthritis and multiple sclerosis.

As we age, the thymus gland, situated in the center of the chest behind the breastbone, can atrophy and lose functional capacity, and our infection-fighting lymphocytes lose potency.

Declining thyroid hormone and DHEA and imbalances in the adrenal hormone cortisol play significant roles in maintaining normal immunity. Lowered levels make us more susceptible to autoimmune diseases such as rheumatoid arthritis.

Enhancement of immune function in aging is critical for cancer prevention, protection against autoimmune disease, and the ability of our body to resist life-threatening infections.

More Physiological Changes That Affect Homeostasis

A number of other changes occur in your cells, tissues, organs, and function during aging. Let's review a few of these that are pertinent to our discussion on prolonging health.

Organ Reserve: When you are young, your body easily adapts to internal and external psychological stress and physiological demands. This ability is due to the capacity of your organs to respond to the increased functional demands of environmental stressors and is called functional or organ reserve. It is that "extra" capacity reserved for beyond-normal needs. As you age, your organs tend not only to decrease in size and volume, but also to lose some of their reserves. Along with that, your capacity to respond to the stress of physical demands, such as aggressive exercise or an infection, is considerably reduced. In fact, after the age of 30 you lose about one percent of your heart's functional reserve each year. Organ reserve is also lost in the kidneys, liver, spleen, and pancreas. One of the keys to successful aging is to maintain and restore these reserves.

Biological Rhythms: All living cellular organisms on Earth have evolved under the influence of the Sun and its effects, the light and dark cycles of day and night, and the phases of the Moon. Over countless millennia, these rhythmic influences patterned our genes to operate on diurnal cycles, and the physiological functions in your body similarly have cyclical patterns of activity. For example, cortisol production is highest in the morning when you need more energy for work and lowest in the afternoon when the body needs to slow down, rest, and prepare for sleep. The body's clock that controls these alternations between rest and activity is thought to be located in the anterior hypothalamus in the brain.

Another example of a biological rhythm is melatonin secretion, a substance produced by the pineal gland that appears to control diurnal rhythmicity. As you age, melatonin production decreases, and in the very elderly, its production is nearly absent. Some longevity researchers consider it the primary hormone responsible for aging and suggest that its age-related decline triggers "aging" genes that go into activity to control aging on the cellular level.

Sleep patterns, also associated with melatonin levels, can change during aging, and the majority of elderly people accept disruption of sleep as part of aging. However, in investigating sleep and longevity, William Dement, M.D., Ph.D., director of Stanford University's Sleep Disorder Center and considered the world's authority on sleep disorders, found that those who live the longest sleep better than other elderly people. These people get an average of eight hours of sleep per night compared to those who sleep less than four hours or who get more than ten hours of sleep (Dement 1999). It is not known exactly why those who sleep well have greater longevity; however, it is well known that deep sleep supports the body's ability to repair. Regular, deep sleep is also an indication of well-functioning biological rhythms and may be reflective of adequate melatonin secretion.

Intercellular Functions and Aging: Age-related changes occur on all levels in the body, including within individual cells and at the tissue, organ, and system levels. But your body's cells also communicate to one another in a highly sophisticated and complex manner, utilizing countless chemical messengers, which include hormones, neurotransmitters (serotonin and dopamine), messenger substances (cyclic adenosine monophosphate [cAMP]), and many other substances. Even essential fatty acids play a role in facilitating intercellular communication. Aging appears to cause a reduction in the ability of our cells to communicate effectively to one another; to function well, they require enzymes, growth factors, and specialized protein substances.

How Aging Effects Homeostasis: For the body to function properly, it must maintain an equilibrium called homeostasis. Though homeostasis is ultimately determined by cellular function, it is also influenced by the environment and regulated by our organ systems. This constant interchange between external environmental forces and the internal functions of the body, which also includes molecular activity and thermogenic processes, is a pivotal aspect of health and aging.

So important and fragile is the homeostatic state that Nathan Shock, Ph.D., considered the "father of gerontology" and one of the founders of the Baltimore Longitudinal Study of Aging of the National Institute of Aging, suggested that homeostasis may well be the *primary* issue in aging—once we lose it, we begin to age (Shock 1984). In *Aging and Human Longevity*, Marie-Françoise Schulz-Aellen says: "Establishing the nature of homeostatic events and the causes of age-related decrease in functional reserves will undoubtedly produce a major breakthrough in

our understanding of the phenomena of aging" (Schulz-Aellen 1997).

It is with this theme that I would like to conclude this chapter. It is central to the development of an integrated theory of aging, as well as for constructing a comprehensive strategy to prolong health and maximize life span, so I discuss it further in part 2. For now, we are certain that unhealthy aging results in disruption of homeostasis, which in turn appears to trigger a cascade of senescence effects that further accelerate aging. Therefore, maintaining homeostasis is the central goal in the *Prolonging Health* program.

You may accomplish this through diet, exercise, stabilizing natural rhythms and restoring the body's biological clock as described above, managing stress, and other lifestyle measures that promote health.

In this chapter, we reviewed the changes that our body experiences while aging and learned several clues about aging. Homeostasis is maintained by the main functional systems, such as the cardiovascular system, in a synergistic relationship with the endocrine and immune systems. The external environment plays a key role in maintaining homeostasis, so it is important to maintain balance between environmental and physiological factors in order to prolong our health. Communication within the cell, as well as between cells, is altered with aging, and these changes participate in a variety of ways that directly influence homeostasis and aging.

• The body ages slowly over a lifetime.

• Environmental and cellular factors are involved.

• All organ systems decline, but there are ways to prevent and reverse these.

• Maintaining normal homeostasis is central to controlling the rate of aging.

3 When We Age

There are many milestones in life, such as your birthday, when you turned 21, and when you got your first gray hair. For women, the distinctive changes that occur in their reproductive cycle, such as their first menstrual period signaling the onset of childbearing potential, having children, or when they reach menopause, the cessation of menstruation, and the end of fertility, define four decades of female life. Yet despite the old saying "over the hill at 40," there is no specific moment when you can definitively state "that was the day I turned old." Aging happens gradually, incrementally, and it is not visible on a daily basis no matter how closely you look in the mirror. A process rather than a single event, aging occurs in many but not all parts of the body with more or less the same timing, though not simultaneously.

In chapter 1, I discussed several theories of aging and explored the importance of environment on aging, including the degradation of cells by oxidation, infections, damage from solar and other natural sources of radiation, and exposure to toxic environmental chemicals, as well as metabolic influences such as when insulin is too high due to long-term dietary imbalances from eating sugars and carbohydrates and not getting enough exercise. These and the other conditions discussed contribute to the cellular changes that influence when and how we age, which eventually manifests in how we look and function. I describe this in chapter 2, where we explored the physical changes that happen to our body as we age.

Now, in this chapter, I explain how and when aging appears, the difference between chronological and biological age, the different aging periods or zones, the concept of an aging axis, and why it is important for you to know when aging begins. The changes that I describe constitute the typical scenario for somebody who has lived a conventional life. You assist senescence and accelerated aging at any time during your adult life with a highly stressful and unhealthy lifestyle, obesity, faulty genetics, abuse of pharmaceutical or recreational drugs, infections, overexercise, and disease. In this conventional scenario, at 30 you can feel 40 and look 50.

It is our goal to defeat this typical scenario through practicing the *Prolonging Health* strategies outlined in part 2. If we start practicing them at age 30, when we are in our fifties, we'll be healthier than those who didn't. If we start in our fifties or sixties, we'll still be healthier in our later decades.

Well before the age of 50, subtle age-related changes have been taking place. Researchers have found that starting around age 30 four variables changed a lot: (1) pulmonary function, defined by maximum respiratory capacity, declined steadily; (2) kidney function, defined by creatinine clearance, decreased significantly; (3) systolic blood pressure rose; and (4) glucose tolerance, defined by measuring blood glucose levels after a high dose of an oral glucose drink (glucose tolerance test), showed a reduced ability to return to normal.

Aging by the Decades

According to longevity researchers, the process of aging and the long road to senescence actually starts shortly after pubescence. Just as you are entering puberty, your body's cells are already aging. For most people, no noticeable changes occur until they are between 28 and 30 years, and even then they don't associate them with aging. By 30 years old, you get tired more easily than when you were younger, and aches and pains are more frequent. For some, the first symptoms of autoimmune illnesses appear, such as swollen joints and fatigue. Neither doctors nor patients associate these complaints with aging, but undetected age-related changes are already occurring.

Typically, it's not until one's fiftieth birthday that people acknowledge the onset of aging. Perhaps it is because we arbitrarily assigned living to 100 as the maximum life span, and 50 is the halfway mark; or it may be because it is around 50 when women cease menstruating, and when men begin to lose muscle and sexual libido, a time that both men and women begin to lose their sexual attraction.

However, well before the age of 50, subtle age-related changes have been taking place. In the Baltimore Longitudinal Study of Aging, four physiological variables of aging were evaluated in 500 volunteers between the ages of 18 and 103. The researchers found that starting around age 30 all four variables changed a lot: (1) pulmonary function, defined by maximum respiratory capacity, declined steadily; (2) kidney function, defined by creatinine clearance, decreased significantly; (3) systolic blood pressure rose; and (4) glucose tolerance, defined by measuring blood glucose levels after a high dose of an oral glucose drink (glucose tolerance test), showed a reduced ability to return to normal.

So don't be surprised to learn that the first signs of age-related changes occur at about age 25, just past the time of peak reproductive maturity (the ages of 16 to 23). These signs include early hair loss in men, the first hints of infertility in women, and the first occurrences of low back pain. Then between 30 and 40, peak athletic performance declines, hormone levels dip, metabolism slows, women gain weight while men lose muscle if they aren't exercising, and both genders feel stiff with more muscle soreness.

By 40, age-related changes are well under way, and we have our "over-the-hill" birthday. We start to visit the doctor not only more frequently but for complaints that we didn't have before, such as chronic back and neck pain, digestive problems, fatigue, and mild depression. If we exercise, we get injured more easily and recovery takes longer. When we go to a conventional medical doctor, he might comment, "Well, what do you expect, you're over 40." We are prone to use over-the-counter analgesics and anti-inflammatory medications (such as aspirin, ibuprofen, and acetaminophen) regularly, and more willingly accept a prescription drug for pain, sleeping problems, or a mood disorder.

Between 40 and 50, fertility in women declines and, as they approach age 50, their menstrual cycle becomes irregular and eventually stops. Bone density that has already been declining since age 30 may show the early stages of osteoporosis, called osteopenia. In women, there are big fluctuations of hormone levels, causing mood swings. Fatigue is more common. Our skin becomes less elastic, sun-damaged areas appear, and brown spots show on the sides of the face and back of the hands. By your late forties, aging reveals itself in an increasing number of gray hairs; some people's hair may have already turned mostly gray. Muscle tone weakens and breasts sag. During this time and into one's early fifties, women experience hot flashes, while men may show the first signs of heart disease.

Typically, by 50, most people's vision and hearing have diminished, and reading glasses are common. Between 50 and 60 women are unable to conceive and men's sexual drive is decreased, and both of these changes are accompanied by sharp drops in sex hormone levels. In your fifties, the force of aging is undeniably present: your body shape changes and organ function declines, both men and women have a tendency to gain weight around the waist, the arches in your feet fall, and the muscles in your buttocks sag. Heart disease becomes more common, energy and endurance are considerably reduced, and your memory begins to slip.

The obvious effects of the pervasive deterioration of the body's structure and function begin after age 60, and include an increase in the incidence of heart disease, heart attack, stroke, Type II diabetes and insulin resistance, mood changes and sleep disturbance, and increased muscle soreness and joint pains including degenerative disc disease. Immune function declines and we become more susceptible to infections, have poorer defenses, and have more difficulty recovering if we do become infected, as with the virus that causes influenza or the bacterium that causes pneumonia. Latent viruses such as herpes zoster (the same virus that causes chickenpox in children) can reactivate and cause the painful condition known as shingles. Cancer becomes more common.

Once you're in your sixties, your skin is thinner and you have less hair; your bones are also weakening and your muscle strength is fading fast. By your seventies, if you have aged well, you may call yourself distinguished, but in your eighties you are feeling frail and all of your sensory organs are ceasing to function: your vision dims and you can't hear as well. If you make it past 85, you most likely have outlived your friends and peers, and are considering where to live out your remaining years, usually in a nursing home, although some may be lucky enough to share their last days with their family.

From these examples we observe that aging, though subversively happening all the time, seems to manifest major changes in each decade of life. I discuss these cumulative effects in the next section, but before that, I want to remind you that the changes I presented in this section and the previous chapters are all based upon how *average* people age, and not on those who practice anti-aging therapies and life-extension techniques.

Two of my patients who started following *Prolonging Health* techniques early are Ron and Bruce. Their cases illustrate the benefits of a natural longevity program and the importance of starting to reverse the course of aging as early as possible.

Ron, an attorney who now serves as the president of a highly successful natural foods company, is tall, with dark hair and a lean muscular body from a lifetime of athletic training. However, at age 34 he began to notice that his energy was not as vital as in the past, and he experienced fatigue for the first time in this life. His family doctor told him that his cholesterol was slightly elevated, but otherwise there was nothing wrong with him. When he came to see me, we discussed how aging begins after age 30 and how the environment, individual genetics, and psychological stress influence aging.

I ordered additional laboratory tests including those to measure his levels of testosterone, DHEA sulfate (DHEA-S), cortisol, and thyroid hormones. The results revealed that Ron's testosterone levels were already lower than normal and his DHEA-S levels were very low, while his cortisol and thyroid hormone levels were normal. Additional test results suggested an increased risk for early cardiovascular disease. I started him on a healthier diet to lower his cholesterol, recommended natural medicines to enhance his testosterone production, and prescribed a low dose regimen of DHEA.

Today, at age 45, Ron has more energy than he had at 30, and looks and feels younger than he did when he first came to see me. His cholesterol level has been in the optimal range for the last ten years, and his risk for cardiovascular disease is nonexistent. His testosterone and DHEA-S levels are in the upper end of the optimal range. If he continues with his *Prolonging*

Health plan, at age 55 he'll likely look and feel much the same as he does now.

When Bruce first came to see me, he was 42 and told me that he felt extremely well and was at the top of his performance. He told me that, as the international sales manager for a major company, his income was in the high six figures, and that he had been taking vitamin and mineral supplements for years, yet he was concerned about the effects of aging on his body and wanted his hormone levels tested.

Hormone tests are expensive and constitute the biggest expenditure for patients evaluating their aging status. Some health insurance plans cover at least some of the tests required, but many are not reimbursed. Laboratory tests are considerably higher in the United States than in other countries. For example, a test for the total amount of testosterone in the blood costs between $60 and $120 in the United States. The same test in Belgium, Germany, or Mexico costs about $8.

Since money was not an obstacle for Bruce, I ordered a comprehensive panel of hormones including total testosterone, free testosterone, DHEA-S, pregnenolone, cortisol, and insulin, several tests to evaluate cardiovascular risks, and immune function tests. The results revealed low DHEA-S and pregnenolone, normal testosterone and cortisol, and some risk for cardiovascular disease. I started Bruce on a complete *Prolonging Health* plan including DHEA and pregnenolone to compensate for his declining hormone production; I made dietary recommendations, outlined a detoxification program, and suggested he add yoga to his exercise regimen.

I see Bruce every year when we reevaluate his hormones, and based on the results of his tests I make adjustments to his plan. He is now approaching 50, and looks and feels as he did when he was 35.

As each of these men enter their fifties, they will probably not experience the effects of lower hormone levels, and they will continue to look and feel young.

The Classic Aging Zones

As discussed in the previous section, aging clusters around certain periods throughout one's life, with significant age-related changes appearing to fall about every ten years. Though aging occurs as a lifelong process, it begins before age 30, manifesting specific changes in body structure and function at each of these times. It is during these times, or aging zones, that the homeostatic balance tips from youthful vigor towards declining function, when the different factors involved in aging start to outweigh the processes that promote tissue repair, and the definitive tissue changes that characterize aging begin to appear.

In this chapter, we explore these specific changes as preparation for part 2, where I explain how to prolong your health. By following the strategies outlined in the second part of this book, you can create the foundation for living a long and healthy life. For now, let's consider the principal influences that occur in the different aging zones.

Metabolic Changes: As our body ages, metabolism gradually changes, and at times starkly. The principal metabolic "fuel" in the body is glucose, but underlying this are neuroendocrine signals and genetic messages that communicate directly to the cells. All of these mechanisms eventually affect the ability of cells to utilize insulin. Disruption in this process can cause metabolic conditions such as Syndrome X, Type II diabetes, and hypo-

Comparison of Anabolic and Catabolic Processes in Aging	
Anabolic Processes (regeneration)	**Catabolic Processes (degeneration)**
cellular regeneration and repair	tissue destruction and inflammation
glucose used as fuel	abnormal glucose use
increased muscle	muscle tissue degradation
healthy regulatory hormone levels: growth hormone, testosterone, estrogen, DHEA, thyroid, insulin	high levels of catabolic hormones: insulin, cortisol, adrenaline, parathyroid

glycemia. Not only is glucose metabolism affected by aging, but the digestion, absorption, and assimilation of macronutrients from food are reduced, causing a decrease in general metabolism. Declining metabolism causes changes in body shape: women gain weight more easily and men develop a potbelly.

Closely related to general metabolism is body thermodynamics. During aging our body is unable to regulate internal temperature as well as when we were young, which is one of the reasons why vasomotor symptoms such as hot flashes and night sweats appear or why we feel the cold more. This is one of the first signs that your thermodynamic system is changing due to aging.

Cellular metabolism is affected as well. The energy-producing powerhouses of cells, the mitochondria, become less efficient, and we are more easily fatigued, have reduced tolerance for exercise, and slower recovery after exercising.

A variety of hormonal changes occur that directly influence metabolism, thermodynamics, and cellular function. During the early phases of aging, hormone production does not decline too much, but the way your body utilizes hormones does. The natural balance between hormones is also altered, including those that affect metabolism, principally cortisol and insulin. A gradual shift occurs from a predominance of anabolic steroid and sex hormones (estrogen, progesterone, testosterone, and DHEA) to hormones that have catabolic effects at higher levels, principally cortisol, insulin, and adrenaline.

Anabolic processes are those that build muscle, strength, endurance, and support metabolic activity, and catabolic are those that take them apart. Normally, catabolic processes balance anabolic activity by breaking down tissue, but when they predominate, more wear and tear—and accelerated aging—occurs.

As discussed, by age 50 the production of nearly all hormones is reduced and levels have either dropped significantly or are in steady decline. This dramatic change in hormone levels and function causes many of the visible age-related changes that occur in our body such as thinning skin, loss of muscle mass and tone, and hair loss. These changes have led the proponents of the neuroendocrine theory of aging to believe that aging can be reversed simply by replacing hormones. Though there is some truth to this, only some of the effects of aging can be improved by taking hormones, which is why it is necessary to follow a comprehensive plan for prolonging your health.

As we age, our neurological system and its intimate relationship with the endocrine and metabolic systems falter. Neurological decline leads to memory lapses, makes it more stressful to navigate new surroundings, causes mood disorders such as depression, and in some people may lead to neurodegenerative conditions such as Alzheimer's or Parkinson's disease.

Strictly speaking, there is no established metabolic aging zone. However, metabolic changes influence so many systems in the body, participate in a variety of disease processes, and color aging to such a degree that for our purposes of prolonging health, we can usefully think in terms of a metabolic zone in which aging processes are accelerated or delayed. This metabolic zone falls roughly between the ages of 30 and 65; it generally occurs before frailty and other aging symptoms manifest; it is largely dependent on diet; and it culminates in a point of no return when the catabolic processes of aging dominate anabolic ones.

Karlis Ullis, M.D., a sports medicine physician at the University of California in Los Angeles and the author of *Age Right*, refers to this time as the "critical point" (Ullis 1999). Drawing from physics and upon principles from the thermodynamic theory of aging, as well as his experiences with overtraining in athletes, Dr. Ullis rightly suggests that as we age catabolic hormones increase and metabolic activity that tears down our body takes precedence over anabolic rebuilding ones. At the critical point, our body's metabolism becomes considerably less efficient in building up muscle and producing energy, and therefore cannot repair injured or damaged tissue as easily as when younger. It is at this time in life when age-related changes occur more intensively.

All changes that affect metabolism significantly disrupt homeostasis, which in turn affects every other system and organ in the body. As an example of how this occurs, let's look at three different times of life when the effects of aging are most evident: menopause, andropause, and somatopause.

Menopause: The most studied of aging zones is menopause, the time that signals the end of the female's reproductive capacity, characterized by the cessation of menstruation. Doctors define natural menopause as the lack of menstruation for 12 consecutive months, in the absence of surgical or hormone therapies that inhibit menses in a woman between the ages of 48 and 52.

All of the major hormones decline sharply

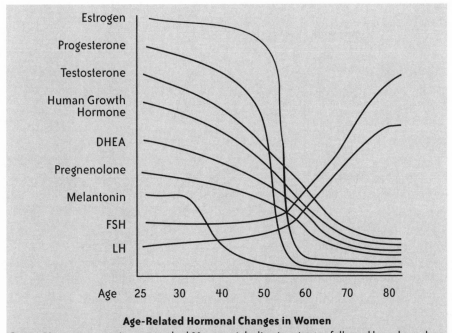

Age-Related Hormonal Changes in Women

By age 50, women experience a gradual 30 percent decline in estrogen followed by a sharp drop after menopause. Progesterone begins to fall off as early as the mid-thirties, with a major drop-off by menopause. Human growth hormone, DHEA, pregnenolone, and testosterone show a steady decline starting in the late twenties, with a 75 percent loss by age 70. Melatonin remains relatively constant until between 40 and 50 years old and then drops off significantly. Levels of follicle-stimulating hormone (FSH) and luteinizing hormone (LH) rise.

around age 50, while follicle-stimulating hormone (FSH) and luteinizing hormone (LH) increase. This is because the pituitary gland is attempting to stimulate ovarian hormone production by increasing those hormones (FSH and LH) that increase estrogen and progesterone secretion. In a similar fashion, thyroid hormone secretion is often reduced while thyroid-stimulating hormone (TSH) increases. Levels of the adrenal hormones DHEA and cortisol decline, but in some cases cortisol may actually rise, creating further imbalances.

Metabolism declines and women either gain weight or become thinner, and in either case have typically less muscle mass. Body temperature regulation becomes imbalanced and

some women experience hot flashes, and may also become more sensitive to the cold. At about the same time that all of these hormonal imbalances are taking place, blood pressure may rise in some women.

The word menopause comes from the Greek root *men*, referring to the moon, and suggests the rhythmical monthly cycle of menstruation. Therefore the menopause is not only, in a sense, the failure of ovarian function and a deficiency and imbalance of female hormones, but also a dysfunction in biorhythms and signals an alteration in the homeostasis of earlier years.

Andropause: The male equivalent of menopause is termed andropause. *Andro* also comes from the Greek and refers to male as in

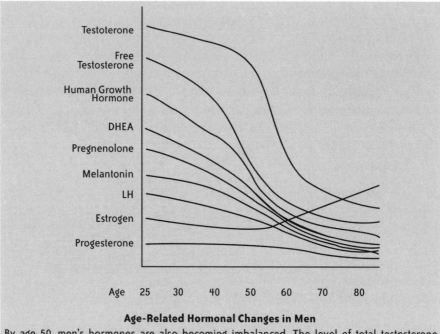

Age-Related Hormonal Changes in Men
By age 50, men's hormones are also becoming imbalanced. The level of total testosterone declines at least 25 percent by age 80, and free testosterone by at least 50 percent. Estrogen may rise and LH fall, and GH and melatonin drop as well.

androgens, which are steroid hormones such as testosterone that cause masculine characteristics. Actually, the male change starts in the late forties and becomes increasingly more apparent by the mid-fifties, and is more progressive and less marked than menopause. It is characterized by reduced muscle mass and tone, reduced strength, fatigue, depression, loss of sexual libido, decrease in body hair, and increase in abdominal fat (Morales 2000).

Blood levels reveal a decrease in both total and free testosterone and DHEA—all androgenic hormones. In fact, an 80-year-old man will have only 25 percent the testosterone of a 20-year-old, and free or available testosterone will have declined by at least 50 percent. Other hormonal changes occur, such as increasing levels of estrogens and sex hormone–binding globulin, and decreasing levels of luteinizing hor-

mone (LH), growth hormone (GH), and melatonin are present in blood samples (Gould, Petty, and Jacobs 2000).

When estrogen levels rise in men, they experience feminizing characteristics including less facial hair and increased body fat. As noted, LH is a hormone released by the pituitary gland in your brain; it controls the release not only of estrogen but also of testosterone. When LH levels are low, there is less production of estrogen and testosterone in the body.

Somatopause: Though sex hormone levels decline sharply for women at the time of menopause, and significantly though gradually for men about the same time, the true aging zone, called somatopause, doesn't happen for at least another decade after menopause and andropause. Blood tests reveal that low growth hormone, low sex hormones, low insulin-like

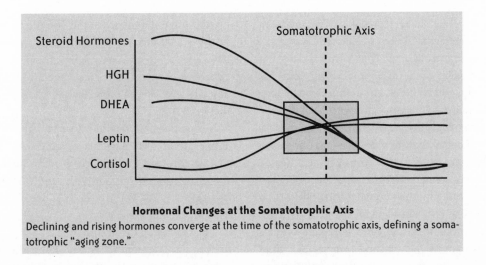

Steroid Hormones

HGH

DHEA

Leptin

Cortisol

Somatotrophic Axis

Hormonal Changes at the Somatotrophic Axis
Declining and rising hormones converge at the time of the somatotrophic axis, defining a somatotrophic "aging zone."

growth factor I (IGF-I, also called somatomedin C), increased sex hormone–binding globulin, and increased levels of homocysteine, which is a toxic amino acid by-product of metabolism, all occur at the somatotrophic axis. This is when you reach the somatopause, or the aging zone.

In addition, cortisol and insulin levels may increase, as well as leptin, a protein released by fat cells that influences weight and blood pressure. The somatotrophic axis is the major hormonal system controlling growth in the body. In aging, it is marked by an irreversible decline in growth hormone (GH) and insulin-like growth factor I (IGF-I). This is thought to cause the typical decreased muscle mass and strength, decreased bone density, and increased body fat generally associated with the aging body.

Longevity researchers believe that aging, largely associated with the progressive decrease in human growth hormone, is best defined as when an individual crosses the somatotrophic axis, characterized by a decrease in skeletal muscle mass and bone density resulting in frailty. Human growth hormone (HGH) is indirectly measured by blood levels of insulin-like growth factor 1 (IGF-1), a

substance produced in the liver related to growth hormone release. Lower IGF-1 levels are due to reduced liver stimulation by growth hormone, secreted by the pituitary gland. Levels of HGH, as measured in the blood and urine, are also lower in older people, with a 14 percent decline between the ages of 21 and 71.

The Age-Point Concept

However, besides the metabolic aging zone and somatotrophic axis, there is another transitional point. In this book, I call this the *age-point* to distinguish it from the somatotrophic axis and Dr. Ullis's "critical point." I coined this term to distinguish it from other age-related transitional points, because to effectively prolong health and extend life span, it is necessary not only to know when aging has taken place, but what is the optimal time to intervene in the aging process.

The age-point is not solely dependent on levels of GH or IGF-I, as in my opinion, when these hormones are low, you are close to the point of no return. After having been in decline for years, levels of HGH and IGF-I alone are not sufficient to evaluate aging, and other biomarkers are necessary, such as DHEA sulfate. The age-point is also not the metabolic critical point, which signifies a shift from anabolism to catabolism that can actually occur at any time in your life depending on your diet, the amount you are eating or not eating, stress, and your level of exercise. From an age-related perspective, there is no doubt that metabolism influences age. Increased catabolism assures that you will age faster. However, though both of these are defining markers of aging they only describe part of the problem, not the entire picture.

In order to understand aging in a more comprehensive manner and to intervene clinically early enough to make the deep changes necessary to prolong health and reach our maximum life span, we have to discover that point in time when our aging first begins, not after it has already happened. We must find the age-point that happens before both the critical point and the somatotrophic axis.

Early Signs of the Age-Point

• Fatigue

• Loss of balance

• Loss of muscle mass and strength, especially in the legs

• Glucose imbalances (sugar craving, weight gain around the middle of the body)

• Chronic low-grade pain (joint pain, headaches, low back or neck pain)

• Reduced tolerance for exercise

When Does the Age-Point Occur? There is no exact science on how to measure this change, nor, as I mentioned earlier, is there an exact moment when it occurs. However, an astute physician who practices anti-aging medicine and life extension practices can determine

if you have entered any of the aging zones, are at the somatotrophic axis or critical point, or have passed it and are experiencing the full effects of senescence. Of course, if you are at any of these stages, you have already passed the age-point.

To better understand where you are on the aging curve, it is necessary to determine how well you are aging, what factors are influencing the aging process in your body, and what your own age-point is. You can do this on your own without the help of a doctor.

Surrounding the age-point is an aging zone of from five to ten years when the different aging factors begin to influence how your body functions, signaling that senescence is at hand. Obviously, the earlier you intervene, the better chance you have of prolonging your health, but it is also true that you can begin your program at any age.

The transitional stages of aging occur earlier than obvious symptoms of aging. Perimenopausal symptoms such as hot flashes and night sweats happen between ages 48 and 50, but hormone decline and imbalances have been taking place for at least a decade before that. Though men don't experience changes as abruptly as women, and there is no medical consensus on when the andropause actually takes place (though most symptoms of testosterone deficiency occur after age 50), gradual hormonal insufficiency starts around age 35. Fluctuations of hormone levels caused by stress and dysfunction in hormone metabolism and utilization by the tissues due to poor diet and lack of exercise contribute further to reaching the age-point early. Therefore, we can say the age-point generally occurs between ages 35 and 45.

Signs that indicate you are near the age-point include generalized stiffness and gradual loss of flexibility, gradual loss of balance, lack of muscle tone and strength, increasing fatigue, low

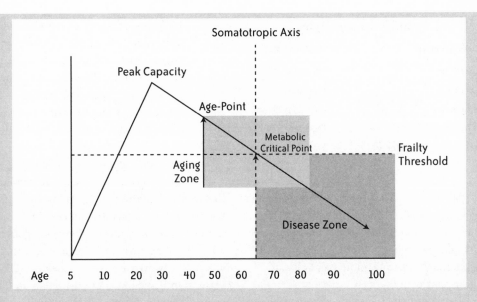

Somatotropic Axis

Peak Capacity

Age-Point

Metabolic Critical Point

Frailty Threshold

Aging Zone

Disease Zone

Age 5 10 20 30 40 50 60 70 80 90 100

Comprehensive Aging Chart

This chart integrates the concept of the **age-point** and other theories of aging zones and axis. The vertical soma-totrophic axis is intersected by a frailty threshold, when physical strength and performance decline, and is sur-rounded by the general aging zone that includes menopause, andropause, and the somatopause. Peak capacity is achieved early in life between the ages of 20 and 30, followed by steady decline. The age-point falls along this line touching the aging zone, and precedes both the "critical point" and somatotrophic axis. A disease zone, where an increasing incidence of illness occurs, roughly follows the critical point and extends towards the later years.

exercise tolerance, and glucose imbalances. All of these are caused by a combination of the con-ditions discussed: declining hormones, thermo-dynamic and metabolic changes, as well as the interplay of evolutionary forces and genetics.

For both men and women, by the time they are in their late forties and early fifties, undeni-able changes occur, including hot flashes and night sweats in women and loss of energy and strength in men. These obvious changes indi-cate that you are well into the aging zone, may have passed the critical metabolic point, and are headed for senescence. Our goal is to pre-vent this from happening, or if it has occurred, to reverse it.

Can the Age-Point Be Influenced? It should be clear by now that how we age is mal-leable and that we have a considerable degree of control over the aging process. We may not be able to stop it, or entirely reverse it, or live for-ever; but we can certainly *influence* it in a posi-tive manner and prevent diseases associated with aging and halt the effects of senescence.

Unfortunately, most anti-aging programs are too generalized in their approach or they concentrate on hormone therapy to relieve some of the major symptoms of aging, without actually reversing the underlying aging process. In order to influence aging in a markedly effec-tive manner, you need to know exactly where you are on the aging curve, adapt the principles discussed in this book, and adjust the specific dosages of the medications that I outline in part 2 to *your* individual situation.

For example, Barry Sears, Ph.D., the best-selling author and father of the "30-30-40 Zone

Influences on Aging

Positive Influences	Negative Influences
Regular exercise	Sedentary lifestyle
Healthy diet	Poor diet
Extra nutrients	Lack of nutrients
Healthy hormones	Deficiency of hormones
Effective stress management	Stress

diet," speculates in *The Age-Free Zone* that by taking omega-3 fish oil and eating more protein and fat, we can enter a zone where aging doesn't take place (Sears 1999). Like most anti-aging programs, this one addresses only part of the aging puzzle. In this case, not only are more omega-3 oils and high-quality protein necessary, but you need a complete healthy diet plan including an abundance of fresh organic vegetables. Yet however important diet is in retarding aging, it is not sufficient only to eat well and remain inside this anti-aging zone. The age-point itself must be reset.

By *resetting the age-point,* you lower your biological age. Biological age measures how old your body is based on aging biomarkers. It may be lower or higher than your chronological age based on your birth date. To prolong health you must delay the onset of the age-point, reset it if you are currently in the early stages of aging, and if past it, reverse as many of the aging factors as possible (see part 2). We also want to lower biological age and remain in the upper end of the aging zone for as long as possible.

Senescence is *avoidable,* even if aging is not. In your seventies, even though visibly older, you can retain youthful vigor and peak energy that allows you to perform physical activities unheard of in people of this biological age in earlier generations.

Gina Kolata, a science reporter for the *New York Times,* covering a scientific convention on the limits of aging at the University of California School of Medicine in Los Angeles in 1999, summarized this point well. She said, "The goal is to allow people to be vigorous and healthy as they age, to stretch out the good years rather than elongate the bad ones" (Kolata 1999).

Older people are becoming more active and remaining productive longer. But to stay healthy during the aging years, the use of natural medicines and keeping a healthy lifestyle become critical. One of my patients at 86 is the active owner of a vegetarian restaurant where she works every day making delicious vegetarian dishes for her customers and counseling them on how to be healthy. Her blood profiles are like that of a healthy person in the prime of life with no abnormalities in levels of cholesterol or glucose.

Consider a few more people who have aged well, such as former astronaut and United States Senator John Glenn, who at 77 returned to space to orbit the Earth for nine days. The oldest skydiver is Herb Tanner from Ohio, who at 92 jumped out of an airplane and parachuted safely to Earth. Science fiction author Ray Bradbury wrote *From the Dust Returned* in his early eighties, and the American artist Paul Cadmus painted into his nineties.

Aging occurs subtly and gradually, starting between the ages of 25 and 30. From there, the signs of aging show up every decade. The years between 45 and 75 constitute an aging zone where the first major age-related changes occur, especially in our reproductive cycle and the sex hormones that maintain fertility, and we undergo menopause and andropause. Within this zone is a critical point where the body's metabolic balance is tipped in favor of age-related changes. The somatotrophic axis, occurring between age 65 and 75, signals significant age-related hormone decline in HGH and IGF-I, and is a definitive marker for senescence.

In order to effectively influence the aging trajectory, we need to find an earlier point—*the age-point*—outside the aging zone, and before both the critical point and somatotrophic axis. We prolong health by preventing disease and controlling the effects of senescence. When combined in an organized way, information on aging zones and points helps in the construction of an effective individual strategy for prolonging our health.

- The first signs of aging appear between the ages of 25 and 30.

- The typical age-point is between ages 35 and 45.

- Age-related changes in reproductivity occur between ages 40 and 50.

- The aging zone is between 45 and 75.

- A metabolic critical point happens in the aging zone and signals accelerated aging.

- Frailty begins at the somatotrophic axis, occurring between ages 65 and 75.

- We must start resisting aging earlier than once thought.

- Knowing your age-point is the best place to begin.

4 How to Determine Your Biomarkers

In this chapter, you will learn how to evaluate the effects of aging by filling out a questionnaire, learning about information found in routine blood profiles, and by visually examining your body. This may be strange for many people used to having a doctor examine them. To prolong your health and achieve maximum longevity, it is necessary for you to become more comfortable with looking at your body and to see how it is aging.

Understanding how your body shapes itself according to the food you eat, your level of exercise (or lack of it), your hormonal balance, and other aging factors provides invaluable information about how *you* are aging and helps in determining *your* biological age, age-point, and how healthy you are in the aging zone. Contained within these tests is valuable information about your health during aging. When put together, an aging profile emerges informing you about your biological age and how well, or poorly, you are aging. It brings the *Prolonging Health* program right into your life and body.

Reversible Biomarkers of Aging

Biomarker is a term popularized in 1990 by William Evans, Ph.D., and Irwin H. Rosenberg, M.D., of the USDA Human Nutrition Research Center on Aging at Tufts University in Boston. This term refers to selected biological markers that indicate critical physiological functions that occur in aging (Evans 1991). In the narrow definition of the term, as used by researchers, biomarkers must be measurable, quantifiable, and universal, applying to all people under similar circumstances.

For example, herpes zoster or shingles primarily occurs in older people due to declining immunity, but it also occurs in younger people and it does not occur in all older people; therefore, it is not universal. The incidence of cancer is higher among older people, but it does not occur universally in this group. However, underlying both cancer and shingles is immune weakness, which does occur in most older people. Therefore, a test that measures immune function may be more useful as a biomarker because of its universal appearance. Besides blood tests, biomarkers reflect physical activity, strength, and other bodily functions such as aerobic capacity that influence fitness, vitality, and wellness.

Originally, Drs. Evans and Rosenberg identified ten reversible biomarkers. These included cholesterol/HDL ratio, blood pressure, and percentage of body fat, and though these are still used by physicians to evaluate biological age, there are many other measure-ments and tests that serve as biomarkers, and which help approximate biological age com-pared to chronological age, as well as determine the age-point. The new biomarkers provide for greater individualized information on how *you* are aging; ultimately, the success of your *Prolonging Health* program is judged by how well you normalize all of these measurements and not just the ten original biomarkers.

Ten Original Biomarkers of Aging

1. Muscle mass
2. Strength
3. Basal metabolic rate
4. Percentage of body fat
5. Aerobic capacity
6. Blood sugar tolerance
7. Blood pressure
8. Cholesterol/HDL ratio
9. Bone density
10. Body temperature regulation

New Biomarkers

In addition to the ten original biomarkers, I propose these additional ones:

1. Balance
2. Skin elasticity
3. Waist-to-hip ratio
4. Albumin
5. BUN
6. Uric acid
7. Iron
8. Fasting glucose
9. Fasting cortisol
10. Blood lipids: cholesterol, triglycerides, LDL, HDL

11. Triglyceride/HDL ratio
12. Lipoprotein (a)
13. Apolipoprotein E4
14. DXA scan for bone density
15. DHEA-S
16. Total testosterone
17. Estradiol
18. IGF-I

Prolonging Health Recommendations Regarding Biomarkers

1–Complete the Biomarker Questionnaire

2–Determine Your Body Measurements

3–Use Common Laboratory Tests As Biomarkers

4–Get Your Second Level Anti-aging Diagnostics Done

5–Evaluate Your Hormone Levels

6–Determine Your Antioxidant, Vitamin, and Mineral Status

7–Know the Condition of Your Immune System

8–Take Five More Tests to Evaluate Your Health: Tests for Chronic Inflammation, Mitochondrial Function, Genomic Status, Neurotransmitter Profiles, and Toxicology Studies

9–Complete the Age-Point Questionnaire

Prolonging Health Recommendation 1— Complete the Biomarker Questionnaire

Biomarker questionnaires are designed to provide detailed information about body func-tions, tissues changes, mood and cognitive changes, and other parameters that change

The *Prolonging Health* Biomarker Questionnaire

Place a check next to each question that pertains to you. A checked box is a yes answer, and an unmarked one is a no. Total the number of check marks. If you answered less than 10 you are aging well; if between 11 and 20, your aging rate is average; if more than 21, your biological age is higher than your chronological age and you are aging poorly. The goal over time is to have fewer check marks each time you complete the questionnaire. I recommend doing it every three months during your first two years on the *Prolonging Health* program.

Changes in Mood, Memory, and Thinking:

___ Do you sleep poorly or is it interrupted?

___ Are you more forgetful than you used to be?

___ Do you have increasing difficulty concentrating?

___ Have you experienced mood changes that you didn't have before?

___ Do you have unexplained depression?

___ Do you have anxiety or panic attacks?

___ Have you noticed a decreased ability to handle stress or increased anger or irritability?

___ Do you have difficulty finding your way while driving or in a large store?

Changes in Skin and Hair:

___ Is your skin or hair drier than before?

___ Is your skin thinner?

___ Do you have more brown or red spots on your skin?

___ Have you noticed more spider veins on the skin?

___ Are you more wrinkled?

___ Do you have brown spots or a brown mask on your face?

___ Do you bruise easily?

___ Is your hair thinner than before?

___ Have you lost a significant amount of hair?

___ Is your hair more than 50 percent gray?

Changes in Appetite, Digestion, and Elimination:

___ Do you have any sensitivity to certain foods that you didn't have before?

___ Has your ability to tolerate alcohol decreased?

___ Do you experience more gas or bloating after meals than when you were younger?

___ Are heavy foods like meats more difficult to digest?

___ Do digestive enzymes improve your digestion?

___ Do you have a greater tendency than before to have constipation or diarrhea?

___ Is your appetite less than it was when you were young?

Hormonal Changes:

___ Is your sex drive and/or performance less than it used to be?

___ Do you have hot flashes?

___ Do you have night sweats?

___ For women: do you have vaginal dryness?

___ For men: do you get up more than one time a night to urinate?

Immune System Changes:

___ Do you experience slow wound healing?

___ Do you easily catch colds or flu, or find them lasting longer than before?

___ Do you have or have you had any of these viral infections:

___ Herpes Zoster (shingles)?

___ Epstein Barr Virus?

___ HIV?

___ HHV-6?

___ Hepatitis?

___ For women: do you have chronic vaginal or bladder infections?

___ For men: do you have chronic prostate infections?

___ Do you have chronic yeast or parasitic infections?

___ Do you have more allergic reactions than when you were younger?

__ Do you have chronic sinus infections?

__ Do you have an autoimmune disorder?

Changes Involving Chronic Inflammation and Pain:

__ Are you stiff in the morning?

__ Do you have chronic pain or inflammation in your joints, muscles, lower back, or neck?

__ Do you have osteoarthritis?

__ Do you have irritable bowel syndrome, colitis, or Crohn's disease?

Cardiovascular Changes:

__ Do you have cardiovascular disease?

__ Do you have high blood pressure?

__ Have you had a stroke?

__ Have you had bypass surgery or angioplasty?

__ Do you easily get out of breath?

Changes in Energy or Carbohydrate Metabolism:

__ Do you have a reduced capacity for physical work and exercise?

__ Is it difficult for you to stay up late?

__ Have you experienced significant weight loss in the last 1–2 years?

__ Have you gained weight?

__ Have you noticed more body fat?

__ Are there more fat deposits on your abdomen and waist?

__ Do you wake up tired?

__ Are you more fatigued?

__ Do you require longer recovery time after exertion?

__ Do you have a craving for sugar?

__ Are you rarely thirsty, or very thirsty?

Changes in Body Composition, Structure, and Posture:

__ Have you experienced a decrease in muscle mass?

__ Is your physical strength reduced?

__ Are you less flexible?

__ Are your muscles flabby, especially under your arms and in the buttocks?

__ Is your spine less flexible?

__ Has your posture changed, or do you stoop forward?

Changes in the Urinary Tract and Sexual Function:

__ Do you have urinary incontinence?

__ Do you have to urinate more than one time nightly?

__ Do you have repeated urinary tract infections?

__ Have you lost more than 50 percent of your pubic hair?

__ Is your interest in sex reduced by more than 50 percent or entirely absent?

Changes of Sensory Function and Balance:

__ Do you lose your balance more easily, or frequently feel dizzy?

__ Do you have ear ringing?

__ Have you fallen down more than two times in the last year and for no obvious reason?

For Women:

__ Have your breasts decreased in size and fallen?

__ Do you have vaginal dryness?

__ Has sexual intercourse become painful?

For Men:

__ Do you have erectile dysfunction or impotence?

__ Do you have feminizing characteristics such as less body hair and breast enlargement?

during aging. The questionnaire provides a complete review of all the body systems and other changes that occur during aging as discussed in the previous chapter. Most biomarker questionnaires are graded by a number system, which I find too time consuming and tedious; also, self-evaluation forms are highly subjective, as the person answering the questions is the one experiencing the condition and therefore the answers are subject to wide individual interpretation. For example, one person may consider joint stiffness and pain a minor inconvenience, but someone else might find the same condition debilitating. I prefer simple "yes" or "no" forms.

In my clinic, I use the biomarker questionnaire. Every new patient fills out this form along with a health and medical history form and a detailed lifestyle questionnaire. After the patients have completed the biomarker form, I discuss the answers with them to define their condition further. Through this, in combination with the family history, a physical examination, and laboratory tests, I determine their aging status. The questionnaire is also useful for follow-up to evaluate the progress of their program, and I ask my patients to fill out the same form six months after their first visit and once a year thereafter. You can do the same, beginning by completing the biomarker questionnaire and other methods of evaluation presented in this part of the book.

A Representative Case Study: To illustrate how the biomarker questionnaire works, let's look at a case study. I vividly recall the first phone call I received from Maurine, a 65-year-old woman who told me that she had advanced osteoporosis. Emotional and with difficulty remaining focused on her condition, she informed me that after years of following a strict health food regimen and what she considered a healthy lifestyle, several bones in her

right foot spontaneously fractured. When she came to my office, her foot was in a cast and she carried a stack of medical records.

In tears, Maurine explained her medical situation, which not only involved osteoporosis but also a progressive degenerative eye disorder, allergies, asthma, and difficulty gaining weight. She was also concerned about Alzheimer's disease since several members of her family had developed dementia.

Her biomarker questionnaire score was 27, which told me that she was already biologically older than her age based on her birth date. Among the questions she checked were fatigue, forgetfulness, poor concentration, sensitivity to cold, thinning and drier skin, and more frequent infections.

I ordered additional blood tests and bone density studies, and reviewed all of her results, after which I formulated my impressions of her condition. Then, I started her on a natural bio-identical hormone prescription and a comprehensive nutritional plan. After six months, Maurine's score had fallen to 18, which suggested an average rate of aging. In one year her bone density was significantly improved, she had more energy, her memory was better, and she could think clearer. At the end of two years, her score was 9, she was feeling better than she had in a decade, and her osteoporosis was reversed as revealed by annual bone density studies.

Prolonging Health Recommendation 2— Determine Your Body Measurements

Though providing useful information for the clinician and patient on a broad range of body systems, questionnaires are only the first phase in evaluating your aging profile. The second method used to determine the effects of age and the degree of senescence involves measurements of various physiological functions and physical changes that occur with aging.

The following six biomarkers are best measured in a clinical setting, but they can also be assessed at home on your own. They provide an estimate of how well you are aging:

• Aerobic capacity

• Balance

• Blood pressure

• Body temperature

• Skin elasticity

• Body Composition

Aerobic Capacity: Observe the carefree movements of children. They play effortlessly for hours because their aerobic capacity is perfectly adapted to their body. However, as we age, the aerobic capacity of most of us declines, with a 30–40 percent decrease by age 65. Some of this decline is due to age-related changes in the function of the heart and lungs, but most loss of aerobic capacity is actually due to poor fitness caused by years of sedentary lifestyle. It can be reversed by exercise and a healthy lifestyle.

Your aerobic capacity is the ability of your lungs and heart to process oxygen, especially under increased demand. In order to do this, the lungs must be able to inhale large volumes of air without difficulty or tiring. Once in the lungs, oxygen is exposed to the blood in the alveolar tissue and the pulmonary capillaries. The oxygenated blood returns to the heart in the pulmonary veins and is pumped by the heart into the arteries, which then supply all the body's tissues and cells. To oxygenate blood and to move the oxygenated blood to all tissues in the body, the lungs and heart must be strong and functioning effectively.

Aerobic capacity is measured in two basic ways, by direct and indirect methods. In the lab or clinical setting, aerobic capacity is measured directly by ergonometric equipment or by a cardiopulmonary analyzer; this measures the volume of air inhaled and the concentration of oxygen in the blood. Direct methods require technical support, and a physician may have to be in attendance. These methods are not to be confused with a treadmill stress test, which records the heart's electrical activity by measuring its rate and rhythm during exercise-induced exertion, in this case while running on a treadmill.

Direct methods for measuring aerobic capacity are costly, and though providing useful information for research purposes and generating a record of your performance, they are not necessary for an evaluation of your aerobic capacity. For this, indirect methods are satisfactory. These are based on the idea that there is a direct relationship between heart rate and oxygen uptake such that the higher your activity level the greater your heart rate and the deeper and faster you breathe, which increases oxygen uptake.

To measure this you need a stationary bicycle, a quarter-mile track (440 yards), or stairs; you ride, walk, or step for a specific time or distance and then measure your pulse rate. Your age and pulse rate are marked on a chart and are scored against averages for your age group. This method is complicated and time consuming, and though it appears to be objective, in reality it only provides a general estimate of your aerobic capacity.

Since our goal is to return your aerobic capacity to a youthful level, I suggest that you use the track at a local high school, college, or fitness center, or measure off a quarter-mile along a safe and level street in your neighborhood. Then walk that quarter-mile at your best and most brisk pace, making sure you can finish it at that pace. If you can safely walk a quarter-mile, then increase it to one mile. You should be able to walk a mile in less than 20 minutes. You also should reach a target heart rate, which the American Heart Association recommends should be 50–70 percent of your maximum heart rate. You can calculate your target heart rate by subtracting your age from 220 and multiplying by 0.75. For example, a 65-year-old person's target heart rate is about 120 beats per minute. (See the appendix for websites that provide target heart rate calculators.)

Immediately after you've completed your walk look at your watch, which you've already used to mark the time it took to complete, and take your pulse rate. To take your pulse rate, place the first three fingers of one hand across the radial artery at the wrist just below the thumb of the other hand. Once you've found your pulse, use your watch to time ten seconds while counting each pulsation. Multiply the total beats per ten seconds by six to obtain how many times your heart beats per minute. See if you are reaching your target heart rate by the end of your walk. If not, and you are not completing the mile in 20 minutes, your aerobic capacity is weak. You may increase your aerobic capacity and endurance by exercising regularly.

Balance: Children delight in balancing tricks, and even something as simple as standing on one leg or walking the lines in a sidewalk provides them with joy and a sense of accomplishment. However, as we age we tend to lose our balance, and older people have a tendency to fall more frequently, often with disastrous results. Hip fractures are common in elderly women and though due to falling, the underlying cause of the fracture is reduced bone density (osteoporosis). These are all conditions associated with the frailty of aging, and are

largely due to lack of fitness and years of inactivity, resulting in weakness of the leg muscles and loss of balance. In the United States, one of every three people over 65 falls once each year (Sattin 1992) and the falls account for 87 percent of all hip fractures (Fife 1985) requiring medical treatment in a year.

Here are three ways to evaluate your balance:

1. Stand upright with your feet six inches apart and your arms by your sides.

   Breathe evenly and relax for a few moments.

   Close your eyes while remaining as steady as possible.

   Time yourself by using the second hand on a clock or watch to see how long you are able to stand still and straight before losing your balance or feeling dizzy. If you can stand without losing your balance for longer than three minutes, you are doing well.

2. Stand with your feet together, large toes and the insides of the heels touching.

   Close your eyes and see how long you can stand without feeling dizzy or losing your balance. If you can stand perfectly still for more than one minute, you are doing well. If you get dizzy or lose your balance immediately, your sense of balance is deteriorating.

3. Finally, stand on one leg by lifting up until the toes are only touching the ground, and then lift it completely off the ground. If you can balance for one minute with your eyes open, you are doing well. You may improve balance through practicing tai chi, yoga, and balancing exercises.

Blood Pressure: Blood pressure tends to rise with age mainly due to reduced heart function and stiffening of the arteries. But it may also be caused by poor kidney function, imbalanced hormonal activity or low production, and other factors such as imbalances in sodium and potassium from eating salty foods or processed foods containing sodium. Though high blood pressure (hypertension) is frequently associated with aging, many older people actually have normal blood pressure.

One of my patients, an 85-year-old man, first came to me with a very high blood pressure reading of 200/100. After he changed his diet and took natural medications for several months, his blood pressure normalized to 140/78. Another patient, an 87-year-old woman, has consistently had normal blood pressure readings with her systolic range between 104 and 140 and the diastolic between 70 and 80. These examples show it's possible for older people to maintain and restore their blood pressure to normal ranges.

The systolic reading is the pressure that the blood exerts on the muscles of the arterial walls when the heart contracts and blood is pumped out of the heart into the vessels; it is the reading most often elevated in older people. The type of high blood pressure in which the systolic reading is elevated and the lower reading is normal or low is called isolated systolic hypertension; it is defined by a systolic pressure higher than 140 mmHg (mercury).

The diastolic reading is the pressure between heartbeats. If the arteries are elastic, the peripheral and major blood vessels are not blocked with calcification or fatty plaques, and the blood volume and viscosity are normal, then a normal diastolic reading for a person over 60 should be about the same as for a younger person: less than 120 mmHg.

Your blood pressure is a reliable biomarker for your cardiovascular disease risk, and indirectly it provides a clue to your fitness level. Elevated blood pressure indicates that your cardiovascular system is in poor physical condition, with an increased risk for stroke, heart attack, and kidney failure. Hypertension can cause headaches and vague symptoms such as fatigue,

but often it causes no symptoms at all—a characteristic that earns it the title of "the silent killer." Your doctor or nurse can take your blood pressure, but you can also easily take it yourself at home with a digital automated blood pressure cuff. You can buy one at your local pharmacy, over the Internet, or through a catalog.

If your blood pressure is high, start active treatments using natural medicines, lifestyle changes including regular exercise, changes to your diet (including eating more vegetables), and eliminating salt. In my clinical opinion, hypertension is a preventable condition that does not have to accompany aging. Many physicians agree. Michael Mogadam, M.D., author of *Every Heart Attack Is Preventable* (Mogadam 2001), and Richard D. Moore, M.D., Ph.D., author of *The High Blood Pressure Solution* (Moore 2001), contend that hypertension and most cardiovascular diseases are preventable with diet and exercise. By keeping your blood pressure within normal to optimal ranges, you may reduce your risk for heart disease, heart attack, and stroke.

If your blood pressure is too low, you will feel tired and often experience dizziness when you stand up too quickly. Although low blood pressure is not associated with stroke, it may be a sign of other body imbalances including low thyroid or adrenal gland function. The necessary tests to evaluate hormones are discussed in the next chapter, but make sure your doctor evaluates you for both high and low blood pressure.

Body Temperature: If you go to the beach on a chilly day don't be surprised to see young children playing contentedly in the cold water for hours. You'll see the same indifference to cold during winter, when children often prefer to play without coats or sweaters and even take off their gloves to play in the snow. Children's body temperature regulatory mechanisms are

Ranges for Blood Pressure Readings

Elevated	greater than 140/90 mmHg
Acceptable	less than 130/85 mmHg
Optimal	less than 120/80, but not lower than 90/60 mmHg

very flexible, but as you age, your body's thermostat doesn't work as well as when you were young. You are more sensitive to cold, as well as heat, indicating that the homeostatic mechanisms in the brain that regulate your internal temperature (thermoregulation) are less functional. That's typically why older people move to Florida, Arizona, or Southern California: to avoid the cold northern winters.

Elderly people also suffer more during hot weather, and extreme heat can even cause death. Dehydration, due to not drinking enough water, changes in the hormones that retain fluids in your body, and poor kidney function are common problems with older people and contribute to poor or inefficient thermoregulation. Older people tend to sweat less, which is one of the body's means of regulating internal temperature, and therefore are more intolerant to heat.

Though the average body temperature (taken with an oral thermometer) is around 98.6° F (37.5° C), there is considerable individual variation. Normal temperatures can range from a low of 97.6° to a high of 99.3° F. Body temperature also follows a circadian rhythm with lower temperatures occurring in the morning and slightly higher ones in the afternoon. To find out your average core temperature, place a common fever mercury or digital thermometer under your tongue twice each day for five days, and at different times during the days; then calculate the average. If it falls within 0.5 degrees of the norm (98.6°), you are doing well.

Another way to measure body temperature

is with a basal thermometer. Basal metabolic temperature (BMT) is the measure of the lowest temperature your body reaches when at complete rest; it provides an estimation of your basal metabolic rate (BMR), which is the minimum amount of energy measured in calories needed to sustain life during complete rest. Children have high metabolic rates, burning energy for growth, but metabolic rate slows during aging. Lower basal metabolism is also an indicator of low thyroid function, a hormone that commonly declines with age. The normal range for basal temperature is 97.8° to 98.2° F.

To take your basal body temperature you need a basal thermometer obtainable from a drug store. Basal thermometers differ from regular mercury fever thermometers in that their bulb ends are rounder and they are calibrated in different increments. Keep the basal thermometer by your bed, and after sleep and before getting out of bed in the morning, place the thermometer under your arm in the armpit for several minutes (up to 10 and no less than 5).

Record the reading in a notebook directly after taking your temperature and before moving about and getting out of bed. It is very important to take your temperature at approximately the same time every morning for at least five days and then calculate the average reading. If your average basal temperature is below 97° F, your metabolic rate is reduced and you may have low thyroid function; these are conditions associated with aging.

Skin Elasticity: Healthy children and young adults typically have a rosy complexion, are wrinkle free, and their skin is plump and highly elastic. As we age, our skin becomes drier, more wrinkled, thin, and considerably less elastic.

To evaluate your skin's elasticity, perform

what doctors call the "pinch test." Pinch the skin on the back of one hand between your thumb and forefinger, holding it about five seconds, and as you quickly release, watch how your skin behaves. If it springs back immediately and flattens out quickly, your skin has retained its elasticity. However, if it flattens slowly or remains ridged, your skin has lost much of its original elasticity. Skin that is slow to flatten can also signify dehydration, which also is accompanied by dry and flaky skin. In this case, drink more water on a regular basis and repeat the pinch test in a few days.

You can tell if you are dehydrated or holding too much water by performing another simple test. Sitting in a chair, place the hand of one arm on your knee, palm down. Observe the veins on the back of your hand, and then slowly lift your arm all the while watching the back of your hand. If the veins gradually disappear by the time your hand is shoulder height, your fluid levels are normal. If they don't disappear at all, even when your hand is over your head, you may be dehydrated. Drink more water.

If no veins are visible when your hand is still on your knee and your hands, fingers, and wrists are puffy and swollen, you are retaining too much fluid. Since water acts as a diuretic, simply drinking more water may cause you to urinate more, eliminating much of the excess fluid in your body. If that doesn't work, employ the natural diuretic effect produced by drinking carrot or watermelon juice.

Body Composition: In this section, we discuss four additional measurable biomarkers under the category of body composition: waist-to-hip ratio, lean muscle mass, muscle strength, and the circumference of the thigh and calf. These serve as valuable biomarkers providing important information on our risk for degenerative disease and life expectancy, and they can help in monitoring the success of our program.

As people age they tend to lose muscle and gain fat, though some lose both muscle mass and fat, becoming abnormally thin and underweight. At the same time, remaining body fat accumulates in the central part of the body. The gradual erosion of lean muscle appears to be universal in advanced aging in both men and women, although women lose less total muscle than men. As noted, this body configuration is called sarcopenia. It is characterized by loss of muscle mass, muscle weakness, increased fatigability, and frailty. Perhaps more than any other condition during aging, sarcopenia plays the greatest role in the overall physical decline that accompanies the aging process.

If you are otherwise healthy, but are gradually losing muscle and gaining fat, even if you are not obese but have a higher fat-to-muscle ratio, you are more prone to all of the age-related degenerative diseases. Insulin resistance and glucose intolerance in particular are associated with the sarcopenic body type.

However, sarcopenia is preventable because it is the result of neuroendocrine imbalances, changes in protein metabolism, and neuromuscular changes that happen during aging. All these are modifiable by following the *Prolonging Health* program, and there is considerable scientific and empirical evidence that physically active older people do prevent and even reverse sarcopenia.

As a general rule, the onset of fat gain and muscle loss begins around age 45; it is largely caused by sedentary lifestyle, improper diet, changes in body metabolism, anabolic and other hormone deficiencies, and a reduced ability to build and repair protein in the skeletal muscles. The main anabolic hormone that builds and maintains muscle mass is testosterone. Though not an anabolic steroid hormone, human growth hormone also increases lean muscle mass.

Having a greater muscle mass to fat ratio improves aerobic capacity because there are more muscle cells and therefore a greater demand for oxygen. It also improves strength, increases bone density due to indirect benefits of resistance training when you build muscle through weight lifting, and improves your appearance and indirectly your self-esteem because you look better.

With age, the percentage of body fat has a tendency to rise while both muscle mass and strength gradually decline. This is largely due to poor diet, sedentary lifestyle, and abnormal insulin regulation. The composition of the average sedentary 65-year-old woman's body is about 43 percent fat (adipose), while that of a 25-year-old is between 22 and 28 percent; female athletes may have less than 12 percent. The average young adult male has about 15–18 percent body fat, and a male athlete may have less than 5 percent; the average elderly American man typically has 35 percent body fat.

Body composition testing measures your percentage of body fat and tells you if you have too much or too little fat compared to lean tissue. There are several ways to determine body composition. Unfortunately, none are highly reliable, but they are the only methods we have at this stage (Clasey 2000). The most accurate (and most inconvenient) involves being completely submerged in a tank of water in order to calculate the amount of water displaced by your body. This method gives a reliable measure of total body fat. Another uses skinfold calipers with measurements taken at several locations around your body. The person performing the test uses the calipers to pinch the skin together; the amount of skin and fat under the skin (subcutaneous adipose tissue) is recorded and your body fat percent is determined by a formula. This method is useful and

relatively easy to perform, but it provides only an estimate of your total body composition.

Other methods include bioelectrical impedance testing and dual energy x-ray absorptiometry. Impedance testing involves connecting you to a small device that sends an electrical current through your body to measure tissue resistance: the slower the signal, indicating increased resistance, the more fat you have. Impedance testing is popular in many clinics because it is easy to perform, but it also provides only an estimate of body composition. Bone density testing by dual energy x-ray absorptiometry (DEXA) can also determine body fat percentage; if you have this procedure done to evaluate osteoporosis, ask for a body fat percentage report as well.

Although it is useful to know your body fat percentage, it is not necessary in order to get started on your *Prolonging Health* program. If you do not have access to any of the methods I've described, you can obtain a general idea of your body fat by observing your own body shape, as discussed in the previous chapter, and by measuring your hips and waist to obtain the hip-to-waist ratio.

WAIST-TO-HIP RATIO: One of the most common changes seen in people over 40, though also noted in unhealthy younger people, is a change in body shape in which fat is deposited around the waist and upwards toward the lower margin of the rib cage. The effect is a greater diameter above the waist than around the hips. In both men and women, a ratio greater than 1.0 increases the risk of cardiovascular disease and diabetes, as well as reduces your general health and fitness; it also increases your biological age and negatively influences your age-point.

Knowing your waist-to-hip ratio is a significant biomarker because it provides information about body composition and insulin regulation. There is a greater tendency to collect fat around and above the waist when insulin and cortisol are elevated. Unlike many of the previous biomarker measurements, the waist-to-hip ratio is easy to measure on yourself.

To measure your waist-to-hip ratio use a non-stretching cloth tape measure like tailors or seamstresses use. Place it around your waist, then measure the circumference of your waist at its natural curve; if lacking that curve, measure at its widest part. When putting the tape around your waist, only touch the skin and do not pull it tight or perform the measurement immediately after eating a large meal. Record the number. Then measure your hips at their widest point above the buttocks. Record that number as well. Now, divide the waist measurement by the hip number. The result is your waist-to-hip ratio.

LEAN MUSCLE: One of the hallmarks of aging is the disappearance of muscle, which in its extreme form is sarcopenia. In order to age well, prolong your health, and reach your maximum life span, you must retain as much muscle as possible and increase your lean muscle as it is essential to attain longevity. Most Americans as they age increase body fat while losing muscle—a sure formula for accelerated aging and increased risk for degenerative diseases.

Body mass index (BMI) has been used for decades to estimate one's degree of obesity, as an estimate for growth and development in children, and recently as a measure for longevity because it has predictive values for mortality (Shiner 2001). The World Health Organization classifies obesity at three levels, with those having body mass indexes of over 30 prone to the most risk.

The Centers for Disease Control (CDC) provides this formula for calculating your BMI: Divide your weight in pounds by twice your height in inches and multiply the result by 703.

$$BMI = \left(\frac{\text{Weight in pounds}}{\text{Height in inches} \times \text{Height in inches}} \right) \times 703$$

For example, if you weigh 100 pounds and are five foot two inches tall, your BMI is about 20. You can also use the precalculated table found on the National Institutes for Health website.[5]

To find your BMI:

- Find your height on the left side of the chart.
- Move across the row to the right until you find your weight.
- Follow the column up to find your BMI at the top of the chart.

The optimal body fat percentage for men should be less than 15 percent, and for women less than 25 percent. For BMI, the dividing line for overweight is 25, with values above 30 indicating obesity. A healthy BMI for both men and women is in the range of 20–25, and for optimal health less than 20.

However, keeping your body fat percentage and BMI within ranges is not enough to prolong your health. To do so requires maintaining and even increasing lean muscle mass, as well as muscle tone and strength. Weight training, certain forms of isometric exercises, and some types of traditional hatha yoga are the only known ways to increase muscle mass. In addition, the steroid anabolic hormones DHEA and testosterone, as well as growth hormone, can markedly improve body composition, lowering the percentage of fat and increasing the size of muscle.

MUSCLE STRENGTH: Since frailty is one of the main characteristics of advanced age, your strength is a central biomarker of aging. It can provide a reliable indicator of how well you will

Body Mass Index Table

Healthy BMI ranges are between 19 and 24; your risk for degenerative disease is low. If your BMI is between 25 and 29, you are overweight with a moderate risk for degenerative disease. BMI above 30 indicates obesity. You have an increased risk for degenerative disease and accelerated aging. Above 35 signifies extreme obesity, very high risk, and very accelerated aging.

	Normal				Overweight					Obese									
BMI	19	20	21	22	23	24	25	26	27	28	29	30	31	32	33	34	35	36	37	38
Height (inches)		Healthy				Moderate					Increased Risk and Accelerated Aging									
58 (4'10")	91	96	100	105	110	115	119	124	129	134	138	143	148	153	158	162	167	172	177	181
59 (4'11")	94	99	104	109	114	119	124	128	133	138	143	148	153	158	163	168	173	178	183	188
60 (5'0")	97	102	107	112	118	123	128	133	138	143	148	153	158	163	168	174	179	184	189	194
51 (5'1")	100	106	111	116	122	127	132	137	143	148	153	158	164	169	174	180	185	190	195	201
62 (5'2")	104	109	115	120	126	131	136	142	147	153	158	164	169	175	180	186	191	196	202	207
63 (5'3")	107	113	118	124	130	135	141	146	152	158	163	169	175	180	186	191	197	203	208	214
64 (5'4")	110	116	122	128	134	140	145	151	157	163	169	174	180	186	192	197	204	209	215	221
65 (5'5")	114	120	126	132	138	144	150	156	162	168	174	180	186	192	198	204	210	216	222	289
66 (5'6")	118	124	130	136	142	148	155	161	167	173	179	186	192	198	204	210	216	223	229	235
67 (5'7")	121	127	134	140	146	153	159	166	172	178	185	191	198	204	211	217	223	230	236	242
68 (5'8")	125	131	138	144	151	158	164	171	177	184	190	197	203	210	216	223	230	236	243	249
69 (5'9")	128	135	142	149	155	162	169	176	182	189	196	203	209	216	223	230	236	243	250	257
70 (5'10")	132	139	146	153	160	167	174	181	188	195	202	209	216	222	229	236	243	250	257	264
71 (5'11")	136	143	150	157	165	172	179	186	193	200	208	215	222	229	236	243	250	257	265	272
72 (6'0")	140	147	154	162	169	177	184	191	199	206	213	221	228	235	242	250	258	265	272	279
73 (6'1")	144	151	159	166	174	182	189	197	204	212	219	227	235	242	250	257	265	272	280	288
74 (6'2")	148	155	163	171	179	186	194	202	210	218	225	233	241	249	256	264	272	280	287	295
75 (6'3")	152	160	168	176	184	192	200	208	216	224	232	240	248	256	264	272	279	287	298	303
76 (6'4")	156	164	172	180	189	197	205	213	221	230	238	246	254	263	271	279	287	295	304	312

Source: Adapted from *Clinical Guidelines on the Identification, Evaluation, and Treatment of Overweight and Obesity in Adults: The Evidence Report.*

age such that those with greater muscle strength generally age better than those with less. Though the cause of age-related muscle atrophy and gradual loss of strength is a sedentary lifestyle, the underlying reason muscles lose mass and strength is a reduction in the total number of muscle cells, leading to shrinkage or reduced muscle cell size. This age-related change affects neuromuscular communication from the nerves to the remaining muscle fibers and leads to increased stiffening of muscle fibers (fibrosis), reduced protein metabolism, and falling levels of anabolic hormones such as testosterone.

Studies have shown that people lose 30 percent of their total number of muscle cells between the ages of 20 and 70. Indeed, many older people often lose so much strength in their leg muscles that they have a hard time walking, finding it difficult even to get back up when they bend down or to rise from a sitting position from a chair.

Loss of muscle mass and function not only affects overall strength, but influences other same weight more times, or to lift a heavier weight.

THIGH AND CALF CIRCUMFERENCE: Since muscle mass, strength, and tone are critical during aging, which muscles or muscle groups are most important? It appears that maintaining the muscles in the legs is very important in overall fitness, cardiovascular health, and in the prevention of age-related erosion of body composition. Also, compressed discs in the lower spine and the accompanying entrapment of the spinal nerves that supply the lower extremities may cause atrophy of the calf muscles.

As you start your *Prolonging Health* program, measure both of your thighs and calves at their thickest width using a cloth tape. Record this number, and as you progress through your program, remeasure and compare

Extreme Obesity

39	40	41	42	43	44	45	46	47	48	49	50	51	52	53	54
186	191	196	201	205	210	215	220	224	229	234	239	244	248	253	258
193	198	203	208	212	217	222	227	232	237	242	247	252	257	262	267
199	204	209	215	220	225	230	235	240	245	250	255	261	266	271	276
206	211	217	222	227	232	238	243	248	254	259	264	269	275	280	285
213	218	224	229	235	240	246	251	256	262	267	273	278	284	289	295
220	225	231	237	242	248	254	259	265	270	278	282	287	293	299	304
227	232	238	244	250	256	262	267	273	279	285	291	296	302	308	314
234	240	246	252	258	264	270	276	282	288	294	300	306	312	318	324
241	247	253	260	266	272	278	284	291	297	303	309	315	322	328	334
249	255	261	268	274	280	287	293	299	306	312	319	325	331	338	344
256	262	269	276	282	289	295	302	308	315	322	328	355	341	348	354
263	270	277	284	291	297	304	311	318	324	331	338	345	351	358	365
271	278	285	292	299	306	313	320	327	334	341	348	355	362	369	376
279	286	293	301	308	315	322	329	338	343	351	358	365	372	379	386
287	294	302	309	316	324	331	338	346	353	361	368	375	383	390	397
295	302	310	318	325	333	340	348	355	363	371	378	386	393	401	408
303	311	319	326	334	342	350	358	365	373	381	389	396	404	412	420
311	319	327	335	343	351	359	367	375	383	391	399	407	415	423	431
320	328	336	344	353	361	369	377	385	394	402	410	418	426	435	443

body functions. These include a slowing of metabolism, bone loss, poor blood sugar tolerance, increased body fat, reduced hormone production, and a reduction in overall fitness with declining aerobic capacity. Your muscle strength is measured by lifting a weight or by repetitive lifting of a weight before and after a period of prescribed weight training. The goal is to become progressively stronger, measured by the ability to lift the

Optimal Body Fat Percentage, Waist-to-Hip Ratio, and Body Mass Index

	Body Fat Percentage	Waist-to-Hip Ratio	Body Mass Index
Men	Less than 15%	Less than 0.90	Less than 20
Women	Less than 25%	Less than 0.80	Less than 20

Optimal body fat percentage, waist-to-hip ratio, and body mass index in both men and women should approximate those of youth.

the results. You are gaining muscle mass if your thighs and calves are thicker. Stronger legs are associated with greater health and longevity.

Prolonging Health Recommendation 3— Use Common Laboratory Tests As Biomarkers

A number of blood tests are contained within the general chemistry tests and blood counts that your doctor may routinely order to evaluate your health and screen for diseases. Several individual tests within both these labo-

Studies have shown that people lose 30 percent of their total number of muscle cells between the ages of 20 and 70. Loss of muscle mass and function not only affects overall strength, but influences other body functions. These include a slowing of metabolism, bone loss, poor blood sugar tolerance, increased body fat, hormone production, and a reduction in overall fitness with declining aerobic capacity.

ratory studies are useful as biomarkers and provide information on how well you are aging, as well as your risk for age-related diseases.

Biomarkers in Your Blood Chemistry: A blood chemistry panel, also called a metabolic panel, is a common laboratory test that evaluates 20 or more different substances in the blood. From this information, your doctor obtains a general idea of your liver and kidney function, the level of your blood sugar, and your blood lipids (fats); he can also tell if any of the

most common disease processes are occurring in your body. Depending on which lab is used, average ranges for normal results can vary slightly, which is why is it a good practice to utilize the same lab each time you have a blood test performed. Physicians practicing naturopathic and nutritional medicine agree that optimal values, those values that best reflect the healthy rather than disease state, often have a narrower range than the averages and provide a better picture of how your body is functioning.

When you have your annual physical, ask your doctor for a copy of these tests so you can evaluate the results. Keep a record of them and follow each of them year by year, or at least every two to three years:

- Albumin
- BUN
- Glucose
- Lipids: cholesterol, triglycerides, low-density lipoproteins (LDL), high-density lipoproteins (HDL)
- Cholesterol/HDL ratio
- Uric Acid

ALBUMIN: Serum albumin is a reliable biomarker to evaluate nonmuscle protein status. It is the major protein that circulates in the blood, and among its other functions it helps to maintain water pressure in the blood vessels, which prevents tissue edema from occurring. Albumin is also a weak but important hormone-binding protein. It is produced in the liver and its levels are dependent on adequate dietary protein intake and liver function. Lower levels are associated with inadequate protein in the diet, diarrhea, fever, infection, liver disease, inadequate iron intake, third-degree burns, and edemas, or low calcium.

When followed over several years, declining albumin levels have been shown to be associated with decreased longevity. The average range is 3.5–5.5 g/dL (grams per deciliter), but the ideal value is 4.0 g/dL in an optimal range of 3.8–4.8. Compare your albumin levels over several years; if you have a declining level, it indicates increased physical senescence. Conversely, albumin levels that are too high do not reduce aging and may even hinder your longevity program since albumin acts as a hormone-binding protein in the blood and potentially prevents hormones from reaching their target sites.

BUN: Blood urea nitrogen is the end product of protein metabolism and serves as a marker for protein breakdown. The average range is 5–25 mg/dL. As you age, protein metabolism is reduced, leading to reduced repair of proteins in your tissues. You may recall that proteins are essential for life and are the structural components of your body. If your BUN is low (5–8 mg/dL), it may indicate that you are not getting enough protein in your diet. If it is near the upper end of the range (20–25 mg/dL), it can mean that you have more protein breakdown than normal. Higher than normal levels (greater than 25 mg/dL) can also mean that you are eating too much protein or that your kidney function is abnormal. If the levels are abnormally high, your doctor may request further evaluation of your kidneys. The optimal level is between 15 and 20 mg/dL.

GLUCOSE: Though maintained within a narrow range (mainly by the hormone insulin but also by other body functions), blood glucose levels can vary widely depending on how much

Useful Tips When Having Your Blood Drawn

Since blood chemistry values are designed to be measured after a 12-hour fast, the best time to take this test is early in the morning.

• Do not eat anything after dinner and do not have breakfast until you have your blood drawn. People who are very hungry in the morning may have low blood sugar and often find it difficult to wait to eat.

• Plan to go into the lab as soon as they open in the morning and bring a sandwich, yogurt, or orange juice with you so you can eat something and raise your blood sugar immediately after you have your blood drawn.

• Drink a glass or two of pure water about an hour before your blood is drawn because if you are dehydrated it is difficult for the lab technician or nurse to draw the blood as it may be too concentrated and thick.

and what types of foods you eat. Therefore, a morning fasting level (not having eaten all night) is the standard measurement to evaluate the levels of glucose (blood sugar). The average range is 65–115 mg/dL; however, a tighter normal range of 70–100 mg/dL serves as a better clinical evaluation. Values below the lower end of the range may indicate low blood sugar (hypoglycemia), protein malnutrition, or low adrenal function.

If you suspect hypoglycemia, a glucose tolerance test (GTT) will confirm the diagnosis. The GTT is performed by testing a fasting sample of blood for glucose and then in hourly increments after drinking a 75 gm glucose solution. In my clinical experience, the two-hour GTT is adequate to evaluate hypoglycemia and other disorders such as insulin resistance; however, some physicians prefer the three- or five-hour GTT. If your glucose levels are above 120, you may have diabetes (hyperglycemia) and will need further evaluation by your doctor. Increased levels may also indicate thyroid dysfunction, adrenocortical hormone excess, or that the test was taken after you ate.

Several hormones that affect aging also influence glucose metabolism, including cortisol, growth hormone, and insulin. This has led some researchers to believe that glucose regulation is one of the key factors in how well and how long you live. For now, keep in mind that your fasting glucose reading should remain within the normal range (65–115) and optimally between 78 and 85 mg/dL.

LIPIDS: Measurements for blood lipids, or fat-like substances, are used to evaluate your risk for cardiovascular disease. They include total cholesterol, tryglycerides, low-density lipoprotein (LDL), very low-density lipoprotein (VLDL), and high-density lipoprotein (HDL). Besides dietary fats, several factors influence the lipid levels, including thyroid function, rate of absorption in the intestinal tract, genetic factors, liver metabolism, and glucose control.

For optimal health and longevity, your cholesterol should be under 185 mg/dL, and better yet, between 145 and 165. Triglycerides should be less than 100 mg/dL, the LDL below 100, and VLDL towards the lower end of the reference range of 5–40 mg/dL. Your risk for heart disease is increased if your HDL is less than 40 mg/dL and greatly reduced if it is greater than 60. In my clinic, in testing blood lipids on patients, I find that older women who follow healthy lifestyle guidelines often have HDL levels above 70, while men in the same age group and even younger often have HDL levels lower than 55, providing a clue as to why women live longer than men: they get fewer heart attacks.

Another common value on your general chemistry panel is the ratio of the total cholesterol to HDL (Chol/HDL ratio). This is calculated by the lab by dividing the total cholesterol by the HDL cholesterol. The Chol/HDL ratio provides an additional risk factor evaluation for cardiovascular disease: the higher the ratio, the greater the risk. Keep your cholesterol/HDL ratio under 3.5 and optimally less than 2.5.

URIC ACID: Serum uric acid measures the main end product of purine metabolism in the body. Purines are organic substances made from amino acids, the same building blocks that create proteins; they are involved in the makeup of nucleic acids (DNA and RNA) that compose your genetic material. Purines also are involved in the synthesis of adenosine triphosphate (ATP), the energy currency of all body processes.

Uric acid is a potent antioxidant, and several studies link uric acid levels in the high normal range to longevity (Cutler 1984). As with many important molecules in the body, uric acid if too elevated can cause problems. One of these is gout, a condition characterized by very painful joints primarily in the large toe or ankle. Also, elevated levels are also associated with liver and kidney disease; elevated serum levels of uric acid are present when cells and tissues break down, as when tumor cells break down during chemotherapy. There is concern that too much uric acid may contribute to coronary artery disease (Fang and Alderman 2000). Values at the lower end or below the normal range have been associated with lowered immune function and chronic yeast infection.

Normal values range from 2.2 to 7.2 mg/dL with optimal ranges around 5.5. Levels in women are generally slightly lower than those in men.

Biomarkers Revealed in Your Complete Blood Count: The complete blood count (CBC) is a standard panel of tests that measures the number of the three main types of cells in a sample of blood: red blood cells (RBC), white blood cells (WBC), and platelets. Red blood cells carry oxygen and are the most common type of blood cell in the body. White blood cells are your body's immune cells to help fight infections and prevent cancer. Platelets are necessary for blood clotting. The

CBC also measures the amount of hemoglobin (Hgb), red cell indices that determine morphology, and hematocrit (Hct), the proportion of packed red cells in a standard volume of blood. The types of the main white blood cells, as measured in a differential blood count, are often included in the test results.

The CBC tells your doctor many things about your health. Too many white cells indicate an infection, and too few mean your immune system is suppressed. Low platelets can cause easy bruising, and may indicate poor liver function or a suppressed immune system. If your red blood count is low, you are anemic; when it is high, it can mean you have hemochromatosis (iron overload).

Though iron is essential for life, too much might kill you. Hemochromatosis is considered a genetic disease of abnormal iron metabolism in the body. Too much iron causes damage to the liver and heart, and disrupts the immune and endocrine systems. The average iron content in the body is about 3–4 g, but in hemochromatosis, iron levels can build up to as much as 20 g.

Approximately one out of every two hundred Americans has this condition, and men tend to have a higher incidence than women. Hemochromatosis can cause chronic fatigue, cirrhosis of the liver, joint pains, and hair loss. It is associated with one form of diabetes ("bronze diabetes," characterized by bluish-gray skin coloring), as well as liver and other cancers. Hemochromatosis can also cause hypothyroidism and headaches, and is associated with a tendency to always feel cold and have abdominal pain and swelling; if iron overload manages to affect the immune system, you are more susceptible to frequent colds and flu.

Blood Chemistry Biomarkers

Test Name	Units	Reference Range	Optimal Level
Albumin	g/dL	3.5–5.5	4.0
BUN	mg/dL	5–25	15–20
Glucose	mg/dL	65–115	78–85
Cholesterol	mg/dL	100–199	145–165
Triglycerides	mg/dL	30–150	under 100
LDL	mg/dL	0-129	under 100
VLDL	mg/dL	5–40	5–20
HDL	mg/dL	30–75	over 60
Uric Acid	mg/dL	2.2–7.2	5.5

It is still unknown why too much iron triggers all these problems, but iron's damaging effects in the body are associated with its ability to react with oxygen to generate excessive amounts of free radical molecules. Excess free radicals predispose us to disease and shorten our life span.

If the long list of diseases associated with iron excess weren't enough, those carrying the *HFH* gene associated with hemochromatosis may have a shorter life span. In a Danish study, 1,784 people (including 183 Danish centenarians) participated in an investigation on life expectancy among carriers of *HFH*. The results of this study suggest that hemochromatosis reduces life expectancy (Bathum 2001). In Europe, one out of ten people carries this gene. So if it is so common and potentially fatal, what can we do about it?

Find out if you have hemochromatosis by having a CBC and iron studies, which include total serum iron level, total iron binding capacity (TIBC), and ferritin levels. If you have more red blood cells than normal, along with an elevated hematocrit and hemoglobin levels, and if the total iron levels are high with abnormal TIBC and ferritin values, you have hemochromatosis. Have the genetic marker test for

Health Markers in Your Complete Blood Count

Test Name	Units	Reference Range	Optimal Level
Red blood cells	X10–6/µL	4.1–5.6	4.5–5.5
White blood cells	X10–3/µL	3.7–10.5	4.5–8.5
Platelets	X10–3/µL	155–385	255–385

mutations in the *HFH* gene; the most commonly tested one is C282Y.

To lower iron levels, the most widely used means is by literally removing blood from your body either by donating blood (if your iron level is not too high) or having the blood drawn in your doctor's office and discarding it. Those with the *HFH* gene mutation need to have blood removed three or four times annually to lower their iron loads. Intravenous chelation therapy is also helpful. This is a procedure done in a doctor's office in which a nontoxic chemical agent is introduced into the bloodstream to capture or bind (chelate) metals such as iron.

Because many dietary substances react with iron, including vitamin C, those with hemochromatosis should avoid overuse of vitamin C, confining their intake to 500 mg, three times daily, taken away from food, to prevent the pro-oxidative interaction with iron. Avoid iron-containing nutritional supplements, do not eat red meats, and increase your dietary fiber to block iron absorption and help prevent iron accumulation. Calcium supplements also block iron absorption, as does drinking black or green tea. Taking the nutraceutical inositol hexaphosphate (IP6) can also lower iron levels (Sardi 1999).

The number of red blood cells in a healthy person ranges between 4.1 and 5.6 million per microliter of whole blood. The normal upper range for adult males is 6.1 million red cells per microliter. To prolong your health, keep your red blood count between 4.5 and 5.5 million red cells per liter. A normal white count is 3.7 to 10.5 thousand white blood cells per microliter. The optimal range for prolonging health is between 4.5 and 8.5 thousand cells per microliter. Normal platelet ranges are 155 to 385 thousand platelets per microliter. Keep your platelets between 255 and 385.

Glucose Tolerance and Insulin Resistance: Though I have already discussed blood glucose levels and the glucose tolerance test, glucose tolerance is such an important biomarker that the topic requires another review. It is well known that unhealthy aging is marked by a progressive decline in the ability of the body to maintain glucose tolerance, which is your body's ability to control blood sugar. It is also known that dysfunctional glucose metabolism (as in diabetes) accelerates aging and predisposes one to all of the other late-onset degenerative diseases.

By the age of 70, at least 20 percent of men and 30 percent of women have abnormal glucose tolerance; some statistics report percentages as high as 50 percent, or greater. Abnormal glucose tolerance not only increases the likelihood of Type II diabetes, previously called adult- or maturity-onset diabetes, and heart disease—at least 50 percent of patients with hypertension have insulin resistance—but it also affects your energy and mood, and reduces your wellness.

The factors that contribute to impaired glucose tolerance are not necessarily the particulars of aging itself, but age-related conditions such as increased body fat, reduced muscle mass and less muscle strength, inactivity, a diet high in refined sugar and excess amounts of starches, declining hormone production and impaired hormonal activity, autoimmune reactions, and stress.

Specifically, glucose tolerance is impaired by a reduced organ reserve of the pancreas, causing erratic insulin production and eventually insulin resistance. In this scenario, insulin resistance increases and glucose tolerance decreases, and you age faster.

Insulin resistance is characterized by increasing levels of insulin needed to control glucose. Excess insulin production (hyperinsulinemia) is one of the primary contributing factors in obesity, with the specific pattern of more abdominal fat around the waist, under the ribs, and in the lower abdomen (greater waist-to-hip ratio). Hyperinsulinemia also imbalances other hormones, contributes to lower HDL cholesterol, and affects liver metabolism.

Excess insulin is associated with Type II diabetes and Syndrome X, and contributes to heart disease, speeds up aging, and is associated with a condition in young women called polycystic ovarian syndrome (PCOS), which is characterized by multiple cysts in the ovaries, increased facial hair, infertility, irregular menstrual cycles, and obesity. Levels of testosterone and DHEA sulfate, a hormone produced by the adrenal gland, are often elevated. PCOS is also associated with skin changes called acanthosis nigricans, in which darkened pigmentation of the skin occurs at the neck, in the armpits, and under the breasts.

Summary of Selected Biomarkers

Test or Measurement	Higher Values Raise Biological Age and Promote Disease	Lower Values Reduce Biological Age and Prolong Health
Biomarker Questionnaire	More than 20	Less than 10
Blood Pressure	Higher then 140/90	Less than 120/80
Body Fat Percentage	Men, greater than 20%; Women, greater than 30%	Men, less than 15%; Women, less than 25%
Waist/Hip Ratio	Men, greater than 1.0; Women, greater than 0.85	Men, less than 0.90; Women, less than 0.80
Body Mass Index	More than 25	Less than 20
Fasting Glucose	More than 110 mg/dL	78–85 mg/dL
Total Cholesterol	More than 240 mg/dL	145–165 mg/dL
Triglycerides	More than 190 mg/dL	Less than 100 mg/dL
Triglyderides/HDL ratio	Greater than 4	Less than 2
Total Cholesterol/HDL ratio	Greater than 3.5	Less than 2.5

This table summarizes biomarkers that tend to rise with age, and consequently increase biological age. Information in this chart is based on several different sources, including the American Heart Association, and my own clinical observations.

Insulin resistance is usually marked by increased levels of insulin in the blood, or an abnormal increase in levels after a two-hour glucose tolerance test. Glucose tolerance is evaluated by several laboratory tests, including fasting insulin and total glucose, glycosylated hemoglobin, and fructosamine. If either insulin or glucose levels are elevated or reveal an upward trend over time, and if glycosylated hemoglobin and fructosamine are high, your glucose tolerance is impaired and your life span will likely be shortened.

Since elevated insulin levels are a strong predictive factor for heart disease, in the absence of insulin levels, you can calculate your triglyceride to HDL (TG/HDL) ratio. This provides an approximation of insulin level. Divide your triglyceride level by your HDL level. The TG/HDL ratio should be less than two and not more than four.

In order to evaluate your starting point and assess the results of your *Prolonging Health* program, establish baseline biomarkers. Measures of your body's composition, blood pressure, and other tests are general but important biomarkers too. Many biomarkers of aging are also found in common laboratory tests, so make use of these when you have your annual physical examination and routine blood tests.

To know if your biological age is increasing or decreasing:

• Complete the biomarker questionnaire.

• Take your blood pressure.

• Determine your body fat percentage.

• Know your waist-to-hip ratio.

• Use the BMI table to find your body mass index.

• Use blood test results: albumin, BUN, uric acid, glucose, blood lipids, red and white cells counts, and platelets.

• Calculate your risk for cardiovascular disease using the total cholesterol to HDL ratio.

• Estimate your risk for insulin resistance with the triglyceride to HDL ratio.

5 Anti-Senescence Laboratory Tests to Assess Your Longevity Status

In the last two chapters, we explored how to evaluate the general effects of aging by examining your body, testing your strength and endurance, assessing other physiologic biomarkers of aging, completing a questionnaire, and reviewing routine laboratory tests that provide information on reversible biomarkers. From these you may obtain a general view of how your body is aging, gain insights about the disease processes you might have or are susceptible to, and learn about your susceptibility to the main risk factors for the common diseases associated with aging, such as cardiovascular disease, diabetes, and autoimmune diseases.

In this chapter, we continue our evaluation of aging parameters (the nine *Prolonging Health* Recommendations Regarding Biomarkers, see p. 57) by discussing laboratory tests that form the core of an anti-senescence evaluation, and provide considerable detail about how well or poorly you are aging. These tests include hormone evaluation, antioxidant status, evaluation of toxic substances that negatively influence health and aging, and key vitamins and minerals. Several of these tests provide information about your risk for cardiovascular disease, the function of glucose and insulin regulation in your body, chronic inflammation, and immune function.

Since these tests are probably different from those that your doctor routinely orders, you'll have to request them. Keep in mind that in many cases a conventional medical doctor may be reluctant to order these tests because of unfamiliarity with them, or the insurance carriers may not consider them medically necessary. In that case, you may have to find another physician who will cooperate with you, or one who already specializes in anti-aging medicine and is knowledgeable about these tests and is willing to work with you on your *Prolonging Health* and anti-senescence program. (See the appendix for an extensive list of medical anti-aging organizations that provide referrals to member physicians.)

Prolonging Health Recommendation 4— Get Your Second Level Anti-Aging Diagnostics Done

Second level diagnostics include blood and radiology tests that go beyond the conventional chemistry panel and complete blood count. These contribute to a more accurate health profile and are important to your overall *Prolonging Health* assessment.

Though more comprehensive than standard panels, these six groups of tests can be

A Note on Laboratories and Tests

Levels for all tests discussed in this book are given in the broadest normal range. However, each laboratory uses different assays with different reference ranges. Therefore, when your test results are completed, use the ranges indicated by that particular lab. I explain each test following the list of selected recommended laboratory studies, but keep in mind that the field of laboratory science is developing rapidly and that new and more sensitive tests become available every few months.

Some may be more useful than or best used in addition to the ones I discuss in this chapter. Consult with your doctor at the time your tests are ordered to see if any new ones are available, or if there are any other tests that he would like to add.

In this book, I use values based on the reference ranges of Laboratory Corporation of America (LabCorp) for all blood testing, except where noted. I use AAL Reference Laboratories values for all urine studies. LabCorp is a national laboratory with offices and draw stations across the United States; I have used them as the primary lab for my clinical work since 1984. Other labs of course are equally professional and provide accurate results. My point here is that by using the same lab each time you test, you establish standards and your results can be more consistent.

easily ordered by your physician; some, such as prostate specific antigen (PSA), are frequently ordered for men at the time of a routine physical examination along with the standard blood tests. For others, you have to request a licensed naturopathic physician or anti-aging doctor to order them. Due to the fact that many conventionally minded medical doctors are reluctant to work with anti-aging testing or programs, and naturopathic physicians are not readily available in many states, members of the Life Extension Foundation can order many of these tests on their own (see the resource section in the appendix).

Selected Second Level Diagnostic Tests

- Cardiovascular Tests: homocysteine, lipoprotein (a), apolipoproteins A1 and B, apolipoprotein E4, fibrinogen, lipid peroxides

- CT Scans: coronary arteries, virtual colonoscopy, and whole body scan

- Breast MRI

- Bone Density: DXA and urinary bone loss markers (NTX and pyrolinks)

- Tumor markers, also called immunoassay for tumor antigens: CA 125, CA 27,29; CA 15-3, NMP 22, PSA (free and highly sensitive)

- Glucose metabolism and insulin resistance

Cardiovascular Tests: In my practice, I often have to remind middle-aged patients with a family history of cardiovascular disease, or those with the early warning signs of heart or circulatory problems such as high blood pressure or high cholesterol levels, that the best anti-aging treatments or cosmetic surgery are unimportant if one suffers a fatal heart attack or stroke before their program takes effect. On the other hand, if your heart is strong, you will probably live long, but ironically, a strong heart without a balanced approach to health doesn't guarantee a good quality of life.

Indeed, some of my elderly patients with a strong heart who didn't have the opportunity to work with me earlier in life suffer from osteoporosis and a crumpling spine, the pain of shingles or arthritis, and other chronic problems that could have easily been prevented if caught earlier. These are cases where metaphorically, the car's engine is still good, but the chassis is falling apart. To live long you must have a strong heart, but you must also take care of your overall health, because a genetically strong heart will help you live longer, but in a weak or diseased body, your quality of later life will be poor.

After you have completed a general physical exam, the biomarker screening tests, and the blood profile measurements, consider a comprehensive screening of your cardiovascular system. This is especially important for men since their risk of early heart disease is much greater than for women. Starting at around age 40 for men with a family history of fatal heart disease, between 50 and 55 for men without a significant family history, and between the ages of 55 and 60 for women, I suggest a comprehensive cardiovascular examination and the comprehensive laboratory profile described below.

As a rule, my recommendation for middle-aged and older people is to have this exam performed by a medical doctor who specializes in internal medicine. At the time of the examination, request that the comprehensive cardiovascular laboratory panel and other tests be added to those your doctor routinely orders. If you are unable to find a cooperative internist, try a licensed naturopathic physician, or a medical or osteopathic doctor who specializes in anti-aging medicine; these practitioners are qualified to order these tests and interpret the results.

I discussed cholesterol, triglycerides, and other common blood lipids in the previous chapter. See the section on lipids for a discussion on those tests.

Tests in the Comprehensive Cardiovascular Panel

- Homocysteine
- Lipoprotein (a)
- Apolipoproteins A1 & B
- Apolipoproteins E 2, 3, & 4
- Fibrinogen
- Lipid Peroxides
- C-Reactive Protein

HOMOCYSTEINE: An intermediary metabolite in the biosynthesis of the amino acid cysteine from methionine, homocysteine is an amino acid involved in cellular metabolism and detoxification pathways. Intermediary metabolites are chemicals produced during the metabolism of a substance, but are not the final product. Increased circulating levels of homocysteine are associated with a greater risk of cardiovascular disease, as well as with a wide range of other health conditions including Alzheimer's disease, osteoporosis, and rheumatoid arthritis.

Your level of homocysteine should be below 9 micromoles per liter (μMol/L). However, naturopathic physicians tend to believe, and I agree, that the lower the homocysteine level the better, preferably below 5 and optimally no detectable level is best. Testing for homocysteine serves as an important biomarker for both health and aging.

LIPOPROTEIN(a) AND APOLIPOPROTEINS A & B: Referred to as "lipo small a," and abbreviated Lp(a), lipoprotein(a) is part of the lipoprotein family of molecules made in the liver and intestines that transport triglyceride and cholesterol in the plasma. Elevated levels of Lp(a) are closely associated with an increased risk of coronary artery disease even in younger people, especially men under the age of 45, and therefore may reflect a hereditary cause for early cardiovascular disease. Levels of Lp(a) should be less then 40 milligrams per deciliter (mg/dL).

Other lipoproteins worth testing include apolipoproteins A-1 (apo A-1) and B (apo B), which, like Lp(a), are part of the lipoprotein complexes in the blood. Apo A-1 is the main component of HDL, so higher levels of this

Okinawan centenarians have lower levels of lipid peroxides than average Americans, a fact suggestive of the importance of antioxidant protection for longevity. Green tea and vitamin C, as well as other dietary antioxidants, have been shown to lower lipid peroxide levels.

lipoprotein are associated with greater protection from cardiovascular disease. Levels for apo A-1 range between 94 and 199 mg/dL. Apo B, on the other hand, forms the major constituent of LDL, the "bad cholesterol," and elevated levels of this lipoprotein indicate a higher risk for cardiovascular disease. Levels of apo B should remain within the general reference range of 55–125 mg/dL for women, and 55–155 mg/dL for men. Clinically, the ratio between apo B and apo A-1 (apoB/apo A-1) is used to define the risk of cardiovascular disease associated with these molecules.

The higher the ratio, the greater the risk, and along with Lp(a) the ratio is considered one of the best predictors of a genetic pattern for coronary artery disease. The reference range of the ratio is 0.30 to 0.90, and a ratio above 1.0 indicates a relative risk that is three times the average. Therefore, optimally your ratio should be lower than the mid-range of 0.6.

APOLIPOPROTEIN E2, 3, AND 4: In the body, the apolipoprotein E family is involved in the metabolism and redistribution of cholesterol. Apolipoprotein E4 (apoE4) is associated with higher levels of LDL cholesterol and triglycerides, and serves as a predictive marker for cardiovascular and Alzheimer's disease. Those with the apoE2 and 3 genes are less likely to have these conditions than those expressing the apoE4 marker. Interestingly, features of insulin resistance are associated with both cardiovascular conditions and Alzheimer's disease, and as a risk factor independent of apoE4, insulin resistance is equally, if not more significant (Kuusisto 1997). (An intermediary metabolite in the biosynthesis of the amino acid cysteine from methionine, homocysteine is an essential amino acid involved in cellular metabolism.) Great Smokies Diagnostic Laboratory offers genomic testing for apoE2, 3, and 4.

FIBRINOGEN: This is a globulin (type of protein) synthesized in the liver that strongly influences blood coagulation. High levels of fibrinogen suggest an increased risk for stroke. The reference range is 185–408 mg/dL. If your levels are elevated, you should also request to have the fibrinogen antigen test performed, as well as the C-reactive protein test (see below), in order to evaluate the status of your immune system's response to fibrinogen. Elevated levels of these substances indicate a significant risk for stroke. Complicating factors include high blood pressure and smoking, both of which greatly increase the risk.

LIPID PEROXIDES: The oxidation of lipids in the body causes significant damage to cells and increases the risk for cardiovascular disease, as well as systemic damage, through the action of free radicals. Therefore, evaluating your levels of lipid peroxides (a product of oxidative action on polyunsaturated fatty acids) provides additional information about your risk for cardiovascular disease, as well as for generalized free radical damage.

Lipid peroxides are easily measured from a urinary sample, though also from blood; the lower the range the greater protection within an average reference range of 3.0–9.0 nanomoles per milligram (nmole/mg). Okinawan centenarians have lower levels of lipid peroxides than average Americans, a fact suggestive of the importance of antioxidant protection for longevity (Willcox 2001). Green tea and vitamin C, as well as other dietary antioxidants, have been shown to lower lipid peroxide levels.

Hormones also play a role in cardiovascular health. The hormones most associated with increased risk for cardiovascular disease are testosterone and estrogen at lower levels, and insulin at higher levels. As different hormones either decline or increase with age, risk of cardiovascular disease increases in proportion to these hormonal imbalances. Inflammatory substances, such as C-reactive protein, also play a role in cardiovascular disease.

C-REACTIVE PROTEIN: A molecule that becomes elevated in the presence of inflamma-

Summary of Tests For Cardiovascular Risk

Test	Levels	Risk
Total cholesterol	elevated	increased
Triglycerides	elevated	increased
HDL (high-density lipoprotein	elevated	decreased
LDL cholesterol	elevated	increased
Cholesterol/HDL	elevated	increased
Triglycerides/HDL	elevated	increased
Lp(a)	elevated	increased
Lipo A-1	elevated	decreased
Lipo B	elevated	increased
Apo B/Apo A-1	elevated	increased
Apo E2 and 3	positive	decreased
Apo E4	positive	increased
Homocysteine	elevated	increased
Fibrinogen	elevated	increased
Lipid peroxides	elevated	increased
C-reactive protein	elevated	increased
Insulin	elevated	increased
Testosterone	lower	increased
Estrogen	lower	increased

This table provides a complete list of important tests that serve as predictive biomarkers for cardiovascular disease and function.

tion and is intimately linked to chronic inflammation, C-reactive protein (CRP) is a protein produced by the liver. It interacts with the complement system (a part of your immune system), and elevations occur in acute inflammation, gum disease, autoimmune conditions such as rheumatoid arthritis or lupus, and in heart disease. Your CRP level is a better predictor test for a heart attack or stroke than LDL cholesterol (Ridker 2002). Researchers found that older people had greater concentrations of CRP than younger individuals.

CRP levels greater than 2.1 mg/L for men and 7.3 mg/L for women indicate an increased risk for cardiovascular and other diseases. To prevent a heart attack or stroke, and prolong your health, keep your levels below 0.5 mg/L. Natural medicines that lower CRP include red yeast rice extract (a naturally occuring lovastatin) and vitamin E.

Preventative CT Scanning: Computerized tomography (CT), or computed axial tomography (CAT), is a radiological procedure developed in the 1970s that combines the much older technology of x-rays with advanced computer technology to generate detailed images of the body's structures including bone, soft tissue, and organs. For a CT scan, the patient lies on a table inside a large tube and small amounts of x-rays are projected to the body part being imaged, or over the whole body in the case of body scans.

Conventional CT scans are used to diagnose spinal disc degeneration, and to detect tumors, sinus problems, brain damage, and other conditions. Newer uses of CT technology include scans of the coronary arteries of the heart and carotid arteries in the neck, the colon, and of the whole body to identify disease conditions before symptoms appear.

Using CT scans as a preventative diagnostic tool is a relatively new approach. It has a promising future though it does involve radiation exposure, which damages genetic material and predisposes one to cancer, and of course it accelerates aging. The radiation dosage for one CT body scan is equivalent to about 1,000 regular chest x-rays (Mitchell 2001), which is an unacceptable amount in my clinical opinion. Although newer CT technology allows rapid scanning with considerably lower levels of radiation, and you can have one without your doctor's prescription, don't run off to have a CT scan without thinking about it carefully. The choice to have a CT scan for early detection should be based upon your individual risk factors, including your medical and family history, the type of equipment used and the amount of radiation exposure you will receive, and your doctor's careful recommendation.

CT technology can be invaluable in the early detection of coronary artery disease and many cancers, so let's review a few of the newer uses of CT technology that can have application in your *Prolonging Health* program.

CARDIAC CT SCREENING: A CT scan of the heart, coronary arteries, and the carotid artery in the upper neck can reveal calcification in the blood vessels, which, if present, is a sign of atherosclerotic disease. Early detection, especially in the high risk group of men ages 40–50 with a family history of fatal heart disease, may greatly improve your chances of arresting and even reversing the progression of coronary artery disease, and prevent an early death from a heart attack or stroke.

The accuracy rate for this procedure is high. It can detect calcification in approximately 85 percent of people with early stage coronary artery disease and 95 percent of those with advanced disease. I routinely recommend this test for my male patients in the highest risk group as early as age 35, and for both men and women between 50 and 65 as a preventive screening test for arterial disease. Remember, if calcification is detected, you will have to have additional scans to evaluate progression or regression of the plaques, which increases your radiation exposure. Do not overuse CT scans, if possible.

CT VIRTUAL COLONOSCOPY: Another potential use of CT technology is for virtual colonoscopy. Statistically, the incidence of colon cancer is rising, though in my clinical opinion this is due to faulty diet and sedentary lifestyle. Insofar as most cancers are preventable, it is important to have your colon evaluated, especially as you get older, which is when most of these cancers occur. In the past, barium enemas with an x-ray of the colon were used. Now, doctors look inside the rectum to view the colon with a colonoscope, a long thin flexible tube attached to a video camera; this is generally recommended for all people over the age of 55.

Most patients have an aversion to having such a device inserted into their body, making the less invasive option of a CT scan to view the colon and surrounding structures desirable. A helical CT scanner is used to obtain two-dimensional slices of the abdomen that are converted by a computer program into a 3D representation allowing for a more comprehensive evaluation of the entire colon and abdomen. If there is a family history of gastrointestinal or colorectal cancer, or if you have polyps or other risk factors for colon cancer, consider having a CT virtual colonoscopy performed.

WHOLE BODY CT SCAN: CT imagery can also scan the whole body. Though the concept of having a painless and comprehensive whole body evaluation to find hidden cancers is appealing, the practice of elective body scans remains controversial. For one thing they are prone to false positive results about 43 percent of the time. This means that about half the time what is found by the scanner is either not there at all or is not cancerous.

For example, a patient of mine, a 73-year-old woman and breast cancer survivor, had a complete body scan. It displayed a shadow in one of her lungs that was suspicious for a cancerous mass. The consulting physician sent her a letter recommending that she follow up with an oncologist. This scared her and she called me, in tears, thinking her previous cancer had returned. I immediately referred her to her oncologist, who had copies of all of her previous tests including CT scans of her chest and lungs. Upon careful examination and comparison of her previous studies, we concurred that the body scan image displayed a false positive that had caused her to worry needlessly and spend more money in other testing.

Another patient, a healthy 54-year-old woman with no risk factors for breast cancer, had a body scan upon the recommendation of a nutritionist. The CT image showed a suspicious mass on her left breast. I referred her for a breast MRI, which confirmed my suspicion that the body CT scan showed a false image.

To complicate matters, 90 percent of whole body CT scans reveal abnormal readings, but the significance of most of these results remains unclear to doctors. Some of these results are "silent" conditions that pose no risk to the patient and never develop into a disease. Still the question is: do these silent conditions reduce life span? Which should be treated? The matter of age-related differences in scans is still not worked out, so keep in mind if you undergo a whole body scan that this technology is not precise; it may show abnormal results that are of undetermined significance, it may show false positives about half the time, and its results are not age-matched.

However, CT technology is advancing rapidly. Based upon greater demand, especially among those following anti-aging programs, more people will likely use this diagnostic procedure. Given this, how can you be sure you are getting the best and safest scan?

Elliot K. Fishman, M.D., a professor of radiology and oncology and the director of Diagnostic Imaging and Body CT at the John Hopkins Hospital in Baltimore, Maryland, suggests that you select imaging centers that use state-of-the-art equipment and are staffed by medical experts in CT scanning who offer a follow-up session to discuss the significance of the findings from your scan.

He also suggests that contrast imaging, rather than non-contrast, should be used to improve detection of masses that might not otherwise show up. To add contrast to the image, an intravenous solution of iodine is injected into the veins. This highlights the tissues and structures, allowing for greater sensitivity in detection. Though many people are concerned about the health risks of the contrast material, with the exception of those with allergies to iodine and those with reduced kidney function, it is generally safe to use.

Though there have been many cases where CT body scans found tumors in their early stages, until such scans are more accurate, the price more affordable, and there is less radiation, there are other, better methods to detect cancer.

My clinical opinion is that basic medical skills need to be improved rather than doctors having yet more expensive technology, at least where radiation is a risk factor. There is no replacement for a competent, experienced doctor.

Breast MRI: Since breast cancer has become so common in women in the developed nations, routine screening, especially for those women using estrogen-based hormone replacement regimens, is an important part of preventive care. Mammography is the method generally used; however, it involves radiation exposure and is a very uncomfortable procedure since the breast must be flattened against a screen in order to have accurate imaging. An alternative, though more expensive than a standard mammogram, is the breast MRI (magnetic resonance imaging).

An MRI is 10 to 100 times more sensitive in imaging soft tissue than either an x-ray or a CT scan, and unlike a mammogram, it involves no radiation. Another advantage is that the breast can be imaged in its natural form allowing for greater viewing of all the structures inside it. Since tumors have their own blood supply, a contrast material (gadolinum) is injected into the bloodstream to highlight a possible cancer. Without it, tumors may be missed. Like the iodine used in CT scanning, gadolinum is injected into a vein, but it is not radioactive and is considered safer than iodine. In my practice, I routinely recommend this test, especially for women with breast implants as it provides considerably better imaging in these cases than do mammograms.

Bone Density Studies: Bone density studies use a small amount of radiation (1/10 that of a chest x-ray) but provide accurate and valuable information about the strength and integrity of your bones. This is an important biomarker in your *Prolonging Health* program: the less dense or weaker your bones are, the greater your degree of senescence. Another way of saying this is that having healthy bones lowers your biological age.

Just as cardiovascular disease is more common in men, and early diagnosis and prevention are necessary to prolong health and prevent early death due to heart attack, osteoporosis prevention is important in women. Men get osteoporosis too, though less commonly than women. Osteoporosis is one of the "silent diseases" like high blood pressure; about 30 percent of postmenopausal women have some degree of osteoporosis and by age 90, the possibility of sustaining a bone fracture due to osteoporosis increases to 50 percent.

DUAL X-RAY ABSORPTIOMETRY: There are several ways to evaluate bone density. The most accurate is by dual x-ray absorptiometry (DXA). This is a painless procedure for which you lie fully clothed on an exam table while an x-ray scans your hips and lumbar spine. The information generated by the scan is sent to a computer that plots your T- and Z-scores, which define your bone mineral density.

The Z-score compares your results to an age-matched control group; the T-scores, developed by the World Health Organization (WHO) for the diagnosis of osteoporosis, estimate the patient's degree of bone mass compared to that of a healthy 30-year-old woman. This age was chosen because bone density peaks in the late twenties and early thirties. It is measured in standard deviations from the normal, and for each standard deviation below the normal value the fracture risk increases.

T- and Z-scores are relative measurements and do not take into consideration individual variability, gender, or differences in populations. A more accurate way of evaluating bone mineral density is the absolute score (like your total cholesterol level) calculated in grams per cubic centimeter (g/cm^3), which translates the

T-score into absolute values referred to as standard deviations.

Bone density measurements can be taken of the ankle, the jaw, or even a finger. X-rays, CT, and MRI imaging can distinguish thinning bones, and while these tests can serve as screening for bone density, in my clinical opinion they are not as useful for defining osteoporosis as the DXA scan.

N-TELEPEPTIDE (NTx) & FREE DEOXYPYRIDINOLINE (PYRLINKS OR DPD): Another method to evaluate bone loss is measuring by-products of bone breakdown in the urine. Bone is composed of 65 percent minerals (mainly calcium hydroxyapatite), and 35 percent organic tissue such as collagen (a type of protein), fibers, blood vessels, and nerves. Since bone is very dynamic, measuring the turnover of bone collagen spilled into the urine provides information about bone metabolism.

Excess amounts of collagen in the urine indicate increased bone turnover and indicate a risk for bone loss. This is very useful in the evaluation of osteoporosis, metastatic bone cancer, abnormal calcium metabolism, and in following the results of treatment for osteoporosis. Called bone resorption markers, these tests involve sending a urine sample to the lab for evaluation.

Though several types of bone resorption marker tests are available, the most commonly used are N-telepeptide (NTx) and free deoxypyridinoline (pyrlinks or DPD). The normal reference ranges for NTx are 9.3–54.3 nanomoles per substance calculated by creatinine excretion (nmol/BCE/mmol-Cr). Optimally, your levels should be below 45 nmol/mmol-Cr. The reference ranges for DPD are 2.8–7.6 nmol/ mmol-Cr, with an optimal

Standard Deviations and Degree of Bone Loss

Standard Deviations	Degree of Bone Loss	Bone Mineral Density in g/cm³
-2.5 to -3.5 or greater	osteoporosis with severe bone loss	less than .648
-2.5	osteoporosis or bone loss	.648
-1.0 to -2.5	osteopenia or low bone loss	.648 to .832
-1.0 or less	low to no bone loss	greater than .833
0	normal bone	.956

Standard Deviations are presented as a negative number representing the degree of bone loss. Osteoporosis is defined as a standard deviation of -2.5 or greater. Absolute values of bone mineral density are calculated in grams per cubic centimeter (g/cm³) of bone.

level of less than 6.5 nmol (Nishizawa 2001). Rising numbers indicate increased and continual bone loss, and correlate with accelerated aging. Falling numbers suggest more stable bone metabolism and improve biological age.

Bone health is important especially during aging, and many factors affect bone health, including minerals, hormones, glucose regulation, and immune substances such as various interleukins that influence inflammation. All of these factors are impacted by age and are worsened by an unhealthy lifestyle. In my clinic, I evaluate body composition including muscle mass, percentage of body fat, and bone mineral density as part of the initial examination. Combining DXA measurements with bone resorption studies provides me with valuable information to evaluate bone loss or health, which is useful as an indicator for the degree of physiological senescence.

In my practice, knowing bone density helps me in deciding estrogen and other hormone dosages in postmenopausal women. The greater the degree of osteoporosis, the stronger the estrogen prescription must be because estrogen slows down and can even halt bone loss. The test allows me easier and more frequent follow-up in these cases so as not to overdose on the estrogen dosage.

Tumor Markers: Tumor markers, also called immunoassays for tumor or cancer antigens, comprise a growing list of acronyms that include AFP, BHCG, B2M, CA 125, CA 27-29, CA 15-3, CA 19-9, CA 72-1, CEA, CYFRA 21-1, NMP 22, PSA, free PSA, highly sensitive PSA, NSE, the BRCA1 and BRCA2 genes, and the CHEK2 gene. Tumor markers are molecules

In my practice, I recommend that men over 60 have the more sensitive version of PSA (third generation) and the free PSA tests performed. These offer more specificity in detecting cancerous activity in the prostate, as the free PSA is more accurate in distinguishing between benign elevation of PSA and cancer.

found in the blood, urine, or tissues that are produced by the tumor itself or by the body in the presence of cancer; they are associated with a higher incidence of certain types of cancer.

Ideally, cancer detection through blood testing should be specific to one type of cancer. When results are "positive," this clearly defines the presence of a tumor. Tumor markers also provide an accurate measure of the stage or activity level of the cancerous process, and reflect the effectiveness of therapy. In other words, if the therapy is effective, the levels of the marker should go down in direct proportion to the decrease in size and activity of the tumor. However, this is not always the case with these tests, as they are not yet at the level of sophistication for wide use among patients.

Though many of these tests remain in the early stages of clinical development, and though many physicians are still skeptical of their value in the early detection of cancer, there is no doubt that genetic testing, especially for cancerous activity and genetic predisposition towards cancer, will have an important role in medicine. These tests are valuable in the screening process for cancer as part of your *Prolonging Health* program. I highly recommend that you have screening performed at least once every five to ten years; if any of these tests are positive, I recommend that you have follow-up studies performed by your doctor at least once a year until the results are normalized as a result of resolving the underlying condition.

Let's look at the few of the tumor markers that may be of value in your *Prolonging Health* program.

PROSTATE-SPECIFIC ANTIGEN (PSA): This antigen (an antigen is any substance that triggers an immune response in the body) is made by the prostate gland in men. It is elevated in cases of chronic inflammation of the prostate (prostatitis), age-related enlargement of the prostate (benign prostatic hyperplasia—BPH), and prostate cancer. An elevated level of your PSA doesn't help your doctor distinguish which condition is causing the increase, and further testing is required in order to determine if you have cancer. The normal range for PSA is 0–4 ng/mL. Optimal levels are as close to zero as possible, and at least less than 1.5 ng/mL.

In my practice, I recommend that men over 60 have the more sensitive version of PSA (third generation) and the free PSA tests performed. These offer more specificity in detecting cancerous activity in the prostate, as the free PSA is more accurate in distinguishing between benign elevation of PSA and cancer. Free PSA is measured as a percentage of the total PSA; the higher the percentage of free PSA the lower the risk of cancer. The cut-off point is 25 percent, with higher percentages suggesting a lower probability of prostate cancer.

CA 125: This tumor marker is increased in women with ovarian cancer. A falling level is useful in managing the treatment for this rare form of cancer, while increasing levels suggest that the tumor is not responding to therapy. CA 125 is elevated in the presence of uterine, cervical, liver, pancreas, breast, lung, and colon cancers. Several noncancerous conditions can also produce elevated levels, including endometriosis, liver disease, and inflammation of the pancreas.

CARCINOEMBRYONIC ANTIGEN (CEA): This antigen is found in small amounts in the blood of healthy individuals, but at elevated levels is associated with inflammatory bowel disease, inflammation of the pancreas (pancreatitis), liver disease, and colorectal cancer. The normal range is less than 2.5 ng/mL.

CA 19-9: This marker is elevated in the presence of colorectal cancers, and is also associated with pancreatic, stomach, and bile duct cancers. Noncancerous conditions of the liver (such as cirrhosis), gall bladder, and pancreas can also cause elevation of CA 19-9.

CA 15-3 AND CA 27-29: These markers are found in people with breast cancer. CA 15-3 is the most commonly used of the two. Elevated levels are indicative of cancer and the test can also be used to follow the effectiveness of treatment.

ALPHA-FETOPROTEIN (AFP): This marker is a protein found normally in the serum of the fetus, which clears rapidly from the body after

List of Selected Tumor Markers and Normal Values

Marker	Normal Values
CEA	< 5 ng/mL
AFP	< 15 ng/mL
PSA	< 4 ng/mL; optimal, less than 1.5
Free PSA	> 25%
CA 15-3	< 40 U/mL
CA 19-9	< 35 U/mL
CA 125	< 35 U/mL
NSE	< 15 ng/mL

birth. Elevated levels are useful in diagnosing hepatocellular (liver) cancer and cancers that affect the germ cells. It is rarely elevated in healthy people, but may be elevated in pancreatic, stomach, and colon cancers. The normal range for an adult is less that 10 µg/L.

NEURON SPECIFIC ENOLASE (NSE): This marker is found only in brain and neuroendocrine tissue, and is used to diagnose cancers of the central nervous system, Wilms' tumor, melanoma, and cancers of the thyroid, kidney, testicle, and pancreas.

OTHER TESTS: Additionally, abnormally high levels of the steroid hormones testosterone and estrogen in older people are suggestive of cancerous processes, as are elevated levels of human chorionic gonadotropin (HCG). The latter is a substance normally produced by the placenta, but it can be elevated in the presence of testicular, ovary, liver, stomach, pancreas, and lung cancer. Abnormal values in your blood chemistry and complete blood count are also used to assess cancer activity in your body.

All these tests just reviewed are available through your doctor's regular laboratory services, though several specialized labs such as Cancersafe, a Swiss company partnered in America with Quest Medical, offer comprehensive tumor marker panels. A negative result from any of these tests does not conclusively mean that you do not have or will not have a specific type of cancer. Likewise, a positive result in an otherwise healthy person does not mean that you have cancer; however, in this case the likelihood of a *cancerous process* is high and warrants further testing from your doctor to confirm or rule out this possibility.

Summary of Tests for Glucose Metabolism and Insulin Resistance and Their Effects on Aging

Test	Risk for Insulin Resistance and Accelerated Aging
Fasting glucose	elevated (greater than 90 mg/dL)
Two-hour GTT	elevated (greater than 120 mg/dL)
Fasting insulin	elevated (greater than 10 µIU/mL)
Hgb A1C	elevated (greater than 8%)
Fructosamine	elevated (greater than 236 µmol/L)
Fasting cortisol	elevated (greater than 10 µg/dL)
DHEA (saliva)	decreased (less than 0.7 nmol/L)
IGF-1	elevated (greater than 350 ng/mL)
T/HDL	elevated (greater than 4)
HOMA	elevated (greater than 3)
Percent body fat	elevated (men greater than 25%; women 39%)
Waist-to-hip ratio	increased (men greater than 0.1%; women 0.85%)

This table summarizes tests and selected indices used to determine glucose metabolism and insulin activity in the body, and at what ranges insulin resistance is suspected. Above those levels, accelerated aging is likely to occur. All tests are from blood sample, with the exception of free DHEA, which is from saliva. [1,2,3,4,5,6]

References:

1. Sears, B. *The Age-Free Zone.* New York: Harper Collins; 1999.

2. Yanick, P. *Manual of Neurohormonal Regulation.* Colebrook, New Hampshire: Biological Energetics Press; 1992.

3. Bralley, JA, and RS Lord. *Laboratory Evaluations in Molecular Medicine.* Norcross, Georgia: Institute for Advances in Molecular Medicine; 2001.

4. Dean, W. *Biological Aging Measurement, Clinical Applications.* Los Angeles: The Center for Bio-Gerontology; 1988.

5. Lukaczer, D. *Functional Medicine Adjunctive Support for Syndrome X.* Gig Harbor, Washington: HealthComm International; 1998.

6. Granberry, M, and V Fonseca. Insulin resistance syndrome: options for treatment. *Journal of Southern Medicine* 1999; 922–14.

Tests for Glucose Metabolism and Insulin Resistance: Since normal glucose metabolism is so vital for healthy body function and abnormal insulin activity is a major predisposing factor for cardiovascular disease, neuroendocrine imbalances, Type II diabetes, and even cancer, and if you are to effectively prolong your health and extend your life span, it is critical that you have testing to determine if you have insulin resistance or are prediabetic. Frankly, you will not likely live a long and healthy life if you have either condition.

Unfortunately, though there are very good tests for assessing blood levels of glucose and other tests that help in the diagnosis of diabetes, there is no simple specific test that can determine degrees of insulin resistance. The hyperinsulinemic euglycemic clamp study is the gold standard for evaluating insulin resistance; however, because it is a complicated and expensive test to perform, it does not have practical clinical use. Therefore, in order to evaluate insulin resistance, you or your doctor have to analyze the results of several different tests to determine your glucose metabolism and insulin status.

These include the fasting glucose test (discussed in the previous chapter), the two-hour glucose tolerance test (GTT) performed before and then after eating, cortisol and insulin levels for both fasting and post glucose challenge, Hgb A1C, fructosamine, and IFG-1. The adrenal hormones cortisol and DHEA are also implicated in the homeostasis of blood sugar. Though not in common usage, a number of specialty laboratory tests are available and useful in evaluating insulin resistance, including increased levels of free fatty acids, increased tumor necrosis factor alpha (TNF-alpha), decreased leptin, increased resistin, and decreased adiponectin (a hormone-like substance found in fat cells) (Salteil 2001).

Since triglyceride levels correspond to how well your body utilizes sugars (triglyceride is an intermediary step in the conversion to fats), the ratio of fasting triglyceride to HDL cholesterol (T/HDL) provides another indirect way of evaluating glucose metabolism. A ratio above four is indicative of insulin resistance, and of course, means you are aging faster than is desirable.

Fasting serum insulin levels can vary greatly and do not allow for a clear picture of insulin status, so scientists use the Homeostasis Model Assessment (HOMA), a mathematical model for calculating insulin resistance. The HOMA index of insulin resistance is defined as the average of three fasting insulin levels multiplied by the fasting glucose divided by 22.5. Values below 2.0 are normal; between 2.0 and 3.0 suggest mild insulin resistance; above 3.0 indicate insulin resistance. The higher the value, the more severe the degree of insulin resistance.

However, this model is controversial even among researchers and does not have wide clinical acceptance. All the methods just reviewed are awkward to use, but can produce a useful picture of your glucose metabolism. When you factor in body measurements, especially the waist-to-hip ratio and overall body fat, you can likely obtain a clear idea of whether you have insulin resistance or not.

Until tests become available for insulin resistance, such as a genomic test for familial predisposition to this condition or antibody studies such as for ICA and GADA antibodies against the body's islet cells in the pancreas, we have to depend on several studies together and body measurements for the determination of insulin resistance. Let's explore each of these tests and their significance for your *Prolonging Health* program.

FASTING GLUCOSE AND THE TWO-HOUR GLUCOSE TOLERANCE TEST (GTT): Blood glucose levels can vary widely depending on how much and what type of foods you eat. Therefore, a morning fasting level is the standard measurement to evaluate the levels of glucose or your blood sugar. The average normal reference range is from 65 to 115 mg/dL, but for optimal health purposes a range of 70 to 100 mg/dL is better, and for those who practice life extension therapies, I suggest keeping the range even tighter with 78–85 mg/dL as optimal.

Once you start to have routine values over 90–100 mg/dL, you may be aging faster. Though a randomly taken (nonfasting) glucose level above 200 mg/dL or a fasting glucose of 126 mg/dL is diagnostic for diabetes, in my clinical opinion, fasting glucose values above 100 mg/dL suggest a *risk* for diabetes. On the other extreme, values below 70 mg/dL may indicate low blood sugar (hypoglycemia), protein malnutrition, or low adrenal function (adrenocortical insufficiency), and should be avoided.

The two-hour GTT is performed by analyzing a sample of your blood for glucose; the blood is taken after you have fasted for at least 12 hours. Then you drink 75 g of glucose syrup and two hours later your blood is tested again for glucose levels. Doctors consider the sugary drink the ideal glucose load for evaluating your body's *response* to increased sugar intake as it causes your insulin levels to rise directly in response to the increased glucose in your blood. Your two-hour glucose level should be between 90 and 140 mg/dL, and optimally below 120 mg/dL. Increased levels indicate abnormal glucose metabolism; diabetes may also be present.

Since excess dietary sugar turns to fat, factoring your lipid levels into the equation provides more information on glucose metabolism and insulin resistance. In other words, some of that fat might once have been sugar. One study in the journal *Atherosclerosis* found that insulin resistance had an effect on the association between lipids and lipoproteins (Friedlander 2000). In metabolic syndromes and insulin resistance, patients may have elevated triglycerides, low HDL, and high LDL levels.

Since the liver is the primary organ for the metabolism of glucose, as well as cholesterol and other lipids, reduced liver function is part of the overall physiological activity that leads to abnormal glucose metabolism and insulin resistance. Slightly elevated liver enzymes, as determined in a blood test, in the absence of organic or viral causes, are also suggestive of the metabolic syndrome with insulin resistance.

INSULIN LEVELS: Next to fasting glucose, your insulin levels are the most important test in determining insulin resistance and if your body is in a heightened catabolic state. Catabolic and anabolic metabolism balance each other in the healthy state. An emphasis on anabolism (upbuilding) as you get older is important to age well, since increased catabolism (breaking down, the more common metabolic state during aging) is associated with accelerated aging.

Determination of your insulin level can be performed from the same blood sample as your glucose test, both fasting and at the time of the two-hour GTT; it's measured in micro international units per milliliter (μIU/mL). A normal fasting insulin range is between 3 and 28 μIU/mL; after the two-hour glucose load it should rise (in response to the increase in glucose) to between 12 and 160 μIU/mL, with an optimal range of 22–79 μIU/mL.

Insulin resistance is usually marked by increased levels of insulin in the blood, or by an abnormal increase in levels after a two-hour glucose tolerance test. Most doctors believe that fasting insulin levels of 15 μIU/mL or higher constitute a positive diagnosis of insulin resistance. Ron Rosedale, M.D., of the Colorado Center for Metabolic Medicine in Boulder, Colorado, suggests that fasting insulin levels above 10 μIU/mL indicate a risk for insulin resistance; he suggests patients keep their insulin levels lower than 10 μIU/mL (Rosedale 2001). Excess insulin production (hyperinsulinemia) is one of the primary contributing factors for obesity, with a pattern of more abdominal fat and a greater waist-to-hip ratio. Hyperinsulinemia also imbalances other hormones, lowers HDL cholesterol, and affects liver metabolism.

Since elevated insulin levels are a strong predictive factor for heart disease, in the absence of insulin levels, you can calculate your triglyceride to HDL (T/HDL) ratio. This provides an approximation of insulin level. Divide the triglyceride level by your HDL level to get the T/HDL ratio. It should be less than two and not more than four.

GLYCOSYLATED HEMOGLOBIN TESTING: Glycosylated hemoglobin (Hgb A1C) are molecules in a red blood cell that become chemically linked with glucose; older red blood cells and those in diabetics have a greater percentage of glycosylated hemoglobin. Hgb A1C testing measures small amounts of sugar left in the blood that attaches to hemoglobin, the part of the red blood cell that carries oxygen, as a result of glycoslyation. It provides a picture of your body's glucose tolerance over a longer period of time (two to three months) than fasting glucose; if you have diabetes or insulin resistance, it gives information on the effectiveness of your glucose management program.

The reference range for Hgb A1C is between 4.4 and 6.4 percent; levels higher than 6 suggest accelerated aging. People without diabetes have Hgb A1C levels of 6 or less, and levels above 8 indicate diabetes. The optimal range for you in your *Prolonging Health* program is less than 5 percent.

FRUCTOSAMINE : Fructosamine testing evaluates your blood sugar control over a shorter period of time than Hgb A1C. Fructosamine, like Hgb A1C, is a product of protein glycosylation, an unhealthy mixture of protein and sugar in the body that accelerates aging. Fructosamine blood testing measures the number of proteins in the serum that are chemically combined (glycosylated) with glucose and reflects an average blood glucose level over a two- to three-week period.

This is a useful test if you already have diabetes or insulin resistance and want to know the effectiveness of your treatment. As with glucose monitors, home testing devices for fructosamine are available. Normal ranges are 0–285 µmol/L, in an optimal range of 122–236 µmol/L. For people taking nutritional supplements, such as on the *Prolonging Health* program, high levels of vitamin C may interfere with the test results, so do not take any ascorbic acid or products containing vitamin C for at least 24 hours prior to your test.

CORTISOL, DHEA, AND IGF-1: Several hormones that affect aging also influence glucose metabolism, including cortisol, growth hormone, and DHEA (as well as insulin, discussed above). This glucose-hormone connection has led some researchers to believe that glucose regulation is one of the key factors in how well and long you live. Your risk for insulin resistance is greater if your cortisol levels are high, your DHEA levels low, and your IGF-1 levels are elevated. Paradoxically, in some women, metabolic syndromes and insulin resistance don't mix and their testosterone levels, in the absence of organic causes such as cancer, and DHEA sulfate levels may be high.

By way of summary of this *Prolonging*

Health Recommendation, abnormal glucose metabolism (glucose intolerance) and insulin resistance regulate the aging process. Diabetes accelerates aging, and even mild insulin resistance reduces your health and increases your risk for cardiovascular disease. To prolong your

Abnormal glucose metabolism (glucose intolerance) and insulin resistance regulate the aging process. To prolong your health and achieve your maximum life span, keep your glucose levels within the optimal range and your insulin low. Higher levels of both make you age faster. Therefore, it is wise to take these tests to assess if you have diabetes or insulin resistance.

health and achieve your maximum life span, keep your glucose levels within the optimal range and your insulin low. Higher levels of both make you age faster. Therefore, it is wise to take these tests to assess if you have diabetes or insulin resistance.

Recommendations for Testing Glucose Intolerance and Insulin Sensitivity

- For healthy people without diabetes or a family history of diabetes, and who are not overweight, take a fasting glucose, insulin, and cortisol test.

- Those with diabetes or a family history of diabetes, and who are overweight or underweight, should also take a fructosamine and Hgb A1C test.

- If you have an increased waist-to-hip ratio and suspect that you have insulin resistance, but are

A Note on Interpreting Hormone Test Results

When calculating the results of hormone tests, laboratories adjust the average ranges for each study according to age groups, called the age-adjusted value, and by gender. Though abnormally low age-adjusted values *suggest* that you may feel better after hormonal enhancement, in most cases even these lower levels do not correspond to disease processes.

Low values indirectly correspond to accelerated aging and increased biological age, and also may contribute to a number of age-related conditions including cardiovascular disease, osteoporosis, and Alzheimer's disease.

But low values of themselves, as a rule, do not indicate disease. Do not treat low hormonal levels with high-dose oral or injectable synthetic hormones. Remind your doctor to treat you and your condition, and not merely the numbers of the test results.

not diabetic, take the two-hour GTT with insulin and cortisol levels before and after the glucose drink.

• Those with hypoglycemia require the GTT, and a fasting glucose, insulin, and cortisol test.

Prolonging Health Recommendation 5— Evaluate Your Hormone Levels

Of all the profiles discussed to this point, comprehensive hormone testing is by far the most valuable because the benefits of taking hormones make you feel better when you're older. More important, because hormone therapy, when individualized and done comprehensively, can provide marked improvements in many of the conditions associated with aging, accurate hormone testing is mandatory and should form the core of your *Prolonging Health* biomarker assessment plan.

It is medically well established that hormone values gradually decline, and in some cases fall steeply, as a normal part of aging. However, the majority of the time, lower values do not mean disease is present, but lower levels of hormones in your body will make you tired, reduce muscle mass, and prevent you from gaining muscle even with exercise. Low hormone levels may reduce strength and endurance, reduce or abolish your sex drive and performance, cause more drying and wrinkling of your skin, weaken your bones, cause graying and thinning of your hair, reduce your memory, and affect your glucose metabolism and cardiovascular function. They are influential in causing many other aging conditions—the complete picture of the aging phenotype. Therefore, even if you choose not to use hormones in your program, testing for at least a few key hormones is essential.

The neuroendocrine theory suggests that the declining physiological function and tissue changes that accompany aging are caused by reduced hormone production and abnormal function. It proposes that there are parallels between the reduced hormone levels and age-related changes; and that healthier older people (the Okinawans) maintain higher hormone levels into advanced age.

However, simply introducing individual hormones into the body does not halt or reverse aging. This is because the body's neuroendocrine balancing system is much more complex than can be addressed by a hormone injection or pill. In other words, when evaluating the results of hormone testing, do not focus on the numbers, but take the whole picture into consideration.

Methods for Testing Hormones: There are several methods and different laboratory techniques for measuring hormone levels, including blood, urine, and saliva tests. There is no consensus on which type of test is best; each has certain advantages the others do not offer, and each has disadvantages. From my clinical experience, the different tests serve different purposes, and should be ordered for their usefulness in providing specific information rather than as a matter of opinion or merely for convenience of use either for the patient or the doctor. Use the right test for the best results for the individual patient. Let's look at the different methods of testing hormones, and see which ones may be best for you.

HORMONE TESTING IN BLOOD SAMPLES: Though there is no current standard for anti-senescence hormone testing, blood testing is the main method used to test hormones. There are several reasons for this. More tests have been performed by blood than by other methods and therefore more is known about blood test results. Also, doctors are more familiar with blood testing methods and are more readily able to evaluate the results of most of the hormones from a blood sample than from urine, saliva, or other methods.

A criticism offered by some doctors and laypeople is that blood tests only provide a snapshot of the total amount of hormone circulating in the bloodstream, and that this does not correlate with levels of the same hormone in the tissues. Therefore it does not measure the bioavailabilty of the hormone.

Though this is a valid criticism, it does not answer this question: how does one obtain a tissue specific level of an individual hormone without taking a live sample of that tissue? Of course, this can't be done, since to take samples of living tissue from all the main sites of the body such as the liver, lungs, brain, breast, heart, and muscle would be not only extremely painful, but also very expensive and risky.

There are other advantages to blood tests besides their convenience. Alan Broughton, M.D., director of AAL Reference Laboratories in Santa Ana, California, suggests that blood values are useful in monitoring peak levels of absorption of hormones (when one is on hormone replacement therapies) or the normal metabolic nadir achieved in the natural cyclic secretion of hormones (Broughton 1999). For example, if you want to see if you are absorbing testosterone from the application of a hormone cream or gel, you can measure your testosterone levels two hours after application. The same applies for thyroid medication: measure your thyroid hormone levels after you have taken your thyroid pill to see if it is absorbing sufficiently.

You can also evaluate natural levels of estrogen or progesterone during their monthly peaks, though this does not apply to women past menopause who no longer have a period. Though most hormones are tested for their total circulating level, many hormones can also be tested in blood in their bioavailable or free form. Saliva and urine studies are not able to test for many hormones such as follicle-stimulating hormone, luteinizing hormone, and thyroid-stimulating hormone. Blood tests are preferred for estradiol and other estrogens, free testosterone, IGF-I, DHEA-S, and thyroid hormones.

24-HOUR URINE HORMONE PROFILES: Hormone testing with urine, in my clinical opinion, does not replace blood testing, though many doctors consider it an equally valuable diagnostic tool for several reasons. It covers a much broader range of hormones, including pro-hormones and hormone metabolites. This provides a more comprehensive hormonal picture. Pro-hormones are the precursors or biochemical building blocks for hormones. Hormone metabolites are the biochemical by-products of hormone metabolism. An example of a pro-hormone is DHEA that converts to testosterone or estrogen, and a hormone metabolite example is the 17-ketosteroids, which are breakdown products from the synthesis of androgens made in the adrenal cortex.

The 24-hour period is necessary to collect all of the hormones secreted by your body during this time. Since higher amounts of hormones are secreted at different times during the day, this gives a picture of the average level of hormone secretion.

Other useful hormone tests are available using the urine, including different subtypes of estrogens, such as 16 alpha (OH) estrone, and urinary metabolites of sex steroid hormones, such as those involved in testosterone and pregnenolone metabolism. To list all of these is beyond the scope of this book, and I refer the reader to an anti-aging specialist, neuroendocrinologist, or laboratory scientist knowledgeable in neuroendocrinology for this purpose.

Thierry Hertoghe, M.D., the author of *The Hormone Solution,* proposes that urinary hormone studies provide the best overall picture of hormone metabolism. He says they are a critical component for evaluating age-related hormonal changes, one that blood studies do not provide, and he suggests a comprehensive 24-hour urinary hormone profile as the initial test to be used in hormone balancing therapy (Hertoghe 2002).

I recommend 24-hour urinary profiles for younger patients, aged 35–45, since abnormal hormone values in the blood are rarely found in healthy adults under age 40. It is also valuable in people between 45 and 55 years old for fine-tuning their hormone regimen.

There are several disadvantages to this test. People with kidney disease do not excrete urine or metabolic products normally, so a urine hormone test is not suitable in these cases. Also, older people are often unable to manage urine collection with accuracy, and for these individuals urine testing may be too cumbersome. Another disadvantage is that this test is complex and difficult to interpret, so you need to consult a physician who is an expert in this type of testing to tell you what it means.

SALIVARY HORMONE TESTING: Testing for hormones in a saliva sample is easy and convenient. For most purposes this can be done at home, making it theoretically the ideal method for hormone evaluation. However, there are drawbacks to salivary hormone testing.

First, not all hormones, such as follicle-stimulating hormone (FSH) or IGF-1 are detectable in salivary tests. Second, the amounts of steroid hormones in blood are significantly higher than in saliva, being 10 to 100 times lower in saliva; this makes the reference ranges in salivary samples often difficult to interpret for their clinical significance. Third, contamination by blood, as from bleeding gums, even in invisible amounts, is common in saliva testing. This results in higher values than expected because of the added blood hormones introduced in the saliva; since there is no easy way to adjust for this kind of contamination, the results must be discarded and another sample taken.

There are advantages to salivary testing. One is that newer technology, such as the Luminescence Immunoassay (LIA) developed in Germany, is more sensitive and therefore more accurate than conventional assays. Hormones secreted at different times during the day, such as cortisol and melatonin, can be measured using multiple samples collected throughout the day and night, allowing for a representation of the normal (or deviation from) cyclical pattern (Rufiange 2002). The main advantage of salivary testing is that it measures the free or bioavailable hormone fraction of the total amount of hormone; free means that the hormone is unbound by binding proteins in the blood such as albumin. Though not the same as specific tissue levels, this method offers an approximation of how much hormone is available to enter the tissues (Hofman 2001).

In general, because of the necessity of evaluating diurnal hormonal rhythms for cortisol and melatonin, I routinely recommend salivary testing for these hormones. Also, cortisol and DHEA levels are normally high enough in saliva to make for accurate testing.

Selected Hormone Tests		
Blood	**24-hour Urine**	**Saliva**
Pregnenolone	Free cortisol	Free cortisol
DHEA-S	Cortisol metabolites	Free DHEA
Total testosterone	DHEA	Melatonin
Free testosterone	Total 17-ketosteroids	
Sex hormone binding globulin		
IGF-I		
IGF binding proteins		
Estrone (E1)		
Estradiol (E2)		
Estriol (E3)		
Progesterone		
Luteinizing hormone (LH)		
Follicle-stimulating hormone (FSH; women)		
Insulin		
Thyroid-stimulating hormone (TSH)		
Thyroxin (T4)		
Triodothyroine (T3)		
Free T4		
Free T3		

Salivary studies are also useful when repeated testing is required, such as monthly monitoring of estrogen or testosterone replacement therapy for those individuals who are sensitive to excess amounts of hormones. Otherwise, I prefer blood and urine tests to establish baselines and to follow patient results of therapy in the long term.

WHICH TESTS ARE BEST? The number of hormones and different kinds of tests discussed may seem complicated, but if you follow the recommendations in this chapter you will get the most useful tests taken for your *Prolonging Health* program. Each kind of test has its advantages and disadvantages, so I emphasize the advantages. I recommend a comprehensive blood hormone profile for everyone between the ages of 45 and 55 years. The 24-hour urinary study gives a useful and comprehensive profile and is best for those between 35 and 45 years. Saliva tests are best used to follow up those using topical hormone creams, and for free DHEA, free cortisol, and melatonin.

Important Hormones to Evaluate in Aging: Let's now consider the most important hormones to evaluate in aging, those which serve as biomarkers and are important to follow during your *Prolonging Health* program. Note that hormone tests in the United States are expensive. Because health insurance pays for basic laboratory tests when ordered by a doctor, people are insulated from the true cost of medical care. Many of the tests discussed in this chapter are usually covered by insurance, but if your insurance company will not pay for any or all of the tests that I recommend, ask the laboratory for the price ahead of time so you won't be surprised with a large bill. Some labs will give a discount if you prepay. Astonishingly, the same tests done in Europe, Mexico, and many other countries cost ten times less on average than in the United States.

Real health care, as I propose in this book, costs a bit, but surely it's worth it if you don't get sick later, even if you have to pay some of the costs up front. Once you're sick, money can't buy back your health. So why not invest in your health now for future benefits in wellness? The *Prolonging Health* recommendations and prescriptions presented in this book give you the advantage necessary to live a long and healthy life.

CORTISOL: Cortisol is the most powerful of the hormones produced by the adrenal glands. Abnormal levels affect blood sugar regulation, indicate abnormal communication between the pituitary gland and the adrenal glands, and adrenal hormone malfunction; if levels are too high, accelerated aging may result. Without cortisol, you cannot live very long, so it's a critical hormone to maintain life.

It is tested in serum from a blood sample, but also is accurately tested in saliva or 24-hour urine. Cortisol levels are best kept within narrow limits. Normal fasting blood levels before 9:00 in the morning are between 4.3 and 22.4 micrograms per deciliter (µg/dL), and between 2:00 and 4:00 in the afternoon, when cortisol secretion is lower, 3.1–16.7 µg/dL. The morning fasting level is the best way to determine adrenal output of cortisol, with optimal values above 10 µg/dL.

If your doctor suspects you have adrenal insufficiency, a condition where not enough cortisol is produced, he may want to perform an ACTH stimulation test. This involves injecting you with adrenocorticotropic hormone (ACTH); in people with a normally functioning adrenal gland, this causes a rapid increase in cortisol, while those with weak adrenal function do not have such an increase. Cortisol levels after the ACTH challenge normally rise at least 7 µg/dL above the fasting level, which is taken before as a baseline, with a peak level greater than 20 µg/dL. The clinical rule of thumb is that cortisol levels should double 30–60 minutes after the ACTH injection. If adrenal function is failing, plasma levels of ACTH will be elevated above the reference range of 9–52 pg/mL.

Salivary testing for free cortisol is accurate and offers several advantages over a blood test. Since cortisol secretion varies during the day, as well as from day to day, a series of samples can easily be taken to obtain an average value. The reference range is 1.0–8.0 in the morning, and 0.1–1.0 ng/mL in the afternoon. Measurement of free cortisol in a 24-hour urine sample is also accurate; with other adrenal steroid hormones, it is one of the preferred indexes for analyzing adrenal function. The reference range is 25.00–120.00 µg/24hr; optimal ranges are above 50 µg/24hr, but not to exceed the upper end of the range.

MELATONIN: Since all people living in modern urban areas are exposed to stress, unnatural lighting, and other conditions that inhibit melatonin synthesis and unbalance our internal clock, it is generally not necessary to test for melatonin levels in order to supplement this important anti-aging and immune-enhancing substance. Blood tests for melatonin are not sensitive to the variations in its circadian secretion, so the best way to test for melatonin is by salivary studies.

At least three samples are taken over a 24-hour period: in the morning, evening, and at midnight. The results are then plotted on a graph and compared to normal values. Evening levels should be lowest (0.0–11.9 picomoles/liter), followed by morning levels collected at 8 A.M. (3.5–33.0 picomoles per liter), with the highest levels at between midnight and 4 A.M. (16–100.0 picomoles per liter).[6]

DHEA AND DHEA-S: The adrenocortical steroid hormone called dehyroepiandrosterone (DHEA) and its metabolite DHEA sulfate (DHEA-S) are perhaps the most useful of all aging biomarkers. Though DHEA is measurable in blood, its levels fluctuate throughout the day, making it unreliable as a biomarker. However, its main metabolite, DHEA-S, is very stable and makes an excellent biomarker for the evaluation of aging. That is because most DHEA in the blood is in the sulfated form, acting as a storage supply for DHEA.

Reference values for a 19- to 29-year-old male are 280–640 micrograms/dL; and for a female of the same age, 65–380 micrograms/dL. An elderly person's DHEA-S levels fall to 28–175 mcg/dL for men, and 17–90 mcg/dL for women. When replacing DHEA, optimal levels should be at least 350 mcg/dL for men, and 250 mcg/dL for women.

Salivary testing for free DHEA is accurate and clinically useful, with a range for 20- to 29-year-olds up to 336 pg/mL; for a person over 70, it's 32–106 pg/mL. When taking DHEA replacement, optimal values should approximate those of the younger person.

Urinary levels of DHEA are also useful, but a better marker for adrenal function is total 17-ketosteroids. That is because it is an end product of both DHEA and DHEA-S metabolism. The range for 17-ketosteroids in a 24-hour urine sample is 6.0–22.2 micromoles/24hr. The optimal range is above 8.0.

PREGNENOLONE: 17-Hydroxypregnenolone is not a hormone, but a pro-hormone because it is the *precursor* for the synthesis of all steroid hormones. The range for women is 10–230 ng/dL, and for men 10–200 ng/dL. Optimally, pregnenolone blood levels should be in the upper end of the normal range for both men and women, as deficient levels can result in lower levels of steroid hormones.

THYROID: To thoroughly test your thyroid gland's function, you need a group of laboratory tests. These must measure total and free thyroid hormone levels, and evaluate pituitary response to thyroid hormone and autoimmune activity against thyroid hormone. In my practice I use both blood and urine testing to evaluate thyroid function; however, blood testing is the accepted standard and provides the most useful information.

Recommended Thyroid Profile

- Highly sensitive TSH (thyroid-stimulating hormone)

- Total T-4 (thyroxine)

- Free T-4 (available thyroxine)

- Total T-3 (triiodothyronine)

- Free T-3 (available triiodothyronine)

- Antiperoxidase antibody (microsomal antibody)

- Antithyroid globulin antibody

As with most of the hormones discussed in this book, optimal ranges for thyroid hormones are frequently different from the standard reference ranges, which are based upon averages of a generally healthy population compared to those with clearly defined pathology. Doctors practicing anti-aging medicine have found that the standard reference ranges are not specific enough for those patients wanting to improve function and ability. Thyroid hormone testing is no exception.

Thyroid Function Test Ranges

Test	Reference Range	Optimal Range	Aging Faster
Thyroid stimulating hormone (TSH)	0.35–5.50 mIU/mL	0.35–2.0 mIU/mL	Below 0.1 mIU/mL
Total thyroxin (T4)	4.5–12.0 ng.dL	5.0–12.0 ng/dL	Greater than 12.0 ng/dL
Free T4	0.70–1.54 ng/dL	1.2–1.5 ng/dL	High
Total triiodothyronine (T3)	60–181 ng/mL	75–181 ng/mL	High
Free T3	2.3–4.2 pg/mL	3.0–4.2 pg/mL	High
Antiperoxidase antibody (thyroid peroxidase–TPO)	Less than 150 mIU/mL	Negative	Elevated
Antithyroid globulin antibody	Less than 200 mIU/mL	Negative	Elevated

List of recommended thyroid function tests with standard reference ranges and optimal values. You age faster if you have excessive thyroid activity, either from hyperthyroidism or overuse of thyroid medication.

For example, the standard reference range for thyroid-stimulating hormone (TSH) is between 0.35 and 5.50 mIU/mL; values higher than 5.50 mIU/mL are diagnostic for hypothyroidism, a condition of low thyroid function. In this case, because thyroid hormone production is low, the pituitary gland produces more TSH in an attempt to stimulate the thyroid to make more thyroxin, the primary thyroid hormone; this thereby raises the level of TSH in the blood. Levels lower than 0.35 mIU/mL are diagnostic for hyperthyroidism, as when the thyroid makes too much thyroxin, pituitary response is reduced, and less TSH is produced.

However, some people can have symptoms of hypothyroidism with TSH levels as low as 2 mIU/mL; others do not have hyperthyroid symptoms (indicative of an overactive thyroid) even when their levels are below 0.35 mIU/mL. This is why it is important to work with a doctor knowledgeable in the many manifestations of thyroid hormone imbalances, at least in the early stages of your program, in order to compare the lab results with symptoms and the overall presentation of the patient.

Though there are no standards for optimal ranges of thyroid functions, anti-aging clinicians generally agree that the optimal range for TSH is between 0.35 and 2.00 mIU/mL; for total T3, greater than 75 ng/mL; free T3, greater than 3.0 pg/mL; total T4, greater than 5.0 ng/dL; and for free T4, greater than 1.2 ng/mL. The optimal result for both TPO and antithyroid globulin is a negative test.

Your doctor may want to include one or more additional tests for thyroid function. Though they generate more clinical information they are not substitutes for the recommended tests discussed above: T-3U (T-3 resin uptake), FTI (free thyroxine index), RT-3 (reverse T-3), TRH (thyrotropin releasing hormone), and TBG (thyroid binding globulin).

Long used in Europe, urinary thyroid tests are only just becoming available in the United States. They are easy to use and are relatively inexpensive; they are useful if frequent monitoring of levels is required. Urinary studies measure free T-3 and free T-4. Values under 1,500 pmol/24h for T3, and 1,800 pmol/24h for T4 are considered low.

Since normal thyroid function is important for health and disease-free aging, I suggest that those using anti-aging therapies and practicing life extension techniques have a complete thyroid profile performed at the *beginning* of their *Prolonging Health* program. If all the results are normal, you need only retest the entire profile once every five to ten years, unless you or your doctor suspect developing thyroid decline or disease. If results are abnormal, I suggest that once you start on correct therapies, you retest only those studies that were abnormal, once every six months until they return to normal.

Several drugs interfere with accurate testing, including estrogens, propranolol used for anxiety and hypertension, benzodiazepine used for anxiety, and steroids. Because of the possibility of inaccurate testing, discontinue any of these medications if possible for several days before testing and consult with your doctor before doing so.

ESTRADIOL, ESTRONE, AND 16-ALPHA(OH) ESTRONE: Since estradiol or estradiol-17 Beta, is the most active estrogen in the female body, it provides the most symptomatic response, as in relieving hot flashes. Thus estradiol is the most important of the estrogens to test. Though all three of the main estrogens can be readily tested in a saliva specimen and the urine, the accepted standard is in serum tested from a blood sample.

Ranges for estradiol vary from 107 to 281 pg/mL through a woman's menstrual cycle during her reproductive years, with the highest levels reached just before ovulation. For menstruating women, estradiol levels between day 13 of the cycle to ovulation of 170 pg/mL or less may indicate deficient estradiol production. Perimenopausal women in the age group 46–52 frequently have wide fluctuations in estrogen levels. There are no standards or established laboratory reference ranges for estradiol levels in these women, but clinically doctors practicing anti-aging medicine contend that ranges below 60–80 pg/mL should be considered low.

For postmenopausal women, once menstruation has ceased and ovarian estrogen production has fallen, estradiol ranges are often lower than 20 pg/mL, and these cases require estrogen replacement. The accepted standard for estradiol levels for women using replacement therapy is 60–100 pg/mL. However, my clinical experience has shown that a safe and effective estradiol range for women ages 55 and older is 35–65 pg/mL. Sharp elevations in postmenopausal women may be associated with cancer and should be brought to the immediate attention of a doctor. In addition, pushing estradiol ranges three or more times above normal postmenopausal levels, as was common when Premarin (an estrogen derived from horse urine) was prescribed, may also trigger genes that cause cancer.

Since estradiol converts to estrone, and both estradiol and estrone convert into other estrogens, such as 16-alpha(OH) estrone, some of which promote cancer, it is wise to evaluate estrone levels periodically. Increased levels may be associated with the conversion of testosterone to estrogen, and may contribute to breast cancer. Menstruating women during mid-cycle can have estrone levels as high as 229 pg/mL; postmenopausal women's estrone levels are generally less than 55 pg/mL.

Some women are overly estrogenic by genetic predisposition or because progesterone is too low, causing a relative excess of estrogen, or due to exposure to high levels of xenoestrogens in the environment or from dietary sources such as hormone residues in meats. In those women with a genetic predisposition to estrogen-sensitive cancers, such as breast and uterine, excess estrogen is detrimental to their health and may reduce longevity.

The 16-alpha(OH) estrone is credited as the "bad" estrogen because of its link to cancer, so evaluating this form of estrogen is advisable in the beginning of your program. It should be followed regularly in women in the high-risk category, as described above. 16-alpha(OH) estrone is measured in a urine sample, and a few laboratories also measure it from blood. Urinary ranges are 1.50–1.90 mcg/24hr. The "good" estrone is 2(OH) estrone with a range of 2.2–10.9 mcg/24hr, and the ratio between 2(OH) and 16-alpha(OH) estrone is predictive of cancer risk. The normal ratio of 2(OH) to 16-alpha(OH) estrone is 1.01 to 2.43.

Estradiol levels in men range from 3 to 70 pg/mL and optimally should be below 35 pg/mL; estrone levels range from 12 to 72 pg/mL, and should also be in the middle of the range or lower. Because some testosterone can convert to estrogen, test your estradiol levels if you have been taking testosterone replacement for over one year, and all men over age 55 should evaluate their estrone levels.

Perimenopause is the time of life just before and after menopause, and generally occurs between ages 48 and 52. Women at the time of perimenopause should have a baseline female hormone study. Include estradiol, follicle-stimulating hormone, progesterone, and, if there is concern about breast cancer, estrone and 16-alpha(OH) estrone. Women over 55 and those on estrogen replacement should evaluate their estrone level at least once every two years. Women over 35 years should evaluate their progesterone levels along with every estradiol test.

Basic Female Hormone Blood Profile

- Estradiol—every year after age 48.

- Estrone—once every two years, or yearly with risk of breast cancer and include 16-alpha(OH) estrone.

- Progesterone—every year after age 35, and with each estradiol test.

- Follicle-stimulating hormone (FSH)—every year starting at age 48, but not necessary after age 55.

PROGESTERONE: The female hormone progesterone plays an important role in balancing estrogen in the body and has important activity as a neuroprotective substance. Changes in progesterone production in women happen earlier than with other female hormones, so I generally recommend that patients begin testing as early as age 35. This is especially recommended if they experience premenstrual symptoms such as headaches, abdominal bloating, mood changes, and cramping before their period.

Like estrogen, progesterone levels vary according to the monthly reproductive cycles, with the highest levels up to 28.0 ng/mL occurring just after ovulation. After menopause, levels of progesterone in the serum drop to 0.0–0.7 ng/mL, which is almost nothing. During perimenopause, progesterone levels can fluctuate a great deal, at times dropping to postmenopausal lows.

For men, progesterone levels range from 0.3 to 1.2 ng/mL. Because progesterone is largely a hormone of pregnancy and declines sharply after menopause, it does not play an important role in men's health. However, for those men with prostate enlargement or whose estradiol levels are elevated, a baseline progesterone level can be helpful. For older men, progesterone levels should not fall below the range. Otherwise, progesterone testing for men is not necessary.

In women between the ages of 35 and 45 and who are still menstruating regularly, progesterone levels less than 10 ng/mL, when tested between day 19 and 21 day of the menstrual cycle, may be too low. The menstrual cycle is counted in days starting with the flow of blood as the first day. Ovulation occurs at about the middle of a 30-day cycle. The time after ovulation, and about ten days before the actual onset of the period, is called the mid-luteal phase. Optimal levels during this time should be towards the upper end of the normal range. For postmenopausal women on progesterone replacement, optimal progesterone levels are between 1.5 and 4.5 ng/mL.

Salivary testing for progesterone is popular among patients, especially women in the 35–45 age group who use over-the-counter natural progesterone creams. Levels of free hormones in the saliva represent about one percent of the total serum levels, and levels of these during the mid-luteal phase are between 0.1 and 0.5 ng/mL. Postmenopausal levels are less than 0.05 ng/mL. For practical purposes this is much too small to be of clinical use, so I do not use salivary testing to establish baseline levels.

However, salivary progesterone testing is an excellent way to follow the effectiveness of transdermal application (through the skin) of progesterone creams. It is easy to do at home, and due to the fact that absorption through the skin is rapid and the hormone enters the bloodstream faster, free hormone levels tend to be higher. In the case of progesterone, the range for those regularly using skin creams is 1.0–10.0 ng/mL. It is important not to apply creams the evening before and the morning of the day you perform the test, as results will be too high because of the rapid absorption effect.

In the urine, progesterone is measured indirectly by testing one of its primary metabolites, pregnanediol. A metabolite is a chemical by-product of metabolism. The reference range for women is 0.3–4.2 micromoles/24hr, and optimal levels are over 2 micromoles/24hr. Urinary progesterone studies are not clinically useful as a direct measurement of progesterone secretion.

TESTOSTERONE, FREE TESTOSTERONE, AND DHT: The male hormone testosterone is impor-

tant for optimal aging in both men and women. It is a very active anabolic hormone that helps to maintain and build muscle mass; it is necessary for the conversion of estrogen, and it promotes a sense of well-being and confidence. The preferred test for testosterone is by blood serum, though salivary and urine tests are also accurate.

Ranges of total testosterone for adult males is 241–827 ng/dL, and for women 14–76 ng/dL. Optimal levels for men are above 600 ng/dL, and for women between 20 and 35 ng/dL. Since the production of testosterone in men is stimulated by luteinizing hormone (LH), testing levels for this hormone is helpful in establishing baseline hormonal function in older men, as is testing for sex hormone–binding globulin (SHBG).

Free testosterone levels in serum are tested in order to know the amount of available, non-protein bond, testosterone, which tends to decline steeply during the aging process. Reference ranges are age-specific: in males 20–29 years old, 9.3–26.5 pg/mL; over 60 years, 6.6–18.1 pg/mL; in women 20–29 years old, 0.0–2.2 pg/mL; for those over 60 years, 0.0–1.8 pg/mL. Optimal ranges for older men are at least 12 pg/ml; for women, free testosterone levels should be in the upper end of the normal range.

Free testosterone can also be measured in saliva, with ranges for young men from 20–29 years old between 42 and 145 pg/mL, and older men over 60 in the range of 32–86 pg.mL. Men over 80 years of age have levels as low as 26 pg/mL. The range for women is 17–52 pg/mL in the 20–29 age group, and 12–34 pg/mL for women over 60 years. Free testosterone levels for women between 60 and 80 years old are more stable than those of men.

Dihydrotestosterone (DHT) is the most potent androgen (male sex hormone) made in the body. It is made from testosterone through the action of the enzyme 5-alpha reductase. The concentration of this enzyme is greatest in the hair follicles and in the skin around the genital area; this is why testosterone creams or gels when applied to the scrotum have a tendency to increase levels of DHT, even sometimes beyond the safe range.

The normal ranges of DHT in blood for adult men is 25.0–99.0 ng/dL; for pre-menopausal women it is 2.4–36.8 ng/dL; for postmenopausal women, 1.0–18.1 ng/dL. Salivary free DHT levels for men are 10–40 pg/mL, and for women are 6–20 pg/mL. Adequate levels of DHT and free DHT are necessary for both men and women during aging, and should be kept in the upper end of the normal ranges, but not higher than the upper limits of the reference ranges.

For men, have a baseline total testosterone blood test at age 35 or younger, then once every five years until age 50, when I recommend annual testing. Include free testosterone after age 45, and include DHT when using testosterone skin creams, gels, or patches. Women should have a baseline total testosterone test at age 50, and then once every two years. For both men and women who have osteoporosis, test testosterone annually.

FSH AND LH: Follicle-stimulating hormone (FSH) and luteinizing hormone (LH) are tested from a blood sample. They are not hormones given as part of anti-aging therapies, but knowing their levels provides useful information about testicular and ovarian function and the degree of age-related decline. FSH and LH are produced in the brain's anterior pituitary gland in response to sex hormones—estrogen and progesterone in women, and testosterone in men. They are referred to as gonadotropic hormones, which are under the control of gonadotropin-releasing hormone produced in the hypothalamus.

In women, FSH stimulates the ovarian follicles to grow, and in men, it promotes the production of sperm. FSH is slightly elevated (3.4–33.4 mUI/mL) during the middle of the menstrual cycle, suppressed during pregnancy (less than 0.2 mUI/mL), and extremely elevated during menopause, with levels ranging from 23.0 to 116.3 mUI/mL.

LH targets specific sites called interstitial cells in the ovary and testes, where it stimulates steroid sex hormone secretion. It is also involved in preparing the uterus for pregnancy. Evaluation of LH provides information useful in evaluating communication between the brain and the gonads (ovaries in women and testes in men). If LH levels are low, especially when accompanied by low growth hormone levels, your pituitary gland may be responsible for your rate of aging.

When you are taking estrogen or testosterone replacement therapy, if LH levels are too low, you may be overly suppressing pituitary function and need to lower your dosage of hormone until LH levels return to the normal range. Increased levels of LH are seen when the ovaries and testes have lost their ability to produce hormones, as during menopause in women and in older men with low testosterone production. This is because if levels of sex hormones are low, the pituitary gland is stimulated to produce more LH in order to rouse the ovaries or testes into making more sex hormones.

The normal reference range for LH in women is 0.0–76.3 mIU/mL, with rhythmical pulsations during the menstrual cycle. For postmenopausal women, the range is 5.0–52.3. For optimal hormonal function during aging, supplementing with estrogens and testosterone helps to maintain LH levels within the reference ranges.

The range for FSH in men is 1.4–18.1 mUI/mL. Testing is not necessary in men. The

LH range for men is 1.5–9.3 mUI/mL between the ages of 20 and 70; over 70, 3.1–34.6 mUI/mL. For men, test LH levels when testosterone values are declining. Low LH levels suggest an age-related weakening of pituitary function.

For women between the ages of 45 and 55, I recommend testing FSH to define menopause. During menopause, the FSH level rises while estrogen and progesterone levels decline. Once FSH is above 35 mUI/mL, menopausal changes are well underway. Test LH levels when estradiol and testosterone levels begin to decline, and every two years when using estrogen or testosterone skin creams.

SHBG: Sex hormone–binding globulin (SHBG) is a carrier protein that attaches to steroid hormones (testosterone, DHT, estradiol, estrone, progesterone, DHEA, and androstenediol), and serves as a transport system in the bloodstream. Knowing SHBG levels is valuable in balancing testosterone in the body, as it tends to increase with age and with estrogen, and to decrease in the presence of high levels of testosterone. The reference range for adult women is 18–114 nmol/L, and for men the range is 13–71 nmol/L. Get a SHBG test as a baseline between ages 45 and 55, then once every two to five years when taking hormone replacement.

HUMAN GROWTH HORMONE AND IGF-I: Human growth hormone (HGH) levels are evaluated indirectly by testing for insulin-like growth factor (IGF-I: formerly called somatomedin C) in blood. Urinary tests that measure growth hormone are also available; however, they are not in common use, and are not considered reliable since growth hormone levels vary greatly and the levels in urine are very small, not allowing for practical use in monitoring HGH levels. IGF-I levels, on the other hand, are more stable and have wide enough age-matched ranges to be useful in evaluating HGH status in the body, as well as in measuring the effectiveness of replacement therapy.

IGF-I is a hormone produced primarily in the liver in response to growth hormone. Plasma levels depend on a person's age and gender, and decrease gradually by about 14 percent every ten years after the age of 30. There is no universal standard for optimal HGH levels, but most anti-aging physicians contend that IGF-I levels approximating those of a healthy 29- to 32-year-old are a reasonable goal. The range for both men and women of this age is 114–492 ng/mL, and for those above 55 years, 71–290 ng. For middle-aged adults (roughly 48–65 years of age) aiming for levels of a 30-year-old may be too high and the therapy to attain them too aggressive, so I suggest more moderate goals.

In 1998, the *Townsend Letter for Doctors and Patients* published an article by two national experts, James Jamieson, Ph.D., a pharmacologist involved in growth hormone research, and Allan Broughton, M.D., who developed the first commercial IGF-I laboratory test and who is the director of AAL Reference Laboratory in Santa Ana, California. They suggested an upper IGF-I limit of 250 ng/dL (Jamieson 1998). In my practice, I have found that patients receive benefits from GH enhancement if their blood levels are functionally low (less than 110–145 ng/dL) and those levels are increased to 165–250 ng/dL. I discourage pushing levels higher than 250 ng/dL due to the increasing risks and side effects of replacing GH with a synthetic compound.

I advise testing for insulin-like growth factor binding protein (IGFBP) in people over 55 or in those whose growth hormone status is in decline. As with other binding proteins, if IGFBP is too low, even in the presence of normal levels of IGF-I, insufficient amounts will be carried to receptor sites, causing low functional activity in the tissues. Likewise, if IFG-I levels increase with replacement, but IGFBP levels are high, too much IGF-I may be locked up in the carrier protein with lower levels of the bioavailable form. Excess levels of IGF-I with high IGFBP may also cause receptor resistance because too much of the hormone is trying to get into the cells.

Prolonging Health Recommendation 6— Determine Your Antioxidant, Vitamin, and Mineral Status

Oxidative damage is ruinous to your body's cells, especially to genetic material such as mitochondrial DNA. Antioxidant status plays such a critical role in both cellular and molecular aging that it affects all other systems in the body. That is why evaluating the levels of key antioxidants in your system is an important part of the *Prolonging Health* laboratory evaluation. Several nutrients that are not antioxidants, principally folate and vitamin B_{12}, but that have other important functions in health and aging, are also useful as biomarkers.

Antioxidant status, meaning the respective levels in your body of various vitamins and minerals that combat toxic free radicals, is measured by several different methods. One is through blood, and other methods include salivary and urinary tests. Only a few labs, such as Genox in Baltimore, Maryland,[7] offer comprehensive testing for the effect of free radicals referred to as oxidative stress.

Some labs, such as AAL Reference Laboratories,[8] Great Smokies Diagnostic Laboratory,[9] and Metamatrix Clinical Laboratory[10] offer antioxidant or oxidative stress panels along with other tests. Pantox Laboratories[11] offers a combined antioxidant and biomarker profile. Functional intercellular testing, pioneered by SpectraCell Laboratories in Houston,

Texas,[12] measures antioxidants and other nutrients; it is a valuable clinical tool to identify nutritional risk factors in a variety of late-onset diseases including cardiovascular disease and cancer (Boerner 2001).

Though home-testing will likely gain more popularity in the future, presently only a few labs, such as Home Health Testing of Grand Rapids, Michigan,[13] provide home-testing kits for antioxidants. (See the resource section in the appendix for complete information on these and other diagnostic laboratories.)

Although testing for antioxidant status is not as accepted by anti-aging doctors as hormone testing is, such tests are useful in determining the underlying risk factors for all of the late-onset diseases. I recommend that you begin with a comprehensive antioxidant and oxidative stress profile when you are 55 or older. Oxidative stress is the destructive load placed upon a cell by free radicals. Use tests that evaluate oxidative stress at the cellular level, DNA damage, the amount of free radical activity present in your body, the levels of pro-oxidants like iron and copper, the levels of individual antioxidants, and total antioxidant status.

Repeat testing once every ten years if no abnormal results were found the first time. Based on abnormal levels discovered in your profile, test them annually until they are within normal ranges. No doubt your doctor will use a laboratory that he is familiar with, or you can introduce him to the labs I mentioned above, which are listed in the resource section of the appendix.

Selected Tests Used to Evaluate Antioxidant and Oxidative Stress Status

- 8-hydroxydeoxyguanosine (8-OHdG)

- Carotenoids (alpha-carotene, beta-carotene, zeaxanthin, lycopene, lutein)

- Coenzyme Q10 (ubiquinone)

- Vitamin C (ascorbic acid)

- Vitamin E (alpha-tocopherol)

- Glutathione

- Glutathione peroxidase (GSH-Px)

- Lipid peroxides

- Oxygen radical absorption capacity (ORAC)

- Iron

- Copper

8-HYDROXYDEOXYGUANOSINE (8-OHdG): This is considered the "gold standard" for measuring oxidative stress inside the cell. It is tested from a urine sample and reflects genetic damage including to chromosomal and mitochondrial DNA (Shigenaga and Ames 1991). Elevated levels of 8-OHdG are thought to contribute to both aging and cancer. Low levels of DNA damage and the body's ability to effectively and speedily repair DNA damage prolong health and promote longevity.

CAROTENES: These are measured in a blood sample and are potent lipid soluble antioxidants, substances that dissolve in fat or oil. High levels are associated with cancer protection and longevity (Bielsalski 2002).

COENZYME Q10, VITAMIN C, AND VITAMIN E: These dietary antioxidants and popular nutritional supplements are measured in blood, and higher levels are associated with reduced risk for cardiovascular disease and increased longevity. The value of CoQ10 as a biomarker in aging is undecided, mainly because of lack of accurate testing, but also because researchers disagree over whether CoQ10 blood levels are associated with cardiovascular disease. Some say that decreased levels are not found in coronary heart disease or Alzheimer's disease (Kontush 1999). Those that support the

idea that blood levels of CoQ10 are associated with heart disease say levels should be at least 2.5 mg/mL (Jones et al. 2002).

Vitamin C is measured as ascorbic acid with a reference range of 0.4-2.0 mg/dL; optimal levels are in the upper end of the range (Lykkesfeldt 1998). Vitamin E is a useful biomarker for cardiovascular health and overall antioxidant status. It is measured as alpha-tocopherol with a reference range of 3.0–15.8 mg/L; optimal levels are in the upper end of the range.

GLUTATHIONE AND GLUTATHIONE PEROXIDASE: These evaluate the body's ability to maintain its antioxidant status; abnormal levels indicate oxidative stress. Glutathione is produced within the body and is measured in whole blood or intracellularly from white blood cells. Glutathione peroxidase is an enzyme found in the cytoplasm and mitochrondria and helps to reduce lipid oxidation. Higher levels favor health and longevity.

LIPID PEROXIDE: Lipid peroxides reflect oxidative damage, and high levels are associated with essential fatty acid deficiency and accelerated aging.

OXYGEN RADICAL ABSORBANCE CAPACITY (ORAC): The ORAC test measures the total antioxidant capacity in a sample of blood serum. It is used to estimate the antioxidant potential of naturally occurring antioxidant substances in your body, such as uric acid, albumin, thiols, and other substances. The higher the ORAC results the greater is your body's antioxidant capacity. The antioxidant capacity describes the chemical ability of an antioxidant to neutralize free radicals. Total antioxidant activity represents a synergistic effect that is greater than the sum antioxidant capacity of individual antioxidants found in food or other substances.

ORAC testing is also used in the food industry to estimate the antioxidant capacity of foods. High ORAC foods such as blueberries and spinach, for example, protect against disease, prolong health, and promote longevity, which is another confirmation of how closely we are interconnected with the food we eat.

IRON & COPPER: Excess iron levels in the body cause increased oxidation and are associated with disease and a shortened life span. Iron, ferritin, and total iron binding capacity (TIBC) are best measured at the time of your annual physical exam. Levels for iron should be within the normal range of 40–180 mcg/dL. Copper is an essential trace mineral and is necessary for numerous metabolic processes in the body. It helps to prevent anemia, arthritis, glucose intolerance, cardiovascular disease, and neurological problems. However, in excess it is toxic and causes oxidative damage to DNA and proteins. Normal ranges in a blood sample are 70–155 mcg/dL. Accurate urine testing for copper is also available with a normal range of 3–35 mcg in a 24-hour sample. Copper levels should be maintained towards the middle of the normal ranges for blood and urine.

Testing for Folate and B$_{12}$: A wide range of dietary vitamins and minerals are necessary for optimal health and normal aging, and as you will see in part 3, supplemental nutrients and nutrient-dense phytofoods form an important part of the foundation of your *Prolonging Health* program. Therefore, laboratory testing for key vitamins and minerals may be critical if you have an age-related disease condition. Many key nutrients are tested in your blood chemistry and antioxidant profile, including vitamin C, vitamin E, calcium, magnesium, and phosphorous. However, two other vitamins important to prolonging your health and promoting longevity are folate (folic acid) and vitamin B$_{12}$.

FOLIC ACID: Folate is measured in serum and inside the red blood cells (RBC folate). Because of its importance in health and

longevity, folate levels should remain high through life, falling in the high upper end or above the reference range, which is greater than 2.6 ng/mL for serum folate, and greater than 130 ng/mL for RBC folate.

VITAMIN B$_{12}$: Measured in serum or plasma, vitamin B$_{12}$ status is important during aging since levels tend to decline and lower levels are associated with neurological weakness and cognitive decline. Also, since supplementing with high dosages of folic acid may cause a reduction in B$_{12}$, it is wise to measure both at the same time. The reference range is 725–2045 pg/mL, with optimal levels in the upper end of the range.

SELENIUM: Selenium is important for immune function and low selenium levels are associated with an increased risk for cancer. Measured in serum or urine, selenium levels also provide clues to your antioxidant status. In serum, selenium ranges are 21–321 ng/mL for men, and 0–420 ng/mL for women. For both men and women, optimal levels are over 150 to the upper end of the normal range.

Prolonging Health Recommendation 7— Know the Condition of Your Immune System

Without a well-functioning immune system, we would all be lethally infected by the myriad infectious microorganisms to which we are exposed, a list that includes viruses, bacteria, parasites, protozoa, and fungi. During aging, our immune system can falter, leaving us more vulnerable to infection, and it can become unbalanced in such a way that we have an increased propensity for autoimmune diseases. Cancer, more common in older people, is associated with immunosenescence, the aging of the immune system and the consequent decline in its function.

They do not serve as universal biomarkers of aging, yet a number of immune function tests are important in evaluating your immune status for prevention and identification of cancer, autoimmune diseases, and chronic infections.

Selected Immune Tests

- Autoimmune and auto-antibody tests: antinuclear antibody (ANA, FANA), anti-thyroid antibody, anti-smooth and striated muscle, anti-mitochondrial antibody (AMA), rheumatoid factor (RF)

- Lymphocyte function: total T cells (CD3+), helper T cells (CD4+), suppressor/cytotoxic T cells (CD8+), total B cells (CD20+), NK cell (CD3-CD16+CD56+) count and function

- Cytokines: IL-2, IL-6, tumor necrosis factor (TN-factor)

- Bacterial antibodies: *Chlamydia, Helicobacter pylori*

- Fungal antibodies: *Candida albicans*

- Viral antibodies: Epstein-Barr virus (EBV), cytomegalovirus (CMV), human herpes simplex viruses (HHSV-I and II), human herpes virus-6 (HHV-6), hepatitis B and C viruses (HBV and HCV), human immunodeficiency virus (HIV)

Autoimmune diseases are more common in elderly people, so a blood test that identifies immune reactions to your body's tissues (auto-antibodies) lets you know if an autoimmune process is active. Although nearly all of the autoimmune and auto-antibody tests listed may show slight elevations in older people, and be considered normal by a medical doctor, in my clinical experience healthy elderly people do not test positive for auto-antibodies.

The most useful immune function tests for the evaluation of immune status during aging are lymphocyte counts and activity tests.[14] Optimal values for all T-lymphocytes are in the mid to upper end of the normal range. Cytokine testing informs you about your immune status, as well as provides valuable information on inflammation in the body. Optimal levels are within the normal reference ranges provided by your laboratory. Levels of IL-2 and NK cells should be towards the upper end of the reference range, as they provide immune protection against cancer, as well as viral infection.

Low-grade bacterial, viral, fungal, and parasitic infections can shorten your life. Tests that screen for low-grade infections that undermine your health, cause increased inflammation, overly stress your immune system, and shorten your life span are useful in your *Prolonging Health* program. These include *Helicobacter pylori*, a common bacterium that causes stomach ulcers; *Chlamydia*, a stealth bacterium that

Low-grade bacterial, viral, fungal, and parasitic infections can shorten your life. Tests that screen for low-grade infections that undermine your health, cause increased inflammation, overly stress your immune system, and shorten your life span are useful in your Prolonging Health program. These include Helicobacter pylori, Chlamydia, and Candida albicans.

is associated with cardiovascular disease and Alzheimer's disease; and yeasts such as *Candida albicans*, which causes candidiasis.

Since viral illnesses weaken immunity, activate autoimmune processes, cause serious damage to the liver and central nervous system, and promote inflammation, screening for the most common latent viruses is also valuable for prolonging health. These include Epstein-Barr virus, cytomegalovirus, herpes simplex viruses, hepatitis viruses, and the human immunodeficiency virus that causes AIDS.

If you're healthy, your auto-antibody test results will be normal. Like autoimmune antibodies, antibodies to viruses and other infectious microbes should be absent in your blood test.

Comprehensive stool studies are useful to test for parasites and to evaluate the health of your large intestine, including the number of healthy flora such as *Lactobacillus acidophilus*. Though a useful clinical test, I only recommend a stool study for people with gastrointestinal conditions such as irritable bowel syndrome and not as part of routine testing.

I recommend a screening panel for each of these tests in those over 65 years old. If you are younger, but have symptoms of autoimmune activity such as fibromyalgia or rheumatoid arthritis, or have chronic fatigue or suspect viral or other infections, I suggest you have tests to determine if an autoimmune reaction or chronic infections are present.

Prolonging Health Recommendation 8— Take Five More Tests to Evaluate Your Health

Chronic Inflammation: One of the hallmarks of aging is chronic pain, which is largely caused by ongoing inflammation in the joints and surrounding tissues. Chronic inflammation may be caused by an intrinsic inability of the tissues to repair themselves; it may also be due to autoimmune activity, low-grade chronic infections, improper diet with an imbalance in essen-

tial fatty acids, and lack of antioxidant activity. Regardless of its cause, chronic inflammation, besides causing the discomfort and debility that constant pain creates, is implicated in a variety of diseases, and it accelerates aging.

Selected Tests to Evaluate Inflammation

- C-reactive protein (CRP)
- Cytokines: interleukins (IL) 2, 6, 12; tumor necrosis factor-alpha (TNF-alpha); nuclear factor kappa B (NFK-B)
- Essential fatty acid profile
- Fasting insulin
- Fasting cortisol
- Sedimentation rate (Sed Rate or ESR)
- Neopterin

I already reviewed CRP, ESR, cytokines, and fasting levels of insulin and cortisol; however, we have not yet explored the importance of essential fatty acids in detail nor discussed how to test for them.

Sufficient levels of essential fatty acids (EFAs) and proper metabolism of EFAs are important for cardiovascular health, cognitive function, and even prevent depression. EFAs play a critical role in regulating inflammatory processes in the body and in insulin dynamics that regulate your blood sugar.

Neopterin, a substance released from macrophages (immune cells) during infection, provides a novel diagnostic tool for evaluation of infectious disease such as AIDS (Sarcletti et al. 2002). In addition to infection, high neopterin levels are associated with increases in free radical activity, cancerous processes, neurodegenerative diseases such as Parkinson's (Widner 2002), autoimmune disease (Forsblad et al. 2002), and periodontal disease (Ozmeric 2002). Neopterin is readily measured in blood and urine, and rising levels are indicative of immune activation.

I recommend testing the ESR, C-reactive protein, essential fatty acids, fasting insulin, and fasting cortisol levels for those over 55 years old, and for younger people if they are at risk for cardiovascular disease or diabetes. For those over 65, I suggest evaluating your cytokine and neopterin levels.

Mitochondrial Function: Since mitochondrial function and repair of mtDNA are among the most important factors in aging, and because the mitochondria are the primary sites for the production of energy in the body, assessing mitochondrial capacity is a necessary part of your *Prolonging Health* evaluation. Great Smokies Diagnostic Laboratory offers a panel that tests organic acids in the urine, such as lactic and citric acids, involved in the mitochondrial metabolism and energy production.[15] Organic acids play important roles in muscle metabolism—just think of the pain you experienced when too much lactic acid built up in your muscles during vigorous exercise. Abnormal levels of organic acids may influence a number of neuromuscular and neurodegenerative disorders such as Parkinson's, and they are associated with the aging process.

Test your mitochondrial function if you have chronic fatigue, difficulty gaining muscle mass even with exercise, or have early signs of neurodegenerative diseases such as multiple sclerosis, Parkinson's disease, or Alzheimer's disease.

Genomic Status: As a result of the accomplishments of genomic research at the turn of the twenty-first century, the early phases of the genomic revolution are upon us. Individualized, targeted, tissue-specific therapy has become the standard of care rather than nonspecific generalized drug therapies as previously practiced.

Predictive profiles or individualized testing for genetic markers, which predispose an individual to specific disease, will one day be routine. We are still years away from wide use of genomic technology, yet several genomic profiles are currently available. These include apolipoprotein E (apo E) and variants apo E2, 3, and 4; TNF-alpha; and ICA and GANA antibodies to islet cells that are genetic markers for Type II diabetes. If you have high iron and ferritin levels, and have been diagnosed with hemochromatosis, test for mutations in the HFH gene (C282Y).[16]

In the near future, predictive genomic testing will likely provide clinical insights that doctors only dream of today, and may develop into the foundation of all anti-aging testing.[17] These tests are easy to carry out, involving a simple mouth rinse performed in the morning. If you are at risk for cardiovascular disease, test apo E2, 3, and 4; if at risk for diabetes, test ICA and GANA antibodies; if you have hemochromatosis, test for C282Y. If you are interested in other tests for genetic markers, discuss your concerns with your doctor.

Neurotransmitter Profiles: Another new area in medicine is the classification of "neurotransmitter deficiency diseases." This is a loosely organized group of illnesses that includes obesity, depression, fibromyalgia (chronic muscle pain), certain inflammatory disorders such as irritable bowel syndrome, chronic fatigue syndrome, and alcohol and drug abuse. Since we know that values of the neurotransmitters dopamine and serotonin change with age, evaluating neurotransmitter levels may be useful in the evaluation of the cognitive decline associated with aging.

My preference for testing neurotransmitters is through a urine test that screens for dopamine, serotonin, GABA, epinephrine, and norepinephrine. If you experience significant memory loss, mood changes, disorientation, and other cognitive changes, consider testing for neurotransmitters.[18]

Toxicology Studies: For nearly everyone, no matter where they are, exposure to toxic chemicals today is unavoidable. For some, continual low-level exposure is a daily concern, and though it goes largely unnoticed, it poses considerable risk for cancer, autoimmune disorders, and chronic fatigue and immune deficiency syndromes; the genetic damage it creates also accelerates aging.

Selected Toxic Substance Tests

• Antibodies to silicone (for those with breast implants)

• Heavy metals and other toxic elements (aluminum, arsenic, lead, nickel, mercury) in both hair and urine samples.

• Screening for pesticides and chemical antibodies.

Heavy metals such as mercury and lead get into your body from breathing polluted air, eating mercury-laden fish, or direct contact with these substances. Heavy metals and other toxic elements are tested in hair, urine, and blood. Hair analysis is easy to perform at home and is an inexpensive screening tool for toxic metals. Though in wide use by alternative health practitioners, it has disadvantages. These include contamination from airborne pollutants, hair dyes, and shampoos. Also, as people get older they have less head and body hair. This makes it difficult to collect enough hair to accurately complete the test. I prefer the urine test because it covers a wider range of toxic elements and is more accurate.

Other chemical contaminants to consider are silicone from leaking breast implants. Research shows that silicone causes immune system reactions in your body, which can cause fatigue, severe allergies, and joint pains. Immune reactivity to silicone is tested in blood samples.

In order to achieve optimal results from your *Prolonging Health* plan, all toxic substances must be eliminated from your body. If you suspect that you have had exposure to toxic environmental substances such as the heavy metal mercury, have a 24-hour urine test for toxic metals performed. If you have had or still have silicone breast implants, ask your doctor to order a silicone antibody study. If the results are positive for silicone antibodies, consider having your implants removed and/or replaced with a less toxic substance. If you have had exposure to industrial chemicals or pesticides, have a blood test for chemical antibodies.

Individualized Comprehensive Anti-Aging Testing

You may be wondering if all of these tests are necessary. The answer is: just about. To effectively evaluate your general health status, reveal major disease processes such as diabetes, define the biomarkers of aging, evaluate hormone levels, and monitor the effects of your *Prolonging Health* program, comprehensive testing is mandatory. Which are the most clinically useful tests? Do you need all of them, or can you get by with basic testing?

This is where individualized testing comes in. In my clinical opinion, if you follow the principles of *Prolonging Health*, you have a high probability of living a healthy life and achieving a normal life span, or better. However, my experience has taught me that most people can live well up until their seventies without the help of either spiritual or material science; but to achieve your maximum life span potential you need all the assistance you can get. Since our goal is to achieve maximum life span, living well until age 95, ultimately to 120, or longer, I propose that functional testing provides the information edge you need to succeed in this. No doubt newer and better tests will appear in time, but the tests discussed here are the basis for state-of-the-art evaluation for the biomarkers of aging and late-onset disease.

When Do I Start Testing? Laboratory testing can be performed at any age and at any time during your *Prolonging Health* plan. However, based upon my clinical experience, my understanding of the research data, and interviews with many anti-aging physicians and gerontologists, the optimal time for your first baseline tests is between age 35 and 39. Let's use one of my patients as an example.

Rob was 35 years old when he first came to see me. He was not only healthy without any major complaints, but his physical fitness level was excellent. He competed in cycling and running events but still had concerns about his general wellness and wanted to optimize his fitness and athletic performance. He heard that changes in hormone levels occur as early as age 30, so he was curious to know whether any of the main hormonal parameters or risk factors for degenerative disease were appearing in him.

Rob's physical examination was normal, and many conventional physicians might have stopped there, citing their findings and encouraging him to continue everything that he had been doing. However, most people don't begin where Rob started, at 35–39 years old, though this is the age I consider optimal to begin prolonging your health and reversing aging.

In Rob's case, a 24-hour urine test uncovered slightly lowered values of testosterone, and his blood tests revealed very low levels of cholesterol. He didn't have enough cholesterol, as odd as that sounds in our cholesterol-obsessed society. Since steroid sex hormones are built from cholesterol, it made sense to start by increasing his dietary intake of essential fatty acids and cholesterol-containing foods. Within three months, he was able to raise his testosterone levels solely from natural dietary sources.

I recommend at least a basic evaluation be performed before you start your *Prolonging Health* program; then have more at regular intervals during the program, with annual, biennial, or once a decade retesting. Your doctor may wish to include other tests that she regularly performs, such as mammography, but the panels listed in this chapter are a template for you and your doctor to design individualized testing procedures.

How Often Should I Have Follow-Up Tests Performed? In general, follow-up, including the *Prolonging Health* annual exam and lab studies, can be performed annually, or once every two to five years if you are very healthy. I suggest that you have the comprehensive *Prolonging Health* and anti-senescence profile once every ten years starting at age 50, with regular follow-up on those specific biomarkers that you are working with on an annual basis, if not more frequently, until they are normalized.

If you have abnormal results on any of these tests, or are working on a particular area of your health or anti-senescence program, you may wish to follow up that particular test as often as once every three months until it is normalized, then annually thereafter. Depending on the type and severity of the condition, some physicians may even want to follow your lab tests monthly until they are within acceptable ranges.

Recommended Test Panels

The *Prolonging Health* Baseline Profile

Starting at ages 35–39, take these tests when you begin your *Prolonging Health* program:

• Comprehensive chemistry/metabolic panel

- Complete lipid panel

- Homocysteine

- C-reactive protein

- Complete blood count with differential count

- Iron and ferritin

- Uric acid

- Vitamin E in serum

- Vitamin B_{12} and folate in serum and red blood cells

- Fasting insulin

- Fasting cortisol

- DHEA-S and pregnenolone

- TSH and total T4

- Cancer markers: third generation PSA and free PSA, and CEA, for men; CA125, CA15-3, and CEA for women

- Salivary cortisol and melatonin

- Urine analysis for toxic metals

Include these other tests by age group and gender:

- Ages 35–45

    Comprehensive 24-hour urine hormone evaluation with metabolites

- Ages 46–50

    For men: comprehensive cardiovascular panel, total testosterone, free testosterone, dihydrotestosterone

    For women: a DEXA bone density study and breast MRI, total testosterone, FSH, estradiol, progesterone

- Ages 50 and older

    For men: total testosterone, free testosterone, dihydrotestosterone, luteinizing hormone, estradiol, estrone, sex hormone–binding globulin, IGF-I and IGFBP, total T3, free T3

    For women: total testosterone, FSH, luteinizing hormone, estradiol, estrone, progesterone, total T3, free T3

The *Prolonging Health* Annual Exam

Take these tests each year, or if you are very healthy, every two to five years:

- Comprehensive chemistry/metabolic panel

- Complete lipid panel

- Homocysteine

- Complete blood count with differential count

- Vitamin E

- Vitamin B_{12} and folate in serum and red blood cells

- Fasting insulin

- Fasting cortisol

- DHEA-S and pregnenolone

- For men: total testosterone, free testosterone, DHEA-S, pregnenolone

- For women: estradiol, progesterone, total testosterone, DHEA-S, pregnenolone

Prolonging Health and Anti-Senescence Comprehensive Profile

In addition to the annual exam and hormone profile, the following panels starting at age 50 and performed every decade thereafter form a record of your progress:

- Antioxidant status

- CT scanning: coronary arteries, or whole body

- Essential fatty acid profile

- Genomic predictive profiling

- Immune function profile

- Inflammatory markers

- Insulin resistance profile

- Mitochondrial function

- Neurotransmitter profile

- Tumor markers

I have reviewed numerous laboratory and radiological tests, and discussed their importance in your *Prolonging Health* program. Because there is no one study, or even a profile of tests, that completely defines and quantifies aging, it is necessary to use multiple tests that register the body's functions and responses to the various aging factors. Evaluating each of these determines if you are aging normally, rapidly, or slowly. Slower aging coupled with good health well into old age provides the basis for prolonged health, which is the prerequisite for life extension.

The most important of these tests for anti-senescence purposes are hormone studies. This is because taking hormones greatly diminishes many of the symptoms of aging. However, taking hormones does not in itself constitute a complete health plan as they have potential side effects, the worst being the stimulation of

tumor growth. A balanced and comprehensive longevity plan entails more than hormone treatment and therefore requires tests to determine disease risk, predictive genomic testing, antioxidant status, immune function studies, and toxicology.

- Get your *Prolonging Health* baseline profile.

- Evaluate the results and see if your results meet the optimal levels.

- If not, proceed to part 2 and follow the advice given to modify your longevity factors.

- If you have high risk for a specific degenerative disease, get a comprehensive test done to evaluate your condition in more detail.

- Get the hormone test appropriate for your age and gender.

- If you are between 35 and 39 years, get a 24-hour comprehensive urinary hormone study.

- If you are over 65 years, get the comprehensive anti-senescence profile.

6 How to Determine Your Age-Point

In this chapter, you'll see how to determine your age-point. The age-point is the time of life when you enter the aging zone, which is defined by an increase in aging factors and the characteristic symptoms of aging. Once you're in the aging zone, your body is subject to the negative influence of all the factors that contribute to aging.

If you do nothing to slow aging, you then arrive at the metabolic critical point. This is when catabolic (tearing down) processes operate more than anabolic (building up) ones in your body. When this happens, and if you do not take care of your health, accelerated aging begins to take place and your body may progress into a disease zone where the degenerative diseases of aging dominate the rest of your life. This typical scenario is the way most Americans age. Even if you escape degenerative diseases, if you do not proactively work to prolong your health by mastering the ten factors of longevity, you will likely become frail as you age.

I propose that this typical scenario is unnecessary. It represents unnatural aging, and is associated with degenerative disease and a shortened life span. According to this conventional aging model, aging is not a disease but is accompanied by unavoidable diseases requiring allopathic medical intervention. Using drugs and surgery only treats the symptoms, and does nothing to cure the underlying causes of these diseases.

Though containing beneficial therapies, the alternative solution is used by doctors who practice anti-aging medicine. It is also an allopathic approach and therefore limited to the symptoms of aging. We have yet to discover an approach that reverses the aging process and restores youth.

What I propose in *Prolonging Health* is an integrated approach utilizing comprehensive strategies that address a spectrum of age-related factors. However, before we discuss these, it is necessary to know if you are aging already. Determining your age-point helps you know how well, or poorly, you are aging.

Prolonging Health Recommendation 9— Complete the Age-Point Questionnaire

Though the optimal time to begin your *Prolonging Health* program is between ages 35 and 39, it is never too late to start. You can improve your health at any age. However, the same outcome applies at any age: lower your biological age, reverse the downward trajectory of aging, and return to your individual age-

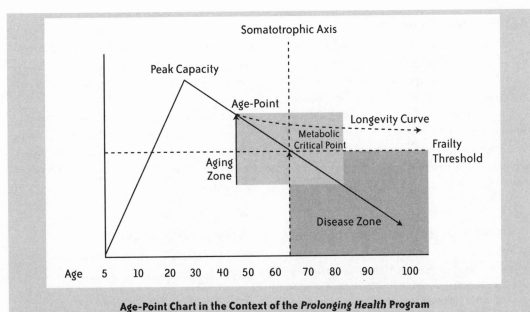

Age-Point Chart in the Context of the *Prolonging Health* Program
This chart illustrates that by modifying the factors that negatively influence longevity, you can improve your health and live longer.

point. By mastering the ten factors of longevity, you can remain at your age-point, biologically speaking, for a long time.

The age-point questionnaire allows you to find your rate of aging. Optimally, you want to keep below the age-point. This means you have a low biological age. Healthy people in their seventies and eighties can have a biological age *half* their chronological age. Though they may have a few wrinkles and gray hair, their body is working efficiently and effectively and is resisting aging.

Let's look at a case to illustrate my point. Walt is a 73-year-old retired entrepreneur who spent the last 12 years working on his health so he can remain active and fulfill his dream of creating a world-class health spa. He considered himself healthy and his medical examination didn't reveal any disease, though his blood tests showed that he was slightly anemic. Otherwise his test results were within the con-

ventionally accepted limits, and many were within optimal ranges.

Here's how they looked: his cholesterol was 117 mg/dL, triglycerides 55 mg/dL, HDL at 34 mg/dL, LDL at 72 mg/dL, cholesterol/HDL ratio 3.4, and the triglyceride/HDL ratio was 2.3. His albumin was 4.2 g/dL, BUN 14.2 mg/dL, TSH 2.8 µIU/mL, free T3 1.4 pg/dL, total testosterone 827 ng/dL, and free testosterone 16.4 pg/mL. His DHEA-S level was 170 ng/dL, cortisol 17.8 mcg/mL, his fasting insulin was 4.6 µIU/mL, and glucose was 85 mg/dL. His IGF-I level was 140 ng/mL. His iron and uric acid levels were within range. He had no infections, degenerative diseases, or cancer, was never tired, had a low PSA of 1.5, a blood pressure of 110/78, low homocysteine levels, and no elevation of C-reactive protein. His body measurements were all within the optimal ranges.

His age-point questionnaire score was 9. That put him right on his age-point, rather than

Age-Point Questionnaire

Place a check next to each question that pertains to you. A checked box is a yes answer, and an unmarked one is no. Total the number of check marks. If you have no check marks, you are before your age-point; if less than 10, you are at the age-point; if between 11 and 20; you have passed the age-point, but are not yet at the metabolic critical point; if more than 20, you are aging poorly.

NOTE: The age-point questionnaire requires that you take the biomarker questionnaire, answer several additional questions, and have results from some of the basic laboratory testing discussed in the previous chapters. When you have taken your blood tests, you can complete the entire questionnaire. If you don't have results yet, you can still utilize the age-point questionnaire. Answer the first six questions. If you answered yes to any of them, you have passed your age-point.

___ I am over 65 years old.

___ My biomarker questionnaire score is more than 20.

___ I have one or more of these conditions: heart disease, diabetes, osteoarthritis, Parkinson's disease, Alzheimer's disease, osteoporosis, or an autoimmune disease.

___ I have chronic fatigue syndrome.

___ I have a chronic viral infection.

___ I have or have had cancer.

___ My PSA (men) level is higher than 3.5.

___ My body fat percentage is more than 15% (men); 25% (women).

___ My waist-to-hip ratio is greater than 1.0.

___ My body mass index is greater than 24.

___ My blood pressure is higher than 120/80.

___ My fasting glucose level is above 85 mg/dL.

___ My total cholesterol is higher than 165 mg/dL.

___ My triglyceride level is more than 100 mg/dL.

___ My HDL is lower than 55.

___ My triglyceride/HDL ratio is higher than 2.

___ My total cholesterol/HDL ratio is higher than 2.5.

___ My homocysteine level is greater than 5.5.

___ I have elevated C-reactive protein levels.

___ My albumin level is less than 4.0 g/dL.

___ My BUN is below or above 15–20 mg/dL.

___ My iron levels are high.

___ My fasting insulin level is higher than 10 μIU/mL.

___ My fasting cortisol level is higher than 10 μg/dL.

___ My DHEA-S level is less than 90 mcg/dL (women); 175 mcg/dL (men).

___ My IGF-I level is less than 145 ng/mL.

___ My testosterone level is less than 400 ng/dL (men); 20 ng/dL (women).

___ My estradiol level (women) is less than 20.

___ My TSH is above 3.5 mIU/mL.

___ My free T3 is below 3.0 pg/mL.

past it, which was consistent with his sense of wellness, energy levels, emotional stability, and physical fitness. Though his chronological age was 73, his biological age was 39. Many of his biomarkers were within the optimal ranges, and some were just outside the ranges. However, his cholesterol and HDL were too low.

I recommended that he eat more fish, be generous with healthy vegetable oils such as olive oil, eat avocados, include more seeds and nuts in his diet, and have two eggs a week from organically raised chickens. I prescribed 20 mg of micronized DHEA and 50 mg of pregnenolone, and recommended that he take 0.1 IU of HGH injections two times weekly. In addition, he took a broad-spectrum multiple vitamin and mineral formula, plus an extra 30 mg of zinc, 200 mcg of selenium, and 500 IU of vitamin E.

At the time of his three-month follow-up visit, he told me that he was able to think more clearly, that he had more energy than before, and felt years younger. After six months on the same regimen, his blood tests improved.

Here's how they looked after six months: his cholesterol was now 145 mg/dL, triglycerides were 73 mg/dL, HDL at 45 mg/dL, LDL at 75 mg/dL, cholesterol/HDL ratio 3.2, and the triglyceride/HDL ratio was 1.6. His albumin was 4.5 g/dL, BUN 16.0 mg/dL, TSH 2.4 μIU/mL, free T3 2.0 pg/dL, total testosterone 725 ng/dL, and free testosterone was 15.1 pg/mL. His DHEA-S level was 223 ng/dL, cortisol 11.4 mcg/mL, his fasting insulin was 4.8 μIU/mL, and glucose was 84 mg/dL. His IGF-I level was 218 ng/mL. This time Walt's age-point score was 5.

Walt's case illustrates how comprehensive testing served as a guide to improve his health and reverse his biological age. Without it, I wouldn't have known that his cholesterol and HDL levels were too low. Though he was eating what he considered a good diet, he was not getting enough healthy fats and oils. By adjusting his diet, enhancing his hormone levels, stimulating his thyroid function, and providing additional nutrients, he lowered his age-point. You can do the same by following the *Prolonging Health* recommendations.

To effectively prolong your health, start your *Prolonging Health* program as early as possible. Optimally, start at the age-point or earlier. The age-point precedes the aging zone and the metabolic critical point, and generally falls between 35 and 39 years. This strategy limits the influences of aging, helps avoid frailty, and you never enter the disease zone. In this scenario, you can live a long and healthy life free of disease and in full command of your body and mind. The goal is to return your health to the level of a 35- to 39-year-old.

- Avoid the aging zone by lowering your biological age and coming closer to your age-point.

- Complete the age-point questionnaire to estimate your aging status.

- Follow the *Prolonging Health* recommendations and strategies.

- Lower your age-point to below 10.

PART II

Ten Modifiable Factors of Aging

"Aging and death do seem what Nature has planned for us. But what if we have other plans?"

—Bernard Strehler, Ph.D.

"The object of living is to live, not merely to exist or grow old."

—Frederic Hudson

"The last time turns love, pain, despair, and habit into poetry."

—James Hillman, Ph.D.

Introduction to Part II

In part 1, we discussed the science of aging and learned how gerontologists study aging. We explored the different ways people try to prevent aging, and learned that aging occurs slowly, though faster in some people and imperceptibly in those who age well. We established that the human life span has been documented to reach about 120 years, but that maximum life span is potentially 150 years or more. We saw that those who reach ages of over 100, and those who lead active and productive lives up to age 100, not only age more slowly, but are also free of infectious and noninfectious diseases, and their bodies remain cancer free.

We also learned that different lifestyle factors such as effective management of stress, a healthy diet, and certain geographical locations influence aging in positive ways and contribute to long life. On the other hand, negative environmental influences such as heavy smoking, sedentary lifestyle, and a poor diet cause degenerative diseases and shorten life span. Further, we noted the importance of staying out of the aging zone, and why it is important to maintain a low biological age.

Now in part 2, I discuss ten factors that significantly influence aging. Though causing considerable damage to the body and shortening life span, remarkably all of these factors are *modifiable* by lifestyle changes and natural therapies. By modifying these factors you can prevent disease, prolong your health, and master longevity.

Bear in mind that each of these aging factors is not a single condition, and even though I present them as individualized causes of aging, they are complex processes that influence aging and disease. When allowed to operate unchecked in your body, they undermine your health and contribute to degenerative diseases; all are enemies of healthy aging. But, by managing or *modifying* these aging factors, we may not only influence age-related conditions, but in many cases significantly minimize the effects of aging. In effect, we slow down the aging process, and in some cases we can even reverse it.

Let's take a closer look at the ten most important aging factors and see how they weaken your health, contribute to disease, and influence aging.

The Ten Most Important Modifiable Aging Factors

- *Prolonging Health* Modifiable Aging Factor 1: Oxidative Damage
- *Prolonging Health* Modifiable Aging Factor 2: Genetic Damage

- *Prolonging Health* Modifiable Aging Factor 3: Impaired Detoxification
- *Prolonging Health* Modifiable Aging Factor 4: Insulin Resistance
- *Prolonging Health* Modifiable Aging Factor 5: Impaired Protein Synthesis and Glycation
- *Prolonging Health* Modifiable Aging Factor 6: Chronic Inflammation
- *Prolonging Health* Modifiable Aging Factor 7: Impaired Cardiovascular Function and Sticky Blood
- *Prolonging Health* Modifiable Aging Factor 8: Declining Hormone Function
- *Prolonging Health* Modifiable Aging Factor 9: Immune System Decline
- *Prolonging Health* Modifiable Aging Factor 10: Neurodegeneration

Here is a quick, preliminary overview of these ten factors:

***Prolonging Health* Modifiable Aging Factor 1: Oxidative Damage:** Oxygen, the main molecule used to create physical energy in our body and derived from the air we breathe, causes unstable destructive chemical reactions. These unstable reactions create biochemical changes that damage our cells and DNA. This leads to disease, and the tissue changes characteristic of aging. However, oxidative damage can be treated with antioxidants, by following the *Prolonging Health* diet, with specialized nutrients, and with other natural medications.

***Prolonging Health* Modifiable Aging Factor 2: Genetic Damage:** Eventually, the result of oxygen utilization accumulates and causes cellular DNA and mitochondrial DNA damage. As these changes accumulate over time, irreparable cellular changes occur, including those that allow for tumor development, cardiovascular disease, and the neurodegenerative changes that lead to Alzheimer's disease. DNA repair substances can help reverse genetic damage.

***Prolonging Health* Modifiable Aging Factor 3: Impaired Detoxification:** Our body attempts to balance processes that build and repair with those that remove and naturally detoxify environmental substances out of our cells. But as we age, toxins and cellular debris accumulate and our body's detoxification systems are unable to keep up with this molecular garbage. In order to prolong our health and prevent aging, we must improve detoxification and cleanse our body.

***Prolonging Health* Modifiable Aging Factor 4: Insulin Resistance:** The hormone insulin drives the rate of aging. It also has an important role in prolonging health; therefore, it is important to keep our blood sugar (glucose) within normal limits. This is accomplished primarily through diet, supplementation with vitamins and minerals, and specialized natural medications, as well as exercise.

***Prolonging Health* Modifiable Aging Factor 5: Impaired Protein Synthesis and Glycation:** Proteins are necessary for life. Abnormal glucose control leads to the gumming up of proteins in a process called glycation; this can be prevented and reversed by controlling glucose metabolism through diet, exercise, and natural medicines. To age well, we must protect proteins from these effects and rebuild them with adequate dietary protein and supplements.

***Prolonging Health* Modifiable Aging Factor 6: Chronic Inflammation:** This plays a key role in the diseases of aging. Preventing the inflammatory changes that accompany aging helps prolong health and extend our life span. We can manage and reduce the effects of inflammation on our body through dietary changes and natural medicines.

***Prolonging Health* Modifiable Aging Factor 7: Impaired Cardiovascular Function and Sticky Blood:** We need a strong heart as we get older and we can protect our cardiovascular system from oxidative damage, toxic buildup, and chronic inflammation with natural medicines.

***Prolonging Health* Modifiable Aging Factor 8: Declining Hormone Function:** Hormones play an important and even central role in aging and by replenishing them we gain some of the strongest benefits available in anti-aging medicine.

***Prolonging Health* Modifiable Aging Factor 9: Immune System Decline:** Without a strong immune system we are more prone to cancer, more vulnerable to infections, and more susceptible to autoimmune diseases; we age faster and die younger. We can strengthen our immune system with natural immune boosters.

***Prolonging Health* Modifiable Aging Factor 10: Neurodegeneration:** Improving neurotransmitter levels, nerve cell regeneration, and brain function is crucial in reversing aging and extending life. We can prevent neurodegeneration and restore our nerve cells with natural brain-enhancing medications and hormones.

These ten aging factors address the main causes and consequences of aging. By controlling or modifying them, we can prolong our health and live longer.

7 *Prolonging Health* Modifiable Aging Factor 1: Oxidative Damage—How to Prevent Degenerative Disease with Antioxidants

The free radical theory of aging, first proposed in 1956, states that over time, random oxidative damage occurs in cells and its cumulative effects lead to age-related diseases, aging itself, and eventually death (Harman 1956). Oxidative damage, also called free radical pathology or oxidative stress, is a product of the natural process of using oxygen for metabolism; in its worst form, it can cause permanent damage to the genetic material, which is why it is considered one of the principal causes of aging. How can oxygen cause such destructive effects?

Oxygen makes up 20 percent of the air we breathe. We take in air through our lungs where the oxygen is separated out from other gases, such as nitrogen and carbon dioxide, then mixed into the blood and pumped throughout the body by the heart. This oxygen-enriched blood is carried in the hemogloblin, an iron-containing molecule within individual red blood cells, to every cell in the body. Cells use oxygen as their primary fuel to produce energy and support life. However, oxygen is a very reactive element and during normal metabolism free radicals are produced from oxygen.

Free radicals are highly reactive molecules released in cells during normal oxidative metabolism, and they can ravage cellular components. The damage they cause breaks chromosomes, cripples DNA replication and inhibits repair, disrupts mitochondrial activity, destroys enzymes, and erodes cell membranes (Halliwell and Mestler 1985). Some cellular components, such as neurons, are more sensitive to oxidative damage than others.

To our advantage, under normal conditions our body effectively manages cellular damage from free radicals, and there are no lasting negative effects to our cells or tissues. However, there are times when too many free radicals are produced. This occurs when immune cells are fighting viruses or other infection-causing microbes, with cancer, and during excessive exercise. At these times, excessive numbers of free radicals escape immune surveillance and control and travel through the body, wrecking tissues and cells.

Additionally, numerous external sources can accelerate free radical damage beyond the body's ability to manage them. These include radiation exposure as from x-rays, environmental pollutants in the air and water, pesticide residues in foods, chemicals used to cure meats, cooking methods that overheat fats and oils (pan-frying or deep-frying), toxic chemicals (pharmaceutical drugs, tobacco smoke), stress, and excessive physical labor or overexercising.

The typical American diet, low in dietary sources of antioxidants and high in processed foods, contributes greatly to free radical pathology, and virtually all of the degenerative diseases associated with aging are linked to free radical damage.

In recent years, scientific evidence has shown that oxidative damage is an underlying cause of most chronic diseases. Researchers in the department of medicine at McMaster University in Ontario, Canada, found that excess free radicals cause severe damage to the endothelium, the inner lining of blood vessels. This kind of damage is associated with atherosclerosis and hypertension, and can lead to a stroke (Walia 2003).

Additional research connects oxidative damage to neurodegenerative disease, and is implicated in Alzheimer's and Parkinson's disease. Cancer patients have increased production of free radicals and less antioxidant protection. This allows for a tumor to overwhelm the immune system (Mantovani 2002). Free radicals also play a major role in how diabetes develops, and high levels of free radicals in diabetics accelerate the development of diabetic complications such as the loss of vision caused by diabetic retinopathy (Maritim 2003). Evidence suggests that free radical pathology is involved in autoimmune diseases such as systemic lupus erythematosus (Ahsan 2003). Other conditions associated with free radical pathology include

cataracts, macular degeneration, arthritis, emphysema, multiple sclerosis, and scleroderma.

When increased free radical production is coupled with reduced antioxidant protection, disease processes accelerate. In addition, insufficient antioxidant intake allows more free rad-

> *The typical American diet, low in dietary sources of antioxidants and high in processed foods, contributes greatly to free radical pathology, and virtually all of the degenerative diseases associated with aging are linked to free radical damage. In recent years, scientific evidence has shown that oxidative damage is an underlying cause of most chronic diseases.*

ical damage to occur, contributing further to the development of degenerative disease.

Most of the time, oxidative damage is neutralized by naturally occurring antioxidants synthesized in our body. Principally, these are glutathione and a variety of antioxidant enzymes such as superoxide dismutase (SOD).

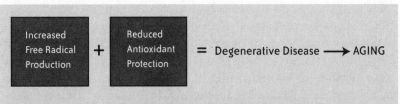

Free Radicals Cause Disease and Aging
In the healthy body, free radical production is neutralized by naturally occurring antioxidants and dietary antioxidants. If not, increased free radical production and reduced antioxidant protection lead to degenerative diseases and accelerated aging.

A Quick Review of Oxidative Damage Essentials

Oxidative damage is the chemical consequence of using oxygen to produce energy in the body and individual cells. Oxygen in the air is converted in the body to energy and water. However, when cells utilize oxygen, electrons are released and toxic by-products called free radicals are formed. Scientists like to call them reactive oxygen species (ROS). Free radicals are molecules that contain one or more unpaired electrons because an electron gets knocked off or added on when oxygen is used to make energy. This process is called oxidation. Molecules are supposed to be electrochemically stable. But when electrons are missing, molecules become unstable and cause destructive reactions in the cell. Free radicals are enemies of healthy cells. Certain substances in the body are more sensitive to oxidative damage, also called free radical damage, than others. Proteins and lipids (fats) are easily damaged by free radicals. Fats that are damaged by free radicals are called lipid peroxides. Lipid peroxides and protein oxidation causes inflammation, leads to cancer, contributes to diabetes and heart disease, and accelerates aging. Antioxidants, also called free radical scavengers, are molecules that stabilize or neutralize free radicals and repair oxidative damage. They stop the destructive chain reaction caused by oxidation.

Other substances found in the body neutralize free radicals, including melatonin, uric acid, and the enzymes protease and peptidase (enzymes that rapidly degrade damaged proteins so that they don't damage tissues).

To prolong our health, we must minimize free radical production, enhance naturally occurring antioxidant synthesis, eat an abundance of fresh fruits and vegetables, and take antioxidant supplements.

Cellular Senescence and Aging

As we age, our cells lose their protective capacity against excessive free radical activity. This combination of reduced antioxidant protection combined with increased oxidative damage from free radicals contributes to degenerative diseases. It's also responsible in part for the aging process. One reason for this may be that free radical activity targets specific substances, the main ones being lipids, proteins, and nucleic acids—all necessary for the continuance of life. Cumulative damage to these substances may overwhelm the antioxidant defenses, with the consequence of accelerated aging.

Lipids, the main material that makes up cell membranes, form a living barrier between the cell and the environment outside of the cell. Lipid membranes are particularly sensitive to oxidative damage. Cumulative oxidative damage weakens the cell membrane, and disrupts the transport of nutrients and other substances between individual cells and the extracellular environment.

Since a large portion of our body is composed of proteins, oxidative damage to proteins causes considerable age-related changes that some researchers believe may even be the hallmark of aging—selective protein oxidation leads to disruption of homeostasis (Starke 1989).

Another target of free radicals is nucleic acids. Excess oxidative damage can cause irreparable DNA damage, which leads to the inability of the genetic material to replicate normally, and this is thought to play a key role in cancer and aging.

Bruce Ames, Ph.D., the 1998 recipient of the National Medal of Science and professor in the graduate school of biochemistry and molecular biology at the University of California at Berkeley, is considered the foremost expert on antioxidants and aging. In laboratory experiments with rats, he has demonstrated that deficiencies of antioxidants and certain nutrients such as vitamins B_{12}, B_6, B_3, and folate contribute to DNA damage. Dr. Ames proposes that, by combining these nutrients with a good diet, oxidative cellular and genetic damage is reversible (Ames 1999, 2001).

An extension of the free radical theory of aging proposes that mitochondria, the powerhouses of cells, perform a central role in aging. Biochemical reactions within the mitochondria are the primary source of energy for all of the tissues and organs. Research performed by Simon Melov, Ph.D, an Australian scientist working at the Buck Center for Research in Aging in Novato, California, informs us that free radical activity within the mitochondria can have a profound effect on life span (Melov 2000). In the body, the main site of free radical production is the mitochondria. Since mitochondria produce the most free radicals, this powerhouse of our cells can suffer significant oxidative damage, in particular to mitochondrial DNA, or mtDNA (Sastre 2000).

Mitochondria have their own genes separate from the DNA in the same cell (chromosomal DNA), and they do not communicate with the chromosomal DNA in the nucleus. As to why mitochondria have their own DNA, scientists speculate that mitochondria were once free-living bacteria that invaded other cells millions of years ago. Mitochondrial DNA was discovered in 1963, and the bacterial origin theory was first proposed in 1992 by Lynn Margulis, Ph.D., a prolific author and distinguished professor at the University of

Massachusetts, Amherst. It was published in her book *Symbiosis in Cell Evolution* (Margulis 1992).

Cellular function depends on the energy-producing activity of the mitochondria. Defects in the mitochondria or decay of mtDNA function affect the whole cell, and potentially the entire organism. Damage to mtDNA can be permanent in cells that are not easily replaced, such as nerve cells in the brain that play an important role in the progression of aging (Austad 1997).

Oxidative damage not only causes mitochondrial and intracellular changes, but it contributes to the accumulation of oxidative end products such as lipofuscin. This is a yellow-brown fluorescent pigment consisting of lipid and protein residues that steadily build up in cells. Kenneth Beckman, Ph.D., a biochemist and expert on mitochondrial aging in the department of molecular and cellular biology at the University of California at Berkeley, suggests that though scientists agree that oxidative damage plays a role in aging, we are still learning the role that free radical damage plays. However, it appears that lipofuscin accumulation impairs mitochondrial efficiency and disrupts other cellular functions (Beckman 1998).

There are several other reasons that more oxidative damage occurs in older people. One of them involves reactions between oxygen and specific metals in the body. Iron and oxygen in particular form a lethal combination. With aging, the body's iron tissue levels rise and this accumulation, along with other toxic substances, greatly increases the degree of oxidative damage. By the age of 80, significant mitochondrial-related damage occurs, principally in the brain, especially in areas high in iron deposits. This is another reason to keep your iron levels within normal ranges (Walter 2002). Though it is not known exactly why iron tends to accumulate, older people should limit their iron intake by avoiding multivitamins that contain iron, not cooking in cast-iron cookware, and minimizing their consumption of red meat.

As we age, our ability to adapt to environmental stresses weakens. Oxidative damage accumulates and antioxidant molecular mechanisms and cellular repair functions falter, and our body's ability to respond effectively to oxidative damage becomes diminished. These adaptive responses are important in the containment of free radical pathology. However, to effectively extend your life span, it is not enough to avoid conditions that cause increased free radicals and to take antioxidants. It is also necessary to increase your oxidative stress tolerance—the ability to withstand and deal with heightened levels of free radicals without your system unduly suffering or its function becoming overly compromised.

Whether genetic or adaptive, some people have better antioxidant defenses than others. Stronger antioxidant defenses more effectively neutralize free radicals and contribute to increased life expectancy (Arking 2001). Gerontologists speculate that this is because certain nontoxic environmental stressors may turn on longevity genes in some people. These genes provide added protection against oxidative damage beyond naturally occurring and dietary antioxidants. One such gene, fittingly called methuselah (mth), was found in 1998 by researchers at the California Institute of Technology in Pasadena (Lin 1998). This gene enhances longevity by 35 percent and increases resistance to a variety of intracellular free radicals (Finkel 2000).

The opposite is also true, and several life-shortening genes have been found, including the cancer gene p53 (Clark 1993) and the apolipoprotein E (apoE) gene that is related to Alzheimer's and heart disease (Schacter 1994). People with these genes are more susceptible to free radical activity. These discoveries suggest an evolutionary role for genes that are influenced by oxidative damage and that play a role as life span determinants. In the future, scientists may find ways to individualize antioxidant programs for people with these different genes.

Ironically, oxygen in the air we breathe that sustains us and promotes life also kills us slowly through the oxidative process. So far in this chapter we've discussed how free radical reactions occur: universally within cells; are cumulative; affect the genetic material inside the cell, the mitochondria; cause cellular changes through gene expression; and participate in the accumulation of destructive end products. The final consequence of free radical activity is disruption of the body's overall homeostasis, and as a result, the gradual loss of cellular function, which in turn causes age-related changes that initiate the aging process.

How Antioxidants Prolong Health

It is well accepted among scientists that free radical damage is an underlying cause of degenerative diseases and a primary aging factor. What is not clear is whether taking oral antioxidants lengthens life span, though there is considerable evidence that antioxidant supplementation *prevents* degenerative and age-related diseases (Yu 1999). However, the link between increased life span and preventing degenerative diseases associated with aging through the use of antioxidants is getting stronger. Researchers have shown that some antioxidants such as N-acetylcysteine and melatonin are capable of extending the life span in experiments with animals (Golden 2001, 2002).

Therefore, for the purposes of our discussion with its emphasis on prolonging health to attain longevity, we now discuss the use of antioxidants and their expected effects on health and aging.

Antioxidants are substances naturally manufactured in our bodies and found in foods that help neutralize free radical damage. Those occurring in the body include a diverse group of chemical substances such as superoxide dismutase, glutathione, the enzyme NADPH oxidase, the hormone melatonin, and uric acid. Though these antioxidants are very powerful, to control free radical activity additional antioxidants must be obtained from antioxidant-rich foods. These are mainly found in brightly colored fruits, dark green leafy vegetables, green tea, and herbs.

Though most antioxidants can be obtained from food, for people under environmental and psychological stress, those with viral infections or cancer, those eating a diet deficient in antioxidants, or when attempting to reduce the effects of aging, the need for antioxidants is higher. Thus supplements are required.

The most valuable nutritional antioxidants include vitamins C, E, B_2, B_6, B_{12}, the carotenoid beta-carotene, the minerals zinc and selenium, and the amino acids arginine, lysine, cysteine, and glutamine. Second-level antioxidants, called this because they were discovered in the last few decades and long after vitamin C and E, are classes of highly potent antioxidant substances that have shown very promising results for their anti-aging effects; these include coenzyme Q10, lipoic acid, N-acetylcysteine, and astaxanthin.

To prolong your health, eating a phytonutrient-rich diet that contains abundant antioxidants and taking supplemental antioxidants is not enough. You must also lower the number of free radicals produced in your body by limiting activities that increase free radical production, such as overexercising, and by avoiding the use of unnecessary pharmaceutical drugs and exposure to environmental toxins in tobacco smoke, pesticides, asbestos, x-rays, and chemical food preservatives. Detoxification practices and calorie restriction can limit free radical production, and therefore help your body fight oxidative damage.

Though there is considerable research under way to find pharmaceutical antioxidants that are better than naturally occurring ones and those found in the diet, these synthetic substances cannot cure the underlying cause or results of oxidative stress. In fact, many drugs deplete the very substances that repair oxidative damage, as you will see when you read about the individual antioxidants. Only naturally occurring substances in foods and natural supplements can help the body overcome antioxidant deficiency and reduce free radical pathology, and thereby restore health and prevent aging.

Prolonging Health Recommendation 10— Eat Foods Rich in Antioxidants

Jean Mayer, Ph.D. (1920–1993), a French nutritionist and former head of the United States Department of Agriculture Human Nutrition Research Center on Aging at Tufts University in Boston, Massachusetts, was the first to suggest that the antioxidant protection from eating fresh fruits and vegetables can slow the aging process. The key is to eat foods that score high on an antioxidant test called ORAC, short for oxygen radical absorbance capacity. This test measures the total antioxidant power of foods and other chemical substances. You can even find the ORAC of blood to determine your own antioxidant power (see below).

By doubling your intake of high-ORAC foods, you can increase the antioxidant protective

The Top Antioxidant Foods

Antioxidant capacity is measured in ORAC units per 100 grams (3.5 oz.) of food. A higher number of ORAC units means more antioxidant power.

Food	ORAC Units
Dark chocolate	13,120
Rosemary	6,000
Prunes	5,770
Blueberries	2,400
Blackberries	2,036
Kale	1,770
Green tea	1,686
Strawberries	1,540
Spinach	1,260
Raspberries	1,220
Brussels sprouts	980
Plums	949
Alfalfa sprouts	930
Broccoli	890
Beets	840
Oranges	750
Red grapes	739
Red bell pepper	710
Cherries	670

powers of your body by 10 to 25 percent. The ORAC value is measured in ORAC units per 100 g (3.5 oz.) of a substance. High-ORAC foods include blueberries, prunes, raisins, blackberries, kale, and spinach. Many condiments such as traditional Japanese or Chinese soy source have high ORAC values. Green and black tea have powerful antioxidant activities, as do herbal teas. A single average serving of fresh fruit or freshly cooked vegetables supplies about 300 to 400 ORAC units. To prolong your health, I recommend at least 5,500 ORAC units each day derived from dried fruits, fresh fruits and vegetables, condiments, and tea.

Evolutionarily speaking, antioxidants in fruits and vegetables are naturally suited to your body. They not only increase your antioxidant protective capacity, but they also have the power to turn on genes that provide additional antioxidant protection. Dietary antioxidants work synergistically with antioxidant supplements.

Prolonging Health Recommendation 11— Get an ORAC Blood Test

At the beginning of your *Prolonging Health* program, have an ORAC blood test. This assay measures the total antioxidant capacity in your blood. The reference range is 3,300 to 5000 µM with a mean value of 4,386. Optimally, your total ORAC score should be above 4,500 µM. Increase your fruits and vegetables and take antioxidant supplements; then have your blood retested after one year on the *Prolonging Health* program. If your score is higher, you are gaining antioxidant protection.

Prolonging Health Recommendation 12— Take Antioxidant Supplements

The antioxidants found in a healthy diet containing plenty of fresh fruits and vegetables are very effective in controlling oxidative damage in the body. Yet to proactively prevent the aging process you need to take additional antioxidants beyond those in your diet. In some cases, a mixture of the basic antioxidants will suffice, such as those found in concentrated fruit and vegetable powders. However, you will run into the same problem that many multivitamin products have: only so much can be packed into one capsule or tablet. Therefore, even in the best of nutritional products, the proper dosage suffers. To get all of the good ingredients into as few capsules as possible, the manufacturer may compromise on dosage. Effective therapeutic dosages are, as a rule, considerably greater than those usually contained in a multivitamin or mixed antioxidant supplement. Therefore, from my clinical experience, it is best to use *individual antioxidants* in sufficient dosages in order to be effective in prolonging your health.

Also, I consider *prescription individualization* according to age, gender, wellness, or disease states the hallmark of knowledgeable nutritional prescribing. So, let's look now at how you can enhance your diet and general multivitamin and mineral supplementation with specific antioxidants and individualize them for different age-related health conditions.

***Prolonging Health* Antioxidant Prescription 1—Begin with Vitamin C:** Vitamin C, also known as ascorbic acid, is the single most important supplemental antioxidant. It is useful in preventing cell death and premature aging. In fact, the results of one British study showed that people who consume vitamin C-rich foods have half the death rate of those who don't. Women seem to get an even greater health advantage from vitamin C. Those women who consume high amounts of vitamin C have a 93 percent decrease in their risk of dying from heart disease compared to those who use the least (Khaw 2001).

Aging is not only associated with increased free radical activity and reduced capacity to repair damaged cells, but also with *a decrease* in as much as 54 percent of ascorbic acid concentration within liver cells (Lykkesfeldt 1998). These findings inform us that optimal levels of vitamin C are necessary to prolong health and to reduce the risk of dying from an age-related disease, and thereby to maximize longevity.

Vitamin C, a water-soluble vitamin that readily dissolves in water, is essential for the normal functioning of the body. It encompasses many functions including the synthesis of collagen, a structural glue-like component of nearly all tissues, especially of the blood vessels, tendons, ligaments, bone, and therefore the joints. It has numerous other functions including immune-enhancing activity, and also assists in detoxification.

It is found in nearly all foods, but is highest in fruits and vegetables. Some tropical sources, like camu camu *(Myrciaria dubia)*, an Amazonian fruit containing 30 times more vitamin C than citrus, and acerola berries *(Malpighia glabra)* from Barbados, make excellent supplemental sources. Broccoli, Brussels sprouts, cabbage, sweet red peppers, parsley, currants, rose hips, all citrus fruits, strawberries, and even potatoes are good sources of vitamin C.

However, the amounts in these foods are not sufficient to treat diseases other than scurvy, the classical vitamin C deficiency disease and the cause of many deaths in previous centuries until the discovery of the antiscorbutic activity of vitamin C as found in limes. Similarly, most multiple vitamins, including some very good ones, do not contain enough vitamin C, or sufficient amounts of flavonoids that complement vitamin C, to counter the effects of aging. To maximize antioxidant protection, higher supplemental dosages of vitamin C are required.

From an evolutionary point of view, most animal species can synthesize vitamin C from glucose and other sugars, but humans, monkeys, guinea pigs, and a few other animals cannot manufacture their own and need to obtain it in their diet. Therefore, it is essential that you include vitamin C-containing foods *and* take supplemental vitamin C every day.

Though vitamin C is used intravenously by physicians to treat acute and chronic viral infections and for heavy metal detoxification, for anti-aging purposes oral forms are sufficient. Vitamin C comes in a variety of forms, the least expensive and most widely used being pure ascorbic acid crystals, a mild acid usually well tolerated by most people taking average dosages of vitamin C (500–2,000 mg).

However, when using very large dosages (above 6,000 mg) for more than two weeks, or for those people whose stomachs do not tolerate acidic foods, I recommend a buffered form of vitamin C. This is gentler on the stomach and does not overacidify the system. To buffer ascorbic acid, manufacturers combine it with sodium, potassium, calcium, magnesium, or a combination of these minerals. Avoid the sodium form as

Today it is medically accepted that, for general health, a moderate dosage of vitamin C in the range of 200–500 mg daily is sufficient. However, most naturopathic physicians, as well as medical doctors practicing natural therapies, recommend higher dosages in the range of 500–2,000 mg daily. Research studies indicate that to treat the free radical damage associated with aging, the minimum dosage for vitamin C should be at least 2,000 mg and upwards to 4,000 mg per day.

it may raise your sodium levels and contribute to water retention; if you are sodium sensitive, it could cause high blood pressure. For these purposes, I recommend powdered calcium-magnesium-potassium ascorbate, a buffered form that provides about 2,500 mg of ascorbic acid per rounded teaspoon, and also provides additional amounts of the buffering minerals.

I also recommend taking ascorbyl palmitate, a fat-soluble form of vitamin C (one that dissolves in oils rather than water). This form of vitamin C is considered to be more accessible to the lipid membranes of cells. It has a history of long use as a food preservative, but its use as an effective form of oral supplemental vitamin C has been overlooked.

In the early 1970s, two-time Nobel prize–winner Linus Pauling, Ph.D., popularized high dosages of vitamin C for everything from the common cold to cancer. Today it is medically accepted that, for general health, a moderate dosage of vitamin C in the range of 200–500 mg daily is sufficient. However, most naturopathic physicians, as well as medical doctors practicing natural therapies, recommend higher dosages in the range of 500–2,000 mg daily. Research studies indicate that to treat the free radical damage associated with aging, the minimum dosage for vitamin C should be at least 2,000 mg and upwards to 4,000 mg per day.

Since optimal blood levels of vitamin C are reached easily with dosages of 200–500 mg, and amounts over that are excreted in the urine, I recommend taking vitamin C in frequent lower dosages: 250–500 mg at a time, two to four or more times per day, providing a daily total of at least 2,000 mg. Take a combination of half pure ascorbic acid or a buffered form for those sensitive to acids, and half ascorbyl palmitate, plus 200 mg of mixed citrus bioflavonoids for each 1,000 mg of vitamin C.

Too much vitamin C can cause uncomfortable abdominal gas, bloating, and watery diarrhea. Called bowel tolerance, a term originally coined by Robert Cathcart, M.D. (Cathcart 1981), these symptoms indicate an acute but temporary gastrointestinal intolerance to vitamin C. It means your gut is saturated with vitamin C and can take no more at that dosage level for the time being. Vitamin C also has pro-oxidant activity. It can work as the opposite of an antioxidant when taken in large amounts or when combined with iron, and can cause oxidative damage to blood vessels, leading to atherosclerosis (Proteggente 2000).

Certainly all substances, when taken in excess, in the wrong combination, or by sensitive individuals, can have adverse effects. However, vitamin C, if taken in moderate dosages and without iron supplements, is considered safe (Proteggente 2001). Remember, the goal is to prolong health by restoring homeostasis, so aim for a stable, sustainable state and avoid extremes.

Other safety concerns have been raised about taking high doses of vitamin C. These include the possibility of increased risk for kidney stones, depletion of vitamin B_{12} leading to pernicious anemia, increased iron absorption, depletion of copper, and increased urinary excretion of uric acid. None of these concerns has been conclusively proven; however, dialysis patients, those with chronic kidney disease, patients with hemachromatosis (an iron-overload disease), gout, or a history of forming kidney stones should avoid taking vitamin C in the higher ranges unless under direct supervision by a physician.

Several drugs deplete vitamin C levels, including estrogen-containing birth control pills, corticosteroids such as prednisone, and frequent use of aspirin. The reverse is less significant: vitamin C has limited or no effect on any conventional drugs. However, patients on anticoagulants, such as Coumadin, should limit their use of vitamin C, as high dosages may interfere with the blood-thinning activity of these drugs. Remember not to take vitamin C with iron or iron-containing supplements because of the potential pro-oxidant effects.

Vitamin C works synergistically with bioflavonoids, N-acetylcysteine (NAC), and vitamin E. NAC is derived from the amino acid L-cysteine and combines well with vitamin C to

modulate cellular changes that cause cancer (D'Agostini 2000). Vitamin E partners with vitamin C and helps to reduce the pro-oxidant effects of vitamin C. Vitamin C assists in regenerating vitamin E after it is used in the body, thus increasing the antioxidant effects of vitamin E.

Vitamin C prepared as a topical ointment, cream, or lotion is helpful in reducing free radical damage to your skin. Regular application removes age spots, corrects sun damage, and restores normal elasticity. Use a product containing between 10 and 20 percent L-ascorbic acid; daily use is recommended until conditions improve.

***Prolonging Health* Antioxidant Prescription 2—Combine Bioflavonoids with Vitamin C:** Bioflavonoids are a group of compounds found in nearly all plants, where they are concentrated in the seeds, flowers, bark, peel, or skin. There are over 4,000 known bioflavonoids and many are present in common beverages such as tea, coffee, beer, wine, and fruit juices. These include red- and blue-pigmented anthocyanidins; the white and pale-yellow compounds rutin, quercetin, and kaempherol; citrus bioflavonoids, and green tea polyphenols, as well the isoflavones in soy, flavans, and flavonols.

Most medicinal herbs are also rich in bioflavonoids, including ginkgo *(Ginkgo biloba)* and milk thistle *(Silybum marianum)*. These compounds have considerable health benefits including anti-inflammatory, anti-allergic, antiviral, antibacterial, anticarcinogenic, and powerful antioxidant activity.

Although most of the better multivitamin supplements contain some bioflavonoids, I recommend taking 250 mg of mixed citrus bioflavonoids for every 1,000 mg of vitamin C. These complement vitamin C and improve its absorption. As people age, their skin thins and often bruises easily. The combination of vitamin

C with bioflavonoids can restore the natural integrity of the capillaries in the skin and eliminate spontaneous skin bruising.

Two flavonoid substances with potent antioxidant activity are also important as anti-senescence medications: quercetin and pycnogenol.

Quercetin is one of the most common flavonoids in the human diet, found in apples, onions, black tea, green leafy vegetables, beans, and other fruits, vegetables, and herbs. It has been studied for its anticancer activity in breast, colon, lung, ovarian, prostate, and other cancers, and has been shown to beneficially affect natural killer cell function (cells that attack and destroy cancer or virally infected cells). Quercetin also has activity that protects cells (cytoprotective) from oxidative damage by increasing the antioxidant capacity of the blood and preventing premature aging (Cesquini et al. 2001).

It is recommended by naturopathic physicians as a natural antihistamine for allergies and is useful in treating hay fever and asthma. It is also useful in the treatment of chronic viral diseases and interstitial cystitis, a chronic urinary tract inflammatory syndrome characterized by severe pelvic pain.

The recommended dosage of quercetin is 250 mg daily, taken with vitamin C. There have been no proven cases of toxicity with quercetin supplementation, and though there is some concern that quercetin may pose a cancer risk, no human studies or clinical evidence have confirmed this.

Originally called pycnogenol by its discoverer, Jacques Masquelier, a professor at the University of Bordeaux, France, oligomeric proanthrocyanidin complexes (OPCs), also called procyanidolic oligomers (PCOs), were first extracted from pine bark in 1951 and later from grape seeds in 1970. These flavonoid substances have powerful antioxidant activity. In fact, grape seed extracts have stronger antioxidant effects than vitamins C and E and beta-carotene. PCOs also exert antibacterial, antiviral, anticarcinogenic, anti-inflammatory, and anti-allergic effects.

They are found in pine bark, grape seeds and skin (and therefore in red wine), tea (both green and black tea), and many herbs, notably bilberry *(Vaccinium myrtillus)*, cranberry *(Vaccinium macrocarpon)*, black currants *(Ribes nigrum)*, and elderberry *(Sambucus nigra)*.

Daily dosage recommendations for PCOs range between 50 and 100 mg. No side effects or interactions are attributed to proanthocyanidin supplementation.

***Prolonging Health* Antioxidant Prescription 3—Get Enough Vitamin E:** Vitamin E is a fat-soluble (dissolves in fats and oils) antioxidant found in polyunsaturated vegetables oils (canola and safflower oil), seeds, nuts, whole grains, wheat germ oil, and soybeans. Leafy greens, such as spinach, also contain small amounts of vitamin E. Like vitamin C, sufficient amounts of vitamin E can be obtained from dietary sources for general health; however, for optimal health and disease prevention benefits, supplemental vitamin E is required.

Research on the anti-senescent effects of vitamin E began in 1976 with Denham Harman, M.D., Ph.D., the father of the free radical theory of aging (Harman 1976). Since then a wide range of properties have been attributed to vitamin E for slowing down the aging process, including antioxidant protection against free radical damage to lipids, proteins, and lymphocytes, and protection of the blood vessels (Grune 2001). Vitamin E has been shown to protect against cancer, improve circulation, speed wound healing, reduce inflammation caused by prostaglandin (inflammation-producing chemicals) activity, and protect the thymus gland in times of stress. Research suggests that vitamin E tends to be low in older people (Requejo 2002).

Actually, vitamin E is not a single substance but a group of compounds called tocopherols and tocotrienols. Though alpha-tocopherol is the most abundant and biologically active form, it is best to take an all-natural vitamin E containing a spectrum of tocopherols. It is best taken with a meal or with some oily food, such as avocado or nuts, to assist absorption. Water-soluble forms are also available, and though more expensive than fat-soluble forms they may be useful in patients who have poor absorption of fats and oils.

The RDA for vitamin E is less than 30 IU, and the generally recommended optimal dose is 200–500 IU; occasionally up to 1,600 IU or higher is required for heart disease or post-mastectomy patients, or for those with fibro-cystic breast disease or Peyronie's syndrome. For anti-senescence purposes, I recommend 500 IU of all-natural vitamin E taken twice daily with food. If your multivitamin does not contain enough vitamin E, supplement the difference to provide a total of 1,000 IU daily.

Vitamin E is generally well tolerated and is safe even in the higher dosage ranges, though some people report headaches and nausea when taking over 1,000 IU. This usually does not occur when vitamin E is taken twice daily in divided dosages of 500 IU. If you experience headaches while taking vitamin E, change from the natural form to a synthetic, as some people are allergic to wheat germ oil; most natural vitamin E is derived from this.

Since vitamin E can affect blood clotting, patients on blood thinners, such as Coumadin or even aspirin, should take only the lower dosages unless under the supervision of a physician. In these cases, vitamin E may interfere with platelet aggregation (clumping of the blood-clotting cells), causing an increased bleeding tendency. Cholesterol-lowering drugs such as cholestyramine resin (Preventalite and Questran) and colestipol (Colestid) can deplete vitamin E levels in the body.

Prolonging Health **Antioxidant Prescription 4—Get Enough Coenzyme Q10:** Coenzyme Q10 (CoQ10), chemically known as ubiquinone, is densely concentrated within the mitochondria, the energy-producing site within cells. Adequate levels of CoQ10 protect the mitochondria from oxidative damage. It is synthesized in all body tissues, and depends on the amino acids tyrosine and phenylalanine, adequate levels of vitamin B_6, and several other vitamins and trace minerals for its production and metabolism. Along with vitamins C and E, CoQ10 is one of the fundamental antioxidants in your body, and is particularly important for proper mitochondrial function.

During aging, your levels of coenzyme Q10 decline (Linnane 2002). You achieve your peak levels at about age 26 followed by a progressive decline (Kalen 1989). Though CoQ10 is principally known as a nutrient for the treatment of heart disease, it has also been found to improve organ reserve in other parts of the body and enhances general immunity in older people and those with chronic illness. Since tissues and cells involved in immune function have a high requirement for energy, CoQ10 may be an important adjunct in maintaining normal immune integrity; it can support an immune system weakened by infections; it may help to reverse immunosuppression related to aging or chronic disease; it also aids in the treatment and prevention of cancer.

CoQ10 is found in all plant and animal cells. Food sources include organ meats, red meat, fish, nuts, vegetable oils, cereal bran, and dark-green leafy vegetables. The basic need for CoQ10 can be met with a healthy diet and a multivitamin and mineral supplement that provide the co-factors necessary for its production. However, since dietary sources only provide about 5 mg per day of this important antioxidant, and due to its expense, most multivitamins do not contain CoQ10; therefore specific supplementation during aging becomes essential.

The basic typical daily dosage of CoQ10 is 30–90 mg, with an average therapeutic range of 120–600 mg daily. For anti-senescence purposes, I recommend 250 mg daily. CoQ10 is a pharmaceutically produced substance and comes as a tablet or capsule. Since it is fat soluble, it absorbs best when taken with a fatty meal or with a little oil. Some manufacturers offer it combined with soybean or palm oil in a soft gel caplet.

Mark C. Houston, M.D., a cardiologist and associate professor of medicine at Vanderbilt University School of Medicine, and many other physicians recommend water-soluble forms such as Q-Gel, which provide improved absorption and higher blood levels (Houston 2002). Idebenone, a synthetic analog and newer form of CoQ10, is considered more easily absorbed than ubiquinone making it more useful for older people. It is taken in the same dosages as CoQ10. Patients with neurodegenerative disorders such as Parkinson's disease often require dosages as high as 1,200 mg daily.

CoQ10 works synergistically with vitamin E to prevent damage to lipid membranes and plasma lipids; it also works well with vitamin C, carnitine, lipoic acid, lycopene, magnesium, and vitamin B_6 (Willis 1999). There are no reported adverse effects of CoQ10 supplementation, though some people find it too energizing and should not take it in the evening before bedtime as it may cause difficulty in falling asleep.

CoQ10 helps to protect against the heart-damaging effects of several drugs, including the anti-cancer drugs Adriamycin and epirubicin, but it should only be used with these drugs with your doctor's approval since these are very toxic chemicals and because drug and nutrient interactions are complicated. CoQ10 is depleted by many drugs, including diuretics, some antidepressants, blood-thinning drugs (warfarin), statin drugs used to lower cholesterol, and blood pressure-lowering medications (Jones 2002). *Candida albicans* overgrowth in the intestinal tract may inhibit CoQ10 absorption as this yeast utilizes it for its own mitochondrial activity (Krone 2001).

Prolonging Health Antioxidant Prescription 5—Take B Vitamins: Nearly all members of the B-complex family are water-soluble and are not appreciably stored in the body. They must be provided daily in the diet. Among the large family of B vitamins, B_2, B_6, and B_{12} have important antioxidant activity. Since B vitamins are synergistic with each other, it is generally advised to take a B-complex or a multivitamin containing sufficient amounts of all the B vitamins rather than individual ones separately. However, there are times when the specific antioxidant B vitamins are required in higher amounts, so make sure that you have sufficient levels of these important antioxidants.

VITAMIN B_2: Vitamin B_2, or riboflavin, is a member of a group of flourescent yellow pigments called flavins; it is the substance that turns the urine bright yellow when you take extra B_2. It acts as a coenzyme necessary for normal energy metabolism of carbohydrates, fats, and proteins; it helps to activate vitamin B_6 and to convert niacin (B_3) into a form more easily utilized by the body. Among its other numerous functions, it has antioxidant activity and assists the function of vitamin E. Low levels of riboflavin can lead to reduced antibody production, resulting in reduced immunity.

It is found in organ meats such as liver and in all red meat, eggs, and dairy products. Unless there are specific symptoms of deficiency, dietary sources and a multivitamin provide adequate levels. However, numerous drugs cause depletion of riboflavin, including thorazine, tricyclic antidepressants (Elavil, Tofranil), oral contraceptives, and many antibiotics (minocycline, the penicillins, tetracycline, and sulfonamides). The basic typical dosage of B_2 is 50 mg daily.

VITAMIN B_6: Vitamin B_6, or pyridoxine, is one of the most important of vitamins. It functions in the formation of proteins and as a coenzyme in more than 100 different metabolic processes in the body. It has antioxidant capabilities and, like riboflavin, a deficiency of pyridoxine can lead to your body having fewer defensive antibodies, a reduction in lymphocytes, and thymus gland atrophy. B_6 helps to lower homocysteine levels and lower blood pressure, and it is an important building block for many neurotransmitters, including serotonin and dopamine. It is found in organ meats, red meat, milk, and eggs, and also in seafood, whole grains, bananas, avocados, soybeans, nuts, seeds, and brewer's yeast.

Since B_6 levels tend to decline with age, additional supplementation of B_6 is needed. It is available in two forms: pyridoxine hydrochloride and pyridoxal-5-phosphate, which is the more active form and the form into which the liver converts pyridoxine in the body. I recommend a combination of both forms of B_6. The basic average dosage is 50–100 mg of pyridoxine hydrochloride daily and 50 mg of pyridoxal-5-phosphate with a therapeutic range up to 500 mg daily. It is best absorbed when taken without food; a B-complex or multivitamin containing B vitamins should be taken at a different time.

B_6 works synergistically in the body with other B vitamins and magnesium, and is required for coenzyme synthesis. Dosages in excess of 2,000 mg or long-term use of daily dosages of 500 mg can lead to nerve damage, with symptoms of numbness and tingling in the hands and feet, and a stumbling gait. Once discontinued, all symptoms clear without any lasting effects. Many of the same drugs that deplete B_2 also lower B_6 levels; conjugated estrogens (Premarin) and esterified estrogens (Estratab) also deplete B_6.

VITAMIN B_{12}: Like B_6, vitamin B_{12} or cyanocobalamin, is necessary for the metabolism of proteins, carbohydrates, and fats. It prevents pernicious anemia, a condition of the red blood cells that occurs mostly in the elderly. Like B_2 and B_6, vitamin B_{12} plays a role in immune function, and low levels can impair natural immunity. B_{12} is essential for the maintenance of the integrity of the nervous system, and along with folate, helps in the synthesis of DNA and RNA. Vitamin B_{12} deficiency mimics many of the symptoms of aging, including depression, memory loss, dementia, loss of balance, loss of bladder and bowel control, hearing loss, poor eyesight, insomnia, fatigue, and impotence.

The best dietary sources are liver, red meat, eggs, dairy products, and seafood. Supplemental B_{12} is available in a wide range of oral pills and tablets, sublingual tablets, nasal sprays, by intramuscular injections, or intravenous solutions. The typical red color of the B_{12} injection solution is due to the presence of cobalt, part of the cobalamin molecule. Unless there is medical evidence of severe B_{12} deficiency or a condition that would benefit from the injectable form, oral administration is effective over time for healthy adults.

Two coenzyme forms of B_{12}, methylcobalamin and adenosylcobalamin, are derived from natural chemical reactions in the body and are manufactured as nutritional supplements.

Since methylcobalamin is more efficiently utilized in the body, it is the preferred form for oral supplementation. A typical basic oral dosage is 1,000–2,000 mcg daily with a therapeutic upper range of 6,000 mcg daily.

For the elderly and patients with chronic disease, most natural medicine doctors still prefer intramuscular injections or intravenously administered B_{12} over oral forms. Injections of 1,000 to 3,000 mg are given in the hip or buttock muscle from one to three times each month.

Many drugs inhibit B_{12} absorption, including oral contraceptives, time-released potassium, histamine-2 blockers used for gastritis and ulcers (Axid, Pepsin, Tagamet, Zantac), proton pump inhibitors (Prevacid, Prilosec), antibiotics, and cholesterol-lowering drugs. There is virtually no known toxicity to B_{12} even in high dosages.

***Prolonging Health* Antioxidant Prescription 6—Boost Your Intake of Antioxidant Minerals:** Several common trace minerals serve as antioxidants in the body. Some are critical for proper immune function, and many are useful as anti-senescence dietary nutrients. There is concern over agricultural practices that deplete the soils, and therefore the prevalence of foods grown on soil depleted of essential trace elements makes supplementation mandatory in immune deficiency states, during healing (recovery from surgery), for cancer prevention, and in aging. A quality multimineral product usually contains trace minerals, but read the label and make sure yours has optimal amounts of the following antioxidants. If it doesn't, supplement them to make up the difference.

SELENIUM: Considered one of the most important trace minerals in the body, selenium functions as a part of the antioxidant enzyme glutathione peroxidase, a substance that works with vitamin E in the body and helps to convert oxidized substances found in harmful fats (margarines, animal fats, processed spreads) into less harmful substances. It also has antioxidant roles of its own and is considered one of the most potent anticancer nutrients. In addition, selenium helps thyroid hormone function, protects against heart attack and stroke, and helps to detoxify mercury and cadmium from the body. Dietary deficiency has a direct effect on lowering immune activity.

As an anti-senescent nutrient, selenium plays a significant role in restoring age-related decline in immune cells (Roy 1995). Like many of the antioxidant nutrients, there is a progressive decrease in selenium status during aging (Olivieri 1994). This, plus the intake of selenium-deficient foods, makes supplementation necessary. The RDA is 55 mcg per day, though optimal protection is achieved at 200 mcg daily. To prolong your health, I recommend 200 mcg of selenium two times daily. Higher dosages may be needed for those with chronic infections or inflammation but should not be used for longer than one month without professional supervision. The preferred oral forms are selenium picolinate or selenomethionine. The best food sources are Brazil nuts, yeast, whole grains, garlic, eggs, liver, and seafood.

Selenium toxicity, which includes symptoms of depression, nervousness, nausea, and vomiting, is rare but can occur when daily supplemental intake reaches 3,500–5,000 mcg, but in some people as little as 900 mcg can result in toxicity. Selenium is synergistic with vitamin E, helping to enhance its antioxidant effect; it is depleted by corticosteroids, such as prednisone, and has been shown to reduce the toxicity of the anticancer drug Adriamycin, without reducing its therapeutic effects.

ZINC: Zinc has powerful antioxidant effects and works with the naturally occurring antioxidant enzyme superoxide dismutase (SOD). It plays a significant role in immunity and healing. Zinc is found in every cell of the body and is a component of over 300 enzymes and involved in over 100 metabolic processes. Zinc supplementation improves age-related low immune status, restores thymus hormone levels, and has antiviral activity.

During aging, hormonal activity is unbalanced and the normal interconversion between estrogen and testosterone is impaired. Optimal amounts of zinc help maintain correct testosterone and estrogen balance by inhibiting aromatase, an enzyme involved in the conversion of testosterone to dehyrotestosterone, and between testosterone and estrogen. Too much dehyrotestosterone and estrogen are associated with prostate cancer. Zinc thus has positive effects on prostate gland function.

Zinc is found naturally in oysters, shellfish, red meat, liver, black-eyed peas, eggs, wheat germ, tofu, and pumpkin seeds. The basic dosage for zinc is 15–25 mg daily, with an upper limit for therapeutic purposes at 150 mg daily. I recommend the picolinate form, zinc bound with picolinic acid, in dosages of 30–60 mg per day as an anti-senescence antioxidant. Zinc is considered nontoxic, but long-term use of zinc above 300 mg can cause copper depletion, resulting in anemia and reduced HDL-cholesterol; in high dosages, zinc may actually depress immune function.

When taking extra zinc in the higher ranges, consider adding 1 mg of copper—best taken in a multimineral—as zinc competes with copper, iron, calcium, and magnesium absorption. Zinc and copper work synergistically as passive viral inhibitors and can prevent autoimmune diseases, allergies, and cancer. Numerous drugs deplete zinc, including corticosteroids, oral contraceptives, and diuretics used to treat high blood pressure.

Prolonging Health **Antioxidant Prescription 7—Fortify Yourself with Lipoic Acid:** Alpha-lipoic acid (ALA), also called thiotic acid, is found in small amounts in the body and in a variety of foods, especially red meat and organ meats. In the body, it is important for energy production, helping to convert carbohydrates into usable energy; for this reason it is often used as an adjunctive treatment for diabetes. ALA is a powerful antioxidant and helps to recycle other antioxidants, principally vitamins C and E. However, it may also replace vitamin E when that is in short supply in the body, since it is both water- and fat-soluble and has a broader range of antioxidant activity than either vitamin C or E. It also functions as a chelating (binding) agent in the removal of excess iron and copper, and toxic metals such as mercury, lead, and cadmium.

As an anti-senescent supplement, ALA prevents age-related decline in mitochondrial function (Hagen 2002), protects against oxidative damage to nerve tissues (Lynch 2001), and enhances the glutathione system, providing increased antioxidant activity (Arivazhagan 2001).

The basic dosage is 25–100 mg, with a therapeutic range as high as 600–1,000 mg. For your *Prolonging Health* plan, take 300–600 mg daily. Though there are no known toxic effects with these higher dosages, as with all nutrients, I recommend that you only take lipoic acid at a dosage over 600 mg under the supervision of a health professional. Since ALA is an acid, it can cause burning in the stomach after swallowing a capsule. Because of this, take ALA with food.

Like vitamin C cream, topical application of lipoic acid lotion can revitalize your skin. Use a product containing 12–25 percent lipoic acid daily.

Prolonging Health **Antioxidant Prescription 8—Go Strong on Carotenoids:** Carotenoids are called pro-vitamins, or precursor forms, because they are converted to vitamin A in the body. This takes place through the action of enzymes in the intestinal tract, a process that depends on thyroid hormone, zinc, and vitamin C to metabolize properly. Besides being converted to vitamin A, carotenoids have useful properties of their own, including powerful antioxidant effects on cancer activity; they are associated with a lower risk of cardiovascular disease, and they have immune-enhancing effects.

Carotenoids are found only in plants; the intense red, blue, purple, yellow, and orange colors in fruits and vegetables are due to plant pigments that have a high carotenoid content. There are over 600 known carotenoids in nature, and though only about 30 to 50 have vitamin A activity, most have antioxidant properties. A diet rich in vegetables and fruits can supply the basic carotenes, but extra supplementation of the full spectrum of carotenoids is often necessary to obtain optimal antioxidant protection. Read the label of your multivitamin and make sure you are getting enough of the following carotenoids:

CAROTENES: A group of carotenoids, carotenes are found in all dark-green leafy vegetables (spinach, collards), yellow- and orange-colored fruits and vegetables (apricots, peaches, carrots, yams, squash), and red fruits and vegetables (strawberries, tomatoes). Beta-carotene is the most abundant of the carotenoids found in human foods. Carrot juice, mixed dark-green leafy vegetable juice, and many of the "green" health drinks containing fresh-water or sea algae (spirulina, chlorella) are rich in mixed carotenes. Indeed, they are so rich in carotenes that if carrot juice or mixed green vegetable juice is included in the diet several times per week, a separate supplementation of beta-carotene is rarely needed.

Carotenes are available commercially in synthetic or natural forms. They are best taken in the natural derived form from palm oil or the algae Dunaliella. Most commercial beta-carotene supplements are the synthetic form, so read labels carefully. The supplemental range is from 25,000 IU up to 300,000 IU (100,000 IU = 60 mg). To prolong your health, take 75,000 IU of carotenes daily.

Carotenes are considered very safe, but should be used with caution in patients with existing liver damage. When taking high dosages or drinking carrot juice daily, the palms of the hands and soles of the feet can take on a distinctive yellow-orange hue. This condition, called carotenosis or carotemia, is harmless and clears up completely once the supplementation or juice intake is discontinued. The same cholesterol-lowering drugs that deplete vitamin A can reduce beta-carotene absorption.

OTHER CAROTENOIDS: Besides beta-carotene, other carotenoids are important in disease prevention. These include alpha-carotene, gamma-carotene, beta-zeacarotene, crytoxanthine, zeaxanthine, lutein, lycopene, and astaxanthine. Lutein, found in peas and cool-weather, green leafy vegetables such as kale, collards, and romaine lettuce, may help to prevent macular degeneration. The red color in tomatoes and watermelon is due to pigmentation from lycopene, which has been shown to reduce the risk of prostate cancer.

Astaxanthine provides the rich pink color found in salmon, lobsters, and shrimp, and is found in the algae consumed by these creatures. It is considered ten times more potent than the standard carotenoids and is able to penetrate the lipid membrane of cells, thereby exerting powerful antioxidant activity within the cell. It is useful in the treatment of some forms of cancer (Tanaka 1994), protects the heart from the negative effects of LDL (Iwamoto et al. 2000), and improves T-lymphocyte function in the co-treatment of bacterial infections (Wadstrom 1999).

These additional carotenoids are best provided in foods or whole foods supplements such as mixed green and algae concentrates.

***Prolonging Health* Antioxidant Prescription 9—Start Consuming Amino Acids:** Amino acids are the building blocks of proteins and enzymes and are necessary for the structural components of the body and maintenance of life. Proteins make up our muscle, tissue, and organs, and even compose part of our bones. The immune system, including immunoglobulins (one of the main components of first-line defense), is also largely made from proteins and is directly affected by how proteins are utilized in the body, how much protein we eat, and the quality of protein we take in.

A full complement of amino acids is found in high-quality protein from seeds and nuts, legumes, whole grains, eggs, fish, poultry, and organic meats, all of which are excellent dietary sources. An amino acid is a compound containing an amino group and having an acidic function. This acidic function makes proteins from meat more acidic in the body; therefore, it is recommended that the majority of one's dietary protein come from plant sources. If one is eating large amounts of animal protein—as in body building—flushing out accumulated acids with plenty of water is essential, along with eating vegetables, which are alkaline, as they balance any acid buildup that develops from eating meat.

Twenty specific amino acids make up all the proteins in the human body: alanine, arginine, asparagine, aspartic acid, cysteine, glutamic acid, glutamine, glycine, histidine, isoleucine, leucine, lysine, methionine, phenylalanine, proline, serine, threonine, tryptophan, tyrosine, and valine. There are other amino acids in the body, such as taurine and ornithine, that have functions not directly related to building protein. These 20 amino acids are divided into two groups, called essential and nonessential amino acids.

This terminology is somewhat misleading as all the amino acids are crucial to life. However, what biologists refer to as the essential group are those that cannot be synthesized in the body and must be obtained through the diet. These eight essential amino acids are isoleucine, methionine, leucine, lysine, phenylalanine, threonine, tryptophan, and valine.

For those with chronic disease and people over age 40, having adequate dietary protein intake is critical. However, people in these categories often are not able to digest and absorb all the amino acids they need for tissue repair and healing. To enhance protein intake, an amino acid supplement is recommended and is best taken in the form of a "protein powder" drink.

To prevent possible gastrointestinal allergic reactions, such as cramping or gas, I suggest avoiding products made from soy, milk casein, gluten (wheat and other grain proteins), and eggs. The amino acids should also be lactose free and have a high biological value, which is measured by the nitrogen retained for growth and expressed as a percentage of absorbed nitrogen.

Like many nutritionists and naturopathic physicians, I specifically recommend hydrolyzed or pure whey as a source of amino acids. This is made up of smaller, more easily digested particles that have less allergic reactivity than conventional whey products. Whey is a byproduct of making cheese from milk. The liquid whey is commercially processed into a dry powder and further purified to make whey protein concentrate. Some whey products are combined with hypoallergenic rice protein to complement the whey. Others, such as MyoSpan, have sustained release whey protein isolates, amino acids that absorb gradually.[19] Many of these hypoallergenic whey products are classified as medical foods and are not available in health stores. Consult with your doctor or see the resource section at the end of this book.

Whey protein includes many other biologically active substances besides amino acids, including beta-lactoglobulin, immunoglobulins, bovine (cow) serum albumin, lactoperoxidases, lysozyme, and lactoferrin (a potent immuno-

People who benefit most from whey protein supplementation are those with a weakened constitution or age-related immune decline, in recovery from a long illness, or who have general immune weakness. The recommended supplemental dosage is 15–20 g per day. Of course, whey is also beneficial for healthy people who want to improve their protein status and increase muscle mass.

modulating substance).

Some whey protein products contain very high levels of immunoglobulin complexes, substances necessary for rebuilding the immune system, and in certain cases may be more beneficial than pure whey. However, it is extremely important not to take whey protein products, especially the immunoglobulin-enhanced products, if you have an autoimmune condition, such as lupus or rheumatoid arthritis, or any chronic inflammatory condition. In such cases,

adding immunoglobulins from milk-based products could cause the immune system to overreact to the foreign proteins, resulting in increased inflammation.

People who benefit most from whey protein supplementation are those with a weakened constitution or age-related immune decline, in recovery from a long illness, or who have general immune weakness. The recommended supplemental dosage is 15–20 g per day. Of course, whey is also beneficial for healthy people who want to improve their protein status and increase muscle mass.

Hydrolyzed whey protein has been shown to effectively boost levels of glutathione, a powerful naturally occurring antioxidant.

Specific amino acids have been shown to improve immune status and enhance glutathione levels. Additional supplementation with these substances can further enhance immunity and prolong health as follows:

ARGININE AS A SPECIAL ANTI-AGING NUTRIENT: This amino acid is referred to as a growth hormone enhancer and is well known in body-building circles as a powerful muscle builder. It is important for cell growth, wound healing, recovery from illness, and during times of stress. It strengthens the immune system by increasing natural killer cell activity; it increases white cell production and stimulates white cell response; and it promotes resistance against infection and stimulates the thymus gland. It is useful in chronic fatigue syndrome and cardiovascular disease, and helps lower age-related systolic high blood pressure (Susic 2001).

The basic dose is 500–1,000 mg daily, but to obtain the growth hormone enhancing effect, dosages as high as 30 g daily are required. Choline, vitamin B_5 as calcium pantothenate, and the amino acid ornithine can enhance this effect. To prolong your health, I recommend taking 1,500 mg of arginine daily. If you are building muscle, take 6,000 mg three times daily.

However, high and sustained dosages of arginine have been shown to activate herpes simplex virus, as arginine acts as an antagonist to lysine, an amino acid that helps to reduce herpes virus activity. In these cases, arginine supplementation should not be used and one should avoid eating arginine-containing foods such as nuts, cheeses, and chocolate. Otherwise, arginine is a safe substance free of side effects.

Since arginine works synergistically with ornithine to stimulate growth hormone, some doctors warn against its use in diabetes, as the growth hormone increase it can cause may overwork the pancreas. Arginine intake should be avoided in cancer patients as high dosages have been shown to increase cancer cell growth.

CYSTEINE: Cysteine is an important amino acid due to its antioxidant activity. It is a nonessential amino acid and one of only a few that contain the sulfur component thiol. Cysteine is involved in many of the body's detoxification pathways, helping to eliminate toxins, drugs, and heavy metals that have a destructive effect on the immune system. It also increases the formation of glutathione.

The recommended supplemental form is N-acetylcysteine (NAC), a derivative of L-cysteine. The basic dosage is 200–500 mg per day, with a therapeutic range up to 5,000 mg. NAC is an important therapeutic nutrient in its own right and is used as a mucolytic, a substance that reduces phlegm, which makes it beneficial in the treatment of respiratory conditions such as chronic bronchitis. It protects cell membranes and liver cells from oxidative damage. NAC has been shown to lower lipoprotein (a), one of the bad blood fats and a genetic marker for early heart disease. NAC is synergistic with other amino acids and vitamin C.

GLUTAMINE: Glutamine is the most abundant amino acid in the body and is important in building muscle and speeding wound healing. It can be used as an alternative fuel by the brain when glucose is low. It also serves as an energy source for the cells of the gastrointestinal tract and is useful in irritable bowel and "leaky gut" syndromes. Glutamine also has immune-enhancing functions; it can increase white cell proliferation and macrophages use it as a source of energy. It is useful for general immune weakness and for those losing muscle mass due to chronic illness or aging. It has antioxidant activity and helps to protect muscles against breakdown during periods of physiological stress.

The basic dosage ranges from 500 to 2,000 mg daily with a therapeutic dosage as high as 40 g daily. If you are engaging in heavy exercise, have cancer or bowel disease, take 4,000–8,000 mg (4–8 g) daily. It is best taken in the powdered form and mixed directly into water or juice, and may be combined with whey protein powder. The exact optimal dosage is not yet known; however, there are no known toxic effects.

Food sources include all meats, fish, and eggs. However, overcooking animal protein foods destroys much of the available glutamine. Slow cooking, pressure cooking, or steaming helps to preserve glutamine as well as other important vitamins and minerals. Glutamine is synergistic with vitamin B_6 and magnesium, and combines with NAC to promote glutathione synthesis.

Prolonging Health Recommendation 13— Restore Your Glutathione

Glutathione was discovered in 1888 by J. de Rey-Pailhade of France, but its chemical structure was not completely defined until the mid-twentieth century by F. Gowland Hopkins, the "father of biochemistry," of Cambridge, England. It was not until the 1980s that its functions and use were elucidated by Alton Meister, Ph.D., of Cornell University in Ithaca, New York. It is now known that glutathione is the most abundant cellular antioxidant, and is involved in a wide spectrum of biochemical processes including the transport of amino acids, the biosynthesis of proteins, enzymes, and hormones, and antioxidant defense against toxic compounds and oxidative stress. Due to this powerful antioxidant activity, glutathione has been referred to as the "master antioxidant."

According to Paris Kidd, Ph.D., a cellular biologist and renowned biomedical nutritionist from Berkeley, California, glutathione can "fine-tune" cells, helping them maintain strong antioxidant protective activity, and thereby guard cells from oxidative damage (Kidd 1997).

Glutathione, referred to as GHS in its reduced form, is a naturally occurring protein composed of three amino acids: cysteine, glutamic acid, and glycine. It is a water-soluble substance found in the cells of all animals and plants. In humans it is stored mainly in the liver, where it is metabolized; the liver is the organ most involved in metabolism and detoxification processes. For these reasons, glutathione restoration is part of a comprehensive approach to revitalizing your antioxidant defense system.

High glutathione status is associated with protection from cancer and the prevention of a wide variety of degenerative diseases, including Parkinson's disease (Kidd 2000). Chronic glutathione deficiency inhibits the natural immune response and is associated with cancer and the progression of HIV and hepatitis C viral infections.

Investigating glutathione's role in heath and aging (Lang 2001), researchers found that higher levels in older adults are associated with better health (Julius 1994) and that lower levels appear to be associated with aging (Lang 1992) and degenerative disease (Lang 2000). The results of these and other studies, plus abundant clinical evidence of the importance of GHS, have led to the idea that the levels of glutathione in the blood and in white blood cells, along with vitamin C and E status, are a prime biomarker of premature aging and immune status. Therefore, restoring glutathione status during aging is a critical component in your *Prolonging Health* program.

Though low glutathione levels are associated with poor health, including lowered immune status, it is unclear if oral supplementation of GSH is of any direct benefit in humans. A few studies have shown that blood levels of glutathione increased with oral dosages, but most of the studies suggest that the body may have a buffering system that makes absorption difficult. However, the importance of glutathione supplementation in maintaining health warrants careful consideration.

As with other important antioxidants, synthetic forms of GHS have been developed (such as the "prodrug" L-2-oxothiazolidine-4-carboxylate called Procysteine), but these substances are not in wide use and it is still uncertain if they can provide consistent results and are safe to use (Moberly 1998). Glutathione can also be administered intravenously and is useful for the rapid elevation of low blood levels in the elderly and those with degenerative diseases. It is also still unclear, though, whether plasma and tissue levels are improved by this method, and even if they are, people are usually unwilling to have intravenous therapy over a long period.

My clinical experience has taught me that to achieve glutathione restoration it is necessary to supplement the diet with several other, related substances. Many of the antioxidants and amino acids discussed in this section increase glutathione levels, including vitamin C, N-acetylcysteine, and glutamine. Vitamin C supplementation in particular appears to significantly raise glutathione levels, with a dose as low as 500 mg (Murray 1996). The amino acid L-methionine and its activated form, S-adenosylmethionine (SAMe), also raise glutathione levels. In addition, take 100 mg of free-form glutathione daily.

To achieve glutathione restoration, you must avoid substances that cause its depletion, including cigarette smoke, pharmaceutical drugs (including over-the-counter ones like acetaminophen), industrial pollutants, pesticides and other toxic environmental substances, and alcohol. Chronic bacterial and viral infections also deplete glutathione status, as does iron overload. Dietary deficiency of methionine, an essential amino acid and a GSH precursor, and vitamin C deficiency can lower glutathione reserves.

At times, the antioxidant defense system cannot keep pace with the amount of oxidation the body endures, and antioxidant maladaptation occurs. Tissue and cellular damage, called free radical pathology, is the result. At this point, even though tissue damage is only just starting, and no specific disease is yet manifest, the person with active free radical pathology may feel tired or vaguely not well, but usually ignores this. However, the stage is being set for illness, and gradually, over time, a wide range of diseases can develop, including cancer, heart disease, allergies, cataracts, macular degeneration, mental impairment and Alzheimer's disease, diabetes, and nearly all of the other chronic degenerative and age-related diseases.

Normally our body has sufficient adaptive mechanisms that automatically restore biochemical stability within the cells by providing extra molecules to neutralize free radicals. However, over time, if the natural adaptive mechanisms falter, or when free radical activity is increased by your exposure to pollution, radiation, smoke, or infection, or triggered by stress or physical trauma including repetitively overexercising, irreparable cellular and genetic damage occurs. This is the type of damage that leads to aging.

Numerous methods are available to improve antioxidant status, including nutritional supplements, intravenous administration of vitamin C and glutathione, diet, herbal medicines, and enhancing the body's adaptive ability with regular exercise and stress modification.

Summary of Antioxidant Recommendations and Prescriptions

- *Prolonging Health* Recommendation 10— Eat Foods Rich in Antioxidants

  Eat at least five to six servings of fresh fruits and vegetables daily.

  Eat more high-ORAC foods. (Get 5,500 ORAC units each day.)

  Use natural condiments that have high ORAC values.

  Drink green tea and herbal teas.

- *Prolonging Health* Recommendation 11— Get an ORAC Blood Test

  Aim for a total ORAC score above 4,500 μM.

- *Prolonging Health* Recommendation 12— Take Antioxidant Supplements

  Prolonging Health Antioxidant Prescription 1— Begin With Vitamin C: Take 2,000–4,000 mg of vitamin C (half as ascorbic acid or buffered vitamin, away from food, and the other half as ascorbyl palmitate with meals) in equal divided dosages two to four times daily. Apply a 10–20 percent topical L-ascorbic acid lotion or cream daily.

Prolonging Health Antioxidant Prescription 2—Combine Bioflavonoids with Vitamin C: Take 250 mg of mixed citrus bioflavonoids with every 1,000 mg of vitamin C. Take 250 mg of quercetin, or 50–100 mg of PCOs, with your vitamin C. Use a 10–20 percent topical vitamin C cream (L-ascorbic acid) daily.

Prolonging Health Antioxidant Prescription 3—Get Enough Vitamin E: Take 500 IU of all-natural mixed tocopherols twice daily with food.

Prolonging Health Antioxidant Prescription 4—Get Enough Coenzyme Q10: Take 250 mg or more daily with food.

Prolonging Health Antioxidant Prescription 5—Take B Vitamins: Get 50 mg of B_2, 50–100 mg of B_6 as pyridoxine hydrochloride, 1,000– 2,000 mcg of B_{12} as methylcobalamin.

Prolonging Health Antioxidant Prescription 6—Boost Your Intake of Antioxidant Minerals: Make sure your multiple vitamin contains trace minerals and take a total of 200 mcg of selenium two times daily, and 30–60 mg of zinc picolinate daily.

Prolonging Health Antioxidant Prescription 7—Fortify Yourself with Lipoic Acid: Take 300–600 mg daily with food. Apply a 12–25 percent topical lipoic acid cream daily.

Prolonging Health Antioxidant Prescription 8—Go Strong on Carotenoids: Take 75,000 IU of carotenes daily, and consume a mixture of other carotenoids containing alpha-carotene, gamma-carotene, beta-zeacarotene, crytoxanthine, zeaxanthine, lutein, lycopene, and astaxanthine.

Prolonging Health Antioxidant Prescription 9—Start Consuming Amino Acids: Drink 15–20 grams of whey protein daily, and add 1,500 mg of arginine, 200–500 mg of N-acetylcysteine (NAC), and 500–2,000 mg daily of L-glutamine.

- ***Prolonging Health* Recommendation 13—Restore Your Glutathione**

  Take 100 mg of free-form glutathione daily.

8 *Prolonging Health* Modifiable Aging Factor 2: Genetic Damage—How to Guard Your Genome Against Aging with DNA Repair Medications

Each of the ten modifiable aging factors influences how we age, the diseases associated with aging, and our potential maximum life span. Oxidative damage, discussed in the last chapter, exerts effects on the whole organism, the cells, and the molecules. These make up the three main levels of the scientific investigation of aging. We've discussed the general aging effects on our body and how free radicals affect our cells. Now, we explore how aging happens at the molecular level.

Scientists who study aging at the molecular level believe that our genes, or genome collectively, hold the key to understanding aging. In fact, recent decades of aging research have largely been devoted to a search for specific genes that might influence aging, cancer, and the diseases associated with aging. The study of aging by exploring how specific genes operate is called the molecular basis of aging.

Several theories have developed around the idea that genetic damage is responsible for aging. The main ones are the DNA damage-repair theory, the telomere theory, and the idea of mitochondrial decay caused by oxidative damage. By studying these, scientists have identified three types of genetic damage that occur during aging:

1) damage to our DNA caused by free radicals (the reactive oxygen species discussed in the last chapter), as well as random errors that happen during the millions of times cells replicate during our life;

2) shortening of telomeres, which are located at the end of chromosomes and are responsible for protecting DNA;

3) mutations to mitochondrial DNA, also caused by free radicals and other cellular issues such as deficiency of micronutrients.

In this chapter, I explain how damage to our genetic material occurs, what the consequences are, how to guard our genome from damage, which natural medicines help repair DNA damage, and how to restore damaged mitochondrial DNA.

Unrepaired DNA Damage Leads to Aging

DNA is damaged in many ways. These include free radical pathology, toxic environmental chemicals, toxic metabolic by-products, radiation, and infections. Accumulated DNA damage combined with inadequate DNA repair can cause improper genetic replication; this leads to abnormal genetic information being passed on from one generation of cells to the next.

The Genome

Cells are the basic functional units of life. The raw material of all genes in every cell on Earth is made of DNA (deoxyribonucleic acid). This, in turn, is made up of thread-like structures found in the nucleus of cells, called chromosomes. A molecule of DNA consists of two chains of nucleotides, called strands, shaped in the form of a spiral—the double helix discovered in 1953 by the genetic scientists James D. Watson, Ph.D., and Francis H. C. Crick, Ph.D., who shared the Nobel Prize in Physiology and Medicine in 1962. Their discovery unlocked the doors to our modern understanding of genetics.

Human DNA is formed by nucleotide pairs made of a molecule of the sugar deoxyribose attached to one of phosphoric acid and a nitrogen-containing base consisting of one of four different chemicals: adenine, cytosine, guanine, or thymine. The complete set of genetic information contained in DNA is called a genome. Though the human genome contains at least 30,000 genes with an average of three billion pairs of DNA, remarkably only two percent of the genome is made up of genes; the remaining portion consists of what scientists call "noncoding regions," the function of which is thought to be to provide chromosome structure and integrity. Chromosomes are made of DNA and proteins, and are composed of a middle section called a centromere, and two tail sections known as telomeres.

Over time, these genetically crippled or mutated cells accumulate in the tissues. Ultimately, protein synthesis is affected, and since proteins are the major structural and metabolic component of all our tissues, inadequate rebuilding of tissue occurs. Abnormal tissue subsequently builds dysfunctional organs and this disrupts normal biological function; disrupted function predisposes us to age-related diseases and increases our biological age, and we age faster. This model of DNA damage is referred to medically as the "instability of the nuclear genome" (Viig 2001).

In the previous chapter we discussed how mutations in the genetic material are largely caused by oxidative damage from free radical molecules. Mitochondrial DNA, the control center in the powerhouse of the cell, is particu-larly hit hard by free radicals. Damage to mitochondrial DNA reduces the efficiency of the cell and over time causes a general deterioration of energy production. With less energy, our body's functions decline and we age.

Besides oxidative damage, toxic environmental chemicals and radiation are well-known causes of genetic damage. In fact, scientists studying cells in laboratory cultures often use toxic compounds to stress cells chemically to see if they age faster. Theoretically, the overuse of pharmaceutical drugs, chemicals foreign to our body, can conceivably cause genetic damage.

Accumulation of metabolic toxins produced within the body also causes DNA damage. Elevated levels of homocysteine, a naturally occurring but toxic amino acid, are an indicator of underlying disease, particularly cardiovascular disease, and a sign of methylation deficiency. Methylation is a metabolic process important in gene activity; for cells to function properly, methylation processes must be balanced. Methylation is a biochemical process important for DNA repair, the growth of new cells, and is involved in the regulation of gene expression. To regulate how genes express information, sets of proteins attach to part of the DNA. One of these protein sets contains a methyl group (a molecule made of one carbon with three hydrogen atoms). Active methylation plays an important role in determining whether a gene is expressed or is "silent" (unexpressed). Reduced methylation (demethylation) causes unhealthy cells. When cells are unable to undergo normal DNA methylation, they are more prone to turn cancerous and age more rapidly.

If DNA methylation is reduced (demethylation), it causes an increase in the expression of cancer-causing (oncogenic) genes. An increase in methylation (hypermethylation) is associated with age-related cellular changes that predispose to disease. Even slightly elevated homocysteine levels, coupled with abnormal methylation, can cause genetic damage and accelerate aging.

Radiation from the sun (you're exposed to it at increased levels at high altitudes during plane flights) and radiation from x-rays and CT scans are well-known mutagens that cause genetic damage and trigger cancer. In fact, even small amounts of background radiation when paired with exposure to foreign toxic chemicals greatly increase the insult to our genetic material and lead to progressive DNA decay.

Viral infections can also damage the genetic material. Viruses are small enough to get inside the nucleus of a cell, where they can damage our DNA and profoundly alter genetic expression; this disruption can lead to cancer and premature aging.

Abnormal hormonal changes triggered by stress, free radical pathology, and aging itself can also affect genomic stability. Hormones are chemical messengers that profoundly influence genetic expression. When hormone function is disrupted, the function of countless cells can

Genetic Expression

Our genetic material, collectively termed genes, is where the instructions are kept for a process known as gene expression. These instructions, in the form of DNA, provide the information that formulates the characteristics for each generation of cells. In order for genes to express the information contained in the DNA, the information must first be copied into another molecule called messenger RNA (ribonucleic acid), used as a template to synthesize proteins from amino acids. Ultimately, genetic expression controls not only the makeup of an individual organism within a representative species, but what diseases that individual is susceptible to, as well as how that individual ages.

be irreparably altered. This has wide-sweeping effects on biochemical processes that run our body; it eventually disrupts homeostasis, which can lead to cancer, other diseases, and a shortened life span.

Despite our living in a complex, often chaotic, and hostile world, our body's cells do a remarkable job of maintaining order. They promote normal growth and repair, resist disease, and keep us healthy. To accomplish this, old cells are continually replaced with new cells in a process called DNA replication. Essentially our cells clone themselves. This is usually done in a controlled and balanced fashion so that the cloned cells do not accumulate and overrun the system. However, there are times when overrun happens; cancer, for example, is essentially the unrestrained replication of abnormal cells: a toxic overrun of cells.

Genetic mutations may occur, but cells have an extraordinary capacity to replicate without mutations most of the time. Considering that each cell must perform this process millions of time during a life span, this is a remarkable accomplishment. In a healthy body, when mutations do occur, they are eliminated by the immune system or through a process of cell "suicide," a programmed cell death called apoptosis. Scavenger immune cells called phagocytes clean up the cellular debris, removing them from the body.

However, not all cancerous, genetically damaged, or mutant cells are removed by the immune system or undergo apoptosis. This reduced DNA repair capacity, combined with insufficient apoptosis and removal of damaged or dead cells, leads to further accumulation of genetic error; magnifying genomic instability, it contributes to degenerative disease, cancer, and accelerated aging.

Shorter Telomeres Means a Shortened Life Span

During replication, individual strands of DNA are altered. Each time DNA replicates itself, telomeres, the tips of each strand, lose some genetic material. In healthy younger people, telomeres rebuild themselves; however, in older people telomeres lose this capacity. Scientists don't know why this happens, but they suspect that telomeres act as molecular clocks regulating the aging process in cells.

Telomeres preserve the integrity of genes during DNA replication. This ensures that no matter how many replications occur, each DNA strand contains the same amount of genetic material. In healthy people, telomeres don't shrink as much as those in older people because telomere length is maintained by the enzyme telomerase.

Thinking that by manipulating telomerase they could extend life, some researchers attempted to enhance telomerase activity in normal aging cells in hopes of promoting longevity. Unfortunately, the relationship between the length of telomeres and activity of telomerase proved more complicated than they expected.

Paradoxically, this same enzyme is present in cancer cells. Scientists, theorizing that telomerase may be the substance that makes cancer cells immortal, found that when telomerase activity was inhibited, cancer cells died. Though inhibiting telomerase stopped cancer

growth, it also shortened life; when they enhanced telomerase, cells lived longer but developed cancer. Such contradictions have confounded researchers, but some are hopeful that further investigation will yield results in retarding aging and in the treatment of cancer.

In complementary and alternative medical research, several investigators are studying the effects of natural medications on the regulation of telomerase. One such researcher is Phillip Minton, M.D., a homeopathic medical doctor and molecular biologist who has put these theories into practice at his clinic in Reno, Nevada. He uses specialized homeopathic preparations of the "immortality enzyme," telomerase, along with other alternative therapies, to treat cancer and slow aging (Minton 2000). A group of scientists at the University of Kalyani in India, found that homeopathic preparations of the herb *Chelidonium majus* were effective in treating liver cancer and protecting genetic material from damage by toxic chemicals (Biswas 2002).

Though it is still too early to tell which direction telomere research will take and what other practical approaches will develop, the current climate in telomere research is heating up and may yield results fairly soon. As a general guideline for protecting your DNA from damage, enhancing DNA repair capacity, and promoting normal telomerase activity, consider using homeopathic and other natural medications, as discussed below.

Mitochondrial Decay Greatly Influences Aging

The theory that mitochondrial DNA may control aging is an extension of the free radical theory of aging. Oxidative damage from free radicals, toxic environmental chemicals, certain antibiotics such as streptomycin and rifampin, and infections directly affect mitochondrial

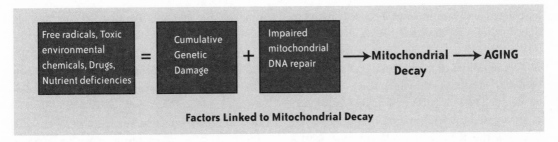

Factors Linked to Mitochondrial Decay

function. Specifically, they interfere with the ability of mitochondrial DNA to produce energy (Sastre 2000). Researchers at the University of Tampere in Finland demonstrated that changes in mitochondrial DNA can result in fatigue, loss of muscle mass, dementia, deafness, difficulty walking, and stroke-like episodes (Pak 2003). As mentioned, mitochondria have their own set of genes that provide the information for their function. Mitochondrial DNA is separate from the DNA in the cell nucleus.

Mitochondria are structures within cells where energy is produced from molecules derived from digested food and inhaled air. The two primary molecules used to make energy are glucose and oxygen. About 90 percent of the oxygen taken in by humans is used by the mitochondria to produce energy.

The universal currency of energy in the body is adenosine triphosphate (ATP). It is produced by the mitochondria in a process called cellular respiration: here the glucose and oxygen are transformed into free energy (ATP), and carbon dioxide and water are released as end products. Nicotinamide adenine dinucleotide hydride (NADH), an important carrier molecule that transports hydrogen between molecules, is produced along with ATP. NADH is a powerful antioxidant and an important nutritional supplement for prolonging health.

Cellular respiration takes place in the inner part of the mitochondria and involves a complex series of chemical events that depend on numerous enzymes. These enzymes catalyze, or boost, chemical reactions and allow them to take place at normal body temperatures. Without them, temperatures higher than the body can withstand would be needed for chemical reactions. Many of these enzymes depend on vitamins and minerals that help in the production of ATP. These include folate, magnesium, B vitamins, amino acids, and lipoic acid.

Mitochondrial decay occurs when there is a breakdown in communication from mitochondrial DNA, with deficiencies of coenzymes, toxic insults from environmental chemicals, and the inability of mitochondrial DNA to repair itself. But how does that cause aging?

Bruce N. Ames, Ph.D., a professor of biochemistry at the University of California in Berkeley, and his colleagues have found that large numbers of damaged mitochondrial DNA appear during aging and that, with increasing age, the mitochondrial ability to produce ATP is greatly decreased (Beckman 1998). Free radicals cause further mutations to the mitochondrial DNA, perpetuating a cycle of mutagenic and degenerative changes. Cellular repair mechanisms eventually are unable to keep up with the rate of decay, and aging results (Beckman 1998).

Certain sites in the body are more sensitive to mitochondrial decay than others, such as the muscles, heart, liver, and brain (Barja 2000). Mutations of mitochondrial DNA are

151

associated with a number of diseases related to aging, such as diabetes, Parkinson's, and Alzheimer's disease. Defects in mitochondrial DNA can influence metabolism and are associated with conditions in which the muscles tire easily, such as mitochondrial myopathy. This is characterized by deterioration of muscle tissue and was the disease that affected the world-class cyclist Greg LeMond. Mitochondrial decay has also been linked to chronic fatigue syndrome, the frailty that occurs with aging, and the reduced immune function characteristic of elderly people.

How to Guard Your Genome Against Aging

Since DNA damage and mitochondrial decay are associated with oxidative damage, you can prevent them by reducing dietary and supplemental iron intake, the main mineral which increases oxidation (Proteggente 2001); through detoxification techniques that remove heavy metals such as mercury (see the next chapter); eating a diet rich in phytonutrients and naturally occurring antioxidants such as carotenoids (Fenech 2002); and supplementing the diet with antioxidants (Sastre 2000).

Calorie restriction lowers metabolism and thus reduces the generation of free radicals in your body. A low-calorie diet can limit the accumulation of oxidative damage to nuclear and mitochondrial DNA (Masoro 1989). Eliminating sugar and refined carbohydrates, and supplementing with the amino acid L-arginine (Bland 1998) and chromium (a nutrient that improves insulin regulation) help to prevent genetic damage (Heydari 1993). Arginine and chromium promote homeostasis and reduce the effects of aging (Hall 2000). Folic acid deficiency is associated with many types of genetic damage; supplementing with folic acid protects mitochondrial DNA and helps

preserve the genome (Branda, O'Neill, Brooks, et al. 2001).

Since chronic infections are a source of significant toxicity to the system and the release of free radicals and cellular debris into the bloodstream leads to DNA damage, accurate diagnosis and timely, effective treatment of all chronic infections is necessary to guard your genome against the effects of aging. Viruses in particular are responsible for destructive genetic insults and should be treated promptly. Many chronic diseases, in particular diabetes and all forms of cancer, cause genetic damage, so proactive prevention of these diseases is mandatory to guard your genome against aging.

Prolonging Health Recommendation 14— Get an 8-Hydroxydeoxyguanosine (8-OHdG) Test

Considered the "gold standard" for measuring oxidative damage inside the cell, 8-OHdG reflects genetic damage to chromosomal and mitochondrial DNA. It is tested from a urine sample. Get this test before you start taking DNA repair medications. Retest one year later. Elevated levels of 8-OHdG are thought to contribute to both aging and cancer. Keep your levels below the mean value of the laboratory's reference range of 0–49 mg/mL. See your physician for details on this test.

Prolonging Health Recommendation 15— Repair Your DNA with Natural Medicines

Every cell in the body contains DNA, and every strand of DNA requires constant repair. This is largely performed by different enzymes that repair specific kinds of damage (Klungland 1999), but you can assist your body's natural repair mechanisms by eating a healthy diet, taking antioxidant supplements, and taking herbal extracts such as *Ginkgo biloba* and medicines prepared from *Uncaria tomentosa*, and other natural substances. Mitochondrial damage can be treated with specialized antioxidants, especially lipoic acid, glutathione, N-acetylcysteine (NAC), coenzyme Q10 (CoQ10), as well as with common antioxidants such as vitamins C and E (Miquel 2002; Lutsenko 2002), and folic acid.

Extensive research has been performed on CoQ10 as a protective substance for the mitochondria and it has been shown to improve mitochondrial activity and gene expression in muscle (Linnane 2002). It can also improve mitochondrial oxidative stress in Parkinson's patients (Ebadi 2001). Lipoic acid is particularly effective in reversing age-related and oxidative damage to mitochondria (Hagen 1999). (Refer to chapter 7.)

The natural medications discussed below provide a valuable addition to the *Prolonging Health* antioxidant recommendations listed in the previous chapter:

***Prolonging Health* DNA Repair Prescription 1—Take Ginkgo Extract:** Ginkgo is one of the top natural medicines for retarding the effects of aging and for that reason I introduce it early in our discussion on how to prolong health. It is best known as a medication for the heart and head. It increases blood flow through the body, especially to the extremities; that is why it is used to enhance memory, treat dizziness and ear ringing, and for intermittent claudication, a condition that causes leg pain every time you walk. However, its use should not be limited to these conditions.

French researchers have shown that ginkgo acts on all levels of the body, from molecules and cells to the entire organism (Christen 2002). Researchers in Spain have shown that ginkgo extract protects mitochondrial DNA from oxidative damage (Sastre 2002a, b) while researchers in the United States demonstrated that it counteracts the effects of free radicals and increases longevity (Wu 2002).

Ginkgo is generally considered safe to take, but those taking blood-thinning drugs should be monitored by a doctor as this combination may cause increased bleeding or bruising. A few patients experience mild stomach upset and some report having headaches when they first start taking ginkgo. These symptoms usually go away in the first week after starting, but if they do not, an allergy to the plant material may be at work and I suggest discontinuing this medication. There are no known interactions with pharmaceutical drugs, and ginkgo is synergistic with nearly all vitamins, minerals, and other herbal medications.

The standardized extract of ginkgo is prepared from the leaf of the Chinese *Ginkgo biloba* tree. Most extracts contain 24 percent ginkgoheterosides and 6 percent terpene lactone, the active constituents, but I recommend products containing higher concentrations: 32 percent ginkgoheterosides and 9 percent terpene lactone. Take 160 mg of the extract twice daily away from food.

***Prolonging Health* DNA Repair Prescription 2—Take Uncaria Extract:** C-MED 100 is a specialized extract of *Uncaria tomentosa* from the South American vine called cat's claw, or uño de gato, found in the Upper Amazon region of Peru. It has been shown to effectively repair DNA damage caused by radiation in experimental animals (Sheng 2000) and in one human study to increase DNA repair (Sheng 2001).

Uncaria extract also has anti-inflammatory, antiviral, and immune-enhancing properties (Williams 2001), making it another top natural medication for treating many of the symptoms associated with aging, and one of my professional favorites. It is a safe medication, though very bitter to taste, and there are no known interactions or side effects.

Take 350 mg of C-MED 100, standardized to 8 percent carboxy alkyl esters, twice daily away from food. If C-MED 100 is unavailable, take 250 mg of a commercial *Uncaria* extract twice daily.

Prolonging Health DNA Repair Prescription 3—Take Nucleic Acids: Though not extensively researched, oral RNA and DNA and injectable nucleic acids, referred to as "live cell therapy," have been used clinically for more than a century as longevity medications. Derived from animal organs, these medications are empirically known to reverse the cellular affects of aging. Health clinics in Germany, Austria, Switzerland, and some other European countries offer injectable live cell therapies. I recommend the German product RN13 (NeyGeront N). It is supplied in 2 ml ampoules and is injected intramuscularly once weekly.

Though injectable live cell therapies are still only available in Europe or Mexico, several companies, such as Atrium Biotechnologies of Quebec, Canada, produce high-quality products for oral use that are available through your doctor in the United States. Take 1 vial of Atrium's NatCell Mesenchyme, derived from organically raised bovine embryonic tissue containing growth factors, on an empty stomach or as directed by your physician.

Dietary sources of nucleic acids include canned sardines and chlorella. A good vegetarian source for RNA and DNA is chlorella *(Chlorella pyrenoidosa)*, a fresh-water algae commercially grown and prepared into a fine green powder. Chlorella is rich in proteins, vitamins and minerals, and growth factors. Take 2–4 tablets daily with food.

Prolonging Health DNA Repair Prescription 4—Take Enough Folate: A member of the B-vitamin family, folate is a col-

lective term for a number of chemically related compounds with similar biological activity. Folic acid is a synthetic form of folate used as a nutritional supplement. Folate is involved in numerous important processes in the body including the synthesis of DNA, RNA, and proteins. It is necessary for DNA repair and the maintenance of the integrity of the genome. Folate deficiency causes megaloblastic anemia, which is similar to the pernicious anemia caused by vitamin B_{12} deficiency. Symptoms of folate deficiency include weakness, fatigue, irritability, headache, poor concentration, cramping, heart palpitations, and depression.

Folate deficiency also appears to allow extensive damage to DNA to occur (Ames 1998), contributing to neurological damage and cancer formation (Blount 1997). Supplementation with folic acid has been shown to guard against genetic defects, counter age-related disease mechanisms (Mattson 2002), prevent genomic instability, and repair damaged DNA.

Folate is found in dark-green leafy vegetables (spinach, kale, beet greens, Swiss chard), oranges, lentils and other dried beans, broccoli, cauliflower, and liver. Since the body only absorbs about 50 percent of folate from dietary sources, supplementation is necessary to prevent degenerative diseases and prolong health. Folate supplementation of 800 mcg daily can prevent neural tube birth defects. It can also lower elevated homocysteine levels.

The basic dosage of folic acid is 400 mcg daily. However, for the prevention of age-related diseases and to improve your health, I recommend 800 mcg daily of L-5-methyltetrahydrofolate, a biologically active form of folate. In addition, I recommend 5 mg of folic acid. These higher dosages of folic acid can deplete vitamin B_{12}; however, since you are also taking extra B_{12} as part of your *Prolonging Health* program, you should not experience any adverse affects. Folate works synergistically with vitamins B_6, B_{12}, and zinc. It is depleted by anticonvulsant drugs, aspirin, and oral contraceptives.

***Prolonging Health* DNA Repair Prescription 5—Take Acetyl-L-Carnitine:** Acetyl-L-carnitine is a compound derived from L-carnitine, itself an amino acid derivative. It has been shown to improve cellular function and reverse many of the age-related mitochondrial defects (Shigenaga 1994; Hagen 1998). Acetyl-L-carnitine's anti-aging effects are attributed to its ability to transport fatty acids across cell membranes and into the mitochondria. Combined with a healthy diet and in the presence of antioxidants, acetyl-L-carnitine is capable of restoring mitochondrial function.

There are no known side effects or interactions with pharmaceutical drugs. Acetyl-L-carnitine is synergistic with alpha-lipoic acid, and they are best taken together. Take 500 mg of acetyl-L-carnitine twice daily with food.

***Prolonging Health* DNA Repair Prescription 6—Take NADH:** As noted earlier, NADH is involved in ATP production within the mitochondria. It is a coenzyme, which is a small molecule that makes up the nonprotein part of an enzyme. NADH is synthesized in the body from the B vitamin, nicotinamide.

NADH increases cellular energy production and is a potent antioxidant playing a role in protecting DNA from oxidative damage. It also assists in DNA repair. The Austrian physician Georg D. Birkmayer, M.D., Ph.D., was the first to use NADH medically for the treatment of Parkinson's disease (Birkmayer 1993) and later for Alzhiemer's disease (Birkmayer 1996).

In my clinical experience, NADH increases energy, reduces depression, and improves the sense of well-being in elderly patients. Take 10 mg of NADH as ENADA once daily two hours away from food and don't eat anything for 30 minutes after swallowing the tablet. (ENADA is the trade name of a patented delivery system for NADH produced in Austria.) NADH can be made into a topical cream by a compounding pharmacist to renew aging skin. Apply a one-percent NADH cream twice daily to the areas of your skin that have had the most sun exposure.

***Prolonging Health* DNA Repair Prescription 7—Take Homeopathic Medicines:** Homeopathic medicines are relatively new as anti-aging therapies. However, they have potential in limiting the effects of oxidative damage to nuclear and mitochondrial DNA, and in stimulating DNA repair mechanisms.

Homeopathic telomerase has not found wide application, but I suspect it will become available fairly soon. For liver protection and detoxification of the entire system, I recommend Heel Chelidonium-Homaccord at a dosage of ten drops directly under the tongue away from food once daily. Other homeopathic formulas I use in my practice include Heel Coenzyme compositum; the dosage is one vial directly under the tongue away from food once weekly.

Extensive oxidative damage in our body not only affects tissues and organs, damaging cell membranes and structural proteins, but it damages DNA and mitochondrial DNA. The cumulative effects from this damage result in genomic instability and lead to aging. Another cause of genomic instability is telomere shortening. Together, both factors produce significant age-related changes including loss of muscle strength, fatigue, neurodegenerative changes, reduced cardiac and liver function, and lowered immunity. All of these accelerate aging and shorten life span. Numerous natural medications guard our genome from these age-related changes, protect against oxidative damage, prolong health, and promote longevity.

In addition to a healthy diet and antioxidants, I suggest that you take folic acid and acetyl-L-carnitine daily. In addition, I recommend that everyone over age 50 take at least one of the other discussed medications on a daily basis.

Summary of *Prolonging Health* DNA Repair Prescriptions

- *Prolonging Health* DNA Repair Prescription 1— Take Ginkgo Extract:
  - Take 160 mg of ginkgo extract (32 percent ginkgoheterosides and 9 percent terpene lactone) twice daily away from food.

- *Prolonging Health* DNA Repair Prescription 2— Take Uncaria Extract:
  - Take 350 mg of C-MED 100, standardized to 8 percent carboxy alkly esters, twice daily away from food.

- *Prolonging Health* DNA Repair Prescription 3— Take Nucleic Acids:
  - Take one ampule of RN13 (NeyGeront N) once weekly as directed by your physician.
  - Take one vial of Atrium's NatCell Mesenchyme once weekly on an empty stomach or as directed by your physician.

- Take 2–4 tablets of chlorella daily with food.

- *Prolonging Health* DNA Repair Prescription 4— Take Enough Folate:
  - Take 800 mcg of L-5-methyltetrahydrofolate *and* 5 mg of folic acid daily. (Also take 2,000 mcg of methylcobalamine daily.)

- *Prolonging Health* DNA Repair Prescription 5— Take Acetyl-L-Carnitine:
  - Take 500 mg of acetyl-L-carnitine twice daily with food.

- *Prolonging Health* DNA Repair Prescription 6— Take NADH:
  - Take 10 mg of NADH as ENADA once daily two hours away from food and don't eat anything for 30 minutes after swallowing the tablet.

- *Prolonging Health* DNA Repair Prescription 7— Take Homeopathic Medicines:
  - Take 10 drops of Heel Chelidonium-Homaccord directly under the tongue away from food once daily.
  - Take one vial of Heel Coenzyme compositum directly under the tongue away from food once weekly.

9 *Prolonging Health* Modifiable Aging Factor 3: Impaired Detoxification—How to Renew Your Tissues and Cells with Cleansing Practices

Your body has elaborate detoxification mechanisms that protect it from naturally occurring toxins created within the body, as well as from exposure to environmental toxic chemicals, whether inhaled or ingested. Unfortunately, modern living exposes us to extremely high levels of toxic chemicals every day, and the accumulated level of these toxic substances is more than the body can effectively process. The toxic burden that this produces not only creates tremendous stress on the liver and the other organs of detoxification and elimination, but the excess toxic substances can accumulate in vital tissues such as the brain, causing neurodegeneration and accelerated aging.

Protecting genomic stability with antioxidants and DNA repair medications is critically important, as is protection against cancer and degenerative diseases, in order to retard aging and achieve your maximum life span. In addition, to effectively prolong your health, you need to renew your body from the inside out and to exchange old cells for new ones. When individual cells are replaced, all tissues are improved; subsequently, organ function can be restored, and only then are we on the healthiest path towards life extension.

As cellular protection begins with antioxidants, cellular renewal begins with detoxification. This refers to cell and tissue cleansing practices, the therapeutic model for facilitating natural detoxification. The body's detoxifica-

> *As cellular protection begins with antioxidants, cellular renewal begins with detoxification. This refers to cell and tissue cleansing practices, the therapeutic model for facilitating natural detoxification. The body's detoxification functions can be improved through a healthy diet, exercise, supplementing with antioxidants such as vitamin C, and using specialized nutrients and herbal medicines.*

tion functions can be improved through a healthy diet, exercise, supplementing with antioxidants such as vitamin C, and using specialized nutrients and herbal medicines.

In this chapter, we discuss the impact of rising levels of environmental chemical toxic substances on our health and how they and naturally occurring biological toxins disrupt homeostasis, lead to disease, and influence aging. We will see how to cleanse and eliminate those toxins through therapeutic cell and tissue cleansing practices. Before we learn the practical aspects, let's discuss some important topics that will help you understand what detoxification is all about.

How Toxic Substances Undermine Your Health

Our modern technological lifestyle continuously pollutes the air, water, and food with extremely hazardous toxic substances. The 2000 Toxic Release Inventory National Report, by the US Environmental Protection Agency's Office of Toxic Substances estimated that seven billion pounds of toxic waste containing over 80,000 different toxic chemicals, including industrial chemicals, drugs, food additives and preservatives, pesticides, herbicides, and other xenenobiotics, have been released into the environment—a staggering amount.[20]

Selected List of Toxic Chemicals and Drugs

- Aromatic Organic Compounds: benzene (in gasoline), styrene (in styrofoam disposable cups), toluene (also in gasoline), and others

- Pesticides: DDT, 1,4-dichlorobenzene (in mothballs and household deodorizers), and others

- Chlorinated Organic Chemicals: PCBs, tetrachloroethylene (dry-cleaning fluid), and others

- Phenols: ethylphenol (in drinking water), butylbenylphtale (in plastics), and others

- Toxic Heavy Metals: mercury, lead, uranium, cadmium, arsenic

- Recreational Drugs: cocaine, amphetamines, heroin

The accumulation of these poisonous substances greatly weakens our neuroendocrine and immune systems, undermining our health and inhibiting natural medical treatments designed to rid us of the underlying causes of disease. Most modern pharmaceutical drugs designed to treat the symptoms of disease actually cause more toxicity in the body.

Fortunately, ever more people are becoming aware of the necessity of using detoxification and cleansing therapies as part of a total health plan, but we must also strive to clean up our environment if lasting health is to be achieved. Even if we were to discover effective anti-aging drugs, synthetic antioxidants, designer molecules that enhance our genomic expression, and high-tech methods to repair DNA damage in older people, none of these medical advances would address the underlying issue of the steadily worsening problem of cellular and genetic damage caused by increasing levels of toxic *environmental* chemicals.[21]

Our constant exposure to chemical wastes predisposes us to all types of disease, including increased susceptibility to viral infection, autoimmune diseases, and cancer. There is significant evidence that environmental toxics reduce our immune capacity by as much as 50 percent, which is enough to make it a major contributing factor in many of the age-related diseases. *Altering Eden*, by Deborah Cadbury, documents the link between the unprecedented rise in incidences of cancer, infertility, and numerous other health conditions with exposure to toxic environmental substances (Cadbury 1997).

Let's begin by defining toxic substances and then find out what harm they cause. The root "tox" comes from the Latin, *toxicum*, for poison. Toxic substances, or toxics, are those that are poisonous, destructive to health, and even deadly; they come from a variety of organic and inorganic sources. Organic toxins are poisonous substances with a protein structure, secreted by different organisms; they include snake or spider venom, and some plants, which cause toxicosis, the pathological state of being poisoned.

The ones that concern us most are *inorganic* toxic chemical substances, or toxics. Xenobiotics are biochemical substances foreign to the body; I use this term interchangeably in this book for toxic environmental chemicals. The prefix "xeno" is from the Greek and Latin *xenos,* meaning "stranger," and it indicates anything foreign. For example, xenoestrogens are biologically active chemical substances from environmental pollutants foreign to the body that disrupt normal hormonal balance (Krimsky 2000). They mimic estrogen, though they derive from a foreign source outside the body.

Xenobiotics have three targets in the body: (1) the immune system, leading to autoimmune diseases, Graves' disease, rheumatoid arthritis, chronic infections, allergies, and cancer; (2) the nervous system, leading to multiple sclerosis and Parkinson's disease; and (3) the endocrine system, causing infertility, menstrual disorders, birth defects, and menopausal symptoms. In the body, they also increase free radical pathology and damage our DNA, which leads to genomic instability as discussed in the last two chapters. All of these damages predispose us to cancer, and significantly influence the aging process.

Selected Chemicals Associated with Hormone Disruption

- Atrazine

- Chlordanes

- Diethylstilbestrol (DES)

- Dioxins

- Lead

- Lindane

- Malathion

- Mercury

- Parathion

- Polychlorinated biphenyls (PCBs)

- Styrene

Toxins are also produced and released within our body, and are called endotoxins. Intestinal bacteria and fungi, viruses, and other microorganisms produce a wide range of toxins that cause poor health and contribute to disease. Even normal metabolism produces a wide range of biological toxins and toxic substances such as lactic and pyruvic acids and urea; certain hormones in excess amounts are toxic, including thyroid hormone and cortisol. However, under normal circumstances in healthy individuals, these substances are effectively and speedily neutralized by the liver, then removed from the body as harmless waste products.

Fortunately, our body has numerous methods for maintaining a stable and toxic-free internal environment. Unfortunately, the overwhelming number and amount of toxic substances that we are exposed to today and that accumulate over time is more than our bodies can manage effectively. Therefore, we have to *assist* the natural detoxification pathways in order to prevent disease, prolong our health, and promote longevity, and we do that through proactive detoxification.

The body is designed by nature to regulate and repair itself, and this includes mechanisms for the removal of wastes and toxins. Referred to as detoxification pathways, these mechanisms are complex, largely carried out by the liver and in the mucous lining of the intestinal tract. These pathways require steroid hormones, fatty acids, amino acids, enzymes, vitamins, and minerals to complete their functions of detoxification.

Though 75 percent of detoxification takes place in the liver, a significant amount of detoxification activity also occurs in the lining of the digestive tract, the intestinal mucosa. Besides our skin, it is at the mucous lining of both the respiratory and gastrointestinal systems that our body is first exposed to xenobiotics and infectious microorganisms; this mucosa provides the body's first barrier against entry of toxics into the body. Since the function of the gastrointestinal tract is also often impaired during aging, which results in poor digestion, reduced absorption of nutrients, and an abnormal intestinal environment (dysbiosis), normal detoxification and neutralization processes may be disrupted as well. Such conditions contribute to the accumulation of toxins and predispose the body to disease, which accelerates the aging process.

Inhibition of the different liver detoxification enzymes may occur through genetic deficiencies, conflict or competition in activity with various toxic substances, and the residues of pharmaceutical drugs. The latter include the commonly prescribed selective serotonin reuptake inhibiting (SSRI) antidepressants such as fluoxetine (Prozac), H-2 blockers (cimetidine), various antibiotics (erythromycin), and HIV protease inhibitor anti-virals (ritonavir). In addition, drug-to-drug interactions can occur, compounding inhibition of detoxification enzymes.

Drug-induced defective detoxification pathway activity cannot only inactivate these important enzymes, but either enhance the drug's effect, causing an overdose, or lead to more rapid elimination of the drug, leading to

lack of efficacy. In our *Prolonging Health* program, the goal is to eliminate all unnecessary drugs, and ultimately to take no pharmaceutical drug at any age.

Therapeutic Detoxification During Aging

During aging, the normal function of the main organs of detoxification—principally the liver, but also the large intestine, lungs, and kidneys—becomes impaired due to oxidative damage, a lifetime of exposure to drugs and other xenobiotics, deficiency of the co-factors necessary for the proper function of the detoxification pathways, and age-related wear and tear due to continuous functioning and the effects of diet and stress. This impairment of the detoxification pathways causes xenobiotics, cellular debris, and metabolic toxins to collect and accumulate in the body's fluids and tissues; this in turn damages cells, causes genomic instability, and leads to reduced physiological function, disease, and accelerated aging.

Therapeutic detoxification therapy is the process of cleansing the body from the inside out using natural methods such as herbs and nutritional supplements. Detoxification helps your body to overcome viral and other microbial illnesses, prevents cancer, promotes health, increases energy, and promotes longevity. Many descriptive terms for detoxification exist, including tissue cleansing, internal cleansing, and simply detox—itself a term referenced to many different processes such as drug and alcohol detox, removal of industrial chemical by-products, and environmental cleanup.

I use the term therapeutic detoxification therapy to refer to cell and tissue cleansing for the removal of the xenobiotic disease-promoting toxic burden from the cells, tissues, and organs for the purpose of prolonging health, normalizing immunity, complementary

Detoxification Precautions

- If you suffer from an autoimmune disorder, cancer, or chronic fatigue syndrome, undertake detoxification *only* if supervised by a naturopathic or other physician skilled in such practices.

- Never practice detoxification when you have a fever.

- If you are chelating heavy metals from your body either by oral DMSA (Captomer, succinic acid) or intravenous DMPS (Dimaval, 2,3-dimercapto-1-propane sulfonate), avoid supplemental minerals for three days before the chelation procedure as these minerals will be removed from your system along with excess calcium and toxic metals. It is critical to add them back immediately after the chelation to replace those lost in the process.

- Never allow yourself to become constipated during the detoxification process. If you have a tendency to become constipated, take extra fiber. Mix one teaspoon of psyllium powder along with bentonite clay in 6 ounces of water; drink this once daily. There are many commercial premixed laxative products that you can buy in a health food store. If you experience constipation, first try increasing your dosage of vitamin C. High dosages of vitamin C, short of those exceeding bowel tolerance, have a laxative effect. If necessary, use an herbal laxative containing cape aloe (*Aloe socotrina*), cassara (*Rhamnus pushiani*), or senna (*Cassia senna*). Commercial products containing these herbs are readily available from health food stores.

- Dark yellow (not bright yellow from B vitamins), brown, cloudy, or frothy urine indicates that you are not drinking enough fluid and your urine has too high a concentration of toxins and toxic substances. If you experience this during your detoxification, increase your water intake; if your urine continues to be colored or has a strong odor, try drinking diuretic juices. If that is not enough to clear the urine, use the diuretic herbal teas while increasing water intake until your urine becomes clear or a very light yellow and without any odor.

- Coffee enemas have a long history of successful use in detoxification therapies. They activate the liver pathways, stimulate the gallbladder to release bile, and act as a laxative. However, I do not recommend using enemas unless you are experienced in the correct manner of administration or are under the supervision of a health care practitioner. Similarly, colonic irrigation can be helpful, but limit use of this to one colonic per detoxification program and only as necessary, as they can be enervating. Older, weaker, and frail patients should not use colonics at all.

- If you have a lot of mercury amalgam dental fillings, have worked in a dental office, or have tested positive for accumulation of environmental mercury, have a 24-hour urine test for mercury. If your mercury levels are high, you will have to undergo chelation therapy. The most effective form is DMPS given in a series of intravenous sessions and administered by a licensed physician. Oral DMSA is somewhat effective for mercury and is equally effective as DMPS or EDTA for other heavy metals such as lead and cadmium. Both of these therapies should be administered only by a qualified health care professional.

- People who are frail, very elderly, and weakened from disease may undergo cleansing therapies and even fasting, but only under the supervision of a qualified health care professional.

- Those with serious viral infections, such as HIV and HCV, should undergo aggressive detoxification only under the supervision of a qualified health care professional. Patients with yeast, fungal, bacterial, or parasitic infections need specialized medications to combat these infections, and that is beyond the scope of this book. (See my *Viral Immunity*, Hampton Roads Publishing, 2002.)

- The excessive die-off of microorganisms that occurs in detoxification can produce flu-like achiness and malaise or a temporary worsening of symptoms. First noticed with the early use of antibiotics, this temporary worsening of symptoms is called the Jarisch-Herxheimer reaction (named after the discoverer). With natural remedies, massive die-off with Jarisch-Herxheimer reactions does not usually occur but is possible. The best way to deal with die-off is to increase your vitamin C by taking 500 mg of buffered C every half-hour until the symptoms disappear. Colonic irrigation can also be extremely useful to limit these reactions.

- If the liver is excessively burdened or unprepared for detoxification, you may experience severe headaches and fatigue, perhaps even dizziness. Increase your fluid intake, reduce solid food, and increase vitamin C. Usually headaches clear in a matter of hours; however, if they persist or are very severe, discontinue the cleansing and start again next month.

treatment of chronic disease, and promoting longevity.

I do not recommend complete fasting for older people or those with a chronic disease or severe viral illness, and I never recommend active cleansing when inflammation and fever are present or for those who are extremely weak such as from chronic fatigue syndrome. These people may experience severe exacerbations of their conditions and should never undergo a fast or lengthy detoxification regimen. In my clinical opinion, fasting any longer than a few days should be done *only* with the approval of and under the supervision of a qualified professional and in a facility with 24-hour care.

For people over 65 years, fasting on water only or juices for too long may weaken their body, which is the opposite of what we are trying to accomplish to prolong health. Long fasting causes muscle loss and reduces organ reserve. However, everyone can benefit from periodic, short-term (one to three days) modified fasting. Remember, the steps to good health begin with a healthy diet and balanced lifestyle, supplementation of micronutrients, especially antioxidants, detoxification, and regeneration therapies to restore organ reserve and promote normal physiological and biological body function. Fasting is only one aspect of a comprehensive approach to aging well.

Detoxification is not a benign process. Naturopathic physicians often refer to detoxification and fasting as "nature's operating table," because of the great demands it puts on your body's reserves and metabolic processes. Chemical toxins and residues are released into the bloodstream, causing the liver to function at an increased level during the cleansing process. Some of these released chemicals are even more toxic than their original form, and sometimes this leads to a detoxification crisis.

Generally, these crises last only a few hours or no more than a day and cause nothing more than headaches, fatigue, and nausea; however, occasionally they can be so severe you will have to discontinue the detoxification process and start again later when your body is more prepared. Do not be discouraged. As long as you persistently move forward, even with a few false starts, you will eventually succeed.

Therefore, before you start any detoxification regimen, you must first eliminate harmful substances from your environment, improve your diet, and strengthen your body with health-giving nutrients and enzymes. By optimizing the key nutritional factors, your body will automatically begin its own intracellular detoxification. You will as a result restore glutathione reserves, improve organ function, restore organ reserve, improve the management of oxidative stress from free radicals, improve gut ecology, build mineral reserves, and improve your strength and endurance.

Prolonging Health Recommendation 16— Follow the Five Rules of Therapeutic Detoxification

There are many cleansing styles and different types of detoxification regimens, so the answer to the question of what approach is best is that it is very individualized. However, to prolong health and for anti-senescent purposes my recommendation is to practice a modified fast one day each week and a three-day modified fast repeated once each month, or at least once every three months. Take a month off if you feel very tired, have an active infection, are overly stressed, or cannot devote three days to healing and rejuvenating yourself.

In general, for longer cleansing diets and detoxification programs, you can begin at any time and go from seven to 21 days. For more intensive detoxification, you need at least seven to nine days, preferably without having to work too hard and with no social functions to attend. For those with serious illness, I recommend that you do the longer and more serious detoxification programs *only* under the direct supervision of a qualified health care practitioner or in a facility that specializes in detoxification therapies with 24-hour care. Several such facilities are listed in the back of this book. Regardless of for how long or when you plan to start your detoxification program, it is important to plan ahead and make it a priority and schedule it into your busy life.

Though many of the body's internal organs, tissues, and cells contribute to detoxification and the removal of wastes, certain organs and physiological processes are more responsible than others for carrying out the detoxification process. Ultimately, it is the cells within the tissues of these organs that perform the bulk of the detoxification processes. To prolong health, live with vitality and energy, and extend your life span, you must address five main rules of modified fasting that promote the natural detoxification process:

1. Reduce the toxic burden on your body.

2. Facilitate the natural detoxifying capacity of the blood and lymph.

3. Improve the liver's detoxification pathways.

4. Cleanse the intestinal tract.

5. Improve the function of the secondary organs of detoxification.

Prolonging Health **Therapeutic Detoxification Rule 1—Reduce the Toxic Burden on Your Body:** For detoxification therapy to be effective, it is first necessary to reduce the toxic burden on your body's organs, tissues, and cells. In general to reduce the toxic load, one must first remove the offending toxins, reduce stress, and take only absolutely essential pharmaceutical drugs. In this way, the incoming burden on the body is reduced and detoxification can more effectively take place. Reduce your exposure to toxic chemicals by eating foods grown without pesticides; eat hormone-free and antibiotic-free meat and poultry; avoid eating swordfish or other fish high on the food chain and that accumulate toxic metals such as mercury; drink pure or filtered water; and avoid indoor air pollution.

Richard Leviton, the author of *The Healthy Living Space*, advocates creating a toxic-free personal environment in your home and immediate surroundings as well to complement the internal cleansing (Leviton 2001). Other ways to improve your immediate environment and reduce your toxic burden include keeping houseplants, planting a garden, and having trees planted near your home to help reduce air pollution.

Gradually, and over time if necessary, change all dietary and lifestyle habits that are not health-promoting. These include reducing (or stopping altogether) smoking, intake of alcohol, coffee, and caffeinated soft drinks and other similar beverages, and any use of recreational drugs including marijuana (cannabinoids, the active component, are liver toxic). It is not wise to start a detoxification program until the negative influences on your health are permanently removed from your lifestyle.

Prescription drugs pose a special problem. Some drugs are critical for controlling symptoms while at the same time they exert a high toxic load on the liver. If you are taking prescription medications, review each with a pharmacist and discuss their necessity with a medical doctor or osteopathic physician who supports your detoxification regimen. You can still perform modified fasting if you are taking prescription drugs; however, I recommend supervision by a physician for your safety.

Limit or completely avoid the use of refined sugar in any form, such as commercial fruit juices, candy, pastries, and sweetened cereals. The same goes for all other refined or processed food; fried and preserved foods, including chips and commercial pickles; and processed fats and oils, such as margarines and including soy spreads. Avoid all dairy and milk products such as yogurt and cheese since dairy products increase intestinal fermentation, increase yeast activity, are highly allergenic foods, and may contain hormones and antibiotics.

***Prolonging Health* Therapeutic Detoxification Rule 2—Facilitate the Natural Detoxifying Capacity of the Blood and Lymph:** Doctors of Chinese medicine and naturopathic physicians know that rejuvenation means complete replacement of diseased cells with healthy ones. To achieve this, they emphasize that cleansing the blood and lymph comes before cleansing the organs of detoxification because without healthy and clean blood the cells can never be renewed.

Signs of Toxic Blood

You may have toxic blood if you:

- Easily have adverse reactions to most drugs, including opposite effects or having effects with small dosages.

- Have adverse reactions to caffeine, including difficulty falling asleep even from coffee drunk in the morning.

- Have pimples, red welts or boils, and easily infected hair follicles.

Making healthy dietary choices, avoiding exposure to environmental toxins, exercising,

and using blood-cleansing herbs are essential steps in detoxifying the blood. Herbs include red clover *(Trifolium pratense)*, yellow dock *(Rumex crispus)*, and echinacea *(Echinacea purpurea, E. angustifolia)*. Mixtures of these herbs along with other blood cleansers have a long history of successful use in natural medicine, including the famous Hoxsey and Essiac formulas. Though these formulas may not be cure-alls for cancer, as their proponents suggest, they are both excellent detoxification formulas and I often recommend them to my patients as part of a detoxification program.

Another body system vital for detoxification is the lymphatic system. This is a network of tiny tubules running through all tissues in the body and through which the lymph, a clear fluid filtered from the blood, circulates. The lymph nodes are filtering stations positioned along these channels and are mostly found on the front and back of the neck (such as the tonsils), in the armpit, along the groin, and in the abdomen. White blood cells are very active inside the lymph nodes, clearing out viruses, bacteria, other infectious microorganisms, and allergens.

Like blood, the lymph must circulate continuously. However, unlike blood that is pumped through the body by the heart, lymph has no pump to keep it moving and has to be moved by physical activity. Exercise helps to move the lymph, especially aerobic types of exercise such as using a mini-trampoline, jumping rope, or calisthenics. Aerobic types of hatha yoga are perhaps the best exercises to move the lymph. Inversion of the body, as done in many yoga postures, is very beneficial for improving lymph circulation as well as providing great benefit for general health. Swedish and lympathic massage are excellent therapies to improve lymph circulation.

***Prolonging Health* Therapeutic Detoxification Rule 3—Improve the Liver's**

Detoxification Pathways: The liver, the primary organ of detoxification, is the most metabolically active organ in the body. It performs an estimated 500 known functions including assisting in carbohydrate, fat, and protein metabolism; maintaining blood sugar levels; producing bile to break down dietary fats; storing vitamins D, A, and B_{12}; regulating the body's use of iron; and filtering viruses and bacteria from the bloodstream. To perform all these functions, liver cells (hepatocytes) are large, and 50 percent of them contain up to eight times the DNA of other cells in the body. This makes hepatocytes more metabolically active and provides them with the energy to carry out detoxification and tissue renewal.

Signs of a Sluggish Liver

- Digestive problems: heart burn, abdominal pain, bloating and discomfort after eating, difficulty digesting fats, intolerance to alcohol, nausea, floating stools, constipation, bitter taste in the mouth, and a thick yellow tongue coating

- Skin problems: acne, rosacea, poor skin tone, swelling and edema, brown spots on the skin ("liver spots"), increased numbers of visible small red blood vessels (spider nevi), and lipomas or lumps of fat under the skin

- Menstrual and hormonal problems: premenstrual tension, painful periods, diarrhea during the period, and reactions to hormone replacement

- Neurological and psychological problems: headaches, irritability, insomnia, depression, poor concentration, overheating of the face and upper torso

- Immune problems: allergies, food and chemical sensitivities, chronic fatigue, fibromyalgia and joint inflammation, systemic infections, and viral hepatitis

- Appearance: sallow or yellowish complexion, yellowing or dullness of the whites of the eyes, dark circles under the eyes, protruding lower abdomen (potbelly), cellulite, accumulation of fat around the upper abdomen under the ribs (liver roll), and overweight

A number of natural substances improve liver function, promote detoxification, and protect the liver cells from damage by toxins and alcohol. These include: liver-protective herbs, such as milk thistle *(Silybum marianum)*, celandine *(Chelidonium majus)*, and dandelion *(Taraxacum officinale)*, and lipotropic nutrients (substances that break down fat in the liver) such as the amino acid methionine, as well as choline, betaine, folic acid, and vitamin B_{12}. These are all essential for restoring liver function. Many foods improve liver function, including beets, radishes, radish seed spouts, dandelion greens, and all green leafy vegetables.

***Prolonging Health* Therapeutic Detoxification Rule 4—Cleanse the Intestinal Tract:** After the mouth, the mucosal lining of the gastrointestinal tract is the next site at which foods, toxins ingested with food, medications, as well as a wide array of infectious microorganisms contact the inside of our body. Since the gut lining provides a physical barrier against toxic substances and organisms entering the body, and since the mucosal membrane inhibits and removes toxins and microorganisms, the second most important organ of detoxification is the large intestine.

Contrary to popular notions, the large intestine or colon is more than a mechanical tube for the removal of feces through defecation. Within it exists a living environment densely packed with anaerobic (non-oxygen-requiring) bacteria, called intestinal microflora; some are "friendly" and some pathogenic. These are all crowded together with parasites, yeasts, molds, tissue cells of various kinds, bile salts, excreted hormones, toxins, drug residues, water, and digested food materials. The intestinal lining itself is biologically active. Composed of the mucous membrane and containing a wide range of immune substances such as secretory IgA, it provides immune protection that neutralizes foreign substances before they enter the liver.

Thus the gut environment and the mucosal

Thus the gut environment and the mucosal lining are integral to effective body cleansing and are as important to health as is a good diet. In general, you can improve the environment of your intestines by eating fresh fruits and vegetables, not consuming much red meat, supplementing with fiber, avoiding antibiotics, and supplementing with acidophilus species.

lining are integral to effective body cleansing and are as important to health as is a good diet. In general, you can improve the environment of your intestines by eating fresh fruits and vegetables, not consuming much red meat, supplementing with fiber, avoiding antibiotics, and supplementing with acidophilus species.

Signs of an Unhealthy Colon

- Constipation, diarrhea, or alternating diarrhea and constipation

- Lower abdominal bloating, gas, or discomfort

- Lower belly distention

- Fatigue

***Prolonging Health* Therapeutic Detoxification Rule 5—Improve the Function of the Secondary Organs of Detoxification:** Though not primary detoxification organs like the liver and large intestine, secondary organs of detoxification are important in successfully detoxifying your body. Included in this group are the kidneys, lungs, skin, and connective tissue.

KIDNEYS: The kidneys are important in helping to maintain normal fluid levels and facilitate the exchange of fresh fluids in body tissues by filtering the blood. They excrete urine in which toxins, hormones, and used-up immune substances are eliminated from the body. Drinking copious amounts of pure water, fresh juices, and herbal teas is an important feature of a cleansing program. Healthy urine is very pale yellow and without any smell. If you do not drink enough water, your urine will be too concentrated and have a strong odor and be dark yellow or even brown. During detoxification, drink enough water to keep your urine clear. However, it is important not to overconsume fluids on a regular basis since they can cause excessive excretion of minerals.

LUNGS: The lungs are responsible for respiration. They are the site in your body where air from the outside interacts with your internal environment. Through a process involving specialized tissue, this exchange of gases occurs in the lungs and eventually oxygen circulates in the blood. Due to the contact with outside air, the lungs are influenced directly by environmental toxins and allergens. Since air must first pass through the nose and then to the lungs via the sinuses, it is not surprising that there is an epidemic today of allergic rhinitis (inflammation of the nasal passages), chronic sinusitis, and asthma due to ever-increasing amounts of toxins and irritants in the air.

Gargling with salt water and using saline rinses or sprays in the nose are necessary acts to cleanse and heal the mucous membranes of the upper respiratory passages. Deep breathing exercises as taught by Chinese *qi gong* and yoga practitioners are very helpful in cleansing the lungs. These are sophisticated methods of moving air through the lungs to heal the body. Of course, most important, one has to stop smoking and avoid indoor air contamination and outdoor pollution as much as possible.

The habit of jogging during lunch hour should be strictly avoided, as the pollution levels are highest around midday, especially in urban areas. This is due to increased automobile exhaust and heat from solar radiation causing an increased release of toxins from plastics and synthetic building materials. When you exercise outdoors, it is best to perform your routine early in the morning when the air is freshest and its oxygen content higher.

SKIN: Toxins are eliminated in the sweat and in secreted oils from the sebaceous glands distributed all over the body's outer protective sheath, the skin (the intestinal lining is the inner one). As part of your cleansing regimen, I recommend showering at least twice daily and taking at least one hot bath in Epsom salt or a detoxifying bath with hydrogen peroxide and sea salt. Dry skin brushing is also helpful, as are saunas, steam baths, or soaking in hot mineral water.

Four Skin Detoxification Tips

How to Have a Detoxifying Bath

1. Epsom salt: add 1–2 cups per tubful of warm water; soak in this for 20 minutes or longer.

2. Hydrogen peroxide and sea salt: add one quart of 3 percent USP hydrogen peroxide and one-half teaspoon of sea salt to a tubful of warm water; soak for 20 minutes or longer.

How to Use Skin Brushing

3. Before your shower or bath: use a dry lufa sponge, a coarse all-natural cotton washcloth, or a dry vegetable bristle brush to gently but briskly rub your entire body. Bathe immediately afterward. Perform dry skin brushing once a day.

How to Make a Floral and Herb Bath

4. Combine: dried rose petals (10 percent), lavender flowers (25 percent), calendula flowers (35 percent), rosemary (15 percent), and thyme (15 percent) and put them into a cotton or cheesecloth bag. Steep the bag in a tubful of hot water for 15 minutes; soak for 20 minutes or longer.

CONNECTIVE TISSUE: According to Dr. Hans-Heinrich Recheweg, a German medical doctor and founder of homotoxicology (a system of medicine using homeopathic remedy combinations to remove toxins and stimulate natural immunity), the connective tissue is one of the branches of what he called "the great defense system." Connective tissue is a group of different tissues and cells that includes collagen, elastin, proteins, and fatty cells. These act as a framework for the body, support organs and fill spaces between them, and form tendons and ligaments. Most connective tissue is composed of intercellular fluid and fibers.

Toxins in the lymph and blood can spill over into the connective tissue, causing it to become charged with toxins and blocked with mucus and fat. Connective tissue is easily damaged by toxins, infection, and bacterial die-off from excessive antibiotic use, and all of these increase inflammation. This contributes to chronic pain and abnormal immune response. Connective tissue is prone to autoimmune diseases such as rheumatoid arthritis, systemic lupus erythematosus, scleroderma, and myositis.

Cleansing the connective tissue is imperative for effective detoxification. Exercise, especially smooth, rhythmic types such as tai chi, dancing, swimming, and hatha yoga, is helpful as it improves blood and lymphatic circulation and clears the connective tissue of toxics. Connective tissue massage, acupuncture, and trigger point therapy are beneficial. Trigger point therapy involves injecting tender points on the body with solutions composed of procaine, vitamin B_{12}, homeopathic medicines, or other substances.

To support the connective tissue repair process, specialized biological medications composed of cellular enzymes and herbal drainage remedies can be used. Drainage remedies are natural herbal medicines or homeopathic preparations that assist the removal of toxins and promote the function of the organs of detoxification, primarily the liver, blood, and lymph, as well as the connective tissue.

Prolonging Health Recommendation 17— Follow the Five Prescriptions for Effective Detoxification

The most important nutrients and supplements for detoxification are outlined here in five prescriptions. Each is mandatory and important for successfully carrying out your detoxification regimen, and together complete my recommendations for modified fasting. Review each prescription carefully to ensure that you understand how to follow them before you start the modified fasting plan.

Prolonging Health Detoxification Prescription 1—Consume Antioxidant-Rich Foods, Fresh Juices, and Herbal Teas: To support natural detoxification, enhance your diet by eating only fresh, seasonal, and organic (if possible) vegetables and fruits. Rice is allowed, but all wheat and other cereal products are out. Animal meats, fish, and poultry are not allowed. Drink one to two glasses of fresh vegetable juice or one to two ounces of a chlorophyll-rich green drink every day. Green drinks include fresh-pressed wheat grass juice, barley grass, spirulina, chlorella, or blue-green algae. Eat foods that support the liver's detoxification functions such as beets, radishes, radish sprouts, daikon, dandelion greens, and endive.

Since many toxic metabolites (by-products of the neutralization of toxic substances) are excreted in the urine, promote your kidney function with natural diuretics (substances that promote urination and water-removal from the tissues) as found in carrots, parsley, watermelon, peaches, and peach leaf tea. Carrot juice (especially with added parsley) or watermelon juice works well as a mild diuretic. During the summer peach season, fresh whole ripe peaches are effective in promoting urination. Pure water is also a diuretic. Drink eight to ten glasses, or more, daily during the detoxification process.

Kidney supportive herbs include uva-ursi *(Arctostaphylos uva-ursi)*, stinging nettle *(Urtica dioica)*, and cleavers *(Galium aparine)*. Green tea is also a diuretic if taken in large amounts; however, during detoxification do not drink strong concentrations of green tea as it may be too stimulating due to the presence of caffeine in its composition.

List of Allowed Foods on a Detoxification Regimen

- Carbohydrates: rice (organic white, jasmine, Thai, basmati, or brown rice)

- Legumes: soy products (tofu, miso, tempeh), mung bean sprouts, aduki beans

- Vegetables: all leafy green vegetables (red, romaine, and other garden lettuces; spinach, endive, kale, Swiss chard, beets tops, bok choy and Chinese broccoli, arugula, mustard green, and dandelion greens); all root vegetables (carrots, beets, parsnips, radishes, fennel root, yams, potatoes—also a carbohydrate—turnips, daikon, gobo, yucca, and rutabagas); cruciferous vegetable (cabbage, cauliflower, broccoli, Brussels sprouts, collards); cucumbers, squashes; onion family (shallots, red and white onions, green onions, leeks, and garlic); asparagus, okra, celery, sweet and hot peppers, and tomatoes.

- Fruits: all fruits, except grapefruit (it contains substances that inhibit liver detoxification); keep acidic citrus intake to a minimum. Do not overdo the fruits. They are high in natural fruit sugar and low in vitamins and minerals compared to vegetables, so do not assist detoxification as much as do vegetables.

- Seeds and nuts: small amounts of raw organic seeds and nuts are acceptable if you get hungry between meals; grind and mix them with juice or make a nut butter for ease of digestion.

- Oils: cold-pressed olive oil is allowed and can be added to cooked vegetables or on salads; evening primrose and organic flax oils are recommended to support omega-3 and omega-6 fatty acid balance.

- Seaweeds: all sea vegetables are allowed and recommended.

- Spices and condiments: vegetable salts, naturally fermented soy sauce or tamari (wheat-free soy sauce), Bragg's liquid aminos; all culinary spices (sage, thyme, basil, cilantro, cardamom, cumin, oregano, marjoram, rosemary, and others), and small amounts of vinegar of all types.

- Teas and herbs: all herbal teas (mint, chamomile, raspberry, and others), chrysanthemum tea, green tea, and jasmine tea are allowed.

- Water: distilled, filtered, or spring water

Prolonging Health Detoxification Prescription 2—Take Antioxidants and Detoxification Nutrients: Increasing your intake of supplemental antioxidants is essential during detoxification. Vitamin C is the main factor here. Take 500–1,000 mg of pure ascorbic acid or buffered vitamin C powder containing ascorbic acid four to five times throughout the day, away from food and up to your bowel tolerance. Take 500 mg of ascorbyl palmitate with each meal.

Take the recommended dosages given in *Prolonging Health* Recommendation 10 for the antioxidant minerals zinc and selenium, and other antioxidant nutrients. In addition, take 500 mg of calcium d-glucarate and methylsulfonylmethane (MSM) two times a day. Calcium d-glucarate is a potent detoxifier of environmental toxins and is useful in the prevention of breast cancer (Walaszek 1986). MSM is an organic sulfur-containing compound and is involved in methionine and cysteine, proteins that assist the detoxification process in your body.

Prolonging Health Detoxification Prescription 3—Take Whey Protein and Amino Acids: According to David W. Quig, Ph.D., a scientist specializing in detoxification processes, cold-processed hydrolyzed whey protein is one of the most important supplements for cleansing (Quig 2000). Whey protein increases glutathione and adds important amino acids that support liver detoxification pathways; it is also high in cysteine and branched-chain amino acids that prevent heavy metals that move into the bloodstream during detoxification from entering the brain. Additionally, antioxidant amino acids and specialty antioxidants that facilitate the liver's detoxification pathways are necessary. These are L-glycine, L-glutamine, taurine, N-acetylcysteine (NAC), and methionine. Mix 10 g (0.15 oz) of whey powder (supplying about 16 g of protein) in rice milk or water; drink two times daily.

You can also use a commercial detoxification product dispensed through a physician's office, such as UltraClear Plus,[22] or MediClear.[23] These products are composed nutrients in a hypoallergenic rice protein base. I regularly recommend both of these for my patients. Use one measured scoop (supplied with the product); add your whey protein powder and drink twice daily.

***Prolonging Health* Detoxification Prescription 4—Take Probiotic Supplements:** Take probiotics during the detoxification process. I generally recommend a combination of *Lactobacillus acidophilus* and *Bifiobacterium infantis,* and both are readily available from health food stores. Probiotics (substances that support "friendly" intestinal bacteria) are measured in viable units of live organisms. Mix an equivalent of five billion viable units into your whey protein drink.

***Prolonging Health* Detoxification Prescription 5—Use Drainage Remedies:** Drainage remedies are important additions to your program as they assist and protect the liver, improve kidney function, activate cellular response, and clean the lymphatic vessels. The original use of the term "drainage" comes from the field of homotoxiocology and refers to medications that drain off toxic waste products.

Herbal medications can also serve as drainage remedies. Herbs commonly used as drainage remedies include red clover blossoms *(Trifolium pratense),* chaparral *(Larrea tridentata),* poke root *(Phytolacca americana),* Oregon grape root *(Berberis vulgaris),* dandelion *(Taraxacum officinale),* burdock root *(Arctium lappa),* and celandine *(Chelidonium majus).* Herbalists call these herbs blood cleansers. Several commercial preparations containing mixtures of these and other herbs with similar effects can be found in health food stores or on the Internet. These include Dr. Christopher's Red Clover Combination, Essiac, and Hoxsey formula. Make an herbal tea from one of them by simmering one tablespoon of the herbal mixture per cup of water for about 20 minutes. Drink one cup three times daily.

Though the herbal teas are effective, my clinical preference is to use homeopathic drainage remedies. My clinical choice is those from the German manufacturer Heel, such as Lymphomyosot, Ubichinon, and Chelidonium-Hommacord.[24] These medications must be obtained from your doctor. In the *Prolonging Health* program, I recommend Chelidonium-Hommacord, a medication prepared from the herb *Chelidonium majus.* Take ten drops directly under the tongue three times daily. Homeopathic medicines absorb best when taken away from food by at least 20 minutes.

Detoxification Nutrient Schedule

- Buffered Vitamin C: 500–1,000 mg of calcium-magnesium ascorbate powder with ascorbic acid, 4–5 times throughout the day, away from food and up to bowel tolerance.

- Ascorbyl palmitate: 500 mg with each meal.

- Vitamin E: 500 IU two times daily, with meals.

- Vitamin B_6: 50 mg of pyridoxine hydrochloride two times daily, between meals.

- Vitamin B_{12}: 1,000 mcg of methylcobalamin two times daily, between meals.

- Folic acid: 5 mg two times daily, between meals.

- Selenium: 200 mcg two times daily, between meals.

- Zinc: 30 mg daily, between meals.

- Lipoic acid: 300 mg two times daily, with meals.

- NAC: 500 mg three times daily, between meals.

- Coenzyme Q10: 250 mg two times daily, with meals.

- Acetyl-L-carnitine: 500 mg two times daily, between meals.

- L-glycine: 1,500–3,000 mg daily, between meals.

- Methionine: 1,000 mg two times daily, between meals.

- Taurine: 500 mg two times daily, between meals.

- L-glutamine: 500–1,000 mg three times daily, between meals.

- Choline: 500 mg two times daily, with meals.

- Calcium d-glucarate: 500 mg two times daily, between meals.

- Magnesium: 250–500 mg two times daily, between meals.

- Niacinaminde (non-flushing form of vitamin B_3, niacin): 500 mg two times daily, between meals.

- MSM: 500 mg two times daily, between meals.

- Whey protein: 10 g (0.15 oz) in rice milk or water two times daily.

- Probiotics: 5 billion viable units *Lactobacillus acidophilus* and *Bifiobacterium infantis* mixed with whey protein.

- Drainage remedies: 10 drops of Chelidonium-Hommacord directly under the tongue three times daily, 20 minutes away from food; drink one cup of a blood-cleansing herbal tea of your choice two times daily.

Your body is inundated by a staggering array of naturally occurring and industrial chemical toxic substances. These have severe consequences on your health, and not only promote cancer but can also shorten your life span. By supporting our natural detoxification processes, these substances can be eliminated from our cells and removed from our bodies. In order to facilitate this process, conduct a detoxification regimen of modified fasting for one day each week or three days every month.

During your detoxification process, get as much rest, stress reduction, peace and quiet as you can. Allow your body to experience the natural cleansing process and give it the opportunity to heal itself. Remember, during the three days of the program, it is your time to rest and recover.

Summary of *Prolonging Health* Detoxification Recommendations

- *Prolonging Health* Recommendation 16—Follow the Five Rules of Therapeutic Detoxification
  - *Prolonging Health* Therapeutic Detoxification Rule 1—Reduce the Toxic Burden on Your Body: remove offending toxics, reduce stress, and take only absolutely essential pharmaceutical drugs.
  - *Prolonging Health* Therapeutic Detoxification Rule 2—Facilitate the Natural Detoxifying Capacity of the Blood and Lymph: cleanse the blood and lymph with herbal medicines, exercise, and therapies like acupuncture.
  - *Prolonging Health* Therapeutic Detoxification Rule 3—Improve the Liver's Detoxification Pathways: take liver-protective herbs and lipotropic nutrients.
  - *Prolonging Health* Therapeutic Detoxification Rule 4—Cleanse the Intestinal Tract: restore your intestinal tract by eating fresh fruits and vegetables, not consuming much red meat, supplementing with fiber, avoiding antibiotics, and supplementing with acidophilus species.
  - *Prolonging Health* Therapeutic Detoxification Rule 5—Improve the Function of the Secondary Organs of Detoxification: improve kidney, lung, skin, and connective tissue function with pure water, natural medicines, detoxifying baths, and exercise.

Simple Breathing Exercise

Thousands of years ago in India, sophisticated breathing exercises called pranayama were developed to increase energy in the body. Practitioners report that pranayama prevent disease and promote longevity. By practicing the essential techniques, we too can improve our health, calm our nervous system, and live longer. Here's a basic guide to simple *Prolonging Health* pranayama:

1. The best time to practice is in the early morning, before breakfast. Stand in a garden or in front of an open window. Face east or south, if practical.

2. Relax your whole body and close your eyes about halfway. This helps to relax the mind.

3. Bring your hands together in front of your chest as in prayer.

4. While opening your arms to your sides, inhale as deeply as you can through your nose. Make loose fists as you bring your arms back.

5. Hold your breath for a count of three.

6. Exhale deeply through your mouth while bringing your arms to the center of your body and your palms together.

7. Do this three to six times. Then put your arms by your sides and rest for three regular breaths.

8. Repeat the deep breathing movements three to six times; then rest.

9. Repeat again.

10. Finally, when you've finished the three sets of deep breathing, lightly tap your skull with your fingertips. Then, tap over your liver (on your upper abdomen, just under your ribs on the right side of your body) and over your kidneys (on your lower back, just below your ribs near the spine).

- *Prolonging Health* Recommendation 17—Follow the Five Prescriptions for Effective Detoxification
  - *Prolonging Health* Detoxification Prescription 1—Consume Antioxidant-Rich Foods, Fresh Juices, and Herbal Teas: enhance your diet by eating only fresh, seasonal, and organic vegetables and fruits. Avoid animal meats, fish, and poultry. Drink 1–2 glasses of fresh vegetable juice or 1–2 ounces of a chlorophyll-rich green drink every day. Eat foods that support the liver's detoxification functions.
  - *Prolonging Health* Detoxification Prescription 2—Take Antioxidants and Detoxification Nutrients: take antioxidants, especially vitamin C. Use calcium d-glucarate and MSM.
  - *Prolonging Health* Detoxification Prescription 3—Take Whey Protein and Amino Acids: consume cold-processed hydrolyzed whey protein, and consider taking a commercial detoxification product.
  - *Prolonging Health* Detoxification Prescription 4—Take Probiotic Supplements: take a combination of probiotics containing *Lactobacillus acidophilus* and *Bifiobacterium infantis*.
  - *Prolonging Health* Detoxification Prescription 5—Use Drainage Remedies: take Chelidonium-Hommacord, or another drainage remedy.

1-Day Prolonging Health Modified Fast

Prepare your body, mind, and spirit the night before.

1. Conduct your normal daily routine, but slow down and mentally prepare for the task ahead.

2. Remove alcohol, unnecessary medications, sugar, sodas, and processed foods from your diet; eliminate milk products.

3. Prepare the cleansing products (see Detoxification Nutrient Schedule).

4. Eat normally in the morning and afternoon the day before starting, but do not eat after dinner in the evening.

5. Take a detoxifying bath and retire to bed early.

Modified Fasting Day:

1. *Morning:* Upon arising drink one cup of the blood-cleansing tea.

   a. Practice breathing exercises for 10 minutes.

   b. Meditate or pray for 10–20 minutes.

   c. Drink 6–8 ounces of water.

   d. Exercise for 10–20 minutes.

   e. Rest.

2. *Mid-morning:* Around 10 A.M., drink 6–8 ounces of pure water and add 0.15 ounces of whey protein. If you are able to obtain UltraClear Plus or MediClear, mix one scoop with the whey protein.

   a. An hour later: drink 6–8 ounces of mixed vegetable juice or a green drink.

3. *Lunch:* Eat a large mixed vegetable salad or steamed vegetables seasoned with olive oil, lemon or lime juice, and a small amount of vinegar for dressing.

4. *Mid-afternoon:* Drink a second glass of vegetable juice.

   a. Exercise for 10–20 minutes, or if you can, take a yoga class of 1–2 hours.

   b. Drink a second cup of whey protein, and if you have them, UltraClear Plus or MediClear.

   c. Rest.

5. *Dinner:* Eat a light dinner of the allowed food groups (see the list of allowed foods):

   a. Carbohydrate (choose one): rice, baked or boiled potato, baked yam, tofu

   b. Steamed vegetables or vegetable soup

   c. Mixed green salad

6. *After Dinner:* Drink another cup of blood-cleansing tea.

   a. Take a cleansing bath.

   b. Go to bed before 9 P.M.

3-Day *Prolonging Health* Modified Fast—For a Weekend

Thursday: Prepare body, mind, and spirit.

1. Conduct your normal daily routine, though slow down and mentally prepare for the task ahead.

2. Follow *Prolonging Health* Detoxification Rule 1: remove alcohol, unnecessary medications, sugar, sodas, and processed foods. Eliminate milk products.

3. Prepare the cleansing products (see Detoxification Nutrient Schedule).

4. Eat normally in the morning and afternoon; have a light dinner from the allowed foods list, but do not eat anything after dinner.

5. Take a detoxifying bath and retire to bed early.

Friday: DAY 1

1. *Morning:* Upon waking, take 10 drops of homeopathic Chelidonium-Hommacord; drink one cup of the blood-cleansing tea.

   a. Practice breathing exercises for 10 minutes.

   b. Meditate or pray for 10–20 minutes.

   c. Drink 6–8 ounces of water.

   d. Exercise for 10–20 minutes.

   e. Rest if you can, or go to work.

2. *Mid-morning:* Around 10 A.M., take the first group of supplements (see Detoxification Nutrient Schedule) with 6–8 ounces of pure water and 0.15 ounces of whey protein. If you are able to obtain UltraClear Plus or MediClear, mix one scoop with the whey protein.

   a. An hour later: drink 6–8 ounces of mixed vegetable juice or a green drink.

   b. Take a second dose of Chelidonium-Hommacord.

3. *Lunch:* Eat a mixed vegetable salad seasoned with olive oil, lemon or lime juice, and a small

amount of vinegar for dressing. Take the supplements that go with meals.

4. *Mid-afternoon:* Take a second dose of the group of supplements for between meals, with a second glass of vegetable juice,

   a. Exercise for 10–20 minutes, or if you can, take a yoga class of 1–2 hours.

   b. Drink a second cup of whey protein with UltraClear Plus or MediClear.

5. *Dinner:* Eat a full dinner, but only from the allowed food groups (see the list of allowed foods):

   a. Carbohydrate (choose one): rice, baked or boiled potato, baked yam, tofu

   b. Steamed vegetables or vegetable soup

   c. Mixed green salad

   d. Take the supplements that go with meals.

6. *After Dinner:* Drink another cup of drainage tea.

7. *Before Bed:* Take the third dose of Chelidonium-Hommacord

   a. Take a cleansing bath.

Saturday: DAY 2

1. Repeat Friday's schedule.

2. Have a massage or acupuncture treatment.

3. Take a yoga class or exercise lightly.

Sunday: DAY 3

1. Repeat Friday's schedule for the morning.

2. At noon have a lunch of vegetable soup and a mixed salad.

3. Repeat Friday's afternoon schedule.

4. Have a full meal in the evening and return to your normal routine on Monday.

10 *Prolonging Health* Modifiable Aging Factor 4: Insulin Resistance—How to Reset Your Insulin Switch with Diet and Natural Medicines

Among the most critical of changes that occur during aging is the reduced ability of our cells to utilize or metabolize glucose, the body's blood sugar and its primary fuel. That something so basic as a molecule of sugar could be associated with the cascade of events that contribute to aging seems too simple. However, from my studies and clinical experience, I know that nature tends to work in just such ways and that simplicity and elegance are in a delicate balance.

In the body, the same principle is true and balance is the rule. Glucose is balanced or regulated by insulin, which is the main hormone secreted by the pancreas. Insulin is responsible for maintaining appropriate blood sugar levels. Diet sources of carbohydrates are the driving force behind glucose metabolism. Fats and proteins also contribute to the body's energy sources, but carbohydrates are the primary source of energy in the body. When glucose metabolism and insulin function are balanced, our body is energetic and healthy. Unfortunately, today we are experiencing an epidemic of diseases associated with unbalanced or abnormal glucose metabolism.

Chronic overconsumption of refined sugar is the leading cause of abnormal glucose metabolism. This eventually leads to a condition called insulin resistance in which receptors located on the surface of the cells inhibit or *resist* the entrance of insulin. Gradually, these cells become desensitized or *resistant* to insulin, causing a condition of improper glucose utilization and control. Insulin resistance is medically defined as when your insulin levels are high when fasting or very high after eating a meal. This causes decreased tissue responsiveness to insulin and produces the tissue changes that result in abdominal obesity and hypertension. Insulin resistance accompanies Type II diabetes.

Four Characteristics of Insulin Resistance

1. If you are overweight by 15–20 pounds and have excess fat around your waist or under the rib cage, or both, you are a candidate for insulin resistance.

2. If you have high blood pressure, you might be a candidate for insulin resistance.

3. If your standard blood chemistry tests reveal that your total cholesterol and triglyceride levels are elevated, and your HDL levels are low, you possibly have insulin resistance as well as abnormal cardiovascular changes.

4. If your fasting insulin levels are above 10 µIU/mL, this is suspicious for insulin resistance.

Though not classified as a medical disease itself, insulin resistance leads to metabolic disorders such as Syndrome X, a condition characterized by weight gain, abdominal obesity, elevated cholesterol and triglycerides, high blood pressure, and dysglycemia or abnormal glucose control. These metabolic disturbances are often accompanied by mood changes such as anxiety or depression, as well as imbalances in other hormones such as estrogen, causing premenstrual syndrome or exacerbating menopausal symptoms.

Characteristics of Syndrome X

Glucose-Related Characteristics:

- Concurrent Type II diabetes

- Insulin resistance

- Glucose intolerance

Cardiovascular Characteristics:

- Hypertension (a blood pressure greater than 140/90)

- High triglyceride levels

- Low HDL

- Increased blood coagulability

Other Characteristics:

- Albumin in the urine

- High uric acid levels in the blood

- Increased blood levels of leptin

Body Pattern:

- Obesity

- Greater waist-to-hip ratio

- Abdominal obesity

Besides Syndrome X, there are a number of other conditions associated with improper glucose control, including hypoglycemia or low blood sugar, and hyperglycemia (high blood sugar) or diabetes.

Hypoglycemia is associated with depression, premenstrual syndrome, migraine headaches, fatigue, poor concentration, sugar cravings, and weight gain. Hypoglycemia is caused by imbalances in how insulin and other hormones regulate glucose so that you don't have of it enough in your blood. It is characterized by too high insulin, low cortisol, and low glucose levels. People with hypoglycemia feel poorly if they miss a meal; often wake up hungry in the middle of the night and can't fall back to sleep; and feel very tired after eating a heavy meal.

Currently 150 million people worldwide have diabetes, but that number is expected to double by the year 2025 (Zimmet 2001). Diagnostically, diabetes is divided into two types. Type I is an autoimmune disease that causes destruction of the pancreatic beta-cells that produce insulin, and is characterized by high glucose and low insulin. It usually requires lifelong administration of insulin. Interestingly, though conventional medical practice believes that all cases of Type I diabetes are incurable, some nutritionally oriented physicians have found that with the correct diet, nutritional supplementation, and exercise the underlying cause is correctable in some patients with late-onset Type I diabetes.

Keep in mind that though some people have been helped, Type I diabetes is a severe condition with potential life-threatening crises if not managed correctly; you should never discontinue your insulin except under the supervision of a qualified physician.

Type II diabetes, as far as insulin is concerned, is the opposite of Type I. In this type, glucose levels are elevated in the presence of higher than normal insulin. High insulin levels are a characteristic of insulin resistance. Type II diabetes makes up 90–95 percent of all diabetic cases (Moller 2001).

Diabetes causes changes in how the blood gets into the tissues and can result in heart and kidney disease, nerve damage, and blindness due to damage to the retina. People with insulin resistance and diabetes have increased risk for heart disease and stroke, and increased risk for colon cancer and breast cancer, while younger women with insulin resistance are more likely to have polycystic ovarian disease (characterized by multiple cysts on the ovaries), plus symptoms of Syndrome X along with signs of excess androgens such as increased facial hair and acne.

The cause of this burgeoning incidence of blood sugar–related diseases is overconsumption of refined sugars and other simple carbohydrates, including staples such as white bread and highly processed white rice, a sedentary lifestyle, overeating, and either a low-fat diet or the wrong kind of dietary fats. An estimated ten to 20 percent of Americans lead sedentary lifestyles and are obese; nine out of ten Type II diabetics are insulin resistant; and 25–35 percent of the population has some degree of insulin resistance (Grimm 1999).

Another condition related to abnormal glucose metabolism and insulin resistance is protein glycation. It is well known that diabetics have increased levels of glycation, a caramelizing effect produced when sugars and proteins combine inappropriately. It is highly likely that those with insulin resistance also have excessive formation of glycosylated proteins; these can cause alterations in immunity, increased inflammation, changes in brain function, and increased biological age. Because of its impor-

tance in the aging process, protein glycation is discussed in detail in the next chapter.

The message of this chapter is simple: to live a long and healthy life, keep your insulin and glucose levels under control. You can improve insulin utilization, manage glucose, and reduce glycation by changing your diet and

> *The message of this chapter is simple: to live a long and healthy life, keep your insulin and glucose levels under control. You can improve insulin utilization, manage glucose, and reduce glycation by changing your diet and managing the total number of calories you eat. Vitamin and mineral supplementation, exercise, and specialized medications also play key roles in controlling these conditions.*

managing the total number of calories you eat. Vitamin and mineral supplementation, exercise, and specialized medications also play key roles in controlling these conditions. But, before I explain how to use these substances to prolong your health and promote longevity, let's understand more about how glucose is metabolized in the body. Since the primary role of insulin is to regulate glucose metabolism, let's start by reviewing its functions and relationship to aging.

Normal Insulin Utilization Is Important for Maintaining Life

Insulin was first identified in 1922 by Sir Frederick Banting, M.D., and Charles Best, of the University of Toronto in Ontario, Canada. Medicinal insulin preparations derived from beef or pork pancreases have been in use since the late 1920s for the treatment of insulin-dependent or Type I diabetes, and in 1923, Dr. Banting won the Nobel Prize in Medicine for his discovery. Due to its importance in the treatment of Type I diabetes, more is known about insulin than any other hormone. Surprisingly, synthesized human insulin, produced from bacteria using recombinant DNA techniques, was only developed in the 1980s; the role of insulin regulation in health, disease prevention, and aging was not recognized until the late 1990s.

Insulin belongs to a family of proteins that include insulin-like growth factors I and II (IGF-I, IGF-II). These substances are produced in the liver and stimulate growth. Categorized as an endocrine hormone, insulin is produced by the beta islets cells in the pancreas; the pancreas is an oblong organ situated on the left side of your abdomen just under the lower ribs and near the duodenum, the junction between the stomach and small intestine. The pancreas also produces digestive enzymes to help prepare food for assimilation, as well as other hormones including glucagon, which is involved in maintaining normal glucose by raising blood sugar levels. To see how this works, let's follow the process by which food is turned into glucose or blood sugar.

When you eat, your digestive system breaks down the ingested food into smaller particles. Carbohydrates such as rice, bread, and potatoes are broken down into simple sugars by specialized enzymes; proteins are broken into amino acids, and fats into fatty acids. The end product of carbohydrate digestion is glucose, the principal energy-promoting substance used by the cells to carry out the functions necessary to maintain life. Glucose is liberated from food in the small intestine, where it is absorbed into the blood; it passes through the liver before entering general circulation in the bloodstream. Through a complex chemical communications system, when glucose concentrations in the blood rise, insulin is secreted by the pancreatic beta cells to lower blood sugar levels.

The main function of insulin is to *regulate* the immediate use of glucose and to store any excess as glycogen, a starchy substance manufactured in the liver and muscles and readily converted back to glucose in a process called glucogenesis. Since every cell in the body requires glucose to function, insulin's activity in glucose metabolism is crucial and depends on the different functions of target tissues. Mainly, insulin facilitates the entry of glucose into muscle cells and adipose tissue.

To accomplish this, cells have biological receptors on their surface that bind with insulin as it circulates in the blood. They activate other receptors and stimulate chemical messengers, such as glucose transporter proteins (Glut4) (Bryant 2002), to draw glucose into the cell, where it is metabolized in the mitochondria into ATP, the primary currency of energy used by cells in the body. The exceptions to this process are liver and brain cells, which have their own mechanisms for transporting glucose into the cells and are not dependent on insulin.

The liver is an important storage site for glucose, and a large portion of absorbed glucose is immediately taken up by the liver and under the control of insulin converted into glycogen. The production of glucose from liver glycogen is carefully regulated by finely tuned mechanisms involving proteins only discovered in 2001 (Yoon 2001). The brain's primary source of energy is glucose, which it can take directly into its cells without the gate-controlling activity of insulin receptors; though it can use ketones as a backup system, it does not function optimally without adequate supplies of glucose. Ketones are substances produced when the body breaks down fats for energy.

Insulin plays additional roles in lipid metabolism, including the synthesis of fatty acids in the liver and the synthesis of triglyceride in the adipose tissue. Paradoxically, it inhibits the breakdown of fat in adipose tissue—one of the reasons why it is so difficult to lose weight once a person has become significantly obese. Insulin facilitates the entry of glucose into muscle, where it is used for energy and stored as glycogen. Once the immediate requirement for glucose is accomplished and any excess stored in the liver and muscles as glycogen, insulin promotes the entry of glucose into adipose cells (called adipocytes), where it is converted to fat.

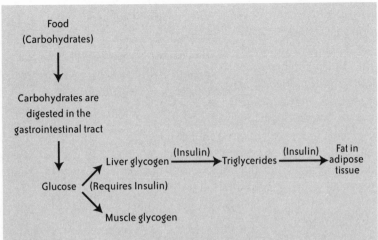

Glucose Metabolism

After food is eaten, it enters the gastrointestinal tract, where it is digested under the influence of various digestive secretions including bile and enzymes. The end product of carbohydrate digestion is glucose, a simple sugar, and some of it is immediately used for energy. The rest is processed into the storage molecule glycogen, with excess amounts converted into triglyceride and cholesterol.

Main Functions of Insulin

- Regulates glucose metabolism
- Stimulates conversion of glucose to glycogen
- Promotes conversion of glucose to fat
- Diminishes breakdown of fat in adipose cells
- Helps regulate blood levels of fatty acids
- Stimulates growth
- Facilitates uptake of amino acids

- Affects estrogen responses
- Increases cell permeability to the minerals potassium, magnesium, and phosphorus
- Modulates genetic transcription, DNA synthesis, and cell replication
- Plays an important role in maintaining homeostasis

Insulin has other effects in the body besides regulating blood sugar. These include facilitating amino acid uptake by muscle cells, regulating levels of fatty acids in the blood, increasing the permeability of cells to potassium, magnesium, and phosphorus, and playing a role in regulating hypothalamic response to estrogen, which is implicated in infertility (Karkanis 1997). Insulin is involved in numerous other biochemical processes, including cell replication, that have implications in cancer cell growth.

Insulin, the primary mediator of anabolic or upbuilding metabolism, is counter-regulated by several other hormones, principally glucagon, cortisol, adrenaline (epinephrine and norepinephrine), and growth hormone, all of which protect against too low a level of glucose.

Fasting Glucose Ranges	
Diabetes	above 126 mg/dL
Pre-diabetes	between 110–125 mg/dL
Normal	between 70–110 mg/dL
Hypoglycemia	below 70 mg/dL

Glucagon (not to be confused with glycogen) is the primary inducer of catabolism or tearing down processes. Insulin secretion is absent when the fasting glucose levels in the blood are between 80 and 85 milligrams per deciliter (mg/dL), and increases in direct proportion to rises in glucose levels, which is directly due to how much you eat.

Therefore, if your fasting glucose levels are consistently above 85–90 mg/dL, it is likely that your metabolism is unbalanced and that more insulin is being produced than necessary, which over time can lead to insulin resistance and glucose imbalance. That is why to prolong your health you must keep your fasting glucose levels within the optimal range of 78–85 mg/dL and your fasting insulin levels less than 10 μIU/mL. Fasting glucose is the amount of glucose in a sample of blood. This requires that you not eat or drink anything but water for eight hours prior to the test and for this reason, it is typically done in the morning before breakfast. Hence, the use of the term "fasting."

Insulin can trigger gene expression in cells that regulate appetite and obesity (Bevan 2001). Consuming carbohydrates rapidly raises glucose levels, and insulin release is triggered as a response to rising glucose. As high-protein foods combined with carbohydrates raise both glucagon and insulin, then overeating both of these foods eventually disrupts the insulin and glucagon balance, weight gain occurs, and homeostasis is disturbed (Hanley 2002).

Insulin plays a role in the female reproductive cycle, which is why, from the clinical point of view, nearly all problems associated with the female hormonal imbalances, such as premenstrual syndrome and menopausal symptoms, are improved with dietary modifications that improve blood sugar regulation. It also influences fertility, which may in part explain some cases of infertility in women who have dieted for years on high-carbohydrate, low-fat regimens.

Researchers found that in a process called molecular signaling insulin communicates chemical messages to cells to exert control over their functions in the body. Before the discovery of signaling molecules, scientists only knew that when glucose and

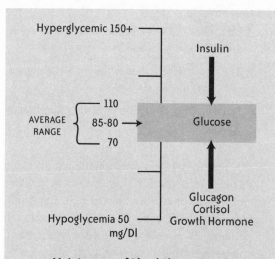

Maintenance of Blood Glucose Levels
The body controls glucose levels within a narrow range by the action of insulin, which lowers glucose, and glucagon, cortisol, and growth hormone, which raise glucose. Insulin secretion is absent when the fasting glucose levels in the blood are between 80 and 85 milligrams per deciliter. Diabetes or hyperglycemia appears when glucose levels rise, and hypoglycemia occurs as they fall.

insulin levels dropped, as in periods of fasting or starvation, levels of the hormone glucagon rose, but they didn't know how the information was communicated to the cells to release glucose-regulating hormones. Now it is known that complex interactions take place between receptors and signaling molecules, as well as hormones and other substances, to regulate glucose utilization.

Several families of proteins that facilitate insulin signaling have been recently discovered, including insulin receptor substrates (IRS 1-4) (Fasshauer 2000), and isp62–a subset of the protein kinase Akt2, discovered by Todd Huffman, a graduate student in the lab of John C. Lawrence Jr., Ph.D., a professor of pharmacology and medicine at the University of Virginia (Cho 2001). These discoveries inform us not only of the complexity and importance of glucose metabolism, but of the sophistication of our body's molecular chemistry; they also hold considerable potential for uncovering more of the secrets of aging.

We previously discussed the important role the liver plays in detoxification, but the liver's function doesn't end there. It also plays a significant part in regulating the body's glucose factory, and therefore directly influences glucose metabolism and ultimately affects homeostasis. According to an article in *Nature* (Vidal-Puig 2001), "The production of glucose by the liver is finely tuned by hormone signals." Let's see how this happens.

Glucagon is a protein composed of 29 amino acids and, like insulin, it is secreted by the pancreatic islets cells. The major activity of this hormone is to increase the level of glucose in the blood by stimulating the breakdown of glycogen (as mentioned, a form of glucose stored in the liver) into glucose. Not only do hypoglycemia or low blood sugar levels trigger the release of glucagon, but high levels of amino acids in the blood (such as are present after consuming a protein-rich meal) also activate the secretion of glucagon.

If carbohydrates or sugar is not consumed at the same time, glucose levels in the blood may be low and amino acid levels high, creating a situation in which both glucagon and insulin are secreted. Body builders strive to maximize this situation with diet in order to enhance their performance and gain muscle. By eating protein-rich foods such as eggs or meat, or a protein shake before weight training, we too can utilize this method to enhance our muscle mass.

Besides glucagon, several other hormones stimulate the liver to break down glycogen and synthesize glucose. These include the adrenal hormones cortisol and adrenaline, often thought of as stress hormones; growth hormone is also involved in glucose metabolism.

Glucose metabolism depends on a biochemical dialogue between muscle and fat. After a meal, simple nutrients (principally carbohydrates and sugars) are broken down into glucose and taken up by the liver, where they are further acted upon in the hepatocytes (liver cells) under the influence of insulin. They then either enter the general blood circulation for use by cells, are stored in the liver, or in the muscle as glycogen, or are converted to triglyericides and then stored as fat in adipose cells (adipocytes).

The "dialogue" between these different organs and tissues is facilitated by a number of messenger molecules such as hormones, signaling proteins, fatty acids, cytokines such as tumor necrosis factor-alpha (TNF-α), and the hormone-like peptides leptin and resistin (Birnbaum 2001). Leptin, a protein manufactured in fat cells, acts upon receptors in the hypothalamus to counteract the feeding instinct, and thereby provides homeostatic control over the amount of food we eat; it is also associated with reproductive function

(Castracane and Henson 2002) and possible longevity (Christou 2002). Though little is known about resistin, researchers believe abnormal levels are associated with Type II diabetes (Sentinelli 2002; Levy 2002).

Insulin Sets the Pace for Aging

In part 1, we reviewed the importance of maintaining metabolic balance, preferably with a slight emphasis on anabolic or upbuilding metabolism. As we age, our body begins a gradual breakdown process where catabolism predominates over anabolism—the more breakdown (catabolism), the faster you age.

Doctors have long known that people with diabetes, a disease characterized by increased levels of blood sugar caused by abnormal control or absence of insulin, suffer from accelerated aging. But the true causes of aging are still unknown, even though it is generally accepted by gerontologists that aging fulfills an evolutionary role in the maintenance of life and that the keys to aging lie at the molecular level. Therefore, all the causes of aging are results of as yet unknown aging processes and contributors to cellular senescence and rapid aging or age-related diseases.

However, some authors and researchers focus on one, or perhaps two, factors with the zeal of religious reformers, professing its primary importance as "the" cause of aging or the key factor in aging. The importance assigned to glucose metabolism and insulin function is a prime example of how this logic operates.

It is well known that, one, glucose is the primary source of fuel utilized by the cells to produce energy in the body; two, glucose is metabolized by insulin, a hormone produced in the beta cells of the pancreas; and three, diabetes is a condition of both abnormal glucose regulation and insulin production, which

results in shortened life span and many of the age-related diseases. So insulin must be the primary factor in determining aging and maximum life span, so the medical logic goes.

This is true, and insulin function is certainly a major aging factor. Yet it is still but one among many determinants in the aging process and not its sole cause. You should not limit your approach to aging to diets or health practices that emphasize insulin alone; rather, it's better to follow a balanced, individualized approach. In fact, managing glucose metabolism requires a *multifactorial* approach involving diet, supplemental nutrients, exercise, and other factors.

Given this qualification, let's now review some of the age-related changes that are caused by abnormal glucose metabolism and insulin resistance before we discuss the methods to normalize and improve this common condition. To begin with, the typical dietary and lifestyle trends of older people affect glucose metabolism. These include increased inactivity, reduced muscle mass, increased consumption of sugar-containing foods such as ice cream and candy, reduced intake of protein foods such as meats and fish, and reduced essential fatty acid and fiber intake. Research has shown that in the general population, fasting glucose levels increase 6–14 mg/dL every decade after age 50. Though this is the trend, it is not necessarily always the case; my elderly patients, for example, have normal glucose and insulin levels.

These same factors (high glucose and insulin levels) cause muscle weakness, greater body fat to muscle mass, greater waist-to-hip ratio, fatigue, and lead to diabetes. It is well known that Type I diabetes is associated with vascular changes that cause poor circulation in the feet, hands, and eyes, and contribute to the causes of heart disease. Type II diabetes is associated with an increased risk for heart disease. Both types of diabetes reduce quality of life and shorten life span. What is less well known is that insulin resistance sets the stage for diabetes, and that nondiabetic people with insulin resistance are at equal risk for cardiovascular disease as are those with diabetes.

Obesity and insulin resistance usually happen together, particularly the accumulation of fat in the midsection of the body and the lower belly, contributing to a greater waist-to-hip ratio; this is also called abdominal or visceral obesity. Lipodystrophy, the body pattern of muscle loss in the arms and legs with fat accumulation in the trunk, occurs with insulin resistance.

Abnormal glucose metabolism and dysfunctional insulin production combined with insulin resistance cause imbalances in several hormones, including estrogen, progesterone, thyroid, and DHEA. The reverse is also true. Long-term use of birth control pills (estrogen and synthetic progesterone), continuous low-dose estradiol and progesterone replacement therapy in menopause, and growth hormone therapy can contribute to an increased risk for insulin resistance.

Insulin resistance occurs when your body cannot respond properly to the insulin it produces and compensates for this by making more insulin. Sustained amounts of insulin can be toxic to cells; therefore, the cell receptors that serve as gatekeepers to the interior of the cell resist insulin entering the cell, so muscle cells cannot take up glucose as easily as they should and fat cells cannot give up their energy stores.

Hormone Changes Associated with Insulin Resistance

- Increased prolactin

- Decreased growth hormone

- Decreased DHEA

- Increased cortisol

- Increased adrenaline

- Decreased thyroid

- Imbalances in estrogen and progesterone

Insulin has dramatic implications on life span. Though abnormal insulin regulation may not be the cause of aging, it does set the *pace* of aging. It does this by its effects on glucose metabolism, its influence on other hormones, its transformation from an anabolic hormone to a catabolic one, its influence on the transport of proteins into the cells, and its ability to act as a signaling molecule triggering abnormal genetic expression. Insulin not only manages how glucose moves from the bloodstream into the cells, but it is also an important chemical messenger involved in maintaining homeostasis.

According to Ron Rosedale, M.D., director of the Colorado Center for Metabolic Medicine in Boulder, insulin appears to be the "common denominator" in many of the age-related diseases, diabetes in particular, as well as cardiovascular disease and cancer. Jeffrey Bland, Ph.D., a nutritional biochemist and director of HealthComm International in Gig Harbor, Washington, says that insulin "plays a principal role in communicating with the genes and altering their expression" (Bland 1999). Barry Sears, Ph.D., the author of the Zone Diet books, considers insulin one of the most important biomarkers of aging, and Diana Schwarzbein, M.D., states: "Prolonged high insulin levels brought on by bad eating and lifestyle habits age the metabolism on a cellular level" (Schwarzbein 1999). Researchers at the University of California at Davis found that the type and amount of dietary carbohydrate significantly affect health during aging and life span (McDonald 1995).

Researchers at Brown University in Providence, Rhode Island, found that reduced insulin signaling increased the life span in all experimental animals (Tatar 2003). Insulin signaling appears to be activated or reduced by specific genes (Hsieh 2002). German researchers at the Max-Planck Institute in Berlin found that insulin signaling is affected by environmental stimuli (Gerisch 2001), and findings by researchers at McGill University in Montreal, Quebec, suggest that environmental stimuli can turn on genes that promote longevity (Hekimi 2003). It appears that insulin signaling affects both ends of life. Gary Ruvkun, Ph.D., of Harvard

The weight of research suggests that insulin may set the pace of aging. It regulates glucose utilization in the body and affects the entire neuroendocrine system. Thus the practical manipulation of aging begins with reducing insulin resistance and improving glucose metabolism.

University, suggests that insulin exerts molecular effects that can regulate fertility, metabolism, and reproduction (Tissenbaum 1998).

The weight of research suggests that insulin may set the pace of aging. It regulates glucose utilization in the body and affects the entire neuroendocrine system. Thus the practical manipulation of aging begins with reducing insulin resistance and improving glucose metabolism.

How to Improve Glucose Metabolism and Reduce Insulin Resistance

The three aspects we will work with to improve glucose metabolism and restore insulin sensitivity are: (1) normalizing insulin utilization; (2) improving liver function; and (3) improv-

ing insulin signaling and reversing the negative gene expression caused by insulin resistance. Normalizing insulin levels and improving liver function through positive lifestyle change indirectly improve insulin signaling.

To effectively lower insulin resistance and improve glucose metabolism, dietary changes and natural medications are necessary. These are supported by stress reduction and other lifestyle changes. Reducing stress and effectively managing stressful circumstances in your life help to normalize adrenal hormone activity and thereby indirectly affect glucose metabolism. Higher than normal levels of cortisol are caused by stress and are associated with insulin resistance. Stress may also indirectly affect leptin and insulin interactions and lead to obesity and diabetes.

After dietary change, exercise is the single most effective method for improving glucose utilization and normalizing blood sugar levels. Sustained physical activity can reduce insulin resistance by improving muscle mass and body fat loss and by enhancing energy utilization in the body. All forms of physical exercise appear to help, including walking; however, an exercise program that supports lean tissue growth, such as resistance training, is optimal.

Researchers found that cigarette smoking aggravates insulin resistance, and that nicotine gum and patches used to help stop smoking are also associated with glucose abnormalities. Though moderate alcohol consumption is associated with improved cardiovascular function and can even improve insulin sensitivity, alcohol can contain up to 10 percent sugar, so if you have insulin resistance I recommend that you avoid alcoholic beverages. Excess alcohol consumption can increase triglyceride levels, cause hypoglycemia, and interfere with weight loss. One drink containing two ounces of 90-proof alcohol has about 200 calories, and one beer contains up to 150 calories. If you are on a calorie-restricted diet, two alcoholic beverages are the equivalent of one-fourth to one-third of the total recommended daily calorie intake of 1,200–1,400 calories.

Insulin sensitivity is necessary to prolong your health and extend your life span. To enhance your insulin sensitivity, start with the lifestyle changes discussed above; then change your diet; continue with nutritional supplements and natural medications; and then improve your liver function.

Prolonging Health Recommendation 18— Get Your Insulin and Glucose Levels Tested

Before you begin using the recommendations in this chapter to modify your glucose metabolism and improve your insulin sensitivity, get your glucose and insulin levels tested, and take the other tests necessary to determine the status of your glucose metabolism and insulin sensitivity. These include blood tests for fasting glucose, insulin, cortisol, and a lipid panel (see Prolonging Health Recommendation 4).

To prevent insulin resistance keep your fasting glucose levels in the optimal range of 78–85 mg/dL; and at least lower than 90 mg/dL and higher than 70 mg/dL. Keep your fasting insulin level lower than 10 mcg/dL; but not lower than 4 mcg/dL, and at least lower than 15 mcg/dL. Your triglyceride to HDL ratio should be less than 2; at least less than 4.

Prolonging Health Recommendation 19— Improve Your Insulin Sensitivity with Smart Dietary Changes

Insulin resistance and its associated metabolic effects are caused by excess consumption of refined carbohydrates, extremely low-fat diets, inadequate protein intake, sedentary lifestyle, and obesity. It is important to remember that underlying these lifestyle issues is a complicated array of biochemical factors including genetic tendencies, DNA and mitochondrial defects (caused by xenobiotics), hormonal imbalances (caused by age-related hormonal decline and dietary influences), cell receptor and transporter messenger dysfunction, abnormal liver function (related to impaired glucogenesis and abnormal insulin clearance), and progressive impairment of the mitochondrial function in pancreatic beta cells. Thus such a multifaceted problem as insulin resistance and abnormal glucose metabolism requires a comprehensive approach, as no single drug or technique will solve it.

For example, the macronutrient content of the diet has direct effects on glucose metabolism. A low-carbohydrate, high-saturated-fat diet is associated with the reduced ability of insulin to lower glucose levels; a high-carbohydrate, low-fat diet is associated with greater insulin production and therefore initial lower glucose levels, but in the long run it causes insulin resistance (Bessesen 2001). Therefore, a balanced approach to the source of your calories, combined with intake of adequate low glycemic index carbohydrates, sufficient unsaturated fats, and complete proteins, appears to be the better dietary plan.

In some cases a higher fat and protein diet, with low carbohydrates, as in the Atkins or 30-30-40 Zone diets, works well as a transition diet from one that is unbalanced and unhealthy to a balanced diet that promotes normal glucose metabolism. However, I do not recommend either of these diets for the long term as they are not individualized to your age, or metabolic and genetic requirements.

It should be clear that the roots of insulin resistance are largely in diet and secondarily in deficiencies of key nutrients. Now, in this section, I discuss how to correct insulin resistance and normalize glucose metabolism with smart dietary changes.

***Prolonging Health* Smart Dietary Change 1—Stop Eating Sugar:** Without a doubt, the first step in improving glucose metabolism and remedying insulin resistance is to remove all refined sugar from your diet. Over my more than 20 years of clinical practice, I have found that nothing undermines health more than refined sugar.

However, since the body quickly becomes addicted to sugar, eliminating it is not as easy to do as it may sound; eliminating sugar without suffering from sugar cravings, fatigue, and mood swings is difficult. Fortunately, these withdrawal symptoms are not dangerous and are only the body's way of readjusting its metabolism; within one to two weeks of avoiding sugar you will feel much better. Of course, you can also gradually eliminate sugar by first replacing it with honey, maple syrup, and ripe fresh fruits, but remember that since they contain natural sugars, these too will eventually have to be reduced if not entirely eliminated if you are to normalize your glucose metabolism, restore insulin sensitivity, prevent disease, prolong your health, and promote longevity.

So avoid overeating fruits and instead eat more vegetables. Fruits are not only largely fructose but they are not as nutrient rich as vegetables, which provide fiber, vitamins, minerals, and many other health-promoting factors.

***Prolonging Health* Smart Dietary Change 2—Manage Your Carbohydrates:** Not only must you eliminate simple sugars, but you also have to manage the type of carbohydrates you eat by choosing foods that break down into sugars more *slowly*. These foods are categorized by their glycemic index, a system of ranking foods by their effect on raising glucose.

The concept of a glycemic index is the result of extensive carbohydrate research; it is accepted internationally as a tool for dietary management for obesity and dysglycemic disorders including Type II diabetes. The Wolever and Jenkins method is the most widely used indexing of foods and the "International Tables of Glycemic Index" is the tool of choice for lists of commonly eaten foods (Jenkins et al. 1994). Choose foods that have a low glycemic index, and completely eliminate foods such as bread and other high glycemic index foods.

Here are some tips to help you choose the right kind of carbohydrates. Substitute whole grain breads for refined flour products like white bread. Avoid commercial breakfast cereals; instead, eat granola or traditional cooked cereals, such as oatmeal made from organic rolled oats. Eat several pieces of whole fruit each day; avoid fruit juices entirely. Eat lots of vegetables of all kinds and prepared in different ways, such as steamed or raw, in salads or soups. Beans of all types are high in fiber and have a low glycemic index, and you should eat more of them, but don't eat too much at one time. Rather, eat small amounts of beans several times a week (Brand-Miller, Wolever, Foster-Powell, et al. 1996).

***Prolonging Health* Smart Dietary Change 3—Restrict Your Calories:** Overall, calorie reduction is necessary to improve insulin sensitivity, normalize glucose metabolism, prolong health, and promote longevity. Restrict your total daily calories with the goal of maintaining a stable level of about 1,200 to 1,400 calories for at least one to three months. Though statistics vary from source to source, the average American eats around 2,200 each day and some as much as 3,800 calories (Cirtser 2003). By way of contrast, an average fast-food meal in America contains 1,876 calories; an average vegetarian eats about 1,600 calories a day.

Calorie restriction is necessary in order to normalize your weight if you are overweight, to reduce the metabolic burden of overeating on your liver and intestinal tract, and to minimize the stimulation of insulin production from the glucose spikes caused by overeating. Remember that when you eat, glucose levels rise and insulin is secreted from the pancreas beta cells.

Prolonging Health
Smart Dietary Change 4—Choose Your Fats Wisely: Avoid eating saturated fats and instead increase your intake of essential fatty acids. Many commercial foods are high in sugars and saturated fats, and eating them results in the greatest insulin and glucose responses—the opposite of healthy balanced metabolic responses. Avoid all commercially prepared foods for this reason.

Let's clarify the difference between types of fats. Fats and oils are essentially the same; both are lipids made up of fatty acids, differing slightly in chemical structure and nature. Fats are very stable chemically and solidify at room temperature (butter); oils such as safflower or olive remain as liquids, are less stable, and therefore oxidize rapidly. There are three types of fats: saturated, monounsaturated, and polyunsaturated. The type found in meat and butter is saturated, while most vegetable, seed, and nut oils are unsaturated. Though oils tend to remain liquid at room temperature, monounsaturated fats such as canola and olive oil become thicker when refrigerated. Hydrogenated oils, such as those found in processed

Glycemic Index of Selected Carbohydrates					
Soybeans	25	Spaghetti pasta	45–61	Bagel	72
Lentils	29	Orange juice	46	Potato, boiled	80
Fructose	31	Grapefruit juice	48	White rice	81
Barley	36	Brown rice	50	Banana	84
Apple	38	Yam	51	Potato, baked	85
Tomato soup	38	Pita bread	57	Sucrose	89
Plum	39	Basmati rice	58	Rye bread	90
Apple juice	41	Corn	59	Whole wheat bread	99
Kidney beans	43	Croissant	67	White bread	100
Lentil soup	44	Carrots	71	Glucose	138

To manage the effects of carbohydrates on insulin levels, choose those with a glycemic index of 55 or lower. Every four days, you can have carbohydrates with a glycemic index of 56–70, but avoid those with a glycemic index of 71 or higher.

foods (margarines), contain trans-fatty acids, which are harmful to health.

Not all saturated fats are bad for you. In fact, meats and milk contain a fatty substance called conjugated linoleic acid (CLA) that actually promotes weight loss and improves insulin sensitivity (Houseknecht 1998). Trans-fatty acids (found in margarines and vegetable shortening) clog arteries and cause heart disease. Monounsaturated fats, as found in vegetable oils such as olive, help reduce the risk of heart disease, benefit Type II diabetes, and exert an overall favorable influence on metabolism (Kelly 2000).

Just as the type of dietary fat you eat is important in managing your glucose metabolism, so is the amount of fat you eat. Many Americans obtain 45 percent or more of their calories from fats, mostly saturated fats from meats and commercially processed foods. Research evidence suggests that diets high in saturated fats promote obesity, increase the risk for cardiovascular disease, and cause insulin resistance. High saturated fat diets also cause more oxidation, which increases free radical damage, which as we know is one of the main causes of aging.

In order to prolong health, eat a diet composed of between 25 and 35 percent unsaturated fat from natural foods. The rule for fats and oils is consume more fish; moderate amounts of red meat and poultry; and more olive oil and avocados; and consume no margarines or processed fats and oils. Remember, sugars and refined carbohydrates such as white flour products readily convert to fat in your body; overeating dietary fats, particularly excess saturated and trans-fatty acids, adds additional calories to your diet. When eaten as part of a balanced diet, fat and oils in themselves do not cause weight gain.

***Prolonging Health* Smart Dietary Change 5—Eat Enough Protein:** Getting enough amino acids from dietary protein is also important. A recommended intake is 65–85 g daily from both plant and animal sources to yield a total of at least 40 percent of the total daily calories from protein sources. In time, as your body becomes more efficient in utilizing dietary energy sources, you can reduce the total percentage; some people as they get older will do well to consider vegetarianism and eliminate all animal products from their diet. However, if you are a vegetarian already, it is still necessary to eat enough high-quality protein foods.

***Prolonging Health* Smart Dietary Change 6—Get Enough Fiber:** Adequate fiber is necessary for the maintenance of health, prevention of cancer, and management of cholesterol. Studies have shown that low-fiber diets increase insulin resistance (Marshall 1997). Though all forms of dietary fiber have some value, oat bran and guar gum help to lower insulin resistance better than psyllium seeds, the most commonly used commercial form of fiber. Although you may be able to obtain up to 25 g of fiber from the type of diet I am describing, optimal fiber levels are only achieved by adding additional fiber to the diet as a powdered supplement. Though commercially available psyllium products are useful in providing bulk fiber, obtain a fiber supplement from your doctor or health food store that contains guar gum and other non-psyllium sources of fiber such as from oats, carrots, peas, or other vegetable sources.

***Prolonging Health* Smart Dietary Change 7—Practice Periodic Modified Fasting:** During fasting, which your body responds to as short-term starvation, glucose levels decline and insulin secretion drops while glucagon, growth hormone, and cortisol levels rise. Glucose concentrations below 50 mg/dL trigger glucagon secretion. The hormones just mentioned stimulate the release of glucose from glycogen stored in the liver and muscle, and glucogenesis is improved. This is why modified fasting helps improve insulin sensitivity (see chapter 9).

Dietary Rules to Restore Normal Glucose Metabolism and Insulin Sensitivity

1. Eliminate refined sugar

2. Go light on fruits

3. Keep your carbohydrate percentage low (30 percent or less)

4. Select low glycemic index carbohydrates (70 or less, and better if 55 or less)

5. Keep your saturated fats low; your unsaturated fats and oils high (30 percent)

6. Balance essential fatty acids (1 to 1 ratio of omega-6 to omega-3)

7. Eat more protein (40 percent or more, providing 65–85 g or more)

8. Maintain high fiber (30–50 g total daily)

9. Keep your total calories moderate (1,200–1,400 calories daily)

10. Eat more vegetables (5–6 large servings daily)

Prolonging Health Recommendation 20— Restore Your Insulin Sensitivity with Nutritional Supplements

Though making changes in your diet is an important step towards improving glucose tolerance, effectively managing insulin resistance, and restoring your metabolism, ultimately you have to include supplemental nutrients and natural medicines to optimize the effects of diet. Among these substances are essential fatty acids and antioxidants such as zinc, vitamin C, coenzyme Q10, and lipoic acid. Herbal medicines and other natural substances include ginseng, cinnamon, and prickly pear cactus. Let's review these and discuss their importance in the treatment of insulin resistance.

Prolonging Health **Insulin Sensitivity Restoring Prescription 1—Supplement Your Dietary Fats with EFAs:** Essential fatty acids (EFAs) are fats and oils that are essential for health and that must be supplied in the diet. EFAs provide the structural material that composes all cell membranes and are necessary to many other functions in the body including the production of eicosanoids.[25] Eicosanoids play a role in nearly every metabolic process in the body, from the control of insulin to serving as autocrine hormones and signaling molecules, and all these roles are critical functions for prolonging health.

Dietary supplementation with essential fatty acids helps restore glucose tolerance and insulin sensitivity (reduces insulin resistance). The most useful types are: (1) gamma-linolenic acid (GLA) from flax and borage oils; and (2) docosahexaenoic acid (DHA) and eicosapentaenoic acid (EPA) from fish oil. The omega-3 fatty acids DHA and EPA exert beneficial effects on the cardiovascular and nervous systems, and may also improve insulin sensitivity. Omega-3 fatty acids are found in fish oils from salmon and other coldwater fish, and in certain types of algae.

The ratio of omega-6 to omega-3 fatty acids appears to be critical in promoting health. Undesirable omega-6 fatty acids are found in processed fats and oils like margarines, and the good or desirable omega-6s are found in vegetable seed oils. The average American diet may have a ratio of six to one, whereas a healthier ratio is two parts omega-6 to one part omega-3 fatty acids; the optimal may be closer to a one to one ratio (Stoll 2000). Eating more fish, particularly salmon, halibut, and other coldwater types; DHA-rich eggs from hens fed algae; and seeds, nuts, avocados, and natural plant oils such as olive promotes essential fatty acid production and helps promote this more favorable fatty acid profile. However, in order to restore the correct EFA balance in your body, improve insulin sensitivity, and prolong your health, it is necessary to supplement the diet with EPA and DHA.

There is no consensus among doctors about adequate daily amounts of EFAs nor about what is the ideal supplemental dosage. In addition, the variety of sources and the percentages of the different types of EFAs make it difficult for one to know what is best. Studies in the use of EFAs in the treatment of depression used at least 9 g daily to obtain results (Stoll 2000). Barry Sears, in *The Omega RxZone*, recommends at least 2.5 g of fish oil daily, gradually increasing the dose until you feel better and experience more mental clarity and enhanced physical performance (Sears 2002).

Jonathan Goodman, N.D., author of *The Omega Solution*, proposes that the total combined amount of dietary and supplemental EFAs be about 10 g daily (Goodman 2001). Given that the optimal dosage varies among individuals, it is reasonable to say that in addition to dietary sources, you should take at least 1.5 to 2.5 g (1,500–2,500 mg) of EFAs daily, with an upper limit of 10 g.

To obtain these dosages, supplement with one teaspoon of flax oil daily with food; one tablespoon of cod liver oil one or two times weekly; and 1,000 to 2,000 mg of EPA/DHA fish oil daily with food (each 1000 mg capsule contains 300 mg of EPA and 200 mg of DHA, the balance being made up of other oils). You may also wish to add small amounts of evening primrose, borage seed, or black currant seed oil. Take all oil supplements with food for better absorption.

Fish oil supplements are considered safe, though some people experience intestinal gas and bloating when taking them. However, if you take too much you may experience excessive or easy bleeding, increased LDL cholesterol, and excess oxidative activity in the body. Be sure to obtain fish oil supplements from sources free of heavy metals and toxic chemical residues.

Recommended Essential Fatty Acid Supplements

10 g daily total from combined dietary and supplemental sources:

- 1 tablespoon of cod liver oil, 1–2 times weekly

- 1 teaspoon of flax oil daily

- 1,000–2,000 mg of EPA/DHA fish oil daily

EFAs are measured in the red blood cells or in serum, though my preference is to determine levels within the red blood cells. If you are using high dosages of EFAs in your program, or to treat depression or cardiovascular disease, or to reduce insulin levels, it is wise to ask your doctor to perform an essential fatty acid profile for you.

***Prolonging Health* Insulin Sensitivity Restoring Prescription 2—Take Trace Minerals:** A number of trace minerals have been shown to improve glucose tolerance and lower insulin resistance. Chief among them is chromium, an essential micronutrient that functions as a cofactor in all insulin-regulating activities in the body. Supplementation with chromium decreases fasting glucose levels, improves glucose tolerance by cells, lowers insulin levels, and helps decrease total cholesterol and triglyceride levels while increasing HDL levels (Dey 2002).

There are numerous forms of chromium, and though the most commonly used form is chromium picolinate, I recommend chromium polynicotinate. In high dosages taken over a long period of time or in sensitive individuals, chromium can be toxic; however, dosages between 200 and 400 mcg taken twice daily with food appear to be safe.

Zinc, an important antioxidant, also plays an important role in the regulation of insulin production in pancreatic tissue, as well as in glucose utilization by muscle and fat cells (Song 1998). Zinc deficiency is common in older people, and research suggests that there is a relationship between low zinc levels and insulin resistance. Zinc picolinate, taken in dosages of 15–30 mg daily, is generally sufficient to improve insulin sensitivity; however, when zinc is used as an antioxidant, higher dosages are frequently called for, and these will enhance its role in regulating insulin.

Vanadium (vanadyl sulfate) helps regulate glucose levels and improve receptor sensitivity to insulin. It is taken in dosages ranging from

75 to 100 mg as an initial starting dose, which is then lowered after several weeks to a maintenance dose of 0.5–2 mg per day.

***Prolonging Health* Insulin Sensitivity Restoring Prescription 3—Get Enough Macrominerals:** The most important of these nutrients for improving insulin sensitivity is magnesium, as deficiency of this mineral is associated with increased insulin resistance. Daily dosages of elemental magnesium range from 250 to 1,000 mg. Supplementation with 500–1,500 mg of calcium and 100–200 mg of potassium also exert positive benefits on glucose metabolism.

***Prolonging Health* Insulin Sensitivity Restoring Prescription 4—Take Antioxidants:** Vitamin C, vitamin E, selenium, and zinc improve insulin sensitivity. The amounts found in a quality multivitamin and mineral supplement along with their use as antioxidants (see chapter 7) are sufficient. CoQ10 in dosages of 120 mg daily combined with other vitamins and minerals assists cardiovascular function in insulin-resistant patients; it may have additional use as a substance to improve insulin sensitivity. Lipoic acid has been shown to improve insulin sensitivity and increase glucose metabolism; if you have insulin resistance or are diabetic, the daily optimal dose for lipoic acid is 600 mg.

Prolonging Health Insulin Sensitivity Restoring Prescription 5—Take Herbal Medicines: Over 400 different herbs have been shown to contain properties that influence glucose metabolism, including the classical Chinese tonic ginseng. Both the Asian variety *(Panax ginseng)* and the American *(P. quinquefolius)* species have shown clinical evidence of lowering elevated fasting glucose levels in diabetics, as well as improving how glucose is metabolized in the body. Though high dosages of ginseng have been shown to cause high blood pressure, anxiety, and insomnia, it is considered an extremely safe medication when taken in the recommended amounts of 200–600 mg daily of the standardized extract.

Other herbs that improve glucose metabolism include goat's rue *(Galega officinalis)*, a guanidine-containing root; bitter melon *(Momordica charantia)*, a commonly used food in Asia; fenugreek *(Trigonella foenum-graecum)*, a widely used remedy for diabetes in India; gurmar *(Gymnema sylvestre)*, also native to tropical India; garlic *(Allium sativa)*; aloe *(Aloe vera)*; the prickly pear cactus or *nopale (Opuntia streptaceantha)* from Mexico (Frati 1988); and a compound found in cinnamon *(Cinnamonum cassia)*, methylhydroxychalcone, or MHCP.

MHCP mimics insulin in the body to encourage cells to take up more glucose in a manner similar to how insulin works (Jarvill-Taylor 2001). MHCP also improves glucose utilization by muscle and liver cells, which facilitates glycogen storage, and it may also have a role in fatty acid metabolism (Jensen 2002). The daily dosage for MHCP is 12 mg, the equivalent to one heaping teaspoon of cinnamon powder. However, it is unlikely that simply adding a teaspoon of ground cinnamon to your daily diet will make a significant difference in your blood sugar levels.

Another Indian herb, *Inula racemosa*, promotes insulin sensitivity and improves glucose metabolism, and is frequently used in combination with other herbs in traditional Ayurvedic formulas for diabetes and heart disease.

Prolonging Health Insulin Sensitivity Restoring Prescription 6—Get Extra Amino Acids: A number of amino acids have shown benefit in improving glucose metabolism, including L-tyrosine, L-arginine, L-carnitine, and taurine. Though additional research is required to document conclusively the beneficial affects

Selected Nutrients for the Treatment of Insulin Resistance

Nutrient	Dose	Comments
Chromium picolinate or polynicotinate	200–400 mcg daily	Up to 1,200 mcg may be necessary in those with imbalanced glycemic conditions.
Zinc picolinate	15–30 mg	The amount in a multiple vitamin and mineral, or antioxidant supplement is usually sufficient.
Lipoic acid	600 mg daily	Lipoic acid is a highly acidic substance, so take with food to buffer it.
Vanadyl sulfate	75–100 mg daily	Higher doses may be necessary in diabetic patients, but increase risk of toxicity.
Coenzyme Q10	120 mg daily	Up to 300 mg or higher are necessary for those with cardiovascular disease and diabetes.
Inositol monophosphate	1,000–2,000 mg	Higher dosages up to 12,000 mg may be necessary in those with a concurrent mood disorder.
Omega-3 fatty acids (EPA/DHA)	500–1,500 mg	Higher dosages up to 6,000 mg are often needed in those with depression, hypertension, and elevated cholesterol.
Magnesium	250–1,000 mg	Dosages above 750 mg may cause diarrhea in some people.

of these amino acids, clinical evidence from naturopathic physicians suggests that they complement other nutrients in improving glucose metabolism and reducing insulin resistance in patients with diabetes and heart disease.

Prolonging Health Insulin Sensitivity Restoring Prescription 7—Include Enough B Vitamins: The B vitamins, particularly B_3, B_6,

biotin, and inositol, improve glucose metabolism. Inositol in particular stands out as a nutritional substance with potential for improving insulin signaling mechanisms; two novel inositol agents have been identified: myoinositol and D-chiro-inositol (Sun et al. 2002). The latter is a substance that occurs naturally in fruits and vegetables, but has been concentrated for investigational use in diabetes and polycystic ovarian syndrome (a condition characterized by multiple small ovarian cysts, weight gain, increased levels of male hormones and imbalanced female hormones, and infertility).

D-chiro-inositol is currently unavailable commercially; however, adding inositol as inositol monophosphate (at dosages of 1,000–2,000 mg daily) may complement your program to improve glucose metabolism. It is safe to take even in high dosages and has no side effects or known complications with other medications.

Prolonging Health Recommendation 21— Improve Your Liver Function to Restore Normal Glucose Metabolism

As discussed in chapter 9, the liver is the main metabolic and detoxification organ in your body, and after the pancreas, the liver is the most important organ for managing glucose in your body. In order to prolong your health and live a long life, you must treat your liver well. Besides antioxidants and the lipotropic substances discussed in chapter 9, and periodic detoxification therapies for improving liver function, several herbs deserve mentioning.

Milk thistle *(Silybum marianum)* improves liver function, protects liver cells from xenobiotic, viral, and alcohol-induced damage, and helps to reduce insulin resistance. Pushkarmoola *(Inula racemosa)* root can contain up to ten percent natural insulin and is useful in improving liver function and normalizing glucose metabolism. Dandelion *(Taraxicum officinale)* supports the liver's detoxification processes and lowers glucose. Inositol, described above, is a lipotropic factor and improves liver function.

Naturopathic physicians have long known the importance of the liver's functions in the body, and some medical doctors are beginning to acknowledge that providing liver-protective substances and improving liver function are among the most important keys to health. Sandra Cabot, M.D., an Australian gynecologist, natural medicine advocate, and author of *The Liver Cleansing Diet* (Cabot 1996), supports the idea of liver cleansing and suggests foods such as carrots, beets, and artichokes as liver restoratives, to be taken along with a high-fiber diet.

In fact, if you follow all the recommendations found in chapters 5–8, with the addition of taking milk thistle, you will likely be well on your way to restoring your liver function. For those with chronic viral hepatitis, primary biliary cirrhosis, cirrhosis due to alcohol or other causes, or hepatocellular cancer, I recommend that you seek the advice of a skilled naturopathic physician, as treatment of these liver diseases is beyond the scope of this book (see also my earlier book, *Viral Immunity*, Hampton Roads, 2002).

In review, after neutralizing oxidative damage with antioxidants (chapter 7), providing DNA repair substances (chapter 8), and detoxifying the liver (chapter 9), the next most important aging factor to understand involves the consequences of abnormal glucose metabolism, including insulin resistance. Insulin is a critical hormone; without it your cells could not access the energy contained in glucose and would starve. As we have seen, insulin has profound effects on carbohydrate and fat metabolism, and it plays a major role in protein and mineral metabolism.

Without insulin we cannot survive for long, and from the evolutionary perspective, our body has developed sophisticated ways of maintaining glucose within tight limits despite daily fluctuations in food intake, types of foods eaten, and periods of starvation or fasting—all under the control of one hormone, insulin.

Glucose metabolism in the body is a highly complex process, primarily involving insulin, which tightly regulates the level of glucose in the blood. It is modulated by a balance between glucose uptake by the muscles and glucose secretion by the liver. When blood sugar levels drop and insulin is less active, other hormones (cortisol, glucagon, growth hormone) drive the liver to break down glycogen (stored glucose) back into glucose. Sophisticated biological signaling molecules provide controlling mechanisms that regulate glucose metabolism on the molecular level. Thus, keeping glucose and insulin within effective and safe ranges helps to prolong health, and without improving insulin sensitivity and restoring glucose metabolism, you can never be truly healthy, nor will you likely live long.

No single drug or simple group of nutrients is likely to reverse advanced abnormal glucose metabolism and insulin resistance. It takes a complete revolution in lifestyle and the way you eat, along with a comprehensive plan of natural medicines to turn this modifiable aging factor around. However, the same dietary principles work in all aspects of the *Prolonging Health* plan, and many of the same natural medications are used to treat other aging factors. Therefore, you can be successful in reversing the aging factors for the purpose of prolonging your health and extending longevity if you learn the principles discussed in this chapter, as well as the other chapters in part 2, then apply them in a manner that fits your way of life.

Summary of *Prolonging Health* Recommendations for Restoring Insulin Sensitivity

- *Prolonging Health* **Recommendation 18— Get Your Insulin and Glucose Levels Tested**
  - Keep your fasting glucose levels between 78 and 85 mg/dL; at least lower than 90 mg/dL and higher than 70 mg/dL; your fasting insulin level lower than 10 mcg/dL, not lower than 4 mcg/dL and at least lower than 15 mcg/dL; your triglyceride to HDL ratio should be less than 2 and at least less than 4.

- *Prolonging Health* **Recommendation 19— Improve Your Insulin Sensitivity with Smart Dietary Changes**
  - *Prolonging Health* Smart Dietary Change 1— Stop Eating Sugar: Eliminate refined sugar completely, and go light on fruits.
  - *Prolonging Health* Smart Dietary Change 2— Manage Your Carbohydrates: Eat only carbohydrates with a glycemic index of 55 or lower; every four days you can have carbohydrates with a glycemic index of 70 or lower.

- *Prolonging Health* Smart Dietary Change 3— Restrict Your Calories: Keep your total daily calories between 1,200 and 1,400 for three months.
- *Prolonging Health* Smart Dietary Change 4— Choose Your Fats Wisely: Keep your dietary fats to between 25 and 35 percent; use unsaturated fats from olive oil, avocados, seeds and nuts; eat more cold-water fish; use moderate amounts of red meat and poultry; and consume no margarines, and no processed fats or oils.
- *Prolonging Health* Smart Dietary Change 5— Eat Enough Protein: Get at least 65–85 g daily.
- *Prolonging Health* Smart Dietary Change 6— Get Enough Fiber: Get between 25 and 50 g daily.
- *Prolonging Health* Smart Dietary Change 7— Practice Periodic Modified Fasting: Follow recommendations for modified fasting in chapter 9.

- *Prolonging Health* **Recommendation 20— Restore Your Insulin Sensitivity with Nutritional Supplements**
  - *Prolonging Health* Insulin Sensitivity Restoring Prescription 1–Supplement Your Dietary Fats With EFAs: Take 1 teaspoon of flax oil daily with food; 1 tablespoon of cod liver oil one or two times weekly; and 1,000 to 2,000 mg of EPA/DHA fish oil daily with food (each 1000 mg capsule contains 300 mg of EPA and 200 mg of DHA).
  - *Prolonging Health* Insulin Sensitivity Restoring Prescription 2–Take Trace Minerals: Take 200–400 mcg of chromium picolinate or polynicotinate daily; 15–30 mg of zinc picolinate daily; start with 75–100 mg of vanadyl sulfate and lower it after several weeks to a maintenance dose of 0.5–2 mg per day.
  - *Prolonging Health* Insulin Sensitivity Restoring Prescription 3–Get Enough Macrominerals: Take 250–1,000 mg of magnesium; 500-1,500 mg of calcium; and 100–200 mg of potassium daily.
  - *Prolonging Health* Insulin Sensitivity Restoring Prescription 4–Take Antioxidants: Get

enough vitamin C and other antioxidants (see chapter 7); 120 mg of coenzyme Q10; and 600 mg of lipoic acid daily.

- *Prolonging Health* Insulin Sensitivity Restoring Prescription 5—Take Herbal Medicines: Take ginseng and other herbal medicines that improve insulin sensitivity; and 12 mg of MHCP daily.
- *Prolonging Health* Insulin Sensitivity Restoring Prescription 6—Get Extra Amino Acids: Take whey protein (see chapter 9) or individual amino acids to supplement your dietary protein.
- *Prolonging Health* Insulin Sensitivity Restoring Prescription 7—Include Enough B Vitamins: Get enough B vitamins (such as in a multivitamin) and take 1,000–2,000 mg of inositol monophosphate daily.

- ***Prolonging Health* Recommendation 21— Improve Your Liver Function to Restore Normal Glucose Metabolism**
Follow the principles of liver detoxification outlined in chapter 9; take the herbs milk thistle, inula, and dandelion.

11 *Prolonging Health* Modifiable Aging Factor 5: Impaired Protein Synthesis and Glycation—How to Undo the Effects of Degraded Proteins Called AGEs

As introduced in the last chapter, glucose reactions in the body don't end with energy metabolism and fat storage, but also involve proteins, the main structural component of all tissues in the body, including muscle, bone, and skin. However, proteins are not the simple structural entities scientists once thought they were. They are dynamic living systems in a state of constant biological activity. They get worn down by use, influenced by hormones and metabolism, and damaged by oxidative processes; the body's protein stores must be replaced as well as repaired.

In fact, thousands of different proteins are necessary in each individual cell for the performance of life-giving functions at any given time, and the combination and activity of these proteins determine the cells' biological behavior. Not surprisingly, proteins are not only important for life, but are involved in aging as well. Here's how they work in your body.

Proteins are synthesized from food, principally foods rich in amino acids such as muscle meats, fish, eggs, dairy products (yogurt and cheese), and plant protein sources such as seeds, nuts, and legumes (soybeans, kidney beans, lentils, and other dried beans). In order for our body to develop structurally and function, sufficient dietary proteins are necessary.

But just how much protein should you eat, from what sources, and what is the optimal form of protein for longevity?

Complete proteins are necessary for the maintenance of life (though vegetarianism provides numerous health benefits for some people). Without sufficient protein, the body cannot repair worn or damaged tissue, cannot build or maintain muscle mass, and has a difficult time regulating glucose. As with all the modifiable aging factors we've discussed, balance is the theme, and in this case it is balance among your body's need for protein, your health and fitness goals, your activity levels, your age, and your dietary sources of protein.

The recommended daily allowance (RDA) for protein is 0.4 g of protein for every pound of body weight. According to the RDA, a 120-pound woman needs 48 g and a 160-pound man needs 64 g of protein each day. Most Americans get more than twice the RDA of protein every day. When you are exercising regularly, as you need to do to maintain muscle mass, your protein requirements increase to 0.6–0.8 g of protein for each pound of body weight per day. Under these circumstances, a 120-pound woman needs 72–96 g of protein daily; a 160-pound man needs 96–128 g of protein per day.

Older people tend to consume less protein and this contributes to the loss of muscle mass commonly seen in the elderly. It is generally thought that as you age, your requirement for protein decreases and that declining kidney and liver function makes your body unable to process higher than the recommended dietary protein intake. This belief is now in question. Researchers have shown that active older people may need more protein and maintain muscle mass when consuming as much as 0.8 g of protein per pound of body weight (Evans 2002). That's the same amount of protein recommended for those who do weight training.

On average, I recommend 65–85 g of protein daily derived from a variety of animal and plant sources. However, to build muscle and repair damaged tissue, your body requires more protein, as much as 125 g or more per day.

Our body absorbs 70–90 percent of the protein from plant sources and 80–100 percent of the protein from animal sources. These percentages suggest that animal proteins are better than plant proteins; however, both sources are good and can satisfy a balanced protein requirement. I recommend eating protein from animal and plant sources at each meal. Try to get at least 80 percent of your protein needs from dietary sources; then supplement the remaining 20 percent with whey protein. Many Westerners are allergic to soy, so I do not recommend soy protein products. Also, soy protein does not absorb well in the gastrointestinal tract; as you get older, it becomes important to consume protein that has 100 percent absorption.

However, we can't absorb much more than 25 g of protein at a time. Nutritional experts say that daily protein consumption in excess of 1.0 g per pound of body weight is too much. Excess protein is excreted in the urine and feces, and can stress your kidneys. It can cause increased excretion of calcium in the urine and that can lead to osteoporosis. Again, balance is the rule. Consume enough protein, but don't overeat protein foods or take too many protein supplements.

In this chapter we discuss the mechanisms that play a role in protein protection and repair, the importance of maintaining protein metabolism during aging, and the effects of protein degradation, as through the glycation process that occurs when glucose molecules bond with

During aging, protein synthesis slows down and becomes less accurate, as evidenced by thinning bones, hair, and skin, and decreased muscle size. Combined inaccurate protein synthesis and unfolding of proteins cause not only structural decline but immune dysfunction, disturbances in neurotransmitters and brain function, and hormonal imbalances.

proteins. We also explore some effective measures to break the cross-linked chain of events that cause protein degradation, and show how to restore normal protein metabolism.

Protein Modifications and Aging

During aging, protein synthesis slows down and becomes less accurate, as evidenced by thinning bones, hair, and skin, and decreased muscle size (Rattan 1991). Distortion of protein architecture, referred to as protein folding, becomes more apparent with age, as does the process by which the body removes damaged proteins. Called protein degradation, this process stalls as we get older. Combined inaccurate protein synthesis and unfolding of proteins cause not only structural decline but immune dysfunction, disturbances in neurotransmitters and brain function, and hormonal imbalances. Let's see how this happens and why proteins are so important for health and in aging. Let's start with a cell.

Cells are, in essence, proteins. Thousands of different proteins are found in each cell. They are not only the building blocks from which cells, and our bodies, are built; proteins also execute nearly all of the functions that run the cell. Proteins make up enzymes that promote chemical reactions, help cell membranes function, and serve as chemical messengers carrying chemical information between cells. In the body, specialized proteins act as antibodies and hormones, and even many toxins are made of proteins.

Proteins are composed of sequences of amino acids. The thousands of proteins in our body are made up of 20 types of amino acids occurring in different variations. To fit into a cell, proteins fold into smaller structures. Folding provides stability to proteins and requires less energy for its maintenance. A protein can be unfolded, which disrupts its function. During aging, large numbers of proteins are unfolded due to oxidative damage, toxic environmental chemicals, and sunlight damage. Sun-induced protein damage affects the outer and inner layers of the skin, causing loss of elasticity, wrinkling, cellular disorganization (which can lead to the formation of skin cancers), and reduced capacity for wound healing, with the end result of loss of youthful tone and vibrancy. However, the influence of proteins on aging goes deeper than cells.

On the molecular level, researchers have found hundreds of proteins that influence aging and, when manipulated in the laboratory,

extend life span. Scientists at the French National Institute of Health in Paris, have found that certain proteins, when biologically manipulated, provide greater resistance to oxidative damage and therefore lengthen life span (Holzenberger 2003).

This research, though still in its early stages, informs us of the importance of proteins on the molecular and cellular levels. It tells us that proteins influence our genes, and not only create who we are biologically, but the rate at which we age. Now, let's discuss the effects of proteins on body structures and how degraded and/or unfolded proteins influence aging. These effects include protein glycation, cross-linking, and AGEs (which stands for advanced glycosylation end products).

Protein Glycation: Referred to as the Maillard reaction or glycation, sugars in the blood and inside cells react with proteins and DNA to form chemical bonds that cause a "browning effect" similar to the browning of the crust on bread or in carmelization. These reactions were first studied by Maillard in the early 1900s, and later by Amadori, both long since forgotten European scientists. More recently, the basic concept was developed into a theory of a new biochemical pathway in the body in which glucose combines with proteins to form permanent sticky structures called glycoproteins (*glyco* for glucose).

It is well known by doctors that damaged proteins are a feature of the accelerated aging associated with diabetes, but even in the absence of diabetes, degraded proteins increase as we age (Ulrich 2001). Poor insulin control and abnormal glucose metabolism contribute to glycoprotein formation, accelerating the aging process. That's another reason why it's important to improve your insulin sensitivity (see chapter 10).

Cross-Linking: The oxidation of glycoproteins results in increased free radical damage to tissues, cells, and DNA in a process called glycoxidation. This breaks the structural backbone that holds proteins together and produces what scientists call cross-linking. Anthony Cerami, Ph.D., of Kenneth S. Warren Laboratories in Tarrytown, New York, based his research on diabetics, who age more rapidly than people without diabetes. He discovered that glucose, although essential for energy in the body, can become "sticky" and act like a molecular glue, forming the glycoproteins that then cause cross-linking of proteins.

Cross-linked proteins are naturally produced yet foreign to the healthy body and can subsequently initiate harmful inflammatory and autoimmune responses to protein molecules such as collagen. Cross-linked collagen reduces the flexibility, elasticity, and functionality of tissues, including your skin. Over time, cross-linked proteins are further converted into advanced glycosylation end products called AGEs. These are brownish fluorescent pigments capable of further cross-linking between proteins.

AGEs: The idea that AGE formation has harmful consequences was first proposed in the late 1980s by Michael Brownlee, M.D., of Albert Einstein College of Medicine in New York, while he was researching a unifying mechanism for the many different complications of diabetes (Brownlee 1988). Since then, Brownlee's ideas have become an important area of aging research.

AGE formation is irreversible. It takes place slowly and its products accumulate in the tissues; over a lifetime, this buildup causes considerable damage to tissues and cells, and participates in age-related diseases, particularly cardiovascular and kidney disease. AGEs may be a contributing factor to atherosclerosis and stiffening of the coronary arteries, and can lead to increased systolic hypertension (high blood pressure), as well as loss of elasticity of the heart muscle—all conditions that are characteristic of the old heart.

Kidney damage is also a common feature caused by AGEs, including thickening of the glomerular walls that constitute the kidney's filtering system and can even lead to kidney failure and death. Other parts of the body affected by AGEs include the lens of the eye and the brain, and AGEs are also implicated in Alzheimer's disease (Dukic-Stefanovic 2001).

Aging is characterized by a progressive buildup of damaged proteins (Ryazanov 2002). Much of the general deterioration and visible physical changes associated with aging are caused by this progressive degradation of proteins in our body. To prolong health, slow aging, and extend our life span, we must prevent protein glycation, improve protein synthesis, and repair already degraded proteins in our body.

How to Improve Protein Synthesis, Prevent Protein Glycation, and Repair Degraded Proteins

Reducing glycoprotein formation starts with preventing insulin resistance and Type II diabetes. Everything we learned in the last four chapters (chapters 7–10) helps prevent glycation, if we apply it. Antioxidants and DNA repair substances reduce the effects of oxidative damage on proteins. Detoxification improves liver function and in the process improves glucose metabolism in the body, which prevents protein glycation. Following a low-carbohydrate diet, as well as taking natural medications that normalize glucose activity and improve insulin sensitivity, lowers the amount of available sugar in the body, and therefore, indirectly helps prevent protein glycation and AGEs. But is there a way to improve protein synthesis? Are there specific medications that prevent the degradation of proteins?

Researchers are actively investigating pharmaceutical compounds that inhibit glycoprotein formation and that restructure cross-linking. Among these are aminoguanidine (Pimagedine) and 3-phenacyl-4,5-dimethylthiazolium chloride (ALT-711) (Borek 2001), both developed by Alteon Pharmaceuticals in Ramsey, New Jersey. Though promising, these medications are still in the developmental stage and are not available yet.

One drug that is available for the prevention of protein glycation is aspirin. We are still finding new uses for aspirin, a product more than a century old, including the prevention of cardiovascular disease and Alzheimer's disease. It may also have uses as an AGE inhibitor (Hadley 2001). The Life Extension Foundation lists aspirin among its "top ten anti-aging drugs," with a recommend dosage of 81 mg daily. If you have questions on how to take aspirin, or if it is right for you, talk with your doctor.

Gerontologists have attempted to slow aging by manipulating diet and restricting different proteins such as tryptophan and methionine in the diet (Zimmerman 2003). These studies have marginally extended the life span of laboratory animals. My clinical opinion is that if supplied enough protein, which is taken with synergistic nutrients, the body will respond by increasing lean muscle, improving organ reserve, and reducing many of the effects of aging. Now that we have examined why proteins are important for health and aging, let's look at some natural ways to improve protein synthesis and reverse protein glycation.

Prolonging Health Recommendation 22— Consume a Regenerative Protein Supplement

Protein from foods can be difficult for some people to digest. Therefore, to help your body regenerate, and to prolong your health, I recommend that you supplement your diet with whey protein fortified with branched-chain amino acids (valine, leucine, isoleucine) and arginine. Branched-chain amino acids, named because of their unique branching structure, are three essential amino acids (valine, leucine, and isoleucine) that make up approximately 70 percent of amino acids in the body. They are readily absorbed and can be metabolized directly by muscle tissue.

Prolonging Health Regenerative Protein Formula

Combine the following ingredients in 8 ounces of water in a blender. Blend to a smooth consistency. Drink once or twice daily, away from other food. If you are exercising heavily, as in weight training, take this mixture twice daily. Other amino acids and nutrients may be added to make a regenerative tonic. With your drink, take a multivitamin and mineral, 250 mg of calcium citrate, and 50 mg of vitamin B_6. If you have difficulty digesting proteins, take a digestive enzyme containing hydrochloric acid with the drink.

- 10 ounces of whey protein (containing about 8 g of protein)

- 4 g of branched-chain amino acids

- 4 g of arginine

- 2 g of L-carnitine

- 2 g of L-glutamine

- 2 ounces of blueberries or other fresh berries

- 1 teaspoon of organic flax oil

Commercial regenerative protein therapies are new to anti-aging medicine. However, as we learn more about how food influences gene expression, how different proteins influence aging, and how caloric restriction slows aging, nutraceutical companies will likely develop protein and nutrient anti-aging formulas. If you are unable to make your own protein regenerative formula, consider using a commercial product like this one. MyoSpan, made up of protein isolates, vitamins, minerals, and antioxidants, is only available from physicians.[26]

Prolonging Health Recommendation 23— Take Vitamin B₆ and Other Synergistic Nutrients with Your Protein Supplement

Protein synthesis in the body requires that synergistic nutrients be supplied at the same time. The most important of these are B vitamins, particularly vitamin B_6. In elderly people, vitamin B_6 levels tend to be lower than in younger people. However, researchers at Purdue University in West Lafayette, Indiana, found that the bioavailablity of vitamin B_6 was not altered during aging (Ferroli 1994). These findings inform us that though people get less vitamin B_6 as they age, our bodies are capable of utilizing dietary and supplemental vitamin B_6 to our benefit as we age.

Vitamin B_6 is found in nutritional yeast, walnuts, sunflower seeds, melons, soy, meats, eggs, and wheat germ. The RDA for vitamin B_6 is 1.3–2.0 mg. Burn and trauma victims, for example, require additional protein for tissue regeneration; in this case 10–15 mg of vitamin B_6 is given to help protein synthesis. My clinical experience suggests that these dosages are too low for prolonging health purposes, so I suggest you supplement your diet with 50–100 mg of vitamin B_6 daily.

It is available in two forms: pyridoxine hydrochloride and pyridoxal-5-phosphate, which is the more active of the two and the form into which the liver converts pyridoxine in the body. I recommend taking a combination of both forms with a multiple vitamin containing a broad spectrum of all the B vitamins. Take these at the same time as your protein supplement. Too much vitamin B_6 (dosages between 200 and 500 mg) can cause peripheral neuropathy, a condition characterized by numbness or tingling in the hands and feet. Otherwise, it is a safe nutrient.

Increased consumption of protein in the presence of calcium and vitamin D can improve bone density and prevent osteoporosis (Dawson-Hughes 2002). Take 500–1,000 mg of calcium citrate and 400 IU of vitamin D_3 daily.

Prolonging Health Recommendation 24— Take Carnosine

So far, only one natural medication, carnosine, has been shown to be an effective inhibitor of protein glycation. Carnosine (beta-alanyl-L-histidine) is a dipeptide molecule formed naturally in human tissues from a combination of two amino acids, ß-alanine and histadine. It exhibits potent antioxidant activity that protects lipids, which make up cell membranes, from oxidative damage (Hipkiss 2000). Other dipeptides occur naturally in the body, such as carcinine, anserrine, homocarnosine, and ophidine; these have not been as well studied as carnosine, but all of them appear to neutralize protein damage.

Researchers have shown carnosine useful as a natural anti-aging medicine beneficial in modifying many of the factors associated with protein glycation and AGEs (Wang 2000). It protects muscle tissue from oxidative damage (Nagasawa 2001), improves cardiac function (Roberts 2000), plays a role in protecting cells from both aging and cancer (Holliday 2000), and acts as a DNA protective substance (Hyland 2000).

Carnosine typically is taken orally at dosages between 50 and 100 mg daily. Its effects may be helped by the addition of other antioxidants such as zinc, vitamin E, coenzyme Q10, and acetyl-L-carnitine. Carnosine is safe and has no known toxicity; it has shown no side effects in studies of people taking more than 500 mg daily (Quinn 1992). Food sources of carnosine include lean red meat and chicken.

Proteins make up who we are biologically. They build our body structure, are present in every cell, and control biological functions by acting as hormones and signaling molecules. Aging is characterized by a gradual decline in protein synthesis and tissue changes caused by protein degradation. Among the most well-studied forms of protein degradation are glycation, cross-linking, and AGEs. Protein degradation is caused by oxidative damage, abnormal glucose metabolism, sunlight damage, and environmental toxics. Sufficient dietary protein is essential for healthy aging. In addition, supplemental protein and synergistic nutrients are necessary. Carnosine is an effective anti-aging medicine. Include it in your *Prolonging Health* plan to prevent and reverse abnormal protein synthesis and glycation.

Summary of Recommendations to Prevent Protein Glycation

- *Prolonging Health* **Recommendation 22—Consume a Regenerative Protein Supplement:** Combine 8 g of whey protein in 8 ounces of pure water, and add 4 g of branched-chain amino acids and 4 g of arginine. Drink once daily away from other food. When exercising heavily, take this mixture twice daily.

- *Prolonging Health* **Recommendation 23—Take Vitamin B$_6$ and Other Synergistic Nutrients with Your Protein Supplement:** Take between 50–100 mg of vitamin B$_6$ daily; a multiple vitamin and mineral; 500–1,000 mg of calcium; and 400 IU of vitamin D.

- *Prolonging Health* **Recommendation 24—Take Carnosine:** Take 50–100 mg of carnosine daily.

12 *Prolonging Health* Modifiable Aging Factor 6: Chronic Inflammation—How to Reduce Accelerated Aging

Chronic inflammation is a hallmark of degenerative disease and unhealthy aging. Along with oxidative damage, it is one of the common denominators for many of the modifiable aging factors discussed in this book. The first five modifiable aging factors with the addition of chronic inflammation form the most destructive group of all of the many biological occurrences during the aging process.

To review, the first five are: (1) oxidative damage caused by free radical molecules; (2) damage to the genetic material and reduced repair mechanisms in mitochondrial DNA; (3) impaired detoxification and the accumulation of toxic chemicals; (4) dysregulation of glucose metabolism and insulin resistance; and (5) advanced protein glycation and degradation.

Chronic tissue inflammation, the topic for this chapter, is an insidiously destructive biochemical and physiological state involving the erosion of a wide range of molecular and cellular processes. These result in gradual tissue damage that causes many of the age-related diseases and accelerates the aging process.

In this chapter, we explore how chronic inflammation participates in these diseases and the aging process. Due to its critical importance in the development and progression of age-related diseases and aging itself, let's first review the processes that contribute to chronic inflammation to understand why it is so devastating and how best to prevent and reduce it.

Acute Inflammation Is a Normal Reaction of Our Immune System

Our immune system responds to infection from pathogenic microorganisms, such as bacteria and viruses, and to tissue damage caused by physical or chemical trauma by a complex process involving inflammation. This is concurrent with a variety of immunological molecular and cellular events such as the activation of lymphocytes—a class of immune cells. Inflammation is closely associated with immune biochemical activity and phagocytosis—the ingestion or "eating" of foreign or diseased substances by macrophages, immune cells involved in innate or first-line immunity, which initiate inflammation. This first immune activity occurs within minutes to a few hours after infection or trauma, and collectively is known as the inflammatory response.

We are all familiar with acute inflammation such as the redness and swelling that occur around the skin when a foreign object (such as a sliver of wood) enters the tissue or when you scrape your knee. We know the swelling, heat, and pain associated with a twisted ankle, or the headache, facial pressure, and fever that can accompany a sinus infection. Acute inflammation is a well-known medical event and is characterized by redness, swelling, heat, soreness, and pain.

As part of the inflammatory response, macrophages secrete immune substances. There are biochemical response mediators called cytokines, proteins that affect the behavior of other cells involved in the immune response. They recruit other immune cells into the infected or damaged area to remove the foreign invader so healing can take place.

Cytokines induce expansion of local capillaries to increase blood flow to the inflamed area, which contributes to the redness and heat and facilitates the movement of fluid into the area, causing swelling. But this allows easier infiltration of immune cells into the inflamed area for the purpose of heightened immune activity. We are just beginning to learn more about the many activities of cytokines, but we are certain that they play significant roles in normal as well as abnormal inflammatory conditions that participate in disease and aging.

The main inflammatory cytokines produced by macrophages are interleukin-1 (IL-1), interleukin-6 (IL-6) (Saito et al. 2000), interleukin-8 (IL-8), interleukin-12 (IL-12), and tumor necrosis factor-alpha (TNF-alpha) (Parham 2000). These potent cytokines, especially TNF-alpha, and other substances such as histamine, are referred to as inflammatory mediators or pro-inflammatory substances. They not only initiate local effects, but can also cause systemic inflammation throughout the body, including fever, fatigue, and malaise. This response is called acute inflammation and is a normal reaction of the immune system against a foreign substance.

Let's look at the effects of one of these pro-inflammatory cytokines. TNF-alpha is a powerful inflammatory mediator that exerts both beneficial and detrimental effects in the body. On the local level during an acute inflammation, it is released by macrophages and induces increased immune cell activity, facilitating resolution of the infection. But when TNF-alpha and other pro-inflammatory substances spread into the bloodstream, they can cause catastrophic systemic effects.

For example, a viral infection in the liver activates macrophages to secrete TNF-alpha, causing local inflammation and activation of other immune cells. Excess amounts of TNF-alpha may spill into the bloodstream, causing inflammation in other parts of the body. The swelling caused by the inflammatory response may decrease blood volume to local tissue in the liver; this results in reduced blood supply and tissue damage or even organ failure. A similar scenario could happen in the brain, heart, kidneys, and other tissues. For reasons such as this, it is necessary to manage chronic systemic inflammation in order to prevent degenerative disease, prolong health, and promote longevity.

Chronic Inflammation Is Destructive to the Body and Causes Accelerated Aging

Unlike simple acute inflammation in response to a bacterial or viral infection, or trauma, the development of chronic inflammation is a complex process. It involves body-wide disruption of normal immune chemistry and hormonal imbalances. It further entails protein glycation, accumulative oxidative stress and accompanying free radical damage, chronic infection, and the disruption of the normal function of fatty acids in the body.

Chronic inflammation is a condition of *ongoing* tissue irritation and may not show obvious symptoms for decades, but it can be more destructive to vital tissue over time than acute inflammation. So to effectively prolong your health and extend your life span, chronic inflammation and its effects must be controlled and eliminated.

Pain and chronic inflammation go together. An example of low-grade chronic inflammation is the typical aches and pains associated with aging, usually involving the joints and ligaments as occurs with arthritis, and that cause stiffness in the knees or hands. These are relatively minor symptoms of underlying chronic inflammation compared with the devastation going on unseen in your blood vessels, brain cells, and other tissues. More active chronic inflammatory mechanisms can cause severe pain.

Unlike acute or minor transitory inflammation, chronic inflammation can trigger complex chemical reactions in your body and is implicated in a number of diseases including heart attack, stroke, many types of cancer, fibrositis and fibromyalgia, arthritis, autoimmune diseases such as rheumatoid arthritis, colitis and irritable bowel syndrome, and Alzeheimer's disease. In fact, conditions associated with chronic inflammation are so common that some researchers call it "the epidemic disease of aging" (Faloon 2002).

The three most studied of the inflammatory diseases are autoimmune diseases such as rheumatoid arthritis, Alzheimer's disease, and atherosclerosis (Brod 2000). Though all of them occur frequently in aging, let's briefly discuss atherosclerosis as an example of the results of chronic inflammation.

Atherosclerosis As an Inflammatory Disease: This is a condition of the arterial walls, characterized by the buildup of fatty plaques and lesions, that eventually leads to heart disease, and it illustrates how inflammatory changes occur in your body. Atherosclerosis was once thought to be simply a process of accumulated fat buildup caused by high cholesterol, but researchers have now discovered that cholesterol has more complicated roles.

Low-density lipoproteins (LDL–the "bad" cholesterol), composed of lipids (fatty substances) and proteins, transport cholesterol from its absorption locations in the small intes-

Chronic inflammation is a condition of ongoing tissue irritation and may not show obvious symptoms for decades, but it can be more destructive to vital tissue over time than acute inflammation. So to effectively prolong your health and extend your life span, chronic inflammation and its effects must be controlled and eliminated.

tine and processing sites in the liver to other parts of the body. Excess LDL and high levels of cholesterol (due to a high fat diet, excess dietary sugars, or faulty lipid metabolism) promote atherosclerosis, which begins when excess LDL particles accumulate in the arteries.

As LDL collects in the inner walls of the arteries, their lipid parts are oxidized and their protein components both are oxidized and undergo glycation (a caramelizing process, see chapter 11). The immune system interprets these changes as harmful and mobilizes the monocytes (a type of white blood cell involved in the initial phase of the immune response) into the area of the oxidized LDL. Immune messenger chemicals called cytokines participate in "telling" the monocytes where the damage is.

When large amounts of LDL are oxidized, the immune system induces the monocytes to enlarge into macrophages. These are large white cells that engulf and digest foreign substances in a process called phagocytosis. If there are large numbers of LDL particles, the macrophages can become so bloated with fatty material that they are called "foam cells," because of their foamy appearance. High LDL blood levels perpetuate this immune activity and cause chronic inflammation.

Other immune activity takes place in response to LDL oxidation. This includes an increased level of T lymphocytes (T cells), immune cells involved in cell-mediated or second-stage immunity. T cells release numerous cytokines, many of which promote inflammation. The combination of immune cell activity and pro-inflammatory cytokine release causes further deterioration of the blood vessel walls. Though this destructive process may go unnoticed for decades, eventually the plaques push inward from the vessel wall, blocking blood flow. Restricted blood flow can lead to more tissue damage. If it occurs in the heart, it may cause cardiovascular disease or a heart attack; if in the brain, a stroke. This example of atherosclerosis shows us that chronic inflammation is tissue destructive, influences disease progression and outcome, and accelerates aging.

Though we still do not understand exactly why chronic inflammation occurs, we are gathering a considerable body of research information about its processes, especially how cytokines, the chemical mediators of the immune response, are involved. Among the most implicated of these is TNF-alpha, which can lead to catastrophic effects when released systemically in the body. One of the initial effects of excess TNF-alpha is on the inner lining of the blood vessels, which participates in the onset of atherosclerosis. Excess TNF-alpha is associated with liver damage, kidney disease, and destruction of brain tissue.

Inflammation may be involved in some aspects of declining brain function during aging (Toliver-Kinsky 1997). Researchers at the University of Rome in Italy found that chronic inflammation is present in the aging brain along with increased levels of TNF-alpha (Casolini 2002). This suggests that the pro-inflammatory cytokines TNF-alpha and IL-6 are present in the brain's blood vessels and nerve cells during aging and may contribute to the progression of Alzheimer's and dementia (Wilson 2002).

Higher cytokine levels, particularly of IL-6 and TNF-alpha, have been found in the muscle tissue of older men and women. The inflammation that they produce is implicated in sacropenia, the loss of muscle mass and strength seen in older individuals (Visser 2002). Leukotriene B4 (LTB4) (Haeggstrom 2002) and interleukin-1 beta (IL-1ß) (Casolini 2002) are other pro-inflammatory cytokines commonly associated with chronic inflammation during aging.

Besides cytokines, several other pro-inflammatory substances are involved in chronic inflammation. These include chemokines, a family of proteins that attracts phagocytes to infected tissue; the interferon family of cytokines such as interleukin-1 beta; as well the pro-inflammatory proteins C-reactive protein, homocysteine, and beta-amyloid. Hormone deficiency, abnormal fatty acid metabolism, and other factors are also involved here. Let's consider these and some other causes of chronic inflammation.

C-REACTIVE PROTEIN (CRP): This is a signaling molecule whose levels become elevated in the presence of inflammation and that is intimately linked to chronic inflammation. CRP, a protein produced by the liver, interacts with the complement system, a group of proteins that circulate in the blood and coordinate or complement the immune response to infection. CRP is generally only present during acute inflammation of the innate immune response, especially in bacterial infections. However, elevations also occur in autoimmune conditions, such as rheumatoid arthritis or lupus, and in heart disease; recent research indicates that elevated CRP may also be associated with Alzheimer's disease, arthritis, and metastatic cancer.

Researchers have found that not only are CRP levels elevated in these diseases, but often older people have greater CRP concentrations than younger individuals (Ballou 1996). I routinely order blood tests for CRP levels in all suspected cases of chronic inflammation, as a screening test for cardiovascular disease, and as a marker for age-related inflammation.

HOMOCYSTEINE: This is a toxic amino acid produced during methionine metabolism, one of the liver's detoxification pathways. Defects in the detoxification of homocysteine result in increased levels of it in the blood, which lead to detrimental effects, including irritation to the lining of the blood vessels and the brain (Myers 2002). Homocysteine actively participates in the process that produces chronic inflammation. Elevated levels of homocysteine are thought to be a sign of malfunction in the liver's methylation cycle.

The methylation cycle has two functions. One of them ensures that cells have enough S-adenosylmethionine, an activated form of the amino acid methionine. S-adenosylmethione works with enzymes that help synthesize hormones, lipids, proteins, and DNA. Methylation is a process important for DNA repair and the growth of new cells, and it helps regulate gene expression. To regulate how genes express information, sets of proteins attach to part of

the DNA. One of these protein sets is a methyl group; it plays an important role in determining whether a gene is expressed or is not.

Unhealthy aging cells are subjected to demethylation, and when unable to undergo normal methylation, they age more rapidly. Homocysteine is thought to participate in the demethylation process, and elevated homocysteine levels are thought to play a role in the chronic inflammation that accompanies heart disease and is associated with unhealthy aging (McCarty 2000).

Excess amounts of the amino acid methionine in the diet can also contribute to elevated homocysteine levels. Methionine is an essential amino acid, but Americans get 60 percent more of it than is necessary. Too much methionine can be difficult for the liver to break down; the remaining methionine is converted to homocysteine via the methylation cycle.

Under normal circumstances, homocysteine is converted into harmless substances such as cysteine. This is a neutral amino acid involved in only a very small percentage of proteins, but critical to the metabolism of a number of essential substances including several antioxidants such as lipoic acid and glutathione. Excess homocysteine is associated with chronic inflammation and is measured in a simple blood test that your doctor can order from any clinical laboratory (SoRelle 2002). I routinely order homocysteine levels on all my patients over 45 years and for younger ones who have a family history of cardiovascular disease.

BETA-AMYLOID: Brain injury from oxidative damage, infections, excess cholesterol, and lack of oxygen to local tissues triggers inflammation as part of an immune response. Amyloid is a protein involved in response to injury. However, too much amyloid can build up in brain tissue and set off a series of biochemical and immunological reactions called an amyloid cascade (Racchi 2003). Amyloid, once deposited in tissues, promotes oxidative damage and protein glycation, and this can cause chronic inflammation. Sixteen different abnormal amyloid proteins have been identified, though beta-amyloid is the most studied of these and is associated with Alzheimer's, cardiovascular disease, and Type II diabetes.

DECLINING HORMONE LEVELS: As we age, our hormone levels decline. Researchers found that as estrogen levels drop, there is a spontaneous increase in the pro-inflammatory cytokines IL-1, IL-6, and TNF-alpha (Bland 2003). Lower testosterone and DHEA levels are also associated with chronic inflammation (Straub 2000, 2002).

ABNORMAL FATTY ACID METABOLISM: Excessive consumption of saturated and trans-fatty acids as found in margarines and processed foods disrupts normal fatty acid metabolism. This causes an unfavorable imbalance between omega-3 (the good fatty acids) and omega-6 fatty acids. High-saturated-fat diets lead to obesity, insulin resistance, cardiovascular disease, and chronic inflammation.

INFECTIONS: Even microorganisms such as viruses in the human herpes virus family, a common infection in humans, and the bacterium *Chlamydia pneumonia,* also quite common, can trigger the immune system's inflammatory response. These are associated with conditions such as cardiovascular disease and Alzheimer's disease in which chronic inflammation plays a key role. Other commonly occurring bacteria, viruses, waterborne parasites such as *Cryptosporidium* and *Giardia,* yeast and fungi such as *Candida albicans,* and the toxins that these microorganisms produce (called endotoxins) are also implicated in chronic inflammation (Saito 2001).

IMBALANCED GASTROINTESTINAL ENVIRONMENT: Many diseases can cause chronic inflam-

mation, the principal one being diabetes, but an imbalanced gastrointestinal environment, especially of the flora in the large intestine, can contribute greatly to systemic inflammation in the body. From the natural medicine perspective, the underlying cause of many chronic diseases is chronic inflammation in the gut and other mucous membrane areas, such as the sinuses.

The mucous membranes that line the nasal and sinus cavities, the respiratory tract, and entire digestive system are the area of first contact for the majority of infectious microbes, allergens, and toxic foreign chemicals. Because of the high level of exposure to these environmental stressors, the mucous membranes have evolved their own complex immunological functions, collectively referred to as mucosal immunity. The primary way to enhance mucosal immunity is through maintaining a healthy gut by supplementing the diet with probiotics such as *Lactobacillus acidophilus,* a naturally occurring "friendly" bacteria found in yogurt or supplied in capsules or powder forms.

PHYSICAL AND EMOTIONAL STRESS: When you overexercise, repetitive tissue and joint trauma trigger the inflammatory response. This results in pain and stiffness in the joints and muscles. Excessive exercise can also increase oxidative damage and contribute to chronic inflammation.

Emotional stress plays a significant role as an underlying condition that sets the stage for inflammation. In response to physical or emotional stress, the pituitary and other hormone-secreting glands in the brain signal the adrenal glands to produce increased levels of stress hormones such as adrenaline. Chronic stress, such as we experience from the fast, demanding pace of modern life, not only causes abnormal levels of adrenaline, but results in imbalances in cortisol, a major hormone produced by the outer cortex of the adrenal gland.

A normal stress hormone response helps modulate inflammation, but high levels of cortisol can produce inflammation and damage sensitive brain tissue in the hypothalamus, one of the body's control centers. These stress-induced changes also cause an activation of immune defenses that can trigger a cascade of other imbalances, resulting in altered gene expression. As a result, chronic tissue inflammation occurs, which further alters gene function and contributes to aging.

This "shift towards inflammation" (Bland 1998) is part of a chain of interlinked metabolic and biochemical events that predisposes us to degenerative diseases, reduces our quality of life, and accelerates our biological aging.

Not only are immunological conditions causes of inflammation, but many of the conditions discussed in previous chapters are linked to chronic inflammation and aging. These include all the conditions caused by oxidative stress, insulin resistance, and protein glycation. The list of inflammatory relationships with aging is thus extensive, suggesting that inflammation accompanies aging and is a causative factor for accelerated aging. In essence, inflammation and its causes disturb homeostasis and precipitate a wide range of conditions associated with aging. In fact, chronic inflammation appears to be one of the characteristic hallmarks of aging. It accompanies all the diseases associated with aging including diabetes, cardiovascular disease, cancer, and Alzheimer's. So to prolong health and achieve maximum life span, it is mandatory to prevent the body's shift towards inflammation.

How to Prevent and Reduce Chronic Inflammation

Acute inflammation results from an obvious and perhaps single event and generally resolves on its own. Chronic inflammation, however, is different. It results from a *combination* of genetic, lifestyle, dietary, immune-driven, neuroendocrine regulated, and cellular mechanisms, and it tends to *persist;* therefore, it requires a comprehensive treatment approach.

As in all diseases, prevention is better than cure, so you may prevent chronic inflammation by following the *Prolonging Health* recommendations and strategies, as these reduce inflammatory activity in the body. You do this by maintaining the correct balance of dietary fats; supplementing with docosahexaenoic acid (DHA) from fish oil; taking antioxidants; improving glucose control; and using hormones such as DHEA, testosterone, and estrogen.

Exercise, effective stress management, getting adequate rest and uninterrupted deep sleep also help manage the effects of chronic inflammation. They reduce the reservoirs of inflammation that occur in the gastrointestinal tract and other mucous membrane areas such as the sinus, and they lower the pathogenic microbial load on the body.

Nutrient supplementation is also helpful. For example, the amino acids arginine and glutamine have anti-inflammatory effects (Kelly 2003). Researchers at the University of North Carolina at Chapel Hill, North Carolina, found that the amino acid L-glycine also has potential as a natural anti-inflammatory. In addition, it can protect cells from toxic chemicals and infections; lessens liver, kidney, and heart damage; and exerts a positive modulating effect on the immune system (Kelly 2003). Let's consider some natural anti-inflammatory medications.

Prolonging Health Recommendation 25— Get Tested for Chronic Inflammation

If you have insulin resistance, Type II diabetes, cardiovascular disease, an autoimmune condition, psoriasis or other skin disorders, osteoarthritis or chronic pain, a chronic viral infection, irritable bowel disease, Crohn's disease, or colitis, get tested for chronic inflammation. These tests include homocysteine, C-reactive protein, and sedimentation rate. Include TNF-alpha and IL-6 if you have a family history of cardiovascular or Alzheimer's disease.

Homocysteine: The general medical consensus for safe homocysteine levels is less than 12–15 micromoles per liter (μmol/L), though some studies indicate that less than 10 μmol/L is a safe upper limit (Andreotti, Burzotta, et al. 1999). However, since higher levels of homocysteine are associated with a greater risk for coronary artery disease and stroke and lower levels with a lower risk, it makes sense that you should keep your homocysteine levels as low as possible.

Drawing on newer scientific evidence, physicians practicing anti-aging medicine or naturopathic-influenced forms of medicine now agree that there are no safe levels for homocysteine. In my practice, I actively work with patients who have elevated homocysteine levels to lower these to less than 5 μmol/L as the optimal goal.

C-Reactive Protein: CRP levels greater than 2.1 mg/L for men and 7.3 mg/L for women indicate an increased risk for cardiovascular and other diseases. To prevent a heart attack or stroke and to prolong your health, I recommend that you keep your CRP levels below 0.5 mg/L.

Sedimentation Rate: The erythrocyte sedimentation rate (ESR or "sed rate") is the most commonly used test to measure generalized inflammatory activity and is useful as a screening test for active inflammation in rheumatoid arthritis and other autoimmune diseases. It is elevated in a wide range of inflammatory conditions and infectious ill-nesses. The ESR measures how fast the red blood cells, or erythrocytes, settle to form sediment in a test tube. Normal values are less than 20 millimeters per hour (mm/hr); however, the lower the value the better. I like my patients to have a level of 0–5 mm/hr.

TNF-Alpha and Interleukin-6: If you have elevated levels of these pro-inflammatory cytokines, most likely you have chronic inflammation. Keep TNF-alpha levels under 8.1 pg/mL and IL-6 levels below 12.0 pg/mL.

Prolonging Health Recommendation 26— Avoid Foods That Promote Inflammation

Do not eat processed spreads and oils, margarines, fatty cuts of meats, organ meats (liver, kidney), or refined sugar and carbohydrates and other high glycemic index foods. Since allergic reactions can trigger inflammation, avoid foods that cause you any gastrointestinal sensitivity or other allergic reactions such as itching or swellings. Though methionine is an essential amino acid and too low levels are related to memory loss and dementia, too much methionine may increase homocysteine. So, be aware of high methionine-containing foods and do not overconsume them. Foods high in methionine include eggs, cheddar cheese, chicken breast, and soy.

Prolonging Health Recommendation 27— Consume Foods That Reduce Inflammation

Studies have shown that foods rich in natural antioxidants reverse the effects of chronic inflammation (Gemma 2002). Consume more fish, cold-processed olive oil, and fresh fruits and vegetables; take one tablespoon of organic flax oil daily with food; eat more avocados, seeds, and nuts; and take green food supplements such as spirulina and chlorella.

Prolonging Health Recommendation 28— Take Probiotics

Enhance your mucosal and general immunity, and lower inflammation in the intestinal tract by replenishing the "friendly" bacteria called probiotics (Erickson 2000). These exert a significant influence on both physiological and pathological processes in the body and can indirectly lower inflammation. Numerous commercial probiotic medications are available from health food stores, compounding pharmacies, or from your doctor's office.

I recommended beginning with a robust species such as *Lactobacillus sporogenes*, a harmless type of bacterium occurring naturally in the intestines, which constitutes a major part of the intestinal environment. *L. sporogenes* is very stable, has a long life, and is resistant to high temperatures, gastric acid, and bile, making it a good choice for re-colonization of the gut with "friendly" bacteria. Take two 150 mg capsules (containing 1.5 billion units each) twice daily with warm water. Other species are also useful: *Lactobacillus acidophilus* and *Bifidobacterium bifidus; Lactobacillus casei;* and *Streptococcus thermophilus* species.

Yogurt is known for its many health advantages including beneficial effects on cancer, chronic infections, gastrointestinal disorders, and asthma, as well as the aging process. It contains numerous probiotic species that promote health (Meydani 2000). The preferred form of yogurt is from natural organic milk without sugar, gelatin, or other additives, and without fruit syrups; add your own flavoring, such as fresh fruit, berries, maple syrup, or vanilla. If you are not allergic to milk products, try a half-cup of fresh natural yogurt daily.

Probiotic microorganisms thrive best in a medium of non-digestible dietary substances called prebiotics. These facilitate the growth and colonization of "friendly" probiotic bacteria. The most-well studied of the prebiotics are inulin and oligofructose (Gibson 1999) derived from a wide variety of starchy grains, vegetables, and fruits such as wheat, onion, garlic, raisins, and Jerusalem artichokes.

Oligofructose is a sweet, pleasant-tasting sub-group of inulin commercially prepared from chicory root or other substances. It is classified as a soluble dietary fiber, which is a dietary substance, but neither a fiber nor carbohydrate, that passes through the small intestine without being absorbed. It promotes normal fermentation in the large intestine. Consume a commercial prebiotic blend when taking probiotics to give your system an initial boost. Follow the manufacturer's directions provided with your choice of prebiotic.

Before you supplement your diet with pre- and probiotics, you may want to ask your doctor to perform a comprehensive stool analysis to evaluate the number of the existing friendly bacteria in your large intestine. Though useful, this is not necessary and you can safely take probiotics without doing this.

Prolonging Health Recommendation 29— Take Fish Oil

Balance omega-6 and omega-3 fatty acids, by eliminating all processed fats and oils (soy margarines, flame-broiled meats, cured sandwich meats, cheese spreads, commercial salad dressings, and fast foods) from your diet. Take 500–1,500 mg daily of fish oil providing at least 300 mg of eicosapentaenoic acid (EPA) and 200 mg of docosahexaenoic acid (DHA) per 1,000 mg of oil. Eat more coldwater fish such as salmon and halibut.

Prolonging Health Recommendation 30— Take Folic Acid, Vitamin B$_6$, and Vitamin B$_{12}$

If your homocysteine levels are above 9 μmol/L, or your levels of C-reactive protein are high, increase your intake of vitamins B$_6$, B$_{12}$, and folic acid. During aging, the absorption and metabolism of these important vitamins, particularly of B$_{12}$ (Carmel 1997), tend to decline. Research has shown that low levels of B$_6$ are associated with inflammation and high levels of both homocysteine and C-reactive protein (Frisco 2001). Take 800 mcg of 5-methyltetrahydrofolate; 50 mg of vitamin B$_6$; and 2,000 mcg of methylcobalamin daily.

Prolonging Health Recommendation 31— Take TMG

Trimethylglycine (TMG) or betaine has methylation functions in the body similar to those of folic acid, vitamin B$_{12}$, and methionine. It is metabolized from choline (tetramethylglycine), a substance also involved in methylation. TMG helps to lower homocysteine levels; it improves liver function; and it plays a role in the synthesis of the amino acid L-carnitine. Take 1,000 mg of betaine hydrochloride following each meal. Other than occasional nausea, TMG has no side effects or contraindications.

Prolonging Health Recommendation 32— Take Niacinamide

A nutritional substance related to niacin but without the typical and often uncomfortable flushing effect caused by the vasodilating activity of niacin, niacinamide is itself a member of the B-vitamin family. It is an antioxidant, helps manage the arthritic inflammation commonly seen during aging, and may also have antidiabetic and anticancer activity. You can take it in dosages up to 450 mg three times daily to reduce joint pain. Niacinamide is a safe substance, but can cause nausea in people with liver disease, in which case it is contraindicated.

Prolonging Health Recommendation 33— Use Red Yeast Rice Extract

Researchers have shown that the cholesterol-lowering statin drugs such as simvastatin (Zocor) lower C-reactive protein levels (Plenge 2002) and may have anti-inflammatory effects in patients with rheumatoid arthritis (Kanda 2002). Unfortunately, these drugs are not free of potential side effects, including liver and kidney problems, making them unsuitable for many patients. For those preferring a natural alternative to synthetic statin drugs, red yeast rice extract, a naturally occurring statin (lovastatin), is useful in lowering C-reactive protein levels (Patrick 2001).

Red yeast rice extract is prepared from the fermented products of the mold *Monascus purpureus* and has a recorded use in China that dates back as far as 800 A.D., when it was first used to ferment rice wine. In addition to its cholesterol-lowering (Heber, Yip, et al. 1999) and anti-inflammatory properties, red yeast rice extract may protect us against some forms of cancer; it also has antioxidant effects.

In general, red yeast rice is a safe substance though some people report heartburn and abdominal bloating when taking it. In sensitive individuals one of its components, the HMG-CoA inhibitors, may cause liver damage; this product should not be taken by people with liver disease.

Red yeast rice extract is not standardized, and some brands contain high levels of citrinin, a potent naturally occurring antibiotic that can cause kidney damage. Only take products without or with low levels of citrinin, and do not use red yeast rice if you have kidney disease. Do not take red yeast rice extracts when using prescription statin drugs. The average dosage is 2,000–3,000 mg, three times daily.

Prolonging Health Recommendation 34— Take Anti-Inflammatory Herbs

A number of Asian herbal medications have anti-inflammatory activity. Traditional Chinese medicine, in particular, has a wealth of herbal anti-inflammatory formulas. What is fascinating about the Chinese method of treating chronic inflammation, especially in older people, is that invariably anti-inflammatory medications are combined with tonic remedies such as small amounts of ginseng, to improve a low energy status that frequently accompanies inflammatory disorders. Since it is impractical to discuss all the Chinese formulas available that treat inflammatory conditions, if you are interested in this form of treatment, I suggest you seek the services of a licensed doctor of Chinese medicine who specializes in herbal formulas for chronic inflammation. Here are two that have proven anti-inflammatory benefits.

Boswellia Extract: Derived from a bush found throughout Asia and known for its aromatic resin containing boswellic acids, boswellia (*Boswellia serrata*) helps to reduce chronic liver inflammation associated with hepatitis, joint inflammation from arthritis, asthma (Gupta 1998), and colitis (Gupta 2001). It has anti-tumor properties (Huang 2000) and may be useful in the generalized inflammation associated with aging. It is considered a safe substance. Take 200 mg of boswellia extract, two times daily.

Curcumin Extract: Another Asian herbal medicine, related to the common household spice turmeric (*Curcuma longa*) that gives Indian curry dishes their bright yellow color, curcumin is a superstar among medicines to manage inflammation. Researchers have demonstrated curcumin's remedial effects in a variety of studies. For example, it protects against nerve cell damage in Alzheimer's disease (Park 2002), and it has been shown to counter the xenoestrogenic (estrogen-mimicking) effects of toxic environmental chemicals (Verma 1998).

However, curcumin is best known for its anti-tumor activity in a variety of cancers including prostate (Nakamura 2002), pancreatic (Hidaka 2002), and leukemia (Han 2002). It is considered a safe herb without side effects when taken in the recommended dosages, and there are no known drug interactions. The typical dosage is 300–600 mg of the standardized extract (containing 90–95 percent curcumin) taken two times daily.

A variety of conditions cause chronic inflammation, and all are associated with declining health, degenerative disease, and aging. The five most common causes of chronic inflammation are: (1) poor diet; (2) dysfunctional glucose metabolism and insulin resistance; (3) deficiency of steroid hormones; (4) insufficient omega-3 essential fatty acids; and (5) abnormal gut flora. Chronic inflammation is associated with elevated levels of homocysteine and deficiencies in vitamins B_6, B_{12}, and folic acid. In order to prolong health and achieve maximum life span, prevent and effectively manage inflammation.

Summary of Prolonging Health Recommendations to Reduce Chronic Inflammation

- *Prolonging Health* Recommendation 25— Get Tested for Chronic Inflammation: If you have chronic inflammation, get a blood test for homocysteine, C-reactive protein, and sedimentation rate. Get tested for TNF-alpha and IL-6 if you have a family history of cardiovascular or Alzheimer's disease.

- *Prolonging Health* **Recommendation 26— Avoid Foods That Promote Inflammation:** Don't eat processed spreads and oils, margarines, fatty cuts of meats, organ meats (liver, kidney), or refined sugar and carbohydrates and other high glycemic index foods. Avoid foods that cause you allergic reactions.

- *Prolonging Health* **Recommendation 27— Consume Foods That Reduce Inflammation:** Eat foods rich in natural antioxidants such as fish, cold-processed olive oil, and fresh fruits and vegetables; take one tablespoon of organic flax oil daily with food; eat more avocados, seeds, and nuts; and take green food supplements such as spirulina and chlorella.

- *Prolonging Health* **Recommendation 28— Take Probiotics:** Replenish the friendly intestinal bacteria in your intestine with probiotics. Take two 150 mg capsules of *Lactobacillus sporogenes* twice daily with warm water. You can take other probiotics such as *Lactobacillus acidophilus, Bifidobacterium bifidus, Lactobacillus casei,* and *Streptococcus thermophilus.* Consume yogurt made from natural organic milk. Take prebiotics such as inulin and oligofructose, and eat more vegetables and fruits.

- *Prolonging Health* **Recommendation 29— Take Fish Oil:** Balance omega-6 and omega-3 fatty acids by eliminating all processed fats and oils (soy margarines, flame broiled meats, cured sandwich meats, cheese spreads, commercial salad dressings, and fast foods) from your diet. Take 500–1,500 mg of fish oil daily providing at least 300 mg of eicosapentaenoic acid (EPA) and 200 mg of docosahexaenoic acid (DHA) per 1,000 mg of oil. Eat more coldwater fish like salmon and halibut.

- *Prolonging Health* **Recommendation 30— Take Folic Acid, Vitamin B_6, and Vitamin B_{12}:** Take 800 mcg of 5-methyltetrahydrofolate; 50 mg of vitamin B_6; and 2,000 mcg of methylcobalamin daily.

- *Prolonging Health* **Recommendation 31— Take TMG:** Take 1,000 mg of betaine hydrochloride following each meal.

- *Prolonging Health* **Recommendation 32— Take Niacinamide:** If you have arthritis, take 450 mg three times daily to reduce joint pain.

- *Prolonging Health* **Recommendation 33— Use Red Yeast Rice Extract:** If you have elevated cholesterol and/or cardiovascular disease, take 2,000–3,000 mg three times daily.

- *Prolonging Health* **Recommendation 34— Take Anti-Inflammatory Herbs:** Take 200 mg of boswellia extract and 300–600 mg of standardized curcumin extract (containing 90–95 percent curcumin), two times daily.

13 *Prolonging Health* Modifiable Aging Factor 7: Impaired Cardiovascular Function and Sticky Blood—How to Strengthen Your Heart

Among my elderly patients, the longest lived and most active—barring cancer or accidents—are those with the strongest hearts. One such patient is Eve, a 99-year-old with arthritis. She recently moved from Southern California to Florida to spend her one hundredth birthday with her retired daughter and family. Another is Pamela, an 86-year-old who continues to drive and remain active with dancing and yoga. My mother, Bernice, is another example, who at 89 continues an active life free of cancer and major degenerative diseases. The common denominator in all three women, though of advanced age, is that they have strong and healthy hearts, normal cholesterol levels, and no signs of inflammation (based on blood tests).

Since your heart is so vital to life, health, and longevity, keep in mind as you read this book and go about your *Prolonging Health* practice that it is not those who take the most nutritional supplements, or who attend the most anti-aging seminars, or who use the strongest hormones who live the longest. It is those whose hearts can sustain the repeated stresses and strains of daily life, are immune to infection, and function efficiently. These are the ones who achieve their maximum life span. I think of it in terms of the '64 Chevrolet I owned

as a young man; nothing much to look at, it served me year after year, and while the seats were worn and the paint peeling, the engine started without fail every time with a single turn of the key. That was a car with a good "heart."

One of the common tenets of *Prolonging Health* is that to achieve your maximum life span your heart must be genetically strong and remain physiologically healthy. However, if your lifestyle does not support health, your quality of life will be poor since the heart will keep pumping even if the rest of your body develops age-related conditions such as osteoporosis, arthritis, and hormonal deficiencies. That is why, even if your heart is strong, you should follow all the other principles and strategies in this book, including taking antioxidant supplements and getting exercise to prolong your health so you can live a long and active life.

People with good cardiac function generally don't have diabetes or suffer from insulin resistance. Conversely, those who prevent and correct glucose-related problems such as insulin resistance have less risk for heart disease. They also have a strong immune system that protects their heart from viral and bacterial infections that damage the vessels, valves, and heart tissue. People with healthy cardiovascular systems have better blood flow to their brain and therefore less Alzheimer's disease, as well as better memory and cognition than older people who have heart problems. Therefore, a strong heart plus a good vascular system is necessary in order to live long and healthily, to be hale and hearty.

A healthy heart is particularly important for Americans, who have one of the highest rates of heart disease in the world. According to the American Heart Association, cardiovascular disease has been the leading cause of death in the United States since 1900, with the exception of 1918 when the Spanish Flu epidemic and loss of life during World War I took more

One of the common tenets of Prolonging Health is that to achieve your maximum life span your heart must be genetically strong and remain physiologically healthy. However, if your lifestyle does not support health, your quality of life will be poor since the heart will keep pumping even if the rest of your body develops age-related conditions such as osteoporosis, arthritis, and hormonal deficiencies.

lives (AHA 2001). Currently, 61,800,000 Americans have some form of cardiovascular disease, which causes 60 percent of all deaths and killed 945,836 people in 2000. The second cause of death is cancer, killing 555,500 (Society 2002), while AIDS only killed 14,802 people during the same time period.

According to the World Health Organiza-

tion, the highest rate of cardiovascular disease in the world is in Finland and the lowest rates are in Catalonia, Spain; Beijing, China; Toulouse, France; and Biranza, Italy. In China, where people eat little red meat, more vegetables and soy foods, and less sugar than Americans, they have the lowest rates of heart disease. Therefore, we should learn from the Chinese example that our food intake shapes our health and to a large degree determines our longevity through the positive expression of our most health-enhancing genes. Okinawans are another example of a people with healthy cardiovascular systems, as they have 80 percent less cardiovascular disease than Americans.

It's true that diet and genes influence our propensity for heart disease, but gender itself is one of the other main determinants. Men are particularly at risk for fatal heart disease; compared to women, men are by far the "weaker" sex with a 1.8 times greater risk of dying from heart disease than women, who have most of their heart attacks after age 75. In contrast, most American men are dead by then, as an average life span for American men is only 73.8 years.

At 40, most men feel that they're "not as young as they used to be," and at 50, that suspicion can be a daily reminder. Remember, these are average statistics and tell nothing about your individual state of health. My patients who practice the life-enhancing *Prolonging Health* strategies typically beat these statistics. For example, Matt is a 45-year-old entrepreneur who not only plays a vigorous game of basketball every week, but also regularly trumps players half his age. Of course, he exercises throughout the week, including weight training under the supervision of a professional trainer, aerobic activity on the basketball court, and salsa dancing several times a week. In fact, each year Matt tells me that he feels better than he used to, instead of worse, like most American men.

Men typically not only have more heart disease than women, but also are at a greater risk for cancer, liver disease, diabetes, and kidney disease, and have a higher incidence of death from accidents and suicide. Therefore, though this book is written for both men and women, it is highly important that men reading this, or wives of men who want their husbands to be healthier, pay close attention to this chapter. If you are male, keep the statistics in mind, but don't let them dictate your life because men can retain their optimal health and vigor, as well as a youthful physique and sexual attraction, well into their late fifties, and even older.

Protecting your heart and circulatory system are vital to your *Prolonging Health* program. In this chapter we explore the cardiovascular system and its importance in maintaining homeostasis, as well as the prevention of age-related cardiovascular diseases, how to keep your heart healthy, and how to improve blood quality and viscosity.

The Cardiovascular System's Role in Homeostasis

The cardiovascular system is composed of the heart, blood vessels, and blood. The heart, a fist-sized muscle situated behind your ribs and breastbone (sternum) to the left of center in your chest and just above the nipple line, is a small powerful muscle that pumps 1.5 gallons of blood per minute throughout your body via the blood vessels. The average adult has about ten pints of blood, made up of a liquid part called plasma and solid components made up of red blood cells, white blood cells, and platelets. The plasma is 92 percent water and contains vitamins, minerals, proteins, lipids, hormones, and other substances, including gases. All of the cells that make up the tissues in your body require oxygen, which is carried to them by the red blood cells.

In order to survive, key aspects of your physiology must be kept within very tight limits, including body temperature, glucose levels, heart rate, and blood pressure. The central and autonomic nervous systems and the endocrine system, collectively referred to as the neuroendocrine system, regulate these functions to maintain homeostasis.

Homeostasis is the equilibrium your body maintains between the external environment and its internal functions in order to survive, reproduce, maintain health, and prolong health for the purpose of maximizing individual life span. Homeostasis is affected by thermodynamics and glucose regulation, but there are cardiovascular implications to homeostasis and aging as well.

Cardiovascular homeostasis involves a healthy vascular system, adequate blood supply to the heart tissue, and regulation of the heart's electrical activity by sodium, potassium, and calcium. Mineral levels are different inside and outside of the cell, and calcium levels are particularly crucial. When calcium builds up inside the cell, referred to as cytosolic calcium, complex signaling events occur that eventually affect heart muscle contraction, such that higher levels of cytosolic calcium are associated with both hypertension and Type II diabetes (Barbagallo 1999).

Until recently, cardiologists used nearly the same paradigm for cardiovascular function as originally developed by the British physician William Harvey and presented in his *On the Circulation of Blood* in 1628. In this model, the heart is seen as a mechanical pump and the vascular system as nothing more than a plumbing system. Medical scientists now know that the vascular system is exceedingly more complex than that, and they agree that we are just beginning to understand its role in health and disease. For example, hypertension is not merely excess pressure in the pipes, but a consequence of complex interactions between genetics, environmental factors such as diet, and the internal environment of bioelectrical activity, hormones, the metabolism and cellular activity of calcium and other minerals, biochemical immune substances, and other factors.

Essentially, as we currently understand it, the heart's role in homeostasis is to maintain the body's internal environment by keeping the blood pressure, blood volume, and blood suffusion of tissues within normal limits in order for the rest of the body and brain to survive.

Age-Related Changes to the Heart, Circulatory System, and Blood

As we age, many changes occur to all components of the cardiovascular system, including the heart muscle, blood vessels, and the blood, as well as disruption of normal calcium metabolism. The three most important cardiovascular changes affecting longevity are irregular heart rate, reduced elasticity of the blood vessels, and sticky (thickened) blood—all work in conjunction to affect cardiovascular homeostasis and reciprocally, the homeostasis of the entire body.

Heart Rate and Pumping Ability Are Reduced During Aging: In aging, the heart rate is reduced during maximum exertion, which causes lack of aerobic fitness. Reduced heart rate results in less oxygen supply to the tissues due to the heart's inability to pump the blood efficiently. The heart may also enlarge, leading to congestive heart failure (CHF); the aorta (the main artery that emerges from the heart) may

increase in diameter and the heart valves can thicken (Kitaman 2000). In this case, blood backs up in the veins, causing a buildup of fluid in the tissues, leading to swelling of the feet and ankles, and in some cases the entire leg; weight gain results from retention of water in the body. Confused thinking and poor memory may also occur due to reduced blood flow into the brain.

Heart rate can also become irregular in older people, resulting in arrhythmias. These cause a variety of symptoms including dizziness, fainting, fatigue, shortness of breath, chest pains, and palpitations, and are also associated with anxiety and confusion. If the heart rate slows down, a condition called bradycardia, less blood is pumped through the body and your tissues receive inadequate amounts of vital nutrients. The opposite problem can also occur. In a condition called tachycardia the heart rate speeds up, the heart is strained by the increase in rate, and tissues receive an erratic supply of blood.

The Blood Vessels Become Less Elastic: During aging the arteries become less elastic and stiffen. Less blood is pumped and is done so more inefficiently. As a result, blood pressure can increase, especially the systolic pressure (the upper number of your blood pressure reading), causing hypertension. This diffuse thickening of the arteries is associated with the accumulation of cholesterol, fibrin, and particularly of calcium deposits along the inner walls of the arteries; it is referred to as hardening of the arteries (arteriosclerosis), which is essentially a problem of the vascular walls affecting the inner surfaces (endothelium) of the arteries.

Arteriosclerosis is thought to be age-related, and is associated with an increased incidence of heart attack and stroke. A term often used interchangeably, but incorrectly, with arteriosclerosis is atherosclerosis; as noted previously, the latter is an accumulation of yellowish cholesterol and fatty substances that form plaques in large to medium-sized arteries and is also associated with high blood pressure, heart attack, and stroke. However, atherosclerosis can occur at any age, and is caused by inflammation, chronic infection, and oxidation of LDL cholesterol. It is a problem that occurs only in focal areas of the endothelium, not in all of the arteries, as with age-related stiffening or arteriosclerosis.

Veins, those vessels that return blood to the heart, become less elastic and stiffen, and when complicated by poor heart and arterial function, vein-related problems can occur, resulting in varicose veins, spider veins and other forms of broken vessels, leg pain and cramps, edema, and ulcers. Collectively referred to as peripheral vascular disease, these conditions become more common as we age. The old saying that "a man is as old as his arteries" has more than a grain of truth to it, so keep your blood vessels elastic as you age by exercising regularly, eating a healthy diet, and taking nutritional supplements.

The Blood Thickens and Becomes Sticky: It is not enough to talk only about the heart's activity and circulation. To prolong health we also must discuss the fluid that the heart pumps and the vessels carry—the blood. Some medical scientists believe that the blood is considerably more than a nutrient-laden fluid, but an organ in its own right, displaying highly complex interactive biological and biochemical functions. Among blood's important qualities are its viscosity (how thick the blood is), its overall quantity and quality of cells, and the amounts of the many suspended substances such as cholesterol and other lipids and lipoproteins. All of this is another important aspect of homeostasis that directly influences aging.

As people age, the level of lipids in their blood changes. When you are over 70 years old, both LDL and HDL cholesterol levels tend to

edge downwards; perhaps this is because older people tend to eat less and have more difficulty eating fatty foods, so they avoid them. But there may be other factors at work, such as gene expression.

Additionally, in people aged 80, the type of LDL present changes. The smaller type, small dense LDL, is generally found in younger people and is very toxic to the lining of the arteries. A bigger, less harmful type, called large buoyant LDL, is less toxic. Though we may not presently understand why these changes occur in the very elderly, we do know that if your blood levels of HDL drop below 35 mg/dL, your risk of having a heart attack is 200 times greater than at 60 mg/dL (Mogadam 2001).

Due to metabolic changes in glucose metabolism, protein glycosylation, lipid metabolism, and blood dynamics, as well as poor hydration from reduced food and water intake and absorption, our blood tends to thicken as we age. This thickening is also accompanied by increased stickiness and is associated with an increased risk of stroke, as well as cognitive decline and dementia (Lowe 2001).

Though a relatively new discovery in Western medicine, this phenomenon has long been known to Chinese medicine, which called it "blood stagnation." This is a syndrome characterized by a dark complexion, dry scaly skin, and localized sharp stabbing pain as experienced in angina; in Chinese medicine it is considered one of the major causes of both disease and aging. Blood stagnation disorders are treated by complex combinations of traditional Chinese herbs.

How to Improve Your Cardiovascular Function

In a study published in the *New England Journal of Medicine* in 2002, researchers found that heart cells can regenerate (Quaini 2002).

These results overturned conventional scientific dogma that heart cells are unable to regenerate. This is good news for life extensionists, since the evidence of this study suggests that humans may have as yet undescribed undifferentiated progenitor cells, parent cells from which other cells develop, situated in organ tissue and possibly freely distributed in the blood. These cells may serve as agents of tissue repair and may even contribute to maintaining organ health in the absence of disease or injury.

The implications of these findings, if proven true, are far reaching. For anti-aging specialists, life extensionists, and gerontologists, it means that if the mechanism of chemical signaling that controls the activation of these progenitor cells is found, organ regeneration might be possible.

Extensive scientific research has focused on nutrients, diet, and exercise in relation to cardiovascular disease, including hypertension, high cholesterol, and other conditions, with positive results (Houston 2002). The outcomes provide strong evidence that lifestyle, diet, exercise, nutritional supplements, and natural medicines can prevent and improve cardiovascular disease, and more important, influence and alter cardiovascular homeostasis.

Let's reiterate the main premise of this chapter: to prolong your health and live long you must have a strong heart, a well-functioning vascular system, and good blood. Since cardiovascular disease is so common in modern America, adjusting lifestyle is the first step to improving your cardiovascular health. So explore the lifestyle factors that influence cardiovascular function and then discuss the natural medications that help improve cardiovascular activity. The four main lifestyle factors that affect cardiovascular function are: (1) diet; (2) exercise; (3) stress; and (4) weight. All of these are largely manageable through lifestyle modification and natural medicine.

Perhaps more than any other cause, dietary factors are the most critical factor in cardiovascular disease. The Siberian Eskimo people of St. Lawrence Island with whom I lived during the winter of 1967–68, and similarly most indigenous peoples worldwide, had virtually no heart disease despite the fact that they ate a diet high in animal protein and fat. Only with the inclusion of sugary foods found in candy bars, canned fruits, and other processed non-foods (which are also high in sodium), which caused diabetes among indigenous people, did cardiovascular disease appear. This informs us of the importance of the quality and type of foods we eat, and also of the negative influences of modern living. It shows us that we too can be completely free of cardiovascular disease.

Prolonging Health Recommendation 35— Eat a Better Diet

To prolong your health, eliminate dietary saturated fatty acids as found in flame-broiled and fried meats; avoid refined sugar and products containing sugar; balance your dietary protein by reducing red meat consumption, increasing fish and poultry, and adding vegetable sources of protein such as legumes, seeds, and nuts; and eat more organic vegetables and fruits in season. Avoid processed omega-6 polyunsaturated fats as found in margarines and commercial vegetable cooking oils. Snack foods such as chips, cookies, and chocolates contain high amounts of these types of fat and should be completely eliminated from your diet. The types of fats that are beneficial to your heart and arteries are monounsaturated vegetable fats, as found in olive oil, and omega-3 polyunsaturated fats found in fish, notably salmon. Reduce your sodium (salt) intake, and

Herbert Benson, M.D., of the Mind Body Medical Institute at Harvard (Benson 1975). Listening to calming music, walks along the seashore or in the woods, writing poetry, painting, and gardening are activities conducive to a meditative attitude and help to unwind the tension caused by stress.

Prolonging Health Recommendation 38—Lose Some Weight

The last major lifestyle factor that influences cardiovascular health is weight. Obesity is a well-documented risk factor for heart disease; however, the distribution of fat rather than the overall weight appears to be the most critical feature. If you have more fat around your waist, as in a potbelly called abdominal obesity (as described in chapter 10 on insulin resistance), your risk for a heart attack is increased; for those with severe abdominal obesity, their risk for coronary artery disease is nine times greater than those who do not have this condition.

Abdominal obesity is determined by measuring your body at the waistline and then at the widest part of the hips, then dividing the measurement of the waist by the one of the hips. The desirable waist-to-hip ratio for men is under 0.90 and for women 0.75 (see chapter 4). Since abdominal obesity is influenced by your metabolism of sugar, as much as, if not more than, the overall amount of food you eat, in order to improve your waist-to-hip ratio you have to not only eat less, but avoid sugar and refined carbohydrates entirely.

Conditions and Lifestyle Factors Associated with Cardiovascular Disease

• Diabetes

• High cholesterol

• Insulin resistance

• Low testosterone and estrogen

• Obesity

• Tobacco smoking

• Sedentary lifestyle

• Increased consumption of refined sugar and carbohydrates

• Excess consumption of saturated fats

• Poor nutrition

• Excess use of alcohol

Prolonging Health Recommendation 39—Take Nutrients That Improve Cardiovascular Homeostasis

Mark C. Houston, M.D., is a distinguished cardiologist, clinical professor at Vanderbilt University School of Medicine, and the director of Hypertension and Vascular Biology at Saint Thomas Hospital in Nashville, Tennessee. He says that combinations of whole foods, antioxidants, vitamins, and minerals are superior to single substances for the prevention and treatment of cardiovascular disease (Houston 2002). To prolong your health, wisely combine nutrients with diet and lifestyle modifications.

After 20 years of clinical practice, and despite the contrary opinions of some doctors, there is no doubt in my mind that nutritional supplements improve cardiovascular health. My clinical experience is validated by a rapidly growing list of scientific studies substantiating the concept of supplemental nutrients for the prevention, treatment, and reversal of cardiovascular disease. This is supported by an increasing number of doctors who are including nutritional therapies in their practice. Among these nutrients are many of the antioxidants discussed in chapter 7, such as vitamin

E. Let's take a closer look at how these improve cardiovascular homeostasis.

Nutrients That Improve Cardiovascular Health

- Alpha lipoic acid
- Coenzyme Q10
- Folic Acid
- L-arginine
- L-carnitine
- Taurine
- Vitamin B$_6$
- Vitamin C
- Vitamin E
- Zinc
- Trimethylglycine

Alpha-Lipoic Acid (ALA): A thiol compound necessary for human health, ALA is a potent antioxidant. It helps to recirculate other antioxidants such as vitamins C and E, and glutathione, the important naturally occurring antioxidants (see chapter 7). Thiols are foul-smelling substances formed when an oxygen molecule, chemically bound in an alcohol compound, is replaced by sulfur; despite their odor, they are important in maintaining the structure of proteins.

Among its actions, ALA helps reduce insulin resistance; improves the structure of the blood vessels; reduces systolic hypertension; improves blood circulation in the kidneys; and helps to improve overall homeostasis by lowering blood pressure; normalizes calcium channels by decreasing cytosolic calcium. The basic typical dosage of ALA ranges from 300 to 600 mg per day; for the treatment of cardiovascular disease and insulin resistance, use upwards to 2,000 mg per day.

Coenzyme Q10 (CoQ10): Used widely by naturopathic physicians and an increasing number of cardiologists, CoQ10 is not only a potent antioxidant, but has significant benefits for the cardiovascular system. It helps to recirculate antioxidants such as vitamins A, C, and E; inhibits the oxidation of LDL cholesterol; reduces total cholesterol and triglycerides; raises HDL cholesterol; improves insulin sensitivity and glucose tolerance; lowers blood pressure; and protects the heart muscle from injury.

Interestingly, CoQ10 is biosynthesized in the body along similar biochemical pathways as cholesterol, which is perhaps one of the mechanisms accounting for its effect on improving the blood lipid profile. An effective daily dose for cardiovascular disease is 250 mg, taken with food, though dosages as high as 600 mg can be required. Allow at least three weeks of daily intake for it to reach maximum blood level, after which time benefits are usually more attainable.

Folic Acid: Folate, in its synthetic form as folic acid, is a member of the B-vitamin family. It is one of a number of related compounds found in the body that are important in many key biological processes including DNA synthesis. It is involved in gene expression and helps to maintain the integrity of the genome; it helps prevent atherosclerosis; and it lowers homocysteine levels.

Folic acid comes in tablet or liquid form, and the recommended basic dosage is 400–800 mcg daily, but up to 5–10 mg daily is often required for the treatment of age-related conditions including cardiovascular disease. L-5-methyltetrahydrofolate, a form of folate involved in the synthesis of homocysteine, should be included in your supplementation of folate, as 10 percent of the population have a defect in the enzyme methyltretrahydrofolate reductase, which catalyzes this process. The dosage for L-5-methyltetrahydrofolate is 800 mcg daily.

L-Arginine: The amino acid arginine functions as the primary precursor for the production of nitric oxide. This is a powerful vasodilator and helps to maintain the tone of the blood vessels; it also inhibits the formation of plaques that cause atherosclerosis and helps to lower blood pressure. Folate and many of the other nutrients mentioned in this section also affect nitric oxide; however, L-arginine in dosages of 10 g or more daily can influence nitric oxide in a positive way. Here it can increase coronary artery flow, reduce angina, improve peripheral blood flow, lower blood pressure, inhibit the oxidation of LDL cholesterol, and exert antioxidant activity and immune-enhancing properties. Though cardiovascular effects can be achieved at 10 g per day, and since it is known the L-arginine promotes growth hormone release at higher dosages, an optimal dosage is in the range of 20–30 g daily.

L-Carnitine: An amino acid derivative found in all cells of the body, carnitine is synthesized in the liver and kidneys. Its primary known function is helping transport long-chain fatty acids across the mitochondrial membrane into the mitochondria, where they are used for fuel. It has significant cardioprotective effects, including lowering triglycerides, reducing angina, normalizing arrhythmia, and lowering blood pressure. It also suppresses oxidative damage during aging. L-carnitine has been successfully used in the treatment of congestive heart failure. The typical dosage is between 1,000 and 4,000 mg daily.

Taurine: A principal free intracellular amino acid, taurine is found in many tissues in the body, particularly the brain, retina, myocardium, platelets, neutrophils, and smooth and skeletal muscle. Taurine is an antioxidant, and exhibits numerous cardiopro-

tective activities including lowering cholesterol and blood pressure. It protects against atherogenesis and reduces symptoms of congestive heart failure; it has a diuretic effect in ascites, a condition characterized by fluid retention in the abdomen, seen in cases of liver and heart disease. The typical dosage is between 2,000 and 4,000 mg daily.

Vitamin B$_6$: Pyridoxine, or vitamin B$_6$, is important in numerous biological processes in the body, including carbohydrate and amino acid metabolism, and hormone and neurotransmitter synthesis. Its cardioprotective effects include lowering blood pressure, reducing homocysteine, and lowering insulin resistance. It is usually combined with vitamin B$_{12}$ and folic acid for its homocysteine lowering affects. The average dosage is 50–200 mg daily.

Vitamin C: Besides its antioxidant effects, this well-known vitamin has cardiovascular benefits including lowering blood pressure; lowering total cholesterol, triglyercides, and LDL while raising HDL; and reducing the risk for heart attack and congestive heart failure. Its actions in cardiovascular disease may work along the lines of the other nutrients mentioned here, including raising nitric oxide levels and decreasing cytosolic (inside the cell) calcium. Vitamin C also improves balance in the sympathetic nervous system and decreases adrenal steroid production, thereby moderating some of the negative physiological effects of stress that damage the heart. The basic dosage is from 2,000 to 4,000 mg daily, with an optimal range upwards to 6,000 mg daily.

Vitamin E: Studies on vitamin E offer compelling evidence of this nutrient's vital role as an antioxidant, cardiovascular protective substance, and longevity medication. Both the United States Female Nurses Study and the United States Male Health Professional Study have shown that vitamin E in dosages above

200 international units (IU) daily lowers the incidence of coronary artery disease by 34–39 percent. In light of the small amount of vitamin E used in these studies, this is an extraordinary achievement by a simple dietary vitamin, and brings up the question of whether higher dosages can produce even greater results. The Cambridge Heart Antioxidant Study found a 47 percent decrease in the incidence of cardiovascular disease with 400–800 IU of vitamin E daily (Emmert 1999).

Vitamin E has been shown to reduce the buildup of pro-inflammatory cytokines such as nuclear factor kappa-B (NFK-B), which induces damage to the arterial wall. Vitamin E can reduce the amount of lipid peroxides caused by the oxidation of fats in the blood; improve insulin sensitivity; inhibit protein kinase C, which is involved in proliferation of smooth muscle cells that contribute to atherosclerotic lesions; inhibit platelet adhesion and aggregation, thereby reducing blood viscosity and preventing sticky blood; and is involved in many other actions that contribute to healthy cardiovascular homeostasis.

The dosage of vitamin E for cardiovascular disease is between 500 and 1,000 IU daily taken with food.

Zinc: Low zinc blood levels are associated with hypertension and other forms of cardiovascular disease. Its antioxidant activity also helps the heart. The dosage for zinc is between 15 and 30 mg per day, and optimally upwards to 60 mg daily.

Trimethylglycine: Also called betaine, trimethylglycine is synergistic with many of the nutrients discussed in this book, including choline, folic acid, vitamin B_{12}, and S-adenosylmethione (SAMe). It is a useful natural medication for liver function, detoxification reactions, the metabolism of lipids, and cancer protection, and it plays a role in lowering homocys-

teine levels. It is a safe nutrient with no known side effects or interactions. The dosage for cardiovascular disease is 1,000–2,000 mg three times daily following meals.

Prolonging Health Recommendation 40— Take Herbs That Improve Cardiovascular Health

A number of natural compounds found in plants have profound effects on the heart. Herbal medicines contain highly complex biochemical ingredients, often in the thousands per plant, making it very challenging to fully understand their actions. Modern pharmaceutical drugs derived from plants usually isolate only the most active compound, which is synthesized and concentrated in the laboratory in order to exert a pharmacological effect strong enough to alter the course of a disease condition.

Used for centuries for the treatment of heart conditions, digitalis, discovered in the foxglove plant (*Digitalis purpurea, D. lanata*) from the Scrophulariaceae family, is one such example. The active constituent digoxin, one of six known glycosides with cardioactive properties found in the plant, was isolated by scientists and then used as the basis for the cardiotonic drug digoxin (Lanoxin) to lower blood pressure in the treatment of congestive heart failure. The plant digitalis is poisonous and should not be used for self-treatment.

However, there are a number of safe natural herbal medications with cardioprotective activity. Among these are ginseng (*Panax ginseng*), hawthorn (*Crataegus laevigata*), mistletoe (*Viscum album*), garlic (*Allium sativa*), and red sage root or salvia (*Salvia miltiorrhizae*), the Chinese medicine *Dan Shen*. Though there are many other herbs that treat cardiovascular conditions, this group not only treats disease but has tonic effects as well, making each an excellent choice as a longevity medicine. All of these herbs are available from a health food store or natural pharmacy, over the Internet, or from your naturopathic doctor.

As a rule, in the clinic I prefer to use standardized extracts, which are high-quality herbal preparations manufactured in Europe by quality controlled laboratories, or in some cases from Asia, prepared in stronger concentrations than tinctures or water extracts. However, you can use all of the herbs listed below as a tea or decoction, with the exception of garlic, which you can eat raw. Remember that though teas are considerably less potent than standardized extracts they still have therapeutic activity, especially when taken over a period of several months.

In general, these herbal medications are safe, but since they all possess cardioactive properties, they should not be used at the same time as pharmaceutical cardiac drugs, antihypertensive drugs, or central nervous system depressants without the approval of your doctor.

Ginseng: Though not known for its direct action on the heart, ginseng is an important longevity medicine. Due to its potent effects on lowering glucose levels as well as being a powerful adaptogenic medicine that normalizes the body's response to stress, it is worth mentioning in this section. It is an important medicine for older people with diabetes, high cholesterol, and fatigue. Ginseng has antioxidant activity, improves organ reserve, and has protective effects on the heart, liver, and lungs. Used as an extract containing at least four to seven percent ginsenosides, the active ingredients, ginseng is often taken in dosages of 100–250 mg daily.

Hawthorn: This herb has a long history as an herbal medicine in Europe for heart conditions. It helps to lower blood pressure, improve arrhythmias, lower cholesterol, reduce angina, and improve the symptoms of congestive heart failure. The German Commission E, the defini-

tive source for scientific knowledge of herbs used in the European Union, also recommends hawthorn as a heart tonic in older people. The recommended dosage is 160 mg three times daily of the standardized extract containing 5–10 mg of flavones or oligomeric procyanidins as epicatechin.

Mistletoe: Another European herb, mistletoe is an evergreen, semiparasitic plant that lives among the upper branches of deciduous trees such as the oak. Though it is found widely in North America and northern Asia, the European varieties are best known for their health-giving effects. In fact, Iscador, a Swiss mistletoe preparation made into an injectable medicine, is widely used in Germany and Austria as immune-enhancing therapy in the treatment of cancer (Grossarth-Maticek 2001).

In my clinical opinion, mistletoe should have broader potential use in the treatment of chronic viral diseases such as hepatitis C, as well as for immune enhancement during aging. The active chemical constituents are the glycoproteins mistletoe lectins I, II, and III, as well as alkaloids, which probably contribute to mistletoe's cardioactive effects.

Regarding mistletoe's cardiovascular effects, it has blood pressure–lowering activity and vasodilating effects, and is used in the treatment of hypertension, atherosclerosis, and tachycardia. The dosage of the 4:1 standardized extract is 100–250 mg daily. When used over the course of several months, mistletoe can be toxic in high sustained dosages and should be used only under the care of a knowledgeable physician.

Garlic: The active component in garlic, which also gives it the characteristic odor and bite when eaten raw, is allicin, a sulfur-containing compound found only in the oil and easily dissipated when cooked. Garlic has mild, but helpful, effects in lowering cholesterol and triglyceride levels, and raising HDL levels. It also improves blood circulation by reducing the platelet aggregation, a cause of sticky blood, and it also helps to lower blood pressure. The daily dosage is at least 5,000 mcg of allicin, or about one medium-sized raw garlic clove.

Salvia: Used in China for several thousand years, salvia was first listed in the *Divine Husbandman's Classic of the Materia Medica* from the later Han dynasty (25–220 A.D.). While completing my hospital rounds in Shanghai in 1986, I had the opportunity to study with one of China's master physicians, Dr. Zhao Yi Ren, a cardiologist and specialist in the use of salvia for heart disease at the Long Hua Hospital. During that time, I learned firsthand the value of this remarkable herbal medicine. Today, I use it regularly in my own health regime and routinely recommend it to my patients.

As a cardioprotective medication, salvia improves blood flow in the coronary arteries, lowers blood pressure, reduces angina, and lowers cholesterol, and can also reduce glucose levels. In addition, it is thought to calm the mind and relieve insomnia. Salvia is taken in a patented form, *Dan Shen Pian,* manufactured in China, and available in Chinese herb stores or from an acupuncturist's office. Take three pills three times daily. Saliva can also be made into a tea: slowly cook 5–15 g of the dried herb in four cups of water for about 40 minutes. Drink one cup of the warm tea twice daily for a course of ten days. For an individualized prescription containing salvia along with other Chinese herbs, I suggest consulting a doctor of Oriental medicine.

The heart and vascular system constitute a critical anatomical component vital to health and longevity. Without a good heart we will likely die young. In addition, arterial disease of the heart predisposes us to a reduced quality of life and shortens our life span, while peripheral vascular disease, common among the elderly, makes life uncomfortable due to leg pain and an inability to walk, or to walk easily.

Lifestyle choices, especially poor diet, greatly affect our cardiovascular health, and though genetic tendencies may predispose us to certain forms of cardiovascular disease, environmental factors trigger negative gene expression. Oxidative stress is a major cause of both cardiovascular disease and aging, so along with a diet rich in naturally occurring antioxidants from fresh fruits and vegetables, supplementing your diet with antioxidant nutrients can improve cardiovascular homeostasis and increase life span.

Natural medicines are an effective first solution for the treatment of mild to moderate and early stage cardiovascular disease. They can act as preventative medications and natural cardiotonics for older people.

Summary of *Prolonging Health* Recommendations for Improving Cardiovascular Homeostasis

Prolonging Health **Recommendation 35— Eat a Better Diet:** Eliminate dietary saturated fatty acids as found in flame-broiled and fried meats; avoid refined sugar and products containing sugar; balance your dietary protein by reducing red meat consumption, increasing fish and poultry, and adding vegetable sources of protein such as legumes, and seeds and nuts; and eat more vegetables, plus organic fruits in season. Avoid processed omega-6 polyunsaturated fats found in margarines and commercial vegetable cooking oils, and eliminate snack foods such as chips, cookies, and candy. Don't add salt to your food, and avoid processed foods high in sodium.

• *Prolonging Health* **Recommendation 36— Get Some Exercise:** Get at least 60 minutes of exercise daily. Take a day off each week for rest and recovery. Promote muscle mass with weight training, resistance training, or isometrics. Do this every other day for between 45 to 60 minutes. Combine weight training with stretching. Consider taking a yoga class. Walk, jog, swim, bicycle, or jump rope for aerobic fitness. Don't overexercise or stress your joints, and guard against injury while exercising.

- *Prolonging Health* **Recommendation 37—Reduce Your Stress:** Practice stress-reducing therapies and activities such as yoga, tai chi, or walking, and consider practicing a form of meditation.

- *Prolonging Health* **Recommendation 38—Lose Some Weight:** Achieve the desirable waist-to-hip ratio: for men under 0.90 and for women 0.75.

- *Prolonging Health* **Recommendation 39—Take Nutrients That Improve Cardiovascular Homeostasis:** For cardiovascular disease take the following nutrients daily:

Alpha-lipoic acid	300–600 mg
Coenzyme Q10	250–600 mg
Folic acid	400–800 mcg
L-5-methyltetrahydrofolate	800 mcg
L-arginine	10–30 g
L-carnitine	1,000–4,000 mg
Taurine	2,000–4,000 mg
Vitamin B$_6$	50–200 mg
Vitamin C	2,000–4,000 mg
Vitamin E	500–1,000 IU
Zinc	15–30 mg
Trimethylglycine	1,000–2,000 mg

- *Prolonging Health* **Recommendation 40—Take Herbs That Improve Cardiovascular Health:** Consider using the following herbs daily:

Ginseng (4–7% ginsenosides)	100–250 mg
Hawthorn (5–10 mg flavones)	160 mg
Mistletoe (4:1 standardized extract)	100–250 mg
Garlic (allicin)	5,000 mcg
Salvia (patented extract)	3–9 pills

14 *Prolonging Health* Modifiable Aging Factor 8: Declining Hormone Function, the Crux of Aging—How to Restore Hormonal Balance

This chapter explains in detail how to use hormones to enhance your health and promote longevity. You'll find it twice as complicated as the rest, but it is crucially important that you understand the basics of hormone therapies. Given the lay misperception and the nonchalance of many medical doctors in prescribing hormone therapies, the information in this chapter may prevent wasted years of imbalanced treatments and has the potential to greatly enhance your health.

Hormones are powerful and potentially dangerous substances. When correctly used as medical treatment, they can restore sexual, cognitive, and metabolic functions. They can revitalize your skin and normalize your body's composition by redistributing fat and increasing muscle. They enhance energy, help you sleep better, and lift mood. When used improperly, they can cause cancer and accelerate aging. Approach them with respect. Study this chapter carefully.

Hormones are among the most important substances in the body. Their functions are diverse and include the promotion of immunity, mediation of inflammation, and involvement in metabolism. They regulate the sex drive to procreate, stimulate appetite and instigate feeding cycles, regulate sleep and waking,

influence moods, are necessary for normal growth and development, and to a large degree dictate body size and shape. Hormones influence aging and play an important role as anti-aging medications.

Hormones are substances produced by the body in small amounts, yet they have remarkable chemical properties and potent biological activity. They act as biochemical messengers providing the signals that facilitate communication between every cell in your body; they are necessary for the maintenance of homeostasis and therefore life itself.

Enzymes, other hormones, vitamins and minerals, and genes tightly regulate hormone production and function. The molecular basis for how hormones work in the body is influenced by the genetic expression of cells, and conversely, hormones are among the many factors that affect how genes operate. A gene, as you recall, is a unit of DNA within a chromosome, which is within the nucleus of a cell; a gene is transcribed into RNA that then builds proteins into structural units that serve specific functions within that cell. Negative gene expression causes disease and accelerated aging, the most feared example being oncogenesis, the development of cancer.

As a modifiable aging factor, hormonal balance can be restored through diet, exercise, nutritional supplements, herbal medicines, and hormone therapy. My aim in this chapter is to show you how to optimize hormonal activity to promote positive genetic expression, which prolongs health, fosters longevity, and minimizes negative gene expression, especially in prevention of cancer.

Though all hormones are necessary for health, some hormones are more important than others. Diana Schwarzbein, M.D., refers to those necessary to sustain life as "major hormones," since without them we would die within a matter of days (Schwarzbein 2002). The two major hormones are insulin and cortisol.

Others, such as human growth hormone (HGH), thyroxin (T4), and dehydroepiandrosterone (DHEA), are "minor hormones," ones that we can live without, though at considerably reduced biological function and with much lower levels of wellness, including fatigue, depression, sleep disturbance, and slower metabolism. Major hormones keep us alive and set the pace of aging while minor hormones help us maintain quality of life, energy, sexual drive, reproductive capacity, and vigor. Abnormal levels of major and minor hormones cause pathological changes in body function and can lead to disease.

For example, Grave's disease (a type of hyperthyroidism, or overactive thyroid gland) results from too much thyroid hormone, and hypothyroidism (underactive thyroid gland) from too little. Too little of a hormone can indirectly cause disease, as seen with osteoporosis when estrogen levels fall during menopause.

The concept of major and minor hormones is extremely important for those utilizing hormone replacement therapies. Keep this in mind as we discuss the use of hormones in your *Prolonging Health* program. Though all hormones are equally necessary for health, some are more important than others. Remember our goal: complete restoration of normal neuroendocrine balance, so do not emphasize one hormone over others.

In this chapter we explore the complex

The concept of major and minor hormones is extremely important for those utilizing hormone replacement therapies. Though all hormones are equally necessary for health, some are more important than others. Remember our goal: complete restoration of normal neuroendocrine balance, so do not emphasize one hormone over others.

and fascinating world of hormone science and find out why hormones are so important in maintaining and sustaining life, and why they are critical to your *Prolonging Health* plan. I will discuss the neuroendocrine theory of aging, explain the significance of hormone decline and its effects on aging, and outline how you can balance your hormones.

Hormones Rule the Intercellular Communications Network

Hormones communicate biochemically with each other and between cells. They do not exist in isolation but interact in multiple ways in all processes and in every site of the body. In particular, hormones intimately interface with the nervous system, which includes the brain,

The Classical Endocrine Glands and Hormones

Gland	Location	Hormones Secreted
Pituitary	frontal lobe of the brain	luteinizing hormone, follicle-stimulating hormone, prolactin, growth hormone, adrenocorticotropin hormone, ß-lipotropin, ß-endorphin, thyroid-stimulating hormone
	intermediate lobe	melanocyte-stimulating hormone, ß-endorphin
	posterior lobe	vasopressin or antidiuretic hormone, oxytocin
Thyroid	front part of neck	thyroxin, triiodothyronine, calcitonin
Parathyroid	in the thyroid	parathyroid hormone
Thymus	behind sternum in center of chest	thymosin fraction 5, thymopoietin, thymopentin, thymulin, thymic humoral factor
Adrenal	cortex	cortisol, aldosterone, dehydroepiandrosterone, androstenedione
	medulla	epinephrine, norepinephrine
Gonads	testes in males	testosterone, estradiol, androstenedione, inhibin, activin, mullerian-inhibiting substance
	ovaries in women	estradiol, progesterone, testosterone, androstenedione, inhibin, activin, follicle-releasing peptide, relaxin
Placenta	in pregnancy	human chorionic gonadotropin, human placenta lactogen, progesterone, estrogen
Pancreas	left mid-abdomen	insulin, glucagon, somatostatin, pancreatic polypeptide, gastrin, vasoactive intestinal peptide
Pineal	within the brain	melatonin, biogenic amines, peptides

The classical list of endocrine glands and hormones secreted by each is well established, as are the diseases caused by abnormally high or low hormone levels.

In fact, the connection between hormones, the nervous system, and neurotransmitters is so close that it is more accurate to describe their function as one elegant neuroendocrine *system,* rather than as separate isolated impulses operating mechanically, as was once thought.

Essentially, the neuroendocrine system helps to coordinate all body functions. It mediates responses from the environment to the body, and therefore plays an essential role in homeostasis. One of the main neuroendocrine system control centers is the hypothalamus. Situated in the brain, the hypothalamus is a gland that stimulates the pituitary gland (also in the brain) to produce hormones that maintain body functions including growth and repair. But the hypothalamus is also considered one of the body's main control centers for homeostasis. It signals hormones to exert regulating effects on appetite and body weight, temperature, blood pressure, fluid and electrolyte balance, and circadian rhythms. All are involved in aging. The interactions among the central nervous system, hypothalamus, and the body's hormonal communications systems

nerves, and a large number of neurotransmitters. These are chemicals that act as messengers to facilitate electrical conductivity between nerve cells.

Some neurotransmitters, such as serotonin, function as chemical messengers and hormones.

are central to how the body maintains homeostasis.

An important feature of neuroendocrine system function in the maintenance of homeostasis is the connection between hormones and the glands that secrete them. These two exist in a complex interdependent relationship referred to as a hormonal axis.

The basis for all hormonal activity in the body is the relationship between the anterior pituitary gland and the hypothalamus, both in the brain. Referred to as the hypothalamic-pituitary complex (HP complex), these form the foundation for the most well-known of the hormonal axes, the hypothalamic-pituitary-adrenal axis (HPA axis).

The HPA axis is central to the body's ability to respond to challenges from the environment such as stress, trauma, and infection (Rabin 1999). It is composed of the HP complex and the adrenal glands. Signals from the hypothalamus and pituitary gland are in continual communication with the adrenal glands. In response to messages from the HP complex, the adrenal glands secrete hormones that help us respond to environmental stresses. Normal HPA axis function promotes health and maintains homeostasis. Abnormal HPA axis function is implicated in stress, chronic fatigue syndrome, mood and sleep disorders, weakened immune reactions to infectious microorganisms such as viruses; it also plays a role in accelerated aging.

Other hormonal axes are present in the body. The most influential of these on aging is the growth hormone/insulin-like growth factor I axis (GH/IGF-I axis), also called the somatotrophic axis. The somatotrophic axis plays a significant role in growth and development during childhood and in aging. In this axis, growth hormone, secreted by the anterior pituitary gland and the main regulator of growth in the body, is stimulated by growth hormone releasing factor (GHRF) from the hypothalamus. This in turn stimulates release of IGF-I in the liver. IGF-I and other growth factors subsequently mediate growth in the tissues, including bone and muscle. This is how we build tissue and grow. Around age 25 our GH and IGF-I levels peak and most growth processes in the body stop; by age 50, they have declined to such a degree that deterioration of tissues begins.

Though scientists are just beginning to understand the complexities of the neuroendocrine system, its importance in aging is so profound that for our purposes in extending life span it would serve us well to explore it in more detail before moving on to discussing how hormones influence aging and what we can do to modify their effects.

The classical model of endocrinology, the study of hormones, is based on the theory that glandular structures in the brain act as control centers and, like a conductor in front of an orchestra, direct hormonal activity in the body from on high. Using the bloodstream as a means of reaching their target sites, the classical hormones are those secreted by the endocrine glands, a group of anatomical structures in the body that include the pituitary gland, thyroid gland, parathyroid glands, thymus, pancreas, adrenal glands, and the gonads composed of the ovaries in women and testes in men.[27]

In order to have a pool of hormones available for use by the tissues and organs, the endocrine glands maintain necessary blood levels of hormones by producing more or less steady amounts controlled by a feedback mechanism between the secreting endocrine organ, the pituitary gland, and hypothalamus. That is why levels of most hormones are readily measured in the serum, the fluid part of the blood

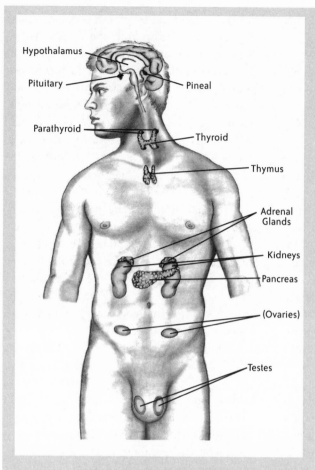

The Classical Endocrine System

The classical endocrine system is composed of discrete individual glands that produce specific hormones, secreting them directly into the bloodstream, through which they act upon cells and tissues in other areas of the body.

Hormones produced by organs other than the endocrine glands are called nonclassical hormones. The organs that produce them include the brain, heart, liver, kidneys, gastrointestinal tract, platelets in the bloodstream, immune cells in the blood such as macrophages and lymphocytes, the arteries, and other parts of the body including fat cells.

The brain, especially the hypothalamus, produces numerous hormone-like substances such as corticotropin-releasing factor and somatotropin-releasing factor, as well as a wide range of growth factors such as transforming growth factor-alpha. The kidney produces the red blood cell stimulating factor erythropoieten; the liver produces insulin-like growth factor I (IGF-I), a substance involved in complex interactions with growth hormone; and the heart, blood vessels, and platelets produce growth factors, immune substances, serotonin, and a wide range of other substances. The intestinal tract synthesizes so many substances and is so complex in its biochemical activities that it has been termed "the second brain" (Gershon 1998); it produces many hormone-like immune substances as well as the neurotransmitter serotonin.

(see chapter 5 for hormone testing). However, the circulating levels of hormones are very minute[28] and remain in the blood circulation for relatively short periods of time, ranging from a few minutes for some of the adrenal hormones to about six days for thyroxin, a thyroid hormone. That is why they must be continuously replaced.

Though useful as a first step in describing the basic functions of the endocrine system, the classical endocrine system model is insufficient for helping us understand how hormones actually work in the body or to help in developing a comprehensive approach to balancing hormones during aging. The classical endocrine model, composed of a few glands and organs that secrete substances directly into the blood, has been replaced by the neuroendocrine system model: intricate, multifaceted, it describes the complex *interrelationships* between hormones and the nervous system, including neurotransmitters, and shows how they influence the body.

Hormones exert a wider influence in the body than medical science previously thought. They interact with the immune system, the cardiovascular system, metabolism, the brain's cognitive abilities, and individual cells; all of these have an impact on how we age. This complexity extends beyond the classical endocrine model, and is even more complex than the neuroendocrine model with its numerous biochemical pathways.

We know now that in addition to the endocrine and non-endocrine hormones, a vast number of cells also exhibit hormonal activity and produce hormones that are diffused throughout the body. These include many of the body's immune cells (mast cells, lymphocytes, macrophages, natural killer cells, and others), epithelial cells in the skin, endothelial cells in the lining of blood vessels, bone and cartilage cells, and many others. The range of hormones and hormone-like substances that they produce covers a broad molecular spectrum including serotonin, melatonin, histamine, endorphins, vasopressin, thymosins, and a long list of additional or presumed substances, many of which we are only beginning to discover.

Among the newly discovered hormones produced in cells is leptin, made in the body's fat cells. Researchers have found that leptin acts on receptors in the hypothalamus, where it counteracts the effects of appetite-stimulating molecules (neuropeptide Y and anandamide). Leptin may be important in controlling weight, as overweight people seem to have too much of it. During aging, leptin levels increase in women and decrease in men.

People with lipodystrophy, a condition where a person's body is unable to make adipose tissue, cannot produce leptin due to the lack of fat cells and therefore have low leptin levels and less appetite. Lipodystrophy is associated with Type II diabetes, and people with insulin resistance are more prone to have this condition when they age. Treatment with leptin has been shown to improve lipodystrophy. Leptin also may play a key role in neuroendocrine adaptation to stress and it is under investigation for its role in alternative signaling pathways that might mediate anti-aging activity in the body during caloric restriction.

This cellular network in combination with the neuroendocrine system is referred to as the diffuse neuroendocrine system (DNES).[29] According to the DNES model, cells are the main regulators of homeostasis, acting through the organs, glands, and hormones of the neuroendocrine system. In this model, the emphasis is placed upon cells and their intercommunication networks.

This expanded hormonal model is essential for our understanding of aging, because it suggests that the body, though composed of various parts, is a *whole* entity such that effects in one part are registered in the entire organism. It also suggests that individual cells are the key components for health and aging; by protecting cell function, the health of the whole organism is improved. The DNES model is important to a main premise of this book: *incremental* disruption of homeostasis on the cellular level is responsible for aging. By reestablishing the normal homeostatic mechanism and reducing ongoing homeostatic damage to cells, we are more likely to prolong our health and achieve our maximum life span.

To understand the DNES concept and its impact on homeostasis and therefore on aging, let's take a closer look at how hormones work in our body. Let's also continue our discussion with the brain, the seat of the central nervous system, and work our way down to hormonal activity in the cells. Keep in mind that the connection works both ways, which we might call the brain-body-mind continuum. Barry Sears, Ph.D., referred in *The Age-Free Zone* to the role of hormones in this connection as the "interconnecting link between mind and body" (Sears 1999).

Within the brain lie several structures that secrete hormones and also influence the synthesis of other hormones in various parts of the body. Among these are the hypothalamus and the pituitary gland, which I introduced earlier, and which together are often referred to as the core of the neuroendocrine system. The hypothalamus, a group a hormone-secreting cells located at the base of the brain, produces six known hypothalamic releasing factors, which are peptide hormones and hormone-like substances. These influence the synthesis of other hormones in the pituitary, which in turn regulate the functions of the thyroid, adrenals, and gonads, as well as control growth, lactation in nursing mothers, and sexual development, among other functions.

The pituitary gland, situated towards the front of the brain, receives the hypothalamic releasing factors through its blood supply. These releasing factors stimulate the pituitary to secrete a wide range of hormones that stimulate the main endocrine glands to produce their characteristic hormones, which are secreted directly into the bloodstream.

While circulating in the bloodstream, hormones are transported by binding proteins, which are carrier substances mainly produced in the liver. During aging, levels of binding proteins, particularly albumin, tend to fall. Changes in thyroid and other hormone levels,

pregnancy, nutritional factors, infections, diseases, and body weight, can directly affect the level of circulating binding proteins. Sex hormone–binding protein (SHBG), which carries estrogen and testosterone, declines when you are overweight, or when there is too much fat around the central portion of your body; both these conditions are associated with insulin resistance.

The bioavailability of hormones is determined predominantly by the percentage of a hormone that is not bound to a carrier protein. The unbound portion of a hormone in the bloodstream is referred to as "free" hormone. Though research is still under way in the field of binding proteins, the accepted thought is that the free levels of a hormone influence its availability. When levels of binding proteins decline, as during aging, a lesser amount of hormone is carried to its target sites; therefore, an overall lower amount of the free hormone is available for use by cells. But less hormone means reduced function, and that can cause age-related symptoms.

During aging, binding proteins can also become elevated. This means that less free hormone may be available because more of the hormone is bound and therefore unavailable to the cells. One of the goals in neuroendocrine balancing is to normalize levels of binding proteins and increase amounts of free hormones, not just to raise total levels of the physiologically active hormones for short-term symptom improvement.

As hormones circulate in the bloodstream, they gravitate towards the target site with which they have the most affinity. There they are taken up by receptors situated on the cell membrane and transported within the cell. Receptors on the cell membrane receive the hormone from the bloodstream and guide it into the cell's interior. The function of a receptor is to recognize a particular hormone needed for its particular purpose among the myriad other chemicals in the blood. Messages within the cell signal the receptor as to which particular hormone is needed. Therefore, a receptor has to have an affinity for a specific hormone, coordinate the binding of that hormone according to the requirements of the cell, and convey the specific molecular information that the hormone encodes into the cell through a biochemical dialogue between the hormone and the cell.[30]

Molecules called second messengers, substances produced by the cell in response to hormonal signaling at the receptor site, carry the hormone's message within the cell. Examples of second messengers include cyclic AMP, cyclic GMP, and calcium. The entire process is a continuous ebb and flow of hormonal activity operating through an elegant communications network between the nervous system and the body's cells and their hormonal activity.

Other parts of the brain also influence neuroendocrine activity and aging, including the hippocampus and the thalamus. These are anatomical areas in the central part of the brain involved in cognition, as well as emotional states, memory, and how we navigate through our physical and psychological environment. The neurotransmitters serotonin and dopamine, as well as a battery of hormones, are involved in these functions.

Due to the complexity of hormonal function, it should not be surprising that there are several other categories of hormones in addition to the classical endocrine hormones, nonclassical hormones, and those just introduced. These include intercellular hormone-like substances produced by cells, such as autocrine, juxtacrine, and paracrine, which entail mechanisms of communication between cells.

Autocrine refers to hormones that act on the same cell from which they were produced.

Juxtacrine refers to the hormonal mechanism in which an adjacent cell interacts with a receptor on a cell next to it and affects only individual or identical cells in the immediate environment.

Interestingly, some cancerous tumors maintain themselves in a similar fashion by producing hormones within the tumor itself, thereby creating self-sufficiency from the surrounding tissues (Graeber 2001). The existence of this mechanism informs us that there are many different biological hormonal communication pathways, and that rather than these pathways being utilized in a destructive way as in cancer, we might be able to activate them in novel ways for the purpose of achieving longevity. It also tells us that in order to control cancerous processes during aging, we need to understand how hormones work within the tissues and specific areas of the body.

Paracrine signaling, the third mechanism, affects cells in the neighboring environment. This is the mechanism by which a hormone or other substance such as a cytokine produced in one cell acts on a neighboring cell, not by direct receptor contact as with autocrine or juxtacrine signaling, or through the blood as with endocrine hormones, but by diffusion through the intercellular space. This type of cellular communication might be seen as short-range signaling. An example of paracrine signaling is the construction and maintenance of the blood vessels (called angiogenesis), which is dependent on paracrine factors such as angiopoietin-1 and -2 (Hanahan 1997). Another example is synaptic signaling between nerve cells (neurons), where neurotransmitters are released and exposed to neighboring neurons in order to activate a nerve.

The intercellular substances that these cells produce include growth factors, immune substances such as cytokines and interferons, interleukins, neurotransmitters, prostaglandins, and eicosanoids. The latter are hormone-like lipid substances important in health and aging, which make up a large group of molecules derived from polyunsaturated fatty acids. Eicosanoids participate in the synthesis of a number of hormonal substances, including prostaglandins, prostacyclins, leukotrienes, and thromboxanes.

The most abundant precursor molecule for these hormones is arachidonic acid. This is a lipid-like molecule present in the plasma membrane of cells and involved in the activation of inflammatory activity in the body. Eicosanoids play an important role in neuroendocrine function, and that is why maintaining normal eicosanoid balance through the inclusion in your diet of omega-3 fish oils and essential fatty acids from olive and flaxseed oil helps improve hormonal balance in the body.

The intricate biochemical wiring between the nervous system and hormones, the complex patterns and rhythms of hormonal secretion, the geometry of the interlaced hormonal axes, the seemingly endless array of intercellular hormones, and the genetic events that influences their molecular origins—all this eventually rests upon the ability of a specific hormone to influence an individual cell. That cell's capacity to function is largely controlled by hormones, and its responsiveness to a hormone is controlled by hormone receptors. Healthy cells help maintain homeostasis; this is necessary to prolong your health and achieve your maximum life span. Now, let's discuss how hormones influence our genes and see their role as an aging factor.

Hormones Serve As Signaling Molecules for Gene Expression

Perhaps the most significant advance in aging research to occur in the last 50 years is the discovery that hormones, particularly insulin and IGF-I, act as signaling molecules.

They trigger genes to express particular functions including growth, cell differentiation, survival, and metabolism. They also have effects on aging and longevity. In the case of insulin and IGF-I, referred to as the insulin/IGF signaling pathway, this mechanism is thought to control the rate of aging.

Insulin helps metabolism through the regulation of glucose, the body's primary dietary fuel source for the production of energy. Likewise, IGF-I also has important functions in the body. These include growth, remodeling of the bones, survival of nerve cells, regulation of cell growth, apoptosis or cell suicide, cell differentiation including of tumor cells, and the promotion of neurogenesis (McCarthy 2001). Since IGF-I shares structural likeness with insulin, these similarities facilitate active molecular "cross-talk" between them.

Gary Ruvkun, Ph.D., a professor of genetics at Harvard University Medical School, experimentally demonstrated that life span is regulated in the nervous system by insulin/IGF-I signaling pathways. These affect the expression of the longevity genes daf-2 and daf-16 (Tissenbaum 1998). Ruvkun and his colleagues also found that the same mechanism affects the life span of fruit flies and mice. They speculate that other mammals, including humans, are equally influenced by insulin/IGF-I signaling mechanisms and have similar longevity genes (Wolkow 2000). This informs us that there is a hormone-to-cell and cell-to-gene connection.

A number of factors influence IGF-I synthesis and its interaction with insulin. These include the amount of IGF-I and insulin produced, interaction with steroid hormones, oxidative activity, and environmental influences. Though most of the body's IGF-I is produced in the liver, substantial amounts are made in other tissues through autocrine and paracrine activity. These tissues include the bone, brain, prostate, muscle, breast, and other sites in the body. Higher than normal levels of cortisol can suppress IGF-I production, while estrogen appears to enhance levels, and testosterone exerts synergistic effects. Too much IGF-I can cause diabetes.

All of these complex interactions in the body eventually find their way into individual cells. Given the right environment, diet, and nutrients, insulin/IGF-I signaling may be able to suppress the aging phenotype and promote longevity. That is why it is important to maintain balanced insulin and IGF-I levels.

Hormones Directly Influence the Symptoms of Aging

Andrzej Bartke, Ph.D., professor and chair of the Department of Physiology at Southern Illinois University Medical College in Carbondale, and one of the world's most distinguished researchers on aging states: "The list of proven, suspected, and potential interactions between the neuroendocrine system and aging is virtually endless" (Bartke 2001).

Hormonal activity begins with fetal development in the womb and extends through one's entire life. This array of potential interactions over a lifetime makes the neuroendocrine system a prime subject for the investigation on the mechanisms of aging. Since hormonal status is a readily modifiable aging factor, this renders hormone therapy as the main medical form for the treatment of age-related changes such as loss of muscle tone and strength, fatigue, depression, memory loss, reduced bone density, reduced skin elasticity, graying of hair, and reduced sexual libido.

Many of the diseases associated with aging

such as cardiovascular disease, osteoporosis, and Alzheimer's disease, are hormone-dependent and thus can be improved by taking hormones. Other more common hormonal deficiency states resemble many of the changes that occur with aging, such as hypothyroidism, and are readily influenced by taking hormones.

Most hormones decline significantly after the peak reproductive years, the time of menopause in women and in the fifties in men. This decline is so well documented in the scientific and medical literature that many scientists and physicians believe this age-related decline in hormones is the critical factor that causes aging. Between the ages of 20 and 80,

Many of the diseases associated with aging such as cardiovascular disease, osteoporosis, and Alzheimer's disease, are hormone-dependent and thus can be improved by taking hormones. Other more common hormonal deficiency states resemble many of the changes that occur with aging, such as hypothyroidism, and are readily influenced by taking hormones.

peak levels of growth hormones progressively decline; IGF-I levels drop off by 40 percent; total testosterone levels are reduced by at least 28 percent; free testosterone levels go down by 54 percent; and the amount of bioavailable testosterone drops off by 62 percent. In women, estradiol falls by more than 20 percent, and free estradiol by nearly 50 percent. Given these statistics, it is not surprising that such steep declines cause numerous symptoms as well as changes in body structure.

Even with all this data, there are many unanswered questions regarding the neuroendocrine theory. The basic, and as yet unanswered, question concerning this hypothesis is whether aging is a direct result of hormonal decline, or if hormonal decline is only *associated* with aging, even when contributing to many of the features of aging. Another unanswered question is this: Is another, perhaps evolutionary, factor at work behind the age-related decline of hormone levels? Yet another issue for researchers concerning age-related hormonal changes is whether aging is an absence of life-giving hormones such as DHEA, or an increase in so-called death-promoting hormones such as cortisol.

Like most dichotomized lines of thinking by scientists working with the biology of living systems, the answer does not lie on one side or the other. In this case, a correct answer only poses more questions and does not provide a definitive therapeutic solution. However, we know that hormonal deficiencies and imbalances between hormones play a role in disease, accelerated aging, and possibly in the aging process itself. For example, progesterone levels in women start to fall in the late thirties and early forties, while estrogen levels remain constant until the late forties or early fifties. This causes a condition of high estrogen relative to the lower progesterone levels, and this is associated with early symptoms of menopause. Once estrogen levels fall, skin becomes thinner and bone density declines.

The neuroendocrine theory of aging postulates that the *interplay* between the nervous and endocrine systems is responsible for the changes seen in aging. It's unfortunate that many anti-aging doctors simplify this theory and bend it to their own purposes by restating it in a basic but incomplete way to say that failure in the production of hormones is the underlying cause of aging and therefore supplying individual hormones reverses aging. It is the contention of this book that nothing could be further from the truth.

However, the neuroendocrine system theory has merit not just for its model of age-related hormone decline, but because the neuroendocrine system initiates and integrates all bodily functions from the reproductive sexual act that created you to the end of your life. During your life, this system is responsible for the adaptive changes necessary in your internal environment needed for your survival and well-being. It is not surprising that any disruption in the smooth operation of this network can have far-reaching consequences on bodily functions and health. Though they may not determine when you will die, neuroendocrine system effects may be a major determining factor for how well you age and how long you'll live.

Another of way of describing the neuroendocrine theory is to say that the deterioration process that appears to be intrinsic and universal in cells, possibly influenced by as yet undiscovered pacemaker genes, acts through neuroendocrine signals that orchestrate the passage of your entire life cycle. So think of the neuroendocrine system as a network, rather than in terms of the older linear model, and imagine that any disturbance in any part of the network, no matter how small, is experienced in the whole system.

Over time, compounded deterioration results in a breakdown of normal hormonal communication, among hormones secreted by the hypothalamus and messenger molecules within the cells. This gradual, subtle breakdown causes the molecular and tissue changes characteristic of aging. Though accumulated over a lifetime, starting before the age of 30, such changes are not evident until we're past our reproductive prime, when the telltale signs of aging indicate we've begun the irreversible march towards frailty and death. However, our primary objective is to transform this morbid picture of aging into a more optimistic scenario in which aging is more malleable than previously thought.

Therefore, the neuroendocrine theory of aging is not one concept but a collection of different ideas about how hormones interact in the aging process. In fact, several potential mechanisms have been proposed to explain how the neuroendocrine theory of aging works. One suggests that aging starts in the brain, and is referred to as the hypothalamic basis of aging. In this model, the hypothalamus control center of the neuroendocrine system is affected by oxidative damage, a lifetime of exposure to cortisol and other damaging hormones, and other factors. This eventually disrupts genetic expression in the hypothalamus, causing a cascade of abnormal neuroendocrine events. The results of these events cause aging. This theory, essentially an extension of the oxidative theory, has merit, but it cannot be the sole way in which the neuroendocrine system affects aging.

Another is the insulin/IGF-I model, discussed above. A similar model, proposed by Marc Tatar, Ph.D., of Brown University in Providence, Rhode Island, postulates a hormone-based aging mechanism based in a gene called an insulin-like receptor (InR). This gene may control overall hormonal secretion, influence insulin signaling, and thereby regulate aging. According to Dr. Tatar, aging may be due to an imbalance between InR and neotenin or juvenile hormone, a youth-promoting hormone (Tatar 2001). Neotenin is an insect hormone secreted by glands near the brain that affects molting, the process of shedding the outer skeleton, but which may have a human counterpart.

Though a similar mechanism in humans has yet to be found, we know that lower than normal levels of insulin in the blood, in the absence of diabetes, are associated with longevity, and that higher levels of insulin are associated with Type II diabetes, insulin resistance, and accelerated aging. Since no human hormone that affects regeneration (such as insects and some animals have, as evidenced during molting) has been found, it is difficult to speculate further on this theory. However, if such a hormone were found, and a method to activate its genetic expression developed, a revolution in the neuroendocrinology of aging would likely occur.

Neuroendocrine Factors Associated with Aging

- Decline in hormone production

- Decreased communication ability between cells

- Cellular resistance and changes in receptor sensitivity and number

- Poor metabolism of hormones and their intermediaries

- Reduced excretion of hormones due to poor liver function

- Reduced amounts of bioavailable or free hormones

- Reduced hormonal activity

- Increased levels of binding proteins

- Reduced function of the HP complex and HPA axis

- Changes in circadian rhythms

- Degradation of enzymes involved in the synthesis of hormones

- Alterations in the ratio of hormones

- Cumulative effects of disease and oxidative processes

- Influences of genetic tendencies and altered gene expression

- Changes in hormone metabolism

- Changes in the responsiveness of target tissues

- Changes in carbohydrate metabolism, and the effects of dysfunctional insulin signaling on neuroendocrine function

- Absence of normal hormonal pulsatile release

- Changes in immune function

The Main Hormones Associated with Aging

We begin our discussion of individual hormones involved in aging with the two major hormones, insulin and cortisol. This is because during aging the levels of both of these hormones tend to rise. According to several researchers, rising levels of insulin and cortisol cause abnormal hormonal signaling and bring imbalance to the entire neuroendocrine system, including a decrease in the levels of other hormones such as testosterone and IGF-I.

After insulin and cortisol, we explore the next three most important hormones: DHEA, pregnenolone, and progesterone. These are the keystones for the conversion of all the other steroid hormones; without normalizing their activity and stabilizing their declining levels, it is difficult to achieve neuroendocrine balance. Next, we discuss thyroid hormones because of their wide-ranging affects in the body; then the sex hormones, estrogen and testosterone. Finally, we consider human growth hormone—the master hormone of anti-aging medicine.

Insulin—The Primary Signaling Molecule: Insulin is a major hormone, one that we cannot live without, and it serves as a signaling molecule for the regulation of several other important hormones. Too much insulin pro-

duction leads to insulin resistance and is associated with Type II diabetes, cardiovascular disease, peripheral vascular disease, neuropathy of the lower extremities, damage to the retina, kidney damage, and reduced cognitive ability. It may not be the entire answer to aging, but without a doubt, insulin resistance is part of the equation for accelerated aging.

Insulin and insulin-like growth factor I (IGF-I) form a signaling mechanism that influences the body's resistance to stress, temperature, and other environmental factors, and the damaging effects of oxidative processes that result in increased free radical damage to vital tissues. Researchers consider the combination of IGF-I signaling and insulin activity to be one of the main influences on the rate of aging.

Features of Insulin Excess
- High triglycerides

- Low HDL

- High blood pressure

- Increased waist-to-hip ratio

- Difficulty losing weight

- Difficulty in stabilizing other hormones

Features of Insulin Deficiency
- Craving for sweets and carbohydrates

- Excessive thirst

- Excessive appetite

- Excessive urination, both in the daytime and at night

- Fatigue

- Difficulty healing

- Changes in body shape with less muscle, and thin buttocks and extremities

The trend during aging is to have rising insulin levels, yet in some cases older people experience falling insulin levels. Decreased pancreatic function is the underlying cause of this; low insulin levels fail to control glucose in the body, and this eventually leads to Type I diabetes, or insulin-dependent diabetes. The outcome of both types of diabetes is similar: increased risk for cardiovascular and other diseases, and accelerated aging.

During aging, insulin levels tend to rise and IGF-I levels tend to decrease. But this is a modifiable hormonal aging factor, so if you can successfully regulate your insulin, manage glucose levels, and moderate IGF-I levels, you may not only prevent accelerated aging but reduce the *rate* at which you age.

Cortisol—The Catabolic Initiator: Cortisol, the most potent of the glucocorticoid steroid hormones produced by the adrenal glands, is also a major hormone. During aging, cortisol levels tend to increase and stress appears to be the main influencing factor on this tendency. One of the first responses by the endocrine system to a stressful challenge is the release of cortisol and other adrenal steroid hormones.

With chronic inflammation, ongoing or repeated infection, and unrelenting stress, the adrenal gland becomes worn down because it is in a constant state of low-level arousal. One of the first symptoms of this imbalanced state is fatigue. This is the body's natural method to remove you from action in order to reset your neuroendocrine homeostasis. If you don't heed this message and continue overworking or other forms of an abusive lifestyle such as drug addiction, pro-

Changes in Hormone Levels During Aging

Hormone	Change During Aging
Growth hormone (GH)	decreased
Insulin-like growth factor I (IGF-I)	decreased
Adrenocorticotrophic hormone	no change
Cortisol	no change, increased, or decreased
Dehydroepinandrosterone (DHEA)	decreased
Dehydroepinandrosterone sulfate	decreased
Aldosterone	decreased
Thyroid-stimulating hormone (TSH)	no change or increased
Thyroxin (T4)	no change or decreased
Triiodothyronine (T3)	decreased
Free T3	decreased
Parathyroid hormone	increased
Calcitonin	decreased
Vitamin D_3	decreased
Luteinizing hormone (LH)	increased
Follicle-stimulating hormone (FSH)	increased in women
Testosterone	decreased
Free testosterone	decreased
Insulin	no change, increased, or decreased
Glucagon	decreased
Prolactin	increased
Melatonin	decreased
Leptin	decreased in men; increased in women

Many serum levels of hormones change during aging. Most decrease, but in unhealthy aging, some increase.

duction of cortisol and DHEA, another adrenocortical hormone, can be severely affected, even diminished, and cause symptoms of adrenal insufficiency. Therefore, for the body to prolong its health, the adrenal glands must function properly.

Cortisol is made in the adrenal cortex or exterior portion of the adrenal gland. Its activity exhibits daily secretion cycles with the highest production in the morning between seven and nine A.M., with lower levels reached by mid-afternoon and the lowest level at about one A.M.; this is followed by a progressive increase during sleep until maximum levels are reached again in the morning.

Cortisol is critical in maintaining appropriate blood levels of glucose, thereby assuring energy production for metabolic activity. If your adrenal glands are unable to respond to an increasing need for cortisol to raise glucose levels, you become hypoglycemic, a condition of low blood sugar characterized by fatigue and poor cognitive ability. Insulin and cortisol are related but have opposite functions: insulin lowers glucose; cortisol increases it.

Increased cortisol participates in damage to the hippocampus (a structure in the brain) and contributes to age-related memory loss and cognitive decline. It causes hypothalamic damage, affects insulin and glucose metabolism, contributes to abnormal changes in body composition (less muscle and more fat) in older people, and destabilizes the central and autonomic nervous systems. Age-related cortisol excess is neurotoxic. It increases catabolic breakdown of the tissues, induces insulin resistance, disrupts metabolism, and causes damage to the skin, immune system, and other parts of the body.

Physical Features of Cortisol Excess

- Thickening of the back of the neck
- Increased waist-to-hip ratio
- Insulin resistance
- Fluid retention

Not all people suffer from increased cortisol with aging. Healthy people typically have no change in cortisol levels, while others, after years of stress, experience lower levels. Low levels of cortisol cause a variety of symptoms including fatigue, feeling exhausted after minimal exertion with poor recovery time, decreased resistance to infections, difficulty handling stress, anxiety, chronic inflammation, hypoglycemia and sugar craving, allergies, a thin body frame, a condition of underweight, difficulty gaining weight, and joint pains.

When cortisol levels are low, you feel very tired, with a profound "flu-like" fatigue, and are more prone to infections. That's because cortisol helps fight off infections and manages inflammation, functions critically important in older people whose immune systems decline with advancing age. In some cases, the adrenal medulla produces increased levels of adrenaline in an attempt to compensate for a stress-induced decline in cortisol. This causes you to feel "wired" and edgy and very tired at the same time, and it is one possible explanation for the crankiness often attributed to the elderly.

Features of Cortisol Deficiency

- Thin face and skinny body
- Chronic fatigue, not relieved by sleep or rest
- Craving for salt and sugar
- Allergies, asthma, eczema
- Low blood pressure
- Increased skin pigmentation
- Easily stressed, and decreased tolerance when stressed
- Mental confusion
- Longer than normal time recovering from common infections
- Dizzy or light-headed when standing up quickly

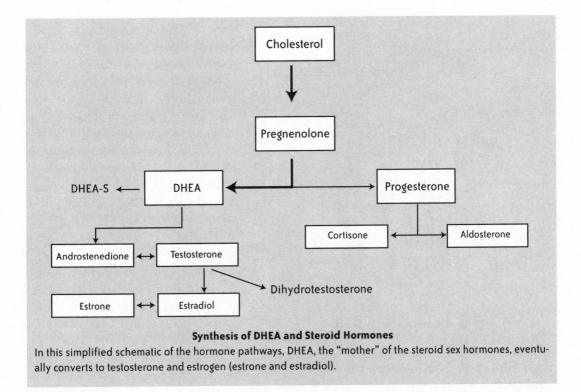

Synthesis of DHEA and Steroid Hormones
In this simplified schematic of the hormone pathways, DHEA, the "mother" of the steroid sex hormones, eventually converts to testosterone and estrogen (estrone and estradiol).

• Lack of interest in life, or a constant mild depression

In order to prolong your health, it is necessary to manage your cortisol levels by improving adrenal gland function and restoring normal neuroendocrine balance between the brain and the adrenal glands. This is a modifiable hormonal aging factor, so lowering cortisol levels prevents excess catabolic activity and slows the rate of aging. When you successfully manage your cortisol levels, you may lower your biological age and reach your optimal age-point.

DHEA—The "Mother" Hormone: Dehydroepiandrosterone (DHEA) is the most abundant androgenic hormone in the body. Androgens are hormones, including testosterone, that cause masculine features such as facial hair growth and increased muscle definition. In fact, DHEA is so abundant that it has

been nicknamed the "mother" of all steroid sex hormones, because, along with pregnenolone, it acts as a precursor or prohormone from which all other steroid hormones derive.

In men, DHEA acts as the precursor for nearly 50 percent of androgens, and in women before menopause it produces up to 75 percent of estrogens. After menopause, DHEA contributes almost exclusively to the formation of the remaining estrogens in a woman's body, producing virtually 100 percent of active estrogens. In men over 50, DHEA may contribute more to estrogen than testosterone production. On average, young adult men have 10–20 percent more DHEA than women; even with aging, older men's levels generally remain higher than those of older women.

Not only does DHEA metabolism account for the majority of the synthesis of androgenic and estrogenic steroid hormones, but DHEA

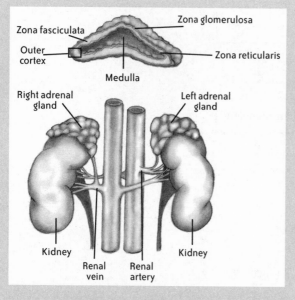

Kidneys and Adrenal Glands

The kidneys are located towards the back just under the last ribs near the spine. The adrenal glands sit atop each kidney. The adrenal gland has two parts: the cortex or outer part and the medulla or inner part. There are three zones of the adrenal cortex. Each of these different zones produces different hormones: the zona reticularis produces DHEA, pregnenolone, progesterone, estrogens, testosterone, and androstendedione; the zona fasciculata produces cortisol; and the zona glomerulosa, the outermost region, produces aldosterone.

sized primarily in the zona reticularis of the adrenal cortex, the same area of the adrenal gland that produces pregnenolone and small amounts of sex hormones. Cortisol is made in the zona fasciculata, a more external region of the adrenal cortex than where DHEA is produced. In women, the synthesis of DHEA occurs almost exclusively in the adrenal cortex, and while men produce most of their DHEA in the adrenal cortex, at least five percent of DHEA-S and 10–25 percent of DHEA is made in the testes. Small amounts are also made in the brain in both men and women, and it is possible that some DHEA is produced in other cells of the body. The total daily adrenal secretion of DHEA is about 4 mg and for DHEA-S about 25 mg.

Levels of DHEA are highest during the developmental years of youth, reaching their peak amounts between ages 20 and 30. After that, DHEA levels gradually decline by about two percent each year. By the eighth decade of life, the cumulative decline in DHEA production leaves it a mere 10–20 percent of its original value. DHEA levels are measured in nanograms per milliliter (ng/mL); youthful highs are 9.5 ng/mL, elderly lows less than 1.0 ng/mL.

According to Thierry Hertoghe, M.D., of Brussels, Belgium, DHEA-S levels provide a better picture of functional activity than DHEA since the half-life, or the time that half of the original amount of a substance remains in the blood, of DHEA-S is considerably longer than that of DHEA.[31] Therefore, the consensus among doctors practicing anti-aging medicine is that the best test for the evaluation of DHEA status is the sulfate form, DHEA-S, measured in micrograms per deciliter (μg/dL).[32]

affects many cells that have receptors for sex hormones. These include the breasts, brain, fat cells, skin, ovaries, prostate, muscles, liver, and cardiovascular cells. Due to this receptor affinity, maintaining DHEA levels during aging improves many age-related symptoms such as fatigue. Some researchers contend that because DHEA readily fits into sex hormone receptors, it prevents overexpression of cells sensitive to stimulation by sex hormones. This makes DHEA a candidate as an anticancer medication during aging.

DHEA, and its principal active metabolite, DHEA sulfate (DHEA-S), are hormones synthe-

DHEA-S Levels in Serum by Ages

Age in Years	Male Levels (μg/dL)	Female Levels (μg/dL)
0–8	3–120	8–112
9–12	16–177	31–187
13–16	39–292	52–308
17–19	76–640	65–380
20–29	280–640	65–380
30–39	120–520	45–270
40–49	95–530	32–240
50–59	70–310	26–200
60–69	42–290	13–130
70 +	28–175	10–90

Not only does DHEA production decline sharply with age, but it drops in response to long-term stress and in autoimmune conditions such as rheumatoid arthritis; it is frequently low in patients with chronic infections and viral diseases. Therefore, DHEA has received wide publicity as a principal biomarker for aging and the diseases associated with aging. But why do we lose DHEA as we age?

There are many reasons for an age-related decline of DHEA. The obvious one is that DHEA plays a primary role in the conversion into sex hormones, which are essential for reproduction. One of the observations of proponents of the evolutionary model of aging is that we begin to age after our peak reproductive period, which might explain why our DHEA then declines: we need less. Another reason is that adrenal production decreases due to the overtaxing of the adrenal gland from the repeated stresses of living; in support of this it has been observed that the zona reticularis, where DHEA is made, atrophies with age.

During aging, enzymes necessary for hormone synthesis and metabolism can become dysfunctional or deficient, or other enzymes that inhibit hormone production can become predominant. The end result is lower hormone levels. In the case of DHEA, the enzyme 17,20 desmolase is essential for the synthesis of DHEA in humans, and there is less of it as we age. As part of the aging process, we experience an overall decline in essential enzymes. Incidentally, this is another reason why a healthy diet and supplemental nutrients, especially trace minerals, are important as part of your *Prolonging Health* program since many of them help to regulate the body's enzyme network.

There also appears to be an inverse

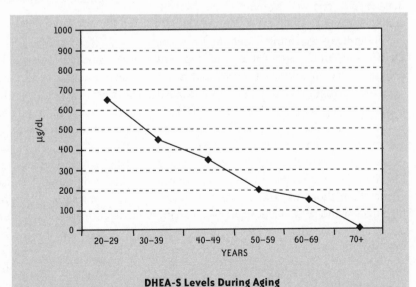

DHEA-S Levels During Aging
DHEA sulfate levels steadily decline during aging until by the age of 70 and older levels are significantly reduced from the peak values of 20–29-year-olds.

relationship between DHEA and the major hormones, cortisol and insulin: as insulin and cortisol go up, DHEA tends to go down. Research in the early and mid-1990s performed by John E. Nestler, M.D., a professor of medicine at the Medical College of Virginia in Richmond, revealed that high insulin levels decrease the concentration of DHEA and DHEA-S in the serum (Lavallee 1997; Nestler 1994). This discovery informs us that insulin acts as a physiological regulator of DHEA. These findings reaffirm my position on the importance of managing and effectively regulating insulin in order to accomplish our goal of prolonging health.

Though exactly how DHEA works in the body is still not completely understood, scientists have found that it plays a role in growth and development, the conversion of steroid sex hormones in both men and women, and fertility. It may have an essential role as part of the body's antioxidant defense system, and it reduces inflammation. DHEA has been shown to inhibit interleukin-6 (IL-6), a pro-inflammatory cytokine that tends to rise with age and in people with chronic inflammatory diseases (Gordon 2001).

In terms of regulating insulin and cortisol, DHEA plays an important role in its apparent ability to lower blood sugar levels, and it has been shown that lower DHEA-S levels parallel elevation in glucose levels (Nihal 1999). DHEA-S also restores the normal ratio of DHEA to cortisol, therefore reducing the negative effects of too much cortisol in the body. Circulating levels of DHEA are on average ten times greater than those of cortisol. As you recall, high insulin and cortisol frequently accompany aging, and along with low DHEA they constitute part of the imbalanced neuroendocrine profile of aging. That is why restoring a more optimal balance between these hormones prolongs health and improves our chances for maximum longevity.

Is DHEA decline a consequence of aging or its cause? Not quite either. Based upon my clinical experience, decreases in DHEA-S levels can be used as a *biomarker* of aging: the lower the level, the greater the biological age. DHEA supplementation has an important role in the treatment of age-related conditions and perhaps in aging itself. However, lower levels are to be looked at as being *associated* with aging, but not as the cause of aging; if they were the cause, then replacing DHEA would have a more profound effect on aging than it does (Osorio 2002).

Features of DHEA Deficiency

- Dry skin, eyes, and hair
- Lack of pubic and underarm hair
- Low energy (but not as profound as in cortisol deficiency)
- Low mood with mild anxiety or depression
- Weak muscles with lack of tone
- Reduced sexual libido
- Intolerance to noise

Since low levels of DHEA and DHEA-S are often found in those with cancer, cardiovascular disease, Alzheimer's, rheumatoid arthritis and other autoimmune diseases, low immune function, and progressive chronic viral infections such as HIV and hepatitis C, some clinicians believe an underlying event in all of these conditions is adrenal exhaustion, or at least low adrenal reserve, which causes imbalances in the secretion of adrenal hormones.

Similarly, the physiological toll that these diseases take on the body itself serves as a significant stressor, so DHEA levels may be low as a consequence of the disease rather than as a causative factor. Also, the use of high doses of cortisone to suppress immune activity (in cases of rheumatoid arthritis and other autoimmune conditions) causes a drastic reduction in DHEA.

Regardless of this chicken-and-egg conundrum, replacing DHEA in cases where DHEA-S levels are low can improve the symptoms of age-related diseases such as Type II diabetes, osteoporosis, and Alzheimer's disease, among others.

Benefits of Replacing DHEA in Aging

The benefits of supplementing DHEA during middle age and in the elder years are many:

- Increase in energy and improved mood

- Improvement in sleep

- Brain and hypothalamic protection from excess cortisol

- Reduction in inflammation

- Management of autoimmune processes

- Improvement in epithelial tissue of the skin, making it thicker

- Improvement in wound healing

- Improvement in the immune response

- Decrease in cardiovascular risk factors

- Improvement in sexual performance

- Improvement in cognitive function

- Promotion of weight loss

- Improvement of adipose metabolism

- Increase in lean muscle mass

- Slowing down of the progression of Alzheimer's and Parkinson's disease

- Possible improvement in prostate function in men and bladder problems in both men and women

- Possible anti-tumor effect against some forms of cancer

Animal models have shown a life-extension effect with DHEA supplementation. Some of these studies were calorie restriction models, which have been shown to conserve optimal levels of DHEA; others were with high dosages of DHEA. The results of these studies showed less graying of hair, more glossy coats on the research animals, and a more youthful look. The animals also had delayed tumor formation, a critical component of our *Prolonging Health* program, and a reduction of atherosclerosis incidence, another important aspect of any anti-aging plan.

DHEA has not been shown actually to reverse the aging process or restore youth, and at least a few studies suggest that it has little or no effect on the parameters of aging (Flynn 1999). But as an anti-aging medicine DHEA is beneficial for its neuroprotective effects, its participation in antioxidant defenses, its ability to improve immunity, positive effects on glucose metabolism, and its remarkable ability to restore well-being.

Pregnenolone—The Overlooked Hormone: In my clinical opinion, pregnenolone is one of the most overlooked anti-aging hormones, the others being melatonin and androstenedione. The reason for this is simple: pregnenolone does not produce the dramatic symptomatic effects that other hormones do, so doctors and researchers find little clinical value in using it. However, since it is the precursor for all the other steroid hormones, including DHEA, and its levels, like DHEA, tend to decline precipitously during aging (60 percent less at age 75 than at age 30), it makes sense that this hormone is also associated with age-related changes in the body. Since pregnenolone is not a steroid hormone, how does it influence age-related conditions? What does it do?

Pregnenolone is directly synthesized from cholesterol in a two-step process within the mitochondria, the cell's powerhouse. It is produced in the adrenal glands and other tissues (including the central nervous system), which rates it an inclusion as a class of hormones referred to as neurosteroids. This is a subclass of steroid hormones synthesized in the central nervous system. Scientists have shown that the brain concentration of pregnenolone is reduced in older animal subjects, as is cognitive performance.

This raises a similar question as with DHEA: are these lower pregnenolone levels a result of age-related changes in the brain or do they have a causative relationship? In this case, at least in research models using rats, memory was improved when pregnenolone was introduced directly to the brain via infusion (Mayo 2001).

Pregnenolone is thought to have a positive influence on neurotransmitters in the brain and to increase neurogenesis, the creation of new brain cells, in particular in the hippocampus, considered the center for memory and cognitive function. A few human studies have confirmed the improved cognitive affects of pregnenolone.

Clinically, my patients often have significant memory improvement when they take pregnenolone for several months. In my clinical experience, supplementing pregnenolone protects brain cells, improves memory, restores youthful appearance, and improves emotional attitude. As the precursor for all steroid sex hormones, including DHEA, pregnenolone must be supplemented to restore neuroendocrine balance.

Features of Pregnenolone Deficiency

- Declining memory

- Stiffness and pain in the joints

- Colors don't seem as bright

- Symptoms associated with lower levels of steroid hormones: fatigue, depressed mood, and sleep disturbance

Progesterone—The Protective Female Hormone: Progesterone was brought to public attention as a protective hormone in the early 1990s by John R. Lee, M.D., author of *Natural Progesterone* (Lee 1993). It is known to reduce the risk of ovarian and uterine cancer, and is considered an important hormone to treat premenstrual cramps and migraine headaches associated with menstruation and to improve bone loss in osteoporosis in postmenopausal women. Progesterone has anti-aging uses as it helps the body balance cortisol and protects it against the negative effects of estrogen.

According to Ray Peat, Ph.D., a researcher and authority on progesterone since 1968, progesterone, like DHEA

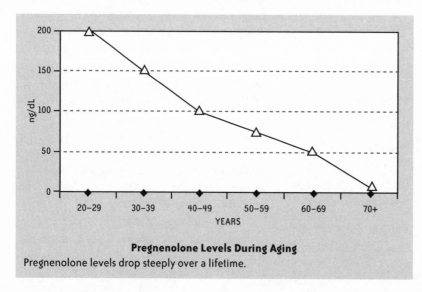

Pregnenolone Levels During Aging
Pregnenolone levels drop steeply over a lifetime.

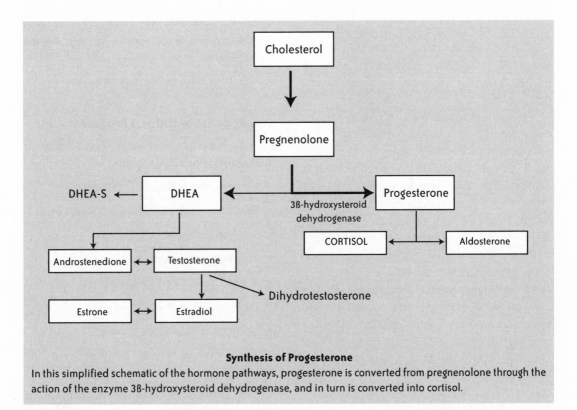

Synthesis of Progesterone

In this simplified schematic of the hormone pathways, progesterone is converted from pregnenolone through the action of the enzyme 3ß-hydroxysteroid dehydrogenase, and in turn is converted into cortisol.

and pregnenolone, is an anticatabolic hormone that protects the body from the destructive effects of cortisol. In his view, overuse of ingested estrogen not only predisposes one to cancer, but also overly excites the nervous system, and in this manner accelerates aging. Progesterone, on the other hand, is a perfect balance to the negative effects of excess estrogen, principally in its estradiol and estrone forms; it has a protective role and functions as an anti-stress and anti-aging hormone (Peat 2001). It is important to understand here that an excess amount of any hormone has its consequences on the body.

Like all steroid hormones, progesterone is converted from pregnenolone, and is principally produced in the mitochondria cells in the ovaries. However, some progesterone is made in the adrenal cortex and other tissues. As with other hormones, the conversion of pregnenolone to progesterone takes place under the influence of enzymes, in this case the principal enzyme is 3ß-hydroxysteroid dehydrogenase. Progesterone is also a precursor hormone for the conversion of other hormones, ultimately forming cortisol, and it participates in the production of testosterone.

Women make considerably more progesterone than men do, with levels rising monthly during the middle of the menstrual cycle. The levels also increase steeply during pregnancy when the majority of progesterone is produced in the placenta; approximately 250 mg is made per day at full term, with plasma levels rising from approximately 10 ng/mL in the first trimester to as high as 420 ng/mL by the third trimester. In contrast, much less is made when a woman is not pregnant, with levels ranging from less than 2 ng/mL to 25 ng/mL at its peak, which occurs during the middle of the menstrual cycle. After menopause, levels of progesterone in women can be barely detectable.

In men, progesterone is so rarely, if ever, measured in plasma or saliva that clinical laboratories don't even chart ranges for men, making it difficult to evaluate declining levels. It is assumed that older men have lower values of progesterone than younger men. Since progesterone competes with testosterone for the 5-alpha reductase enzyme, which converts testosterone to dihydrotestosterone (the hormone associated with prostate and other cancers), older men using testosterone should consider supplementing with natural progesterone cream. This contrarian view, in which men use progesterone, is supported by John Lee, M.D., Carl Urlis, M.D., and a growing list of well-respected physicians.

Features of Progesterone Deficiency

- Abdominal cramping before menstruation
- Feeling nervous or anxious
- Fibrocystic breasts
- Heavy or uncontrolled menstrual or vaginal bleeding
- Increasing symptoms of premenstrual syndrome (moodiness, cramping, and headaches before a menstrual period)
- Malaise and fatigue
- Migraine headaches before the onset of menstruation
- PMS mood changes the week before menstruation
- Restless and light sleep
- Sugar cravings the week before menstruation

- Swollen and sore breast before a menstrual period, or when starting estrogen replacement therapy
- Water retention before menstruation

The Benefits of Natural Progesterone

The benefits of natural progesterone as an anti-aging hormone are numerous:

- Improvement in adaptation to stress
- Protection against uterine and breast cancer
- Improvement in mood
- Improvement in sleep
- Activity as a natural antidepressant
- Improvement in thyroid function
- Normalization of blood clotting
- Restoration of sexual libido in men and women

Progesterone is a neurosteroid that protects the brain from damage caused by excess levels of cortisol and estrogen. It is an antitoxin that protects cell structure and function; a preserver of mitochondrial efficiency; a cardiovascular tonic improving heart rate and vascular tone; and an enhancer of immune function by its protection of the thymus gland (Peat 1997). In fact, the brain contains more DHEA, pregnenolone, and progesterone than all other organs do, and levels of all three of these hormones in the brain, as well as in the blood and other tissues, progressively decline during aging. Since the central nervous system, including the brain, plays a significant role in the aging process, neuroendocrine balance depends on keeping levels of insulin and cortisol from increasing and in maintaining optimal levels of DHEA, pregnenolone, and progesterone.

Melatonin—The Neuroendocrine Regulator: Melatonin was first isolated and characterized in 1958 by A. D. Lerner (Karasek 1999). It is mainly produced in the pineal gland, situated deep within the brain, but other tissues such as bone marrow cells and the intestinal tract also make melatonin.

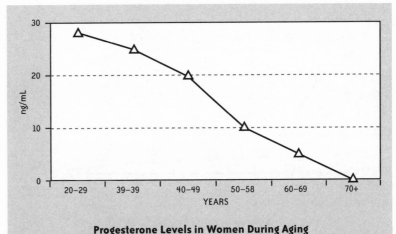

Progesterone Levels in Women During Aging

Progesterone levels drop steeply in women during aging, with undetectable levels by age 70.

The pineal gland has two known functions. It controls circadian rhythms that are linked to the sleep-wake cycle, feeding and drinking, sexual activity, and fertility, and it influences three critical periods of life. These are: (1) the perinatal event when the fetus is in the womb, and its growth and development immediately after birth, which is the time of preparing for life; (2) puberty, when the body prepares for breeding and reproduction; (3) senescence, when the body is preparing for old age and death. Pineal gland research is still in its infancy, but I suspect we have just begun to scratch the surface of our knowledge of this structure and its influence on aging.[33]

Melatonin is chemically related to the neurotransmitter serotonin, which is converted in the pineal gland to melatonin in a two-step process (involving the enzymes N-acetyltransferase and hyroxyindole-O-methyltransferase). Like serotonin, it requires the amino acid tryptophan as a precursor, which is then converted in the pineal parenchymal cells to 5-hydroxytryptophan (5-HTP). 5-HTP, by the way, is a substance now popular because of its ability to improve serotonin levels and thus mood and sleep.

Melatonin is suppressed by light but increased in darkness, which is why it has been called the "hormone of darkness." Peak melatonin production occurs during the darkest hours of the night from between two and four A.M., when it reaches an average level in the plasma of 70 picograms per milliliter (pg/mL) in adults; it declines to nearly undetectable levels during the day.

During the life cycle, melatonin production is highest when we are young, topping off at more than 120 pg/mL per day. Starting around puberty, it declines steeply so that by age 75 our nighttime melatonin levels are so low they are barely detectable in both men and women. Because this decline appears to correlate with nearly all the physiological changes that occur during aging, researchers have long taken a great interest in melatonin as a biomarker of aging, as well as an anti-aging medication.

Features of Melatonin Deficiency

- Difficulty falling asleep

- Abnormal sleep-wake pattern

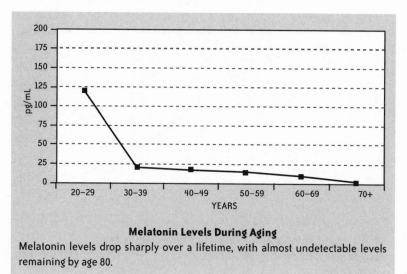

Melatonin Levels During Aging

Melatonin levels drop sharply over a lifetime, with almost undetectable levels remaining by age 80.

- Waking up and finding it hard to fall back to sleep, or falling asleep in the daytime and finding it hard to wake up

- Hard to get going in the morning

- Premature aging, looking older than your age

- Premature gray hair

- Body and extremities are either too hot or too cold at night

- Reduced thyroid function, especially low T3 hormone

- Difficulty normalizing hypothyroid conditions even when taking thyroid hormone

- Excessive symptoms of jet lag

- Feeling out-of-sync with the world

Researchers are still not in agreement as to whether melatonin is a hormone, in the sense that cortisol or estrogen are, or if it is in a separate class of its own. William Regelson, M.D., author of *The Superhormone Promise*, refers to it as a "buffer" hormone (Regelson 1996). Unlike other hormones that have specific target sites, melatonin indirectly influences all cells, tissues, and organ systems in the body, and exerts a synergistic effect on many different hormones at the same time, he says. Walter Pierpaoli, M.D., Ph.D., considered by many aging experts to be the world's leading authority on melatonin, proposes that melatonin is not a hormone in the classic sense. Instead it is a mediator of our biological clock, and therefore directly influences health and aging.

From my clinical experience, I agree with Dr. Pierpaoli. Melatonin is a subtle but powerful neuroendocrine *regulator* that works by normalizing the body's internal clock in ways that we are just beginning to understand. This is why melatonin features high on the list of natural medications in the *Prolonging Health* program.

Supporting this concept of melatonin as a neuroendocrine regulatory substance rather than a classical hormone is the theory that melatonin is an ancient molecule found in all living things on Earth, from single-celled algae to complex biological organisms such as humans, and that in each plant or animal, the structure of melatonin is identical. From this evolutionary view, the ubiquity of melatonin suggests that it evolved in response to the light and dark cycles regulated by the rotation of the Earth on its axis, its rotation around the Sun, and the rotation of the Moon around the Earth. This activity has parallels in sleep, reproductive, and aging cycles. Therefore, melatonin is essential for life and has a role in the aging process, and as such we could rightfully call it an *internal hormonal pacemaker.*

From the point of view that melatonin is a hormonal pacemaker and may even control the rate of aging, scientists theorize that the pineal gland controls the body's biological clock and that melatonin is its messenger molecule. In this model, melatonin is a signaling molecule communicating with melatonin receptors found in all body tissues; conveying information to every cell of the body, it helps to synchronize the neuroendocrine system (Cardinali 1998).

Melatonin is associated with sleep induction and has been shown to improve the quality of sleep and increase blood circulation in the hands and feet while lowering core body temperature during sleep. It influences fertility; levels too high in a woman's body may cause infertility. Melatonin improves thyroid function and has a balancing effect on other hormones. It improves HPA axis activity, and protects the brain and pineal gland against excess cortisol (Sewerynek 1999). Melatonin has powerful antioxidant properties and has been shown to protect against protein damage, lipid peroxidation (Kim 2000), and to protect DNA from oxidative damage (Reiter 1999).

Melatonin inhibits viral replication, protects the body against infection, and has anti-cancer activity. It provides protection against breast cancer and improves the immune activity of cytokines such as interleukin-2 (IL-2) in the treatment of some forms of cancer (Zhang 1997). The types of cancer most successfully treated with melatonin are solid tumors and conventionally untreatable metastatic cancers (Lissoni 2000). Dr. Pierpaoli has shown that inhibition of the synthesis of melatonin suppresses normal immune response. Could it be that another link in the immune deficiency puzzle is abnormal melatonin synthesis, itself another consequence of modern living?

The mechanisms by which melatonin acts as an immune-modulating molecule may be through lymphocyte receptors. As discussed, lymphocytes are cells that play a vital role in immune defenses. Another mechanism might be interactions with various cytokines that produce inflammation, such as tumor necrosis factor-alpha. It may also work through the stimulation of cytokines that promote a favorable immune response such as IL-2 (Lissoni 1999), a cytokine produced in T lymphocytes and essential in stimulating other immune cells to fight infection. The potential for melatonin to stimulate more IL-2 production is important because during aging our T cells make only half as much IL-2 as when we are young, leaving us more vulnerable to the effects of infections.

Due to its neuroprotective effects, anti-inflammatory activity, and its ability to regulate sleep patterns, melatonin also has potential in the treatment of Alzheimer's disease. Though melatonin does not cure Alzheimer's, it helps improve sleep and cognitive function in these cases (Brusco 2000). Inhibition of normal pineal gland activity due to stress, long hours spent under artificial light, lack of daylight exposure, and the use of drugs that deplete melatonin (e.g., indomethacin, beta-blockers, steroids, and many antidepressant and antianxiety drugs) contribute to disrupted melatonin secretion.

In summary, though melatonin is largely thought of as a sleep aid, it is much more than that. Its primary use is to restore neuroendocrine function, and it is an important anti-aging medication to include in your *Prolonging Health* program.

Thyroid Hormone—The Great Imitator: The thyroid is an endocrine gland in the neck. Thyroid hormones control virtually every chemical reaction in your body. The gland has been called the "great imitator" because low thyroid hormone levels cause a wide array of symptoms that mimic other diseases. If your thyroid function is even slightly out of the normal ranges, it

Most experts concur that many of the symptoms of low thyroid (hypothyroidism) resemble the effects of aging, such as drying and thinning of the skin, hair loss, fatigue and muscle weakness, poor sleep, decreased memory, and lowered sexual libido.

will cause your metabolism to waver, your immunity to falter, and your energy to decrease. You will gain weight and your memory will lag. Frequent bacterial, yeast, or viral infections can be the result of low thyroid function, and the risk of cancer increases as well.

Though there is some disagreement among researchers about changes in thyroid hormone production during aging, most experts concur that many of the symptoms of low thyroid (hypothyroidism) *resemble* the effects of aging, such as drying and thinning of the skin, hair loss, fatigue and muscle weakness, poor sleep, decreased memory, and lowered sexual libido.

Hypothyroidism is the most common thyroid disorder in the United States and one of the most common of all endocrine conditions worldwide. It is characterized by a well-recognized set of symptoms and very specific abnormalities in lab testing, the gold standard of this being an elevated thyroid-stimulating hormone (TSH) level. Its opposite condition, hyperthyroidism, involves excess amounts of thyroid hormones. Hypothyroidism is becoming more common as are autoimmune-related thyroid conditions such as Hashimoto's disease (thyroiditis resulting in thyroid hormone deficiency) and Grave's disease (thyrotoxicosis). Though both of these conditions can occur during aging, age-related thyroid hormone dysfunction is mainly characterized by symptoms of low thyroid gland function.

The most common symptom of an underactive thyroid is usually fatigue, yet this is not the typical feeling of being tired. Fatigue caused by low thyroid creates a sense of utter exhaustion, both mentally and physically. An underactive thyroid function can cause many other complaints, such as anemia, heavier than normal menstrual bleeding, constipation, dry skin, and hair loss.

Features of Thyroid Deficiency

- Exhausted feelings that are not related to stress or amount of work or exercise

- Morning tiredness, even after a full night's sleep

- Depression that does not respond to antidepressants, diet, or exercise

- Unexplained anxiety and panic attacks

- Moving as if in slow motion

- Taking too long to respond to questions

- A frequently low or hoarse voice (for a woman)

- Mental sluggishness and difficulty focusing

- Low sex drive, no significant sexual arousal

- High cholesterol level unresponsive to diet or medications

- A tendency to feel cold even in warm weather

- Chronic aches and pains not due to accidents or exercise

- Problems with allergies

- Difficulty losing weight and keeping it off

- Very dry skin, acne, or eczema

- Puffy face and swelling under the eyes

- Thick swollen tongue with teeth marks along the edges

- Swelling of the ankles and feet

- Yellowing of the face and palms

- Slow heart rate

- Diabetes, anemia, rheumatoid arthritis or other autoimmune condition

- Problem with periods, including abnormal menstrual bleeding

- Infertility or a history of frequent miscarriages

- Significant menopausal symptoms

- A tendency to have chronic constipation even with a high-fiber diet

- Lots of hair falling out or brittle hair

- Depigmentation of patches of skin (vitiligo)

- Trembling of hands or stumbling for no reason

Low thyroid function also causes imbalances in the production of other hormones, and it can disrupt the hypothalamic-pituitary complex and other hormonal axes. For example, when thyroid function is low, the adrenal glands may attempt to compensate by producing more adrenaline, which can approach levels as much as 30 to 40 times more than normal. This in turn can cause insomnia, agitation, increased heart rate, and abnormal glucose metabolism.

Low thyroid is also associated with abnormal production of cortisol, melatonin, estrogen, progesterone, and growth hormone.

On the other side of the thyroid equation, hyperthyroidism (too much thyroid activity), even if induced by excess use of thyroid hormone drugs to treat hypothyroidism, can cause osteoporosis, increase heart rate, increase oxidative processes in the body causing more free radical damage, and create an intolerance to heat. In the elderly, hyperthyroidism also causes mental confusion, lack of appetite, and irregular heart rhythms.

The primary hormone secreted by the thyroid gland is thyroxin (T4). It is converted to triiodothyronine (T3) in the peripheral tissues, the liver, and kidneys. Technically speaking, T4 is actually a prohormone for the active form of thyroid hormone, T3, which is used by the body's cells. After T3 is formed, it is released into the bloodstream. The bioavailable form of T3 is called free T3, and it is this free and available form that is picked up by cell receptors and transported inside the cell. Free T3 levels are a biomarker of aging.

As with other hormones, powerful enzymes help the synthesis of the various

Actions of the Different Hormones Involved in Thyroid Metabolism

Hormone	Site of Secretion	Action
Thyroid-releasing hormone (TRH)	Hypothalamus	Stimulates release of TSH
Thyroid-stimulating hormone (TSH)	Pituitary	Stimulates the thyroid gland to produce T4 and other hormones
Thyroxin (T4)	Thyroid	Serves as a prohormone for the conversion of T3; inhibits TSH and TRH
Triiodothyronine (T3)	Liver and Kidneys	Biologically active thyroid hormone
Free T4	Converted in tissues	Bioavailable form of T4
Free T3	Converted in tissues	Bioavailable form of T3
Reverse T3 (rT3)	Peripheral Cells	No known biological activity

thyroid hormones, and their breakdown for reuse or excretion from the body. Like other hormones, thyroid hormones depend on transportation by proteins to move them through the blood.[34] Cell receptors link up with free T3 where it is carried into the cells.

Though most T4 is converted to T3, an alternative product of the metabolism of T4 is reverse T3 (rT3). This form of thyroid hormone is considered to have low biological activity in the body. Due to abnormal thyroid metabolism, as often happens during aging, greater levels of rT3 than free T3 can build in the blood. This buildup of rT3 can produce a form of hypothyroidism called Wilson's syndrome, in which too much rT3 is formed and not enough free T3 is available.

During aging, thyroid function, complicated by environmental effects and stress, can become progressively abnormal. However, most gerontologists agree that under normal circumstances, thyroid function can remain relatively stable during the aging process, but that low thyroid function does contribute to senescence. Though the number of thyroid cells does not decrease with age, a number of changes occur in the structure of the thyroid gland. These include swelling and the development of abnormal structural shapes inside the cells, such as in the mitochondria. In addition, there are fewer thyroid hormone receptors in the body; this, when coupled with increased resistance to thyroid hormone, causes a reduction in thyroid hormone activity.

Since normal amounts of T4 and T3 in the body are dependent on the interaction of the hypothalamus, pituitary, and thyroid gland, any age-related disruption of the hypothalamic-pituitary complex can cause disruption in the neuroendocrine relationship between these glands.[35] Abnormal activity in this relationship causes a decrease in thyroid hormone production, but also can make the thyroid gland less responsive to thyroid-releasing hormone and thyroid-stimulating hormone, and both result in low thyroid function.

The thyroid gland can store large amounts of hormone and release it as needed, even over several weeks. Therefore, plasma levels of thyroid stimulating hormone (TSH), total thyroxin (T4), and total triiodothyronine (T3) can remain relatively stable during aging. But the production of both T4 and T3 declines with aging; T4 drops by approximately 25 percent and T3 by at least 30 percent. There is a reduced conversion of T4 to T3, and this results in reduced amounts of the bioavailable forms, so free T3 levels declines steadily with age.

Though plasma levels of thyroid hormones may be within the normal reference ranges, the tendency in older people (this can show up as early as middle age) is to have slightly rising TSH (suggesting hypothyroidism). However, some have decreasing amounts of TSH. In the absence of hyperthyroidism (low TSH and increased T4), this suggests declining pituitary function. In this case, thyroid-releasing hormone secreted by the hypothalamus may also be low and fail to stimulate TSH production. When pituitary function is diminished, other pituitary hormones, such as growth hormone, tend to be low; this is a sign of accelerated aging. Autoimmune-induced hypothyroidism may occur more frequently in people as they age, and blood tests (antiperoxidase antibody) for this may be positive even in the absence of normal TSH, T4, and T3 levels.

If you suspect that your thyroid might be low and your blood tests keep returning within the normal ranges, consider a 24-hour urine test for thyroid hormone levels. This test measures a sample of urine collected over a 24-hour period and tests for the average thyroid hormone activity during an entire day. It can detect changes that a blood test might miss.

Slightly low thyroid function occurs frequently in older people, but many diseases common to aging, such as cancer and autoimmune disease, cause alterations in thyroid function and changes in levels of thyroid hormones. Other causes of borderline hypothyroidism include loss of muscle mass, adrenal insufficiency, protein malnutrition, and low levels of B vitamins, especially folic acid. Due to the difficulty in clinically assessing borderline low thyroid function in the elderly, and because of the possibility of complication with other medical illnesses, if you are diagnosed with a low or high thyroid condition, be sure to ask your doctor what the cause is. Do not assume that it is simply age related.

Other conditions of aging that may have a basis in low thyroid function are a decrease in growth hormone and a decrease of natural killer cells involved in defense against viruses and cancer (Kmiez 2001). Low thyroid can exert a hormone-lowering effect on estrogen and abnormal activity between estrogen and progesterone, especially during menopause. This is why perimenopausal women should always have a TSH test along with testing for FSH, estradiol, and progesterone levels.

Paradoxically, scientists have found that animal subjects tend to live longer with low levels of thyroid hormones. This is probably because of the lower metabolic rate that is concurrent with reduced thyroid function. However, a similar paradoxical situation occurs with growth hormone—lower levels are associated with longevity—as well as with IGF-I, corti-

General Levels of Thyroid Hormones in Older People	
TSH	increased or unchanged
T4	normal or slightly low
T3	slightly low
Free T4	normal or slightly low
Free T3	low
Reverse T3	normal or high

sol, insulin, and prolactin, all which have less to do with metabolism and thermodynamics than thyroid hormones do. Why does this occur?

We know that high levels of cortisol and insulin accelerate aging and that lower levels of some hormones are associated with longevity, but the reason for this still eludes researchers. For our purposes, keep in mind that the intention is to restore neuroendocrine *balance*. If you add hormones to your *Prolonging Health* program to do this, do not use excessive amounts that push levels above normal physiological ranges; otherwise, you could be trading off short-term improvement in symptoms for a shorter life span. As a general rule, to prolong your health and promote longevity, keep your thyroid gland healthy.

Estrogen—The Aging Woman's Friend, or Foe? Estrogen participates in initiating the menstrual cycle, prepares the uterus for conception, and promotes fertility. In its most active form, estradiol, it affects nearly every type of cell in the female body. Low estrogen is implicated in hot flashes, night sweats, thinning skin, facial pallor, thinning vaginal tissue, lack of body fluids, lack of vaginal lubrication, insomnia, poor concentration, reduced bone density, and fatigue.

Features of Estrogen Deficiency

• Thinning head hair, and increased facial hair

• Dry eyes

• Hot flashes and night sweats

• Tiredness and depression

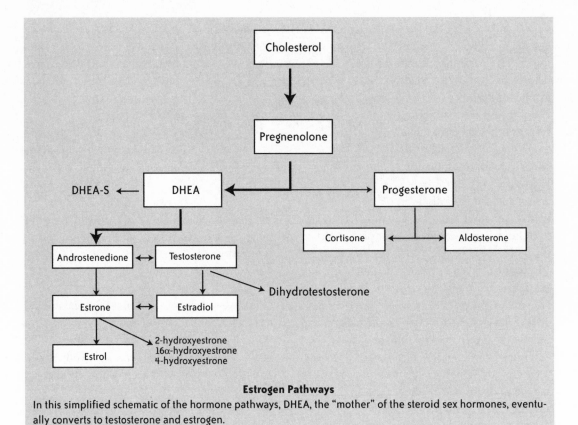

Estrogen Pathways

In this simplified schematic of the hormone pathways, DHEA, the "mother" of the steroid sex hormones, eventually converts to testosterone and estrogen.

- Poor sleep

- Decreased sexual desire

- Fine facial wrinkles, especially around the mouth and lips

- Vaginal dryness, itching, and soreness

- Increased frequency of urinary tract infections

In premenopausal women, most estrogen synthesis takes place in the ovaries. Like all steroid hormones, estrogen's precursors include cholesterol and pregnenolone, and it follows the pathway using DHEA as a prohormone to make testosterone, which is then converted into estradiol (E2), then into estrone (E1) and estriol (E2). Estrogen can also be produced by the adrenal gland, by way of the con-version of androstenedione, with additional conversion in the fat, skin, muscle, and endometrium of the uterus. In older women, as well as older men, estrogens are produced in the peripheral tissue from androstenedione, made in the adrenal glands, and converted primarily to estrone.

Estrone comes in several forms. One, 2-hydroxyestrone (2OHE), is synthesized in the liver, and may provide anticancer activity. Two others, 16α-hydroxyestrone (16OHE) and 4-hydroxyestrone (4OHE), are thought to be cancer inducing and have been shown to promote cell proliferation and induce DNA damage (Liska 2002). The ratio between 2OHE and 16OHE appears to influence cancer activity. Women who predominantly converted more

2OHE have a 40 percent reduced risk of developing breast cancer (Meilahn 1998), so keep your 2OHE/ 16OHE ratio higher than 2.

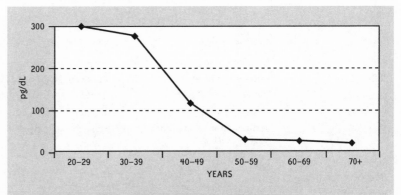

Estradiol Levels in Women During Aging
Estradiol levels drop steeply in women, with continuous lower levels after menopause and values less than 20 pg/dL by age 70.

Estrogen's neuroendocrine relationships are complex. Neurotransmitters produced in the hypothalamus influence estrogen metabolism and activity in the body. They also influence hormones that work closely with estrogen, such as follicle-stimulating hormone (FSH), luteinizing hormone (LH), and prolactin, in complex patterns of complementary and antagonistic actions; these include adrenaline, dopamine, endorphins, and serotonin.

All influence aging and age-related conditions, and have a close connection with carbohydrate metabolism, insulin resistance, body weight, and cognitive effects such as memory, mood, and sleep. Thyroid hormones, growth hormone, and melatonin also play interactive roles in estrogen's neuroendocrine dance, influencing and stimulating production, receptor sensitivity, and metabolism (Maran 2000).

Estradiol (E2) levels in women of reproductive age vary through the month according to the stage of their menstrual cycle. As it is the predominant active estrogen in women, E2 is the one physicians follow when testing for estrogen levels in your blood. During the first week of the monthly cycle, the early follicular stage or beginning of the proliferative phase when the uterus is preparing for possible pregnancy, E2 levels range from about 40 picograms per deciliter (pg/dL) upwards to 80 pg/dL; and during the second week, the mid-

follicular stage, E2 levels surge up to as high as 300 pg/dL. At mid-cycle, when estradiol is at its peak, a 36-hour ovulatory phase occurs when the ovum or egg is ripe for fertilization. If pregnancy doesn't take place, over the next two weeks, the early and late luteal phases, E2 levels gradually fall to their lows of around 40 pg/mL.

During menopause, ovarian function declines and hormonal imbalances occur, redefining a woman's hormonal life. During the years between 35 and 45, many women can experience increased levels of premenstrual discomfort. This is often due to the fact that progesterone levels begin to decline well in advance of age-related changes in estrogen production. By the late forties, many women experience perimenopausal symptoms including hot flashes, night sweats, reduced interest in sex, vaginal dryness, and other symptoms of estrogen deficiency. At this time, E2 levels may be erratic and levels begin to decline.

Then when a woman ceases menstruating, usually between the ages of 48 and 52 (though some women continue into their mid-fifties), progesterone levels are barely detectable and E2 levels have sunk to a constant range, often

Estrogen Ranges

Test	Reference Range	Optimal Range	Aging Faster
Estradiol-17 Beta (E2) in pg/mL	Women: preovulatory, 107–281; postmenopausal, less than 20. Men: 3–70	Women: perimenopausal, 60–80; postmenopausal, 35–65. Men: less than 35	Women: less than 20. Men: more than 70
Estrone (EI) in pg/ml	Women: mid-cycle, up to 229; postmenopausal, less than 55. Men: 12–72	Women and Men: close to mid-range	Women and Men: excessively high
16-alpha(OH) Estrone (mcg/24-hour urine)	1.50–1.90	Within range	Higher than range
2(OH) Estrone (mcg/24-hour urine)	2.2–10.9	Upper end of range	Lower than range
2(OH):16-alpha(OH) Estrone Ratio	1.01–2.43	Higher than 2	Lower than 1.5

below 20 pg/dL. Concurrent with declining estradiol levels, FSH and LH levels increase.

Postmenopausal women who retain their ovaries produce mostly androstenedione and testosterone, though at much lower levels than before menopause. The adrenal gland also continues to secrete some androstenedione, which is converted to testosterone and then into estrogens in the peripheral tissues.

From the clinical view, though there is no defining moment, postmenopause may be declared to have started when a woman has had no menstruation for at least 12 months, and when her estradiol levels decline to below 20 pg/ml, and FSH and LH levels are greater than 20 IU/L and 30 IU/L, respectively (Speroff 1999). It is at this time, and in the few years preceding menopause, that estrogen deficiency symptoms begin to appear, increasing with time as a woman ages.

Keep in mind that these hormone values are textbook numbers, and though giving us general ranges, they do not define hormonal variations and the various degrees of change experienced by individual women. Each woman's neuroendocrine rhythms are slightly different from the next. FSH levels, for example, can range as high as 95 IU/L or higher, while in some women estradiol levels may plateau at about 30 pg/mL and never reach the "textbook" low.

The benefits of estrogen replacement in women just before and after menopause are well established, but so are the risks. Chief among them is breast cancer, but improper use of estrogen in higher than physiological amounts leads to a host of other adverse conditions, including excitation of nerve cells, which can lead to agitation, mania, and neurotoxicity in the brain; fluid retention; the promotion of inflammation in the body; and an increase in oxidative processes and free radical damage. High, continuous levels or bursts of estrogen may contribute to accelerated aging.

Symptoms of Estrogen Excess

- Extreme agitation
- Wild mood swings
- Fluid retention
- Migraine headaches

- Breast pain and swelling

- Vaginal bleeding

There is no doubt that estrogen has its bad points, but the question that most concerns us is: can we isolate the good and limit the bad, or do they always come together?

On the plus side, *appropriate* amounts of estrogen promote central nervous system adaptability and renew nerve cells in the brain. They help to regulate the immune response and the expression of cytokines and growth factors that are involved in development. They increase the synthesis of growth hormone; act as an antioxidant; prevent bone loss; help control autoimmune processes; and prevent many of the symptoms of aging.

Researchers have gathered evidence that estrogen may directly influence the aging brain such that low levels of estrogen appear to accelerate aging. Replacing estrogen has been shown to prevent age-related cognitive decline, reduce the risk of Alzheimer's, and improve memory (Norbury 2003). It does this by protecting brain nerve cells from neurotoxins and oxidative damage, and it may even promote neurogenesis, the creation of new neurons (Azcoitia 2003).

Estrogen being the most commonly prescribed hormone for women, when used properly it gives significant benefits, but when used unwisely, it causes major harm. For example, estrogen has been shown to improve immune function. However, it also can stimulate oncogenes in susceptible tissue such as the breast and uterus, and it can create an "immune sanctuary" in the body, allowing cancers to develop protected from the general immune system. This may explain why cancer patients are often mystified as to why they have cancer when they thought they were healthy.

In their older years, as their hormone production declines, men and women have about the same levels of sex steroid hormones. Older men in general who gain more body fat and lose muscle as they age are predisposed to have more estrogen than testosterone; that is because they aromatize more androstenedione and testosterone to estrogen. Aromatization is the process by which the enzyme aromatase converts androgenic hormones to female hormones.

A younger man has a testosterone-to-estrogen ratio of 50:1, while an older man's ratio drops to about 8:1 (Bland 2001). This decrease in testosterone may not be beneficial, as there is some evidence that men receive some cancer protection from maintaining a balance among estrogen, progesterone, and testosterone, as do women, and that they have an increased risk from prostate cancer if their estrogen levels go too high. Too much estrogen is not good for younger men, but does estrogen play any beneficial role in older men?

There is little consensus that estrogen provides any anti-aging benefits to older men. The exception is the practice of some medical practitioners who use short-term bursts of estradiol in men to increase sexual responsiveness and energy. In my clinical opinion, it is best not to use estrogen in men, even to temporarily lower age-related symptoms, until we understand estrogen's role in the aging male, and to use it sparingly and with caution in women.

For women, correct estrogen replacement returns a youthful appearance, fills out wrinkles, restores sleep, improves mood, improves memory, and increases sexual enjoyment. It helps lower biological age and assists you in staying at your age-point.

Testosterone—The Hormone of Power: As an anti-aging hormone, testosterone is a star performer with many benefits for men and women. It enhances the effects of growth hormone by increasing muscle mass and strength, it balances estrogen and other female sex steroid hormones, improves cardiovascular function, improves energy, lifts the mood, and deepens sleep, among other effects. Like nearly all of the other hormones we've discussed, testosterone has its proponents who link its declining levels with aging. Despite the continuing debate of whether some hormones are the cause or are associated with aging, hormones such as testosterone significantly improve many of the features associated with aging.

Features of Testosterone Deficiency

- Decreased muscle size and tone, reduced strength

- Increased flabbiness

- Increased abdominal fat

- Hair loss in women, balding in men

- Fatigue and weakness, lack of stamina

- Depression

- Increased anxiety and irritability

- Decreased sex drive, loss of interest in the opposite sex

- Decreased body hair

- Decreased aggressive drive

- Occasional night sweats

Andropause, the "male menopause," is a term used to encompass the changes that men experience as their testosterone levels decline during the aging process. Alternatively, this decline has also been termed "androgen decline" in the aging male, or ADAM (Morales, 2000). The onset of these changes is slower than women experience during menopause, so this clinical syndrome is characterized by obvious changes in physical features and cognitive function, and it affects men *and* women.

The normal plasma total testosterone range for younger men is between 241 and 827 nanograms per deciliter (ng/dL). The majority of younger males fall in the upper end of the range with at least 650 to 800 ng/dL, though some young men have natural levels as high as 1,200 ng/dL. As men approach age 45, their testosterone levels have already fallen off by about half their youthful peak levels, and decline further as they pass the age of 55. It has been estimated that at least 50 percent of men over 50 years of age have low testosterone levels compared to peak levels of younger men, and that they have fallen as much as 90 percent from peak levels by the seventh and eighth decade of life.

In my practice, I routinely check for total testosterone and free testosterone, and I also request the percentage of free-to-total testosterone in men over the age of 45, and in some cases earlier. I recommend testosterone supplementation for men when levels of total testosterone fall below 400 ng/mL or when levels of free testosterone fall below the reference range. Free testosterone, also referred to as bioavailable testosterone, is measured in nanomoles per liter (nm/L) or picograms per milliliter (pg/mL) depending on which laboratory you use. Therapeutically, aging men may feel better when their testosterone reaches optimal ranges, those that are within, or in some cases above, the normal age-matched values, and those that approximate youthful levels. For aging men, optimal free testosterone levels are 21–26.5 pg/mL.[36]

In women, testosterone production also declines with age, but the decrease in estrogen levels is much steeper, so it is not uncommon for some women around menopause to show signs of testosterone excess. These signs may include a leaner body with more muscle than fat, a deeper voice, more aggressive behavior, and increased facial hair; this happens because the ratio of testosterone to estrogen is temporarily higher.

Of course, not all women develop these features, as many experience a drop in both estrogen and testosterone at about the same time, with the production of testosterone falling from 25–75 per-

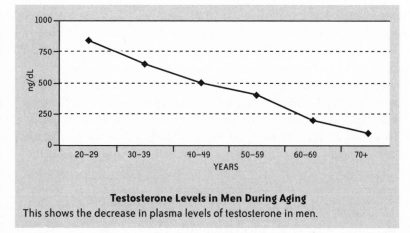

Testosterone Levels in Men During Aging
This shows the decrease in plasma levels of testosterone in men.

cent between the reproductive and post-menopausal years. Some women experience drops in testosterone before their estrogen and progesterone levels decline, and this causes them to feel fatigued. Before menopause, women synthesize androgens, androstene-dione and testosterone in the adrenal glands and ovaries; after menopause more testosterone is made in the ovaries, if they haven't been surgically removed. DHEA, also an androgen, is made largely in the adrenal glands, before and after menopause.

The reference range for total testosterone in women is between 20 to 80 ng/dL. Since hormonal secretion varies with the individual, some menopausal women can have testosterone levels either above or below this range, which extends the normal range from lower than 20 ng/dL to as high as 100 ng/dL, or even higher. After menopause, testosterone levels fall only slightly, but in women over 65 years of age, levels decline further and may approximate the falling levels of men. As a rule, I am clinically satisfied if menopausal women have total testosterone levels between 35 and 55 ng/dL.

The risks of testosterone replacement are small when using low physiologic dosages that maintain plasma levels in acceptable ranges, and when used within the context of an overall neuroendocrine balancing plan. However, the "dark side" of testosterone can be significant and deserves careful consideration before you embark on a testosterone replacement regimen. Foremost among the concerns for men is a possible increased risk of prostate cancer.

European physicians tend to disagree with American doctors that testosterone triggers prostate cancer and believe that testosterone replacement actually lowers the risk for prostate cancer. My clinical experience confirms that the vast majority of men on testosterone have improved prostate function; still, it is best to be careful. In individuals with a family history of prostate or breast cancer (both are hormone-dependent cancers), or in those whose prostate specific antigen (PSA) is above 3.5 ng/mL, I advise *not* using testosterone.

Standardized laboratory values for PSA are 4.0 to 10.0 ng/mL.[37] Studies show that a PSA above 4.0 ng/mL increases exponentially the chances of contracting prostate cancer. Therefore, the medical consensus is that safe ranges for PSA are below 4.0 ng/mL. Some experts believe that the upper limits of PSA values should be age-matched with the PSA for those in their fifth decade and be 2.5 ng/mL; in the sixth decade, 3.5 ng/mL; the seventh, 4.5 ng.mL; and 6.5 ng/mL for those 80 years and older. This is a sensible method, but it is not good enough.

For my patients, I am comfortable only when their PSA levels are well below these age-matched upper limits. I prefer that for men of all ages their PSA be below 2.5 ng/mL. Many doctors might contend that this is an unrealis-

For my patients, I am comfortable only when their PSA levels are well below these age-matched upper limits. I prefer that for men of all ages their PSA be below 2.5 ng/mL. I assure you that this is realistic and attainable, as my male patients routinely have PSA values even lower.

tic or highly optimistic clinical goal for older men. However, I assure you that this is realistic and attainable, as my male patients routinely have PSA values even lower.

I attribute the difference between most of my male patients, who are beating the statistics, and the average American male, who isn't, to the fact that my patients eat a diet that does not promote cancer but does promote strength and vitality. It is a diet that has adequate protein, an abundance of fresh vegetables and fruits, moderate carbohydrates, and enough of the right types of fats. These men also exercise daily and live a lifestyle that is health enhancing, and they take nutritional supplements and herbal medicines.

However, there is more to the testosterone connection than preventing age-related decline or supplementing testosterone when levels fall below the optimum threshold. Additional fac-

tors are involved in testosterone metabolism, in particular how much testosterone, and the other androgens DHEA and androstenedione, are converted into estrogen and dihydrotestosterone (DHT).

In his book *The Testosterone Syndrome*, Eugene Shippen, M.D., calls estrogen "the forgotten side of masculinity" (Shippen 1998). As we discussed in the section on estrogen, as men age, not only does their testosterone level sink, but their estrogen metabolism becomes abnormal at the same time. This is not a good scenario for older men who want to retain their sexual zest and the other features that testosterone provides. The problem appears to lie with the aromatase, an enzyme that helps to convert testosterone to estrogen.

Estrogen plays a number of important roles during aging, including ones to do with sexuality and memory, and it may have a cancer-protective role; but too much causes a host of problems. As noted earlier, a man's level of estrogen throughout life typically is low with a considerably greater testosterone-to-estrogen ratio of about 50 to 1; during aging, that ratio changes to about 8 to 1. Maintaining a ratio similar to that in younger men helps prevent those features associated with hormonal deficiency.

When the balance between the male and female hormones is disrupted, a variety of conflicting symptoms may occur. This might manifest in a man with too much estrogen but normal testosterone levels; functionally, it's as if his testosterone levels were low, because the estrogen molecules interfere with the testosterone receptors. At the same time he may develop features of high estrogen such as more body fat, flabby muscles, water retention, or gynecomastia (flabby enlarged breasts).

Beneath the surface of these feminizing features, in susceptible men too much estrogen may participate in the development of chronic enlargement of the prostate, called benign prostatic hyperplasia (BPH).

The other complication of disrupted testosterone metabolism in aging is the excess conversion of testosterone into too much DHT. The enzyme involved in this process is 5-alpha reductase. There are two types of 5-alpha reductase. One type is found mainly in the skin, where it stimulates sebum in the oil glands, and is also involved in hair growth, or loss, as too much DHT is associated with early balding. The other type is found in the prostate; too much conversion of testosterone to DHT in the prostate is associated with BPH and also with a greater cancer risk.

Another has to do with binding proteins. Sex hormone–binding protein (SHBG) can increase during aging as levels of sex hormones decline. Higher SHBG levels can make testosterone unavailable to attach to cell receptors. In this case, low testosterone with high SHBG causes increased symptoms of testosterone deficiency.

For men, restoring testosterone levels prolongs health by preventing cancer, cardiovascular disease, and eliminating fatigue. It renews the sense of youthful vigor, enhances libido, and improves muscle mass and strength. For women, it improves energy and increases sexual interest. When testosterone levels are restored, you feel and look younger and you can maintain a biological age at your age-point.

Human Growth Hormone—The Master Anti-Aging Hormone: In the public mind, and even with many doctors, growth hormone deficiency has become synonymous with aging. However, this is only partially true. The importance of growth hormone in anti-aging programs makes it necessary to explore it in

some detail here before discussing how to boost levels of growth hormone. The fact is: stimulating too much growth hormone may *reduce* your life span.

Medically speaking, it's true that in a condition endocrinologists call complete hypopituitarism (the absence of pituitary hormones), human growth hormone (HGH) is severely deficient. But so are a wide range of other hormones produced by the pituitary, all of which mimic the signs of aging. We need to ask the same question as with DHEA and thyroid hormone: is the decline in HGH levels during aging the cause of aging? Or is it a phenomenon associated with aging but not directly causative? Answering this question will help us define our strategy for HGH therapy. Let's now discuss what HGH is, what it does in the body, and how it relates to aging.

HGH is a peptide hormone secreted by the anterior pituitary gland in the brain in response to stimulation by the hypothamalic substance called growth hormone releasing hormone (GHRH). Again, we are reminded of the importance of the hypothalamic-pituitary complex as the hinge for all other hormone axes. HGH in turn stimulates the release of IGF-I (somatomedin-C) from the liver.[38]

In the blood circulation, IGF-I is bound to specific binding proteins, but only about one percent is in the free bioavailable state. HGH is secreted predominantly at night in a pulsatile manner, while daytime levels remain relatively constant; HGH pulses decrease with age. Like other hormones, HGH synthesis is regulated by enzymes and other hormones, and it has receptors primarily in muscles and bones.

HGH and IGF-I act as synergistic anabolic, or upbuilding, hormones to stimulate growth in childhood. They stimulate muscle and bone growth, increase lean muscle mass, redistribute

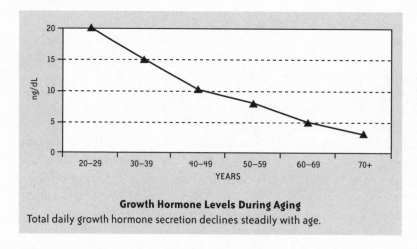

Growth Hormone Levels During Aging
Total daily growth hormone secretion declines steadily with age.

aerobic capacity, increased percentage of fat to muscle, reduced bone mass and density, and smaller organ size. Other features include redistribution of fat to the central part of the body, thinning of the extremities, reduced muscle strength, and a reduction in total body water stores. Though still under investigation, the most likely candidates as the cause for these particular changes are the anabolic hormones such as DHEA, testosterone, and HGH.[40]

fat away from the abdomen and trunk of the body, induce deep sleep, and exert immune-enhancing activity by stimulating thymus gland activity and enhancing natural killer cell activity. HGH and IGF-I may directly affect brain function, including age-related changes, by improving blood flow in the brain (Sonntag 2001).

It has been well documented in the scientific literature that both growth hormone and IFG-I levels decline steadily with age, making them valuable biomarkers for evaluating biological age and for monitoring the effectiveness of anti-aging therapies. HGH secretion declines by an average of 14 percent each decade between the ages of 20 and 70; levels of IGF-I (used as an indirect method of measuring growth hormone secretion) at 30 years are 240 ng/mL and about 40 ng/mL at age 80.[39] This decline appears to be automatic and universal, and is seen in animals as well as humans.

Declining levels of these two hormones appear to correlate with distinct age-related changes. The most notable of these are loss of muscle mass or sarcopenia, and increased frailty. Reduced muscle mass, especially in the legs, is accompanied by measurable changes in fitness and body composition such as reduced

Features of Human Growth Hormone Deficiency

• Sagging cheeks, triceps, and buttocks

• Loose skin

• Thinning hair and skin

• Smaller receding jawbone

• Thinning lips

• Loss of muscle tone

• Exhaustion

• Lack of assertion

• Desire to avoid social interactions, preference to be alone

• Receding gums

• Flabby lower abdomen

• Continual anxiety without cause

• Increased total cholesterol, decreased HDL, and increased LDL

The researcher responsible for the idea that growth hormone deficiency contributes to aging is Daniel Rudman, M.D., considered the father of HGH therapy as an anti-aging medicine (Rudman 1990). He developed this theory as a result of his work with 12 men (60 and 81 years old) who were given HGH for six months. Improvements were noted in nearly all of the biomarkers of aging, including a significant decrease of fat, increased lean muscle, increased bone density, and increased skin thickness.

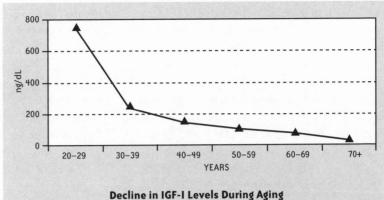

Decline in IGF-I Levels During Aging
IGF-I levels decline sharply after age 25 and continue to decline steadily with age.

Growth hormone deficiency disorders, such as seen in dwarfism, exhibit many characteristics remarkably similar to body changes that occur during aging and were shown to be reversible to some degree with the administration of injectable HGH. That plus Dr. Rudman's research led medical doctors to start using human growth hormone on aging patients (Martin 1999). This clinical trend started in the early 1990s and is now widespread. In fact, the clinical specialty of anti-aging medicine is built on HGH therapy.

The question is: does growth hormone decline because nature intended that, or is it a modifiable aging factor? Many people and a growing number of anti-aging doctors think the latter. But is HGH truly the master hormone of anti-aging practice? Or is it an important part of a comprehensive neuroendocrine balancing program?

Based on a review of the scientific literature, discussions with numerous knowledgeable and ethical physicians practicing anti-aging medicine, interviews with gerontologists, and my own clinical experience, I suggest that GH decline is associated with aging and participates in senescence, but is not the direct cause of aging.

The proof of this lies in the fact that injecting high dosages of human growth hormone does not reverse the aging process. That is not to say that HGH therapy is without benefit, as it definitely improves most of the most common age-related conditions, works synergistically with other hormones, and therefore reverses a wide spectrum of age-related conditions, even though it may not turn back the clock of age.

When HGH is administered in subcutaneous (just under the skin) injections, most of the features and maladaptive conditions of growth hormone deficiency improve. HGH replacement improves both diastolic and systolic blood pressure; it has a beneficial effect on the contractility of heart muscle fibers. It also reduces resistance in the peripheral vascular system, which stiffens with age, and increases nitric oxide production, helping to lower blood pressure. HGH has beneficial effects on blood flow and helps to reverse atherosclerosis (Walker 2001).

Severe HGH deficiency, as seen in some older people and in cases of hypopituitarism, is associated with an increased incidence of cardiovascular disease and early death. Anti-aging physicians report that HGH therapy reverses congestive heart failure and therefore prolongs life in patients with cardiovascular disease. Maladaptive changes such as fatigue and depression, both common symptoms in the elderly, are improved with HGH therapy. Changes in physical features, principally muscle loss and sagging facial skin, are also improved when HGH is given.

Among the two most commonly cited, and most visible, of the benefits of HGH replacement are the increase in muscle volume, tone, and mass, and the loss of excess fat. The overall effects are undeniable changes in body composition that restore a more youthful body shape. In men the physical change includes a smaller waist, more muscular legs, and larger chest with broader shoulders; in women, a smaller waist, less body fat and a better distribution of body fat. In both men and women, HGH therapy lifts sagging cheeks, and tightens underarm and buttocks muscles. It improves mood and reduces fatigue. Though it is still questionable whether HGH helps to increase muscle strength, some studies have shown an increase in maximum strength (Brown-Borg, Borg, et al. 1996). My patients taking growth hormone therapy report increased strength in their weight training, greater endurance, and enhanced sexual ability.

Another beneficial effect of HGH replacement is improved hydration. A common feature of aging is dry and wrinkled skin. Some of this is caused by the inability of tissues to hold water. With an increase in HGH levels, more water is retained in the tissues; there is also an increase in plasma volume, and both improvements appear to be due to increased sodium

retention. Proponents of HGH therapy point to the fact that HGH improves the effects of other hormones. For example, it improves the conversion of thyroid hormone T4 to T3; it modulates cortisol metabolism; and it works synergistically with estrogen and testosterone.

In my clinical experience, most patients receive some, but not all, of these benefits. However, these benefits are usually not as marked as the supporters of HGH replacement suggest.

Opponents of HGH therapy cite the lack of consistent results in the scientific studies. For example, not all researchers find that muscle strength is improved, and those that do find it difficult to explain whether the strength gained is due to the exercise regimen that the study subjects performed or the effects of HGH by itself. However, the majority of papers report favorable results with HGH administration, so this argument is not strong enough to deter proponents of HGH therapy (Johannsson 2001).

The next argument points to a number of potential risks with long-term use such as irreversible acromegaly (abnormal enlargement of the bones), diabetes, edema, and cancer. Fluid retention following HGH administration was known as early as 1959. It is associated with sodium retention and accumulation of fluid in the tissues, and appears to be caused by IGF-I mediated activation of hormones such as aldosterone. These promote changes in kidney function and on how fluids are metabolized in the tissues.

Thus, rather than improving normal hydration, this effect causes abnormal fluid buildup. Some people taking HGH injections experience carpal tunnel symptoms (tingling of the forearms, inside of the wrists, and palms of the hands) severe enough to cause them to discontinue therapy. Sodium retention may also have negative effects on the cardiovascular system, including an increase in blood pressure rather than a decrease (Theusen, Jorgensen, et al. 1994), and it may contribute to kidney degeneration.

These side effects are considered dose-dependent, and do not appear when dosages are kept between 0.5 and 1.0 IU/m², an average daily dose that approximates normal physiological levels. Joint pain, another common side effect of HGH therapy, is also dose-dependent; its symptoms disappear when you adjust the dose downwards or discontinue therapy.

Another side effect is an increased level of insulin—posing a greater possible risk for Type II diabetes. Ray Peat, Ph.D., proposes that though HGH has an important role in growth and development during puberty, once its usefulness is over, levels decline because of its tendency to promote insulin resistance (Peat 2000). This is a condition incompatible with health and longevity.

However, some researchers found that adults with HGH deficiency had some form of increased glucose intolerance, and that HGH therapy, by reducing abdominal obesity, actually improves insulin sensitivity (Beshyah 1994). Though it appears that excessive levels of IGF-I caused by overuse of HGH may cause insulin resistance and glucose intolerance in a few patients, careful regulation of HGH dosage and length of therapy eliminates this risk.

It is well accepted that overstimulation of growth caused by higher than normal levels of growth hormone is unquestionably detrimental to the body. Acromegaly, a syndrome characterized by supraphysiological levels of growth hormone resulting in greater than normal bone and body size, is associated with reduced life span and a wide range of diseases including kidney failure. People overdosing on HGH over long periods of time have displayed acromegalic features.

Also on the negative side, lipoprotein(a), the blood lipid associated with an increased risk for cardiovascular disease, can increase as much as 100 percent with HGH treatment. In susceptible individuals, this outweighs any modest improvement in HDL cholesterol levels that has been reported with HGH administration.

Though not yet fully defined, the possibility that HGH therapy could induce cancer in some individuals makes its use a considerable risk. In this scenario the prize of rejuvenation is won at a high price. Increased levels of IGF-I appear to activate genes that protect cells from apoptosis (programmed cell death) and may activate oncogenes that promote tumor growth. This lethal combination of inhibition of apoptosis (that might otherwise kill a tumor cell) and increased oncogenesis (cancer cell formation) might be enough to trigger aggressive cancers in susceptible individuals.

This brings us back to one of the main conundrums when attempting to extend life. The cellular processes involved in aging and cancer appear to be mutually antagonistic, such that if we find a way to live longer it gives us cancer. It seems that we can't have our cake and live to eat it too. The types of cancers associated with increased levels of HGH and IGF-I include prostate, hypothalamic-pituitary tumors, breast, and colorectal (Shim 1999, Ben-Shlomo 2001).

Very important here is the issue of accelerated aging due to HGH and IGF-I enhancement. The consensus among gerontologists is that animal subjects live longer when calorie restricted, as this causes a stabilization of the levels of many hormones but not a sharp increase. In fact, longevity appears to be commonly associated with *lower* than normal levels of HGH, IGF-I, thyroid hormones, insulin, and prolactin (the hormone that produces milk secretion from the same family of proteins as HGH).

In light of these findings, increasing HGH and IGF-I levels, though offering relief of some of the symptoms of aging, may shorten your life span (Bartke 2001). Since a few deaths have been reported when severely ill patients were given HGH, clearly those with insulin-dependent diabetes, advanced cardiovascular disease, respiratory failure, kidney disease, and those with a history of cancer should not use HGH (Carroll 2001).

While the scientific and medical community remains divided over the human growth hormone issue, researcher William E. Sonntag, Ph.D., a professor of physiology and pharmacology at Wake Forest University in Winston-Salem, North Carolina, suggests that growth hormone and IGF-I have the ability to "reverse the aging phenotype" (Sonntag 2002). Sonntag is one of the leading HGH researchers in the United States and I spoke with him while attending a meeting at the Buck Institute for Aging Research in Novato, California.[41]

He informed me that his research with mice provided strong evidence for rejuvenation effects from growth hormone. However, he acknowledged that more research was necessary before we know if HGH therapy will work safely in humans when taken over a span of several decades as would be necessary to treat a person in their sixties until their eighties, or longer.

Proponents of HGH therapy say that the medical profession is slow to recognize the benefits of many so-called "unproven" but useful medications. European endocrinologists and physicians who practice hormone balancing therapies are convinced that HGH is safe and restores body composition, improves overall health, and brings a sense of well-being to its users. American physicians who practice anti-

aging medicine also agree that HGH replacement lowers biological age and reverses the main features of the somatopause. But don't weight training, yoga, meditation, and proper diet do the same?

These are the basic arguments defining the link between HGH deficiency and low levels of IGF-I and aging. Proponents of HGH replacement point to the benefits of HGH administration, which requires a licensed medical or osteopathic doctor's prescription. Opponents list the potential dangers and caution against its use.

To prolong health and foster longevity, it appears that HGH replacement plays an important role as a symptomatic medicine, but not as a curative therapy. Therefore, it cannot be called a true anti-aging substance. It helps as long as you are taking it, but symptoms return when you stop; it doesn't permanently halt or reverse the aging process. Also, though it may be useful as part of an overall anti-aging plan, it may not be so for everyone, as some individuals are more susceptible to the risks and side effects caused by HGH.

Though researchers are still working out the details of the HGH puzzle, it appears that IGF-I may be the missing modifiable factor. Lower levels of IGF-I are associated with longevity and lower risk for cancer. This is the key we are looking for. The therapeutic direction would be to discover how to increase natural secretion of HGH without overly raising IGF-I levels.

Therefore, if our goal is to prolong health in order to live a longer, healthier life, and not just to be treated as a patient with a medical disease and given more and more physician-administered drugs, then we must approach the use of HGH with caution. Rather than focusing on increasing low levels of IGF-I, we might better attempt to improve the overall *function* of HGH and IGF in the body—the entire HGH/IGF-I axis.

How to Restore Natural Hormonal Balance

Hormones work synergistically with each other. Any treatment aimed at restoring hormonal function works most effectively if the aim is balance rather than merely replacing single hormones that are at low levels. By carefully manipulating this dance of molecules, skilled doctors who use natural biological hormones combined with nutrients and other natural substances obtain better results with lower dosages than conventional physicians using synthetic hormones in high dosages. Not only do hormones work well *together*, but also by using a synergistic model there is less risk of overdosing and a lower incidence of side effects. Nature planned to have hormones work together, so it is our responsibility to find the way in which they work best in our body.

Examples of How Hormones Work Together

- Melatonin helps thymus and thyroid function.

- HGH and thyroid help each other's function.

- DHEA can raise HGH levels.

- Estrogen improves HGH levels.

- Testosterone and HGH work together to build muscle.

- Progesterone counteracts the negative effects of estrogen.

- DHEA helps counter the negative effects of insulin and cortisol.

I generally recommend at least two natural hormones, and usually several at the same time, and never in high dosages. I also recommend diet, exercise, nutritional supplements, and herbal medications that complement hormone therapy. Correct hormonal balance takes place in the context of restoring overall neuroendocrine function. Though the goals of neuroendocrine balancing are numerous and difficult but not impossible to attain, if you follow the principles of integrated longevity medicine as presented in this book and practice the *Prolonging Health* program, your chances of a longer life are greatly increased.

Primary Goals for Restoring the Neuroendocrine System

- Reduce high levels of the catabolic hormones insulin and cortisol.

- Restore the body's biological clock with melatonin.

- Restore thyroid function.

- Protect hormone-sensitive tissues (breasts, uterus, prostate) from damaging effects of sex steroid hormones (estrogen, testosterone).

- Enhance steroid sex hormones (estrogen, testosterone).

- Enhance anabolic hormones (DHEA, testosterone).

- Restore growth hormone levels without causing an excessive increase in IGF-I.

Several methods of hormone therapy are used clinically as well as in anti-aging medicine. However, few practitioners take a comprehensive integrated approach based upon the biology of the neuroendocrine system, advances in aging research, nutrition, and the other concepts reviewed in this book.

The conventional medical practice is to use high-dose synthetic hormones, prescribed based on two criteria: one, the presenting symptoms of the patient; and two, if a particular patient fits a standardized protocol. For example, if a woman is in her late forties, has stopped menstruating, and complains of severe hot flashes, the standard hormone therapy for at least the past three decades has been Premarin, an estrogen compound derived from the urine of pregnant mares. However, in 2002 that model changed when the Women's Health Initiate study was halted three years before its completion date due to increased cancer risk to the participants taking Prempo, a combination hormone containing Premarin and synthetic progesterone (Provera).

In contrast to the previous one-size-fits-all model, doctors practicing anti-aging medicine rely on monitoring hormone levels through laboratory tests. However, that treatment still primarily uses high doses of prescription-strength hormones with little individuality in formulation. The exception to that model is one based on the comprehensive assessment of multiple hormones and a balanced approach to hormone replacement.

This was proposed by Thierry Hertoghe, M.D., of Brussels, Belgium, and presented in his book *The Hormone Solution*. In this model, not just the blood test results but the patient's entire symptom profile as well as physical presentation is taken into consideration (Hertoghe 2002). I had the privilege of studying under Dr. Hertoghe for several years, and found his model to be refreshing and his patient-centered approach to be consistent with naturopathic practice.

Though hormones have considerable physiological effects, and in the hands of a very knowledgeable and skilled physician they are integral to longevity therapies, they can also be very dangerous. They are known to cause cancer, diabetes, stroke, and other undesirable conditions—just the opposite of our desired longevity results! These methods do not take into consideration the complexity of the neuroendocrine system and its diffuse effects throughout every cell in the body; nor do they individualize hormone replacement based upon the needs of the patient, their constitution, physiological makeup, or biochemical individuality.

Supplying excessive amounts of hormones to older people exactly when their own levels are steeply declining disrupts their neuroendocrine system, even further preventing it from ever reaching a healthy balance. Research on calorie restriction suggests that longevity is associated with a global reduction in metabolic and steroid hormones. Taking this into account, the wise approach is to use diet, exercise, and natural substances such as adaptogenic herbs, before launching into a regimen involving only hormones in the belief that they will reverse aging. We need to keep our goals clear to achieve the desired outcome: preventing disease, prolonging health, and fostering longevity.

Therefore, when working with hormones, our primary goal must be to restore normal hormonal balance to the entire neuroendocrine system. This is not merely a matter of adding one or two hormones or pushing hormone levels beyond what the body can tolerate in an attempt to achieve levels that resemble youthful values as determined by blood tests. In my clinical experience, pushing hormone levels ever higher causes further imbalances in all cases, and over time creates other problems. These problems will shorten life, rather than lengthen it.

That is not to say that supplemental hormones don't work, because they certainly have marked effects in the body. Hormones are very powerful substances. In fact, they create the most symptomatic response of all the anti-senescence medications currently available. Since pharmaceutical agents for the treatment of age-related conditions such as cognitive decline are still in their infancy, and until other treatments are available, the use of hormones is necessary to improve many of the symptoms of aging, but they should be treated with considerable respect.

But consider the number of negative effects of improper use of hormones: shortened life span with too much HGH; weakened immunity and neuron damage from cortisol; cancer from HGH, estrogen, and testosterone; excess facial hair growth in women from DHEA and testosterone; and osteoporosis from too much cortisol or thyroid hormone. These are side effects not to be taken lightly.

Now let's review the positive benefits of hormones. These include increased muscle mass and strength; improved energy, sleep, mood, and memory; stronger bones; prevention of anemia and cardiovascular disease; improvement in fluid metabolism and glucose tolerance; and many other important effects. All greatly reduce many of the symptoms of aging.

My approach, as mentioned, is based upon the science of the neuroendocrine system, evolutionary theory, and naturopathic principles—a medical philosophy that says nature knows best. We only have to find a way of working with nature. This is the model of integrative longevity medicine presented in this book. You are already practicing it by following the *Prolonging Health* recommendations.

There are several ways to balance hormones. These include the use of nutritional and herbal substances through what is called nutritional neuroendocrinology to improve insulin signaling mechanisms, to stabilize cortisol activity, and to reset the hypothalamic-pituitary-adrenal axis. If the neuroendocrine system does not fully respond to these ways

and hormone levels remain low, take natural hormones to enhance neuroendocrine activity.

Then, if specific hormone levels still remain low, or your symptoms have not improved, replace deficient hormones with bio-identical hormones to a level that promotes healthy function according to your body. I sug-

When working with hormones, our primary goal must be to restore normal hormonal balance to the entire neuroendocrine system. This is not merely a matter of adding one or two hormones or pushing hormone levels beyond what the body can tolerate in an attempt to achieve levels that resemble youthful values as determined by blood tests. In my clinical experience, pushing hormone levels ever higher causes further imbalances in all cases, and over time creates other problems.

gest that you first proceed through each of the *Prolonging Health* recommendations in this chapter and do not immediately rush to replace deficient hormones. Be patient: you have the rest of your life to get this right.

Prolonging Health Recommendation 41— Get Your Hormones Tested

Before we look at how to restore hormonal balance, and if you haven't done so already, I recommend that you have your hormone levels tested. To establish a baseline for your hormone levels, I recommend blood testing. However, for cortisol, I recommend blood levels plus either salivary testing or 24-hour urine testing. Urinary tests are performed by taking a sample of the total urine excreted (collected in a large plastic container) over a period of 24 hours. This provides an average value of hormone secretion. A good time to start hormonal testing is between ages 45 and 50. However, you can take these tests when you are younger or older than this. When you have your results, compare yours to the optimal ranges (see the tables in chapter 5). Work with your doctor to achieve optimal results.

Baseline Hormone Testing

Take the following blood tests to obtain a basic understanding of your hormone levels:

- Fasting insulin
- Fasting cortisol
- DHEA-S
- Pregnenolone
- Thyroid-stimulating hormone (TSH)
- Luteinizing hormone (LH)
- Insulin-like growth factor I (IGF-I)

For women, take these additional blood tests:

- Follicle-stimulating hormone (FSH)—every year starting at age 48, but not necessary if you're postmenopausal
- Estradiol
- Estrone
- Progesterone
- Total testosterone

For men, take these additional blood tests:

- Total testosterone
- Free testosterone

For a comprehensive baseline, take these additional blood tests:

- Albumin
- Sex hormone binding globulin (SHBG)
- IGF binding protein-1 (IGFBP-1)
- Androstenedione
- Total T4
- Free T3
- For men: estrone, estradiol, dihydrotestosterone (DHT)
- For women: estriol, 16-alpha(OH) estrone, prolactin

For a complete cortisol profile, take these additional tests:

- Salivary free cortisol, four samples over 24 hours
- 24-hour urine free cortisol
- 24-hour urine total 17-ketosteroids

For melatonin:

- Salivary melatonin, four samples over 24 hours

Prolonging Health Recommendation 42— Improve Insulin Signaling with Nutritional Medications

Insulin, as I've emphasized in this book, is a critical hormone in the body and is responsible for the maintenance of normal blood sugar levels. Without the right level of insulin, we suffer from diabetes and increased risk for cardiovascular and other diseases, accelerated aging, and even death. Insulin is also a key signaling molecule, and is responsible in part for controlling the rate of aging. In light of insulin's importance, and for our purposes in *Prolonging*

Health and achieving maximum life span, normalizing insulin sensitivity is the first step to neuroendocrine balance.

Insulin resistance results from consuming refined sugar and excessive amounts of simple carbohydrates, especially white flour products such as pastries; from overeating; from not eating enough protein and essential fatty acids; and from a sedentary lifestyle. The solution is to change your lifestyle from one that causes insulin resistance and glucose intolerance to one that prolongs health (refer to chapter 10 for details).

In addition to diet and exercise, several nutritional supplements are valuable in promoting normal glucose metabolism: vitamin C, vitamin E, coenzyme Q10, lipoic acid, essential fatty acids, magnesium, vanadium, and chromium. Let's briefly discuss these.

Since increased oxidative effects and free radical damage are associated with insulin resistance, antioxidants such as vitamins C and E help to reduce the damaging effects of increased oxidative stress (Ceriello 2000), including inflammatory activity linked to cardiovascular disease (Upritchard 2000). Researchers found that vitamins C and E significantly improve insulin sensitivity even in Type II diabetics (Paolisso 1994). Lipoic acid (Shapiro 2002) and coenzyme Q10 (Izumi 1980) also provide substantial benefits in decreasing blood sugar levels in diabetics and improving insulin sensitivity. Follow the recommendations for supplementing vitamins C and E, as well as lipoic acid and coenzyme Q10 (see chapter 7), as this will provide sufficient levels of these important nutrients.

Essential fatty acids help to decrease insulin resistance and lower blood sugar. They may have other benefits in the treatment of diabetes such as preventing cardiovascular disease, including hypertension, and preventing numbness in the extremities associated with diabetic neuropathy (Goodman 2001). Providing sufficient amounts of essential fatty acids in the diet and through fish oil supplements (see chapter 10) helps to improve insulin sensitivity.

Several minerals are also important in glucose metabolism, and these are magnesium and the trace mineral vanadium. Tissue levels of magnesium tend to be low in diabetics and supplementing with magnesium helps cells process glucose (Lukaczer 1998). Though the exact mechanism is unknown, vanadium salts in diabetes mimic insulin and improve glucose metabolism in conditions of both low and high insulin, and result in improved insulin sensitivity (Cusi 2001).

Adequate levels of magnesium are in the range of 500–1,000 mg daily. Too much magnesium can cause diarrhea, so if that happens reduce the dosage. The dosage for vanadium, supplied as vanadyl sulfate, for the treatment of insulin resistance is between 50 and 100 mcg (Murray 1996). Though vanadium is safe and without drug interactions, there is concern of toxicity in dosages higher than the recommended amounts.

The most important nutritional supplement for managing glucose metabolism is chromium. Though chromium is an essential trace mineral in human nutrition, the average American diet is deficient in this important nutrient. The mechanism is not completely understood, but chromium helps regulate glucose metabolism and is frequently referred to as the "glucose tolerance factor" (GTF). There are many forms of chromium available, including chromium picolinate now famous for its reputed weight-reducing ability. The best form of chromium for improving insulin sensitivity and lowering glucose levels is that derived from brewer's yeast, and labeled GTF chromium.

Newer forms of highly bioavailable chromium are also available, including the patented UltraChrome (chromium 4 oxopyridine, 2,6-dicarboxylate, arginate) from Thorne Research.[42]

The typical recommended daily dietary amount of chromium is 50–200 mcg (most multiple vitamins and mineral supplements contain 200 mcg). For the treatment of insulin resistance, take up to 600 mcg daily. Since kidney and liver damage have been reported with dosages above 1,200 mcg, do not use chromium in dosages higher than the recommended range without the supervision of your doctor. There are no known direct negative interactions with drugs, and chromium is synergistic with vitamin C.

Prolonging Health Recommendation 43—Achieve Neuroendocrine Balance by Neutralizing Excess Cortisol

The second step in restoring normal neuroendocrine balance is to manage excess cortisol. During aging, the function of the adrenal glands may deteriorate and, compounded by stress, this may cause significant alteration in the HPA axis, with excess amounts of cortisol released into the bloodstream. In this scenario, the pituitary gland is unable to shut down the production of cortisol produced in the dysfunctional adrenal glands. Excess cortisol causes a wide range of damage in the body, particularly to the hypothalamus, and is also associated with cognitive decline and shortened life span.

Excess cortisol, even at marginal elevations, may instigate autoimmune reactions and trigger negative genetic expression. Both can contribute to and worsen the symptoms of multiple sclerosis, Alzheimer's disease, several forms of cancer, osteoporosis, and retinitis pigmentosa (an eye condition characterized by excessive levels of cortisol being synthesized in the retina, which causes progressive vision loss).

Of course, some people experience the opposite condition of low cortisol, which I'll address below. For now, let's focus on the disruption to our neuroendocrine system caused by excess cortisol, an insidious condition and a much more difficult problem to remedy than low cortisol.

Though there is no specific natural medication that normalizes cortisol, strive for overall hormonal balance by reducing stress and taking neuroprotective hormones such as progesterone, melatonin, and DHEA, to minimize the damage done by excess cortisol. Among the natural medicines useful here are a few that I have discussed, including vitamin A, zinc, acetyl-L-carnitine, and *Ginkgo biloba*. Here are three additional compounds that help to neutralize excess cortisol levels: DHEA, phosphatidylserine, and Gerivitol.

DHEA: As a rule, though not in all cases, when cortisol levels in the body are elevated, adrenocortical function is disrupted and DHEA levels are reduced. This can be easily evaluated by a saliva test measuring both free cortisol and DHEA-S. Since DHEA has protective effects, if your cortisol levels are high, consider supplementing with DHEA to balance these two important adrenal corticosteroid hormones. An average dosage for DHEA for balancing purposes is between 5 and 25 mg daily. Higher dosages are used during replacement therapy for extremely low levels of DHEA, and this method is discussed in detail in a following section.

Phosphatidylserine: This nootrophic neutraceutical has been shown to relieve exercise-induced cortisol production. It appears to exert a balancing effect on the hypothalamic-pituitary adrenal axis during periods of stress, which are times when cortisol levels tend to rise (Grossman 2000). The typical dosage is 100–300 mg daily, taken as 100 mg three times daily if you have been diagnosed with cortisol excess.

Gerivitol: This is a medication developed by Ana Aslan, M.D., in the late 1940s at the National Geriatrics Institute in Bucharest, Romania, for the treatment of age-related disorders such as arthritis and fatigue. Gerivitol (GH3) has an illustrious history among anti-aging enthusiasts. Actually, Dr. Aslan's formula is a stabilized form of procaine, a common anesthetic first discovered in 1905 by the Austrian biochemist Alfred Einhorn. It contains procaine hydrochloride, benzoic acid, potassium metabisulphite, and disodium phosphate. Interestingly, though few major studies have been performed on GH3 since the 1950s, and the American medical establishment lost interest in it in the 1970s (Ostfeld 1977), and even tried to discredit this medication, Gerivitol continues to sell to large numbers of people worldwide.[43]

Reported to be able to regenerate tissue and enhance cellular metabolism, GH3 has been shown to have regenerative effects on the liver, kidneys, and bone marrow. It helps promote wound healing; enhances immunity; reduces inflammation and treats osteoarthritis; lowers the allergic and asthmatic symptoms; prevents formation of lipofuscin, and lifts depression due to inhibition of the enzyme monoamine oxidase (MAO); and is considered to normalize excess cortisol.

Though not currently available from pharmacies in the United States, GH3 can be legally obtained for personal use from offshore pharmacies or in Mexico. I recommend the original trade-named medication rather than generic brands. Gerivitol comes in 100 mg tablets or 5 ml ampoules for injectable use. To manage chronic excess cortisol, I typically suggest one tablet one or two times daily for two weeks; take an intermission from this for two to four weeks; then repeat the regimen until your cortisol levels are stabilized as demonstrated by a salivary test.

A few variations of GH3, including several German versions, are available in Europe, notably KH3. This is procaine with vitamins and has been shown to improve several age-related parameters such as strength (Hall 1983). An American variation, Gerovital GH3, manufactured by Nutraceutics, is based upon Dr. Aslan's formula and contains vitamins B_6, B_{12}, folic acid, pantothenic acid, and adaptogenic herbs along with p-aminobenzoic acid and other substances.[44]

Since injectable medications enter the bloodstream directly, bypassing the intestinal tract and liver, for anti-senescence therapy I recommend a course of intramuscular injections. Take these three times each week for four weeks, with an intermission of four to six weeks, and then repeat the regimen until symptoms improve. At that point, you may find that one injection every one to two weeks maintains the improvement.

Regardless of degree, excess cortisol is a consequence of physiological and psychological stress, including the stress induced by chronic disease, as well as aging. It will weaken your immune system, cause disease, destroy tissue, and shorten your life span. Thus, restoring cortisol to normal levels is a critical part of your neuroendocrine balancing program.

Prolonging Health Recommendation 44— Achieve Neuroendocrine Balance by Restoring Synchronicity with Melatonin

This is the premier natural substance for resetting the body's biological clock and restoring synchronicity to the neuroendocrine system. For this purpose, I typically recommend that everyone over age 45 take small doses of melatonin nightly, directly before going to sleep but after the lights are out, in ranges of 0.5 to 3.0 mg. Higher dosages may be necessary in some people, such as those with cancer. Dosages between 5 and 8 mg can be used to ease the effects of jet lag after a long-distance flight. Its half-life in the body is 30–60 minutes; it is rapidly absorbed when taken orally, and it reaches peak plasma levels within two hours after ingestion. Melatonin is safe in low dosages and without toxicity.

However, some people report increased dreaming or very vivid dreams when taking melatonin, and in some cases of depression, taking melatonin has aggravated the condition. Also, in high doses, between 150 and 300 mg, melatonin can suppress the production of testosterone, luteinizing hormone, estradiol, and progesterone (Yilmaz 2000). This effect may be desirable when treating cancer with melatonin, but for anti-aging purposes in people without cancer, such dosages are too high and should not be taken.

Restoring melatonin production helps to regulate not only sleep, but mood as well, lowering depression. The key to remember here, as promoted by Russel J. Reiter, Ph.D., author of *Your Body's Natural Wonder Drug: Melatonin,* is: "High serotonin in the day, and high melatonin at night" (Reiter 1995). This means that effective neuroendocrine regulation is dependent on the harmonious activity of sufficient amounts of these two key substances.

Melatonin appears to act synergistically with pyridoxine (vitamin B_6) and zinc, so it should be taken with a low-dosage multivitamin and mineral preparation containing these two nutrients, or in a specially prepared combination containing melatonin, 5 mg of zinc, and 10 mg of pyridoxine. The synergistic effect among these three substances promotes pineal synthesis of melatonin and serotonin and supports melatonin's immune function. You can further enhance melatonin's effects in the body by supporting your neurotransmitters. Take 50–150 mg of 5-HTP and 400 mg of SAMe, after the evening meal.

Supportive lifestyle changes help your body restore its natural synchronicity by maximizing *zeitgebers*. This is a German word used by chronobiologists, scientists who study biorhythms and their significance on health, signifying "time givers," or those practices that restore the body's biological clock and normalize its response to light and dark cycles. Examples include going to bed and waking at the same time each night and morning; allowing rest periods during the day, but without napping, which can disrupt your sleep cycle; not overworking or overexercising; and eating meals regularly. You can raise your melatonin levels and help restore your diurnal rhythms by getting at least four hours of sunlight exposure daily. This helps to suppress melatonin production during the day. You could also completely darken your bedroom as darkness stimulates the secretion of melatonin.

Melatonin is completely safe and nontoxic even in the higher ranges. As noted, it can cause strange effects in some people, including vivid dreaming or nightmares. Like the paradoxical effects of many medications, some people taking melatonin experience stimulating effects and are unable to sleep—as mentioned, this is exactly the opposite effect that most people experience, which is improved sleep.

Also, since melatonin is closely related to the neurotransmitter serotonin, a substance that profoundly influences mood, people sensitive to serotonin or those taking selective serotonin reuptake inhibiting (SSRI) antidepressants (Prozac, Paxil, Celexa) can experience exacerbations of depression and mental illness when taking melatonin. I do not recommend taking melatonin while you are using these or other antidepressant drugs.

Prolonging Health Recommendation 45— Achieve Neuroendocrine Balance by Regulating Your Hormonal Pathways

As you age, and especially in individuals who have the genetic tendency for hormonal imbalances, it is important to assist the body to utilize key enzymes such as aromatase and alpha reductase because it helps to regulate the pathways between the sex steroid hormones. It also prevents hormone-related tumors such as breast and prostate cancer. Aromatase is the enzyme that converts testosterone to estrogen, and too much estrogen is potentially cancer promoting in both men and women. Alpha reductase is the enzyme that converts testosterone into dihydrotestosterone (DHT), the active form of testosterone. Several nutritional and herbal substances naturally inhibit these enzymes and prevent excessive conversion of testosterone into estrogen or DHT. The four best-known of these are isoflavones, lignans, indole 3-carbinol (I3C), and saw palmetto.

Both men and women can use soy products, isoflavones, and lignans from flax. I3C is best for women, though it is also useful in men who are converting testosterone into too much estrogen. Saw palmetto is for men who have prostate problems or excess DHT production.

Soy Isoflavones: Among the most well-studied of the phytoestrogens (plant-derived estrogens), soy isoflavones are known for their ability to inhibit cancer cell growth by a variety of mechanisms. These include decreasing estrogen receptor activity and the inhibition of 5-alpha reductase, the enzyme that helps convert testosterone to dihydrotestosterone (Evans 1995).

Isoflavones also help restore neuroendocrine balance by modulating sex hormone-binding globulin. Soy also has a favorable influence on bone health, another important concern during aging (Brynin 2002). This informs us that soy isoflavones are not only good for you, but contribute to three of the most important features necessary to prolong health: they promote neuroendocrine balance, reduce cancer risk, and promote longevity.

What makes soy so versatile in regulating hormones is the complexity of its constituents. These include protease inhibitors that reduce carcinogenesis, among them lignans; phytosterols that bind cholesterol and prevent its absorption; coumestrol, a phytoestrogenic substance that inhibits the conversion of good estrogen into the undesirable types; and a number of other compounds in addition to the activity of its major isoflavones, genistein and daidzein (Head 1997).

Soy isoflavones may be obtained from naturally fermented soybean foods such as tempeh, miso, and soy sauce. I never recommend soymilk or commercial soy products such as soy hot dogs or soy cheese, as in my clinical opinion, these products are too different and altered from the forms that have been proven safe and health-promoting through generations of use in Asia. Soy isoflavones are also available in concentrated nutraceutical preparations, which I use with my patients in typical dosages of 50–100 mg twice daily with food.

Lignans: Found in the highest concentration in flaxseed, lignans, like soy isoflavones, are considered phytoestrogens. They antagonize the estrogen cycle in a positive way similar to the action of isoflavones. Lignans have anticancer effects, and are known to inhibit aromatase, the enzyme that converts testosterone to estrogen, as well as 5-alpha reductase.

Lignans are synergistic with the naturally occurring omega-3 essential fatty acids in flaxseed oil, which we discussed in the last chapter. Women who use flaxseed meal regularly report improved menstrual cycles. Take one to two tablespoons of fresh ground flaxseed meal daily as a food supplement.

Indole 3-Carbinol (I3C): A chemical substance found in cruciferous vegetables, a family that includes broccoli and cabbage, I3C has antioxidant properties; inhibits breast, prostate, and cervical cancers; prevents DNA damage; and enhances the formation of 2(OH) estrone over 16(OH) estrone, the so-called "bad" estrogen. A patented form of I3C, 3,3'-Diindolylmethane (DIM) is reported to be more absorbable than from plants directly, but since research is still in progress to evaluate its effectiveness compared with I3C, I suggest increasing cruciferous vegetables in the diet first, and then taking I3C.

The typical recommended dosage is between 200 and 800 mg daily; there are no reported contraindications or side effects. Since I3C's effectiveness comes from its conversion in the stomach to DIM and indole 3,2,b carbazole, which only occurs in the presence of hydrochloric acid, conversion and absorption may be improved in older people, who often have lowered secretion, by taking a hydrochloric acid supplement at the same time as I3C, along with a little food. I3C is synergistic with the drug tamoxifen in protecting against breast cancer.

Saw Palmetto: Used to treat benign prostatic enlargement in men, the lipid fraction is derived from the berries of saw palmetto (*Serenoa repens*), a dwarf palm in the *Acrecaceae* family that grows abundantly in Florida. The substance improves urinary flow due to possible 5-alpha reductase inhibiting activity. The recommended dosage is 320 mg daily of the lipophilic extract containing 85 percent fatty acids and sterols. Side effects are rare and there are no contraindications or known interactions with drugs.

Prolonging Health Recommendation 46— Use Herbal Adaptogens to Reset the Hormonal Axis

For several millennia in Asia, humans have used herbal medications to prevent the effects of aging. Though no medication ever reversed or halted aging, adaptogens are very effective in normalizing many of the effects of aging, preventing late-onset diseases, improving biomarkers, and improving quality of life in older people.

Adaptogens are substances that help the body's adaptive processes to stress and therefore promote homeostasis. They promote neuroendocrine communication, normalize adrenal function, stabilize the hypothalamic-pituitary-adrenal axis, and support all neuroendocrine balancing therapies. The four premier herbal adaptogens for neuroendocrine balancing are ginseng, Siberian ginseng, ashwagandha, and rhodiola. A fifth, though technically not an herb but considered a traditional Chinese medicine, is velvet deer horn.

Ginseng: Asian (*Panax ginseng*) and American (*Panax quinquefolius*) ginsengs are superior adaptogens and play an important role in preserving and prolonging health during aging. Historically, wild ginseng was prized for its medicinal and life-giving properties, and as such was referred to in traditional Chinese medicine as a *qi* and *yang* tonic. Qi (pronounced "chee" and sometimes spelled chi) is the vital animating life force present in all living things, but it declines sharply as we age. Yang refers to the quality of energy that is warming, protective, strong, robust, and aggressive. It is due to these two qualities that ginseng usage has been mainly recommended for men; however, post-menopausal women can also take ginseng.

The active principles contained in ginseng root, a complex of numerous compounds collectively called ginsenosides, treat mental and physical fatigue, and depression and other mood disorders; they help regulate glucose, making them useful in the treatment of Type II diabetes; and they are good for immune deficiency conditions. Ginseng has antioxidant properties, and may therefore have undiscovered cellular protective activity. It is because of this broad array of uses that ginseng is so potentially beneficial in the treatment of age-related conditions.

There are three main types of ginseng: American, red Asian, and white Asian. American ginseng is considered cooling and more tonic to the *yin*—those energies in the body that are soft, moist, and nourishing, the balanced opposite of *yang*—making it an excellent choice for women during perimenopause, for stress and anxiety, and to improve sleep; it is also used for its overall calming effect on the neuroendocrine system.

Red Asian ginseng is considered the strongest of the three types and is classified in Chinese medicine as "hot," due to its ability to restore the yang energy. It is most useful in older people who are very weak, pale, and have a tendency to feel cold. The characteristic red color is caused by processing the white root with other herbs to enhance its effect.

In terms of its effect in the body, the ginseng whose qualities fall between American and Asian red, is the white Asian variety from northern China. It is used for its more general tonic effects on the qi, especially for people who are only moderately fatigued and are neither too hot nor too cold; it also works as a general preventative tonic.

Choose American ginseng if you have a tendency to agitation and insomnia; the red form if you are fatigued, have a poor appetite, and tend to feel cold; and Asian white ginseng if you are already generally healthy but want a general tonic. The typical dosage for all three types is 100–250 mg, one to two times daily, of the standardized extract; take it away from food in the morning and midafternoon. It can also be prepared as a tea by slowly simmering 1–2 g of the dried sliced herb for an hour in one quart of water; drink one cup of this once daily in the morning.

Cooking ginseng along with your chicken soup is a centuries-old Asian folk remedy for fortifying the body; it can help modern people as well. Add 0.5 g of ginseng, equivalent to a few sliced pieces, to your soup while cooking and simmer for at least 30 minutes before eating.

Ginseng is considered safe in the recommended dosages, but in some individuals, especially when using higher than recommended dosages, it can cause nervousness or overstimulation and insomnia. It is contraindicated for people with high blood pressure or with fever during an active infection.

Siberian Ginseng: This is not a true ginseng and is only named Siberian ginseng (*Eleutherococcus senticosus*) because of the location where it is found—northeastern China, Siberia, Korea, and Japan—and for its value as an adaptogen and tonic. Even so, it is so highly prized that one of my Chinese medicine professors referred to this herbal medicine as "more valuable than gold."

It increases athletic performance, improves energy level and reduces fatigue, enhances immune function, minimizes the effects of stress, counteracts the effects of radiation, and may be used as a complementary medicine during radiation treatment of cancer, in chronic fatigue, diabetes, and all age-related symptoms.

In addition, Siberian ginseng helps support the liver's detoxification function, and as an adaptogen it promotes normal adrenal gland function. It is not as stimulating as ginseng, so it makes an excellent general tonic and adaptogen and can be used by both men and women.

Though Siberian ginseng can be taken as a tea, it is best used as a liquid or dry extract standardized to eleutherosides B and E; a typical dosage is 250–500 mg daily, taken away from food. A British-made standardized extract, Sibergin, is available in health food stores as 500-mg soft-gel capsules; the recommended dose is one capsule daily, taken in the morning.[45] The Chinese patented liquid extract *wu jia ju*, available from traditional Chinese pharmacies or an acupuncturist, is an excellent and convenient way to obtain the benefits of this adaptogen. Drink 10–15 drops in four ounces of water once daily before bed.

Ashwagandha: A widely used *rasayan*, or tonic, in Ayurvedic medicine, the traditional medical system of India, ashwagandha (*Withania somnifera*) is used to improve overall health and to promote longevity—the basic goals of this book. Due to these effects, it has been referred to as the "Indian ginseng."

Like many traditional Asian medicinal herbs, ashwagandha has a history of use spanning thousands of years, but it has only recently been put under scientific scrutiny. It has anti-inflammatory activity and antioxidant effects, and is useful as an adaptogen that can preserve adrenal function under stress. Ashwagandha improves thyroid function, regulates glucose metabolism, and restores neurotransmitter function (Mishra 2000). The recommended dosage is 150–300 mg daily, in a standardized formula containing 2 to 5 mg of withanolides, the active constituents. Ashwagandha is a safe herb without any known contraindications or drug interactions.

Rhodiola: Another adaptogen with potential for managing a wide range of symptoms related to aging is *Rhodiola rosea*. The plant is found in Russia, China, and parts of Asia, as well as Tibet, where a highly prized variety grows, called *Rhodiola sacra*. It enhances memory, improves exercise performance, and promotes the body's resistance to physical, chemical, and biological stressors (Kelly 2001). Rhodiola has cancer preventive properties, enhances immunity, and has antioxidant activity. It is also cardioprotective and has antidepressant activity.

Twenty-eight active compounds have been identified in the plant, including 12 compounds completely new to medical science. The active constituents are the glycosides salidroside (Rhodidoside) and rosavin, which are components used in the commercially prepared extracts. The recommended daily dosage of a product containing one percent rosavin is 360–600 mg; with 3.6 percent rosavin, the dosage is 100–170 mg. To make a tea, use 5 g of the dried powdered root per cup of water; pour boiling water over the herb, and let it steep for several hours before using. Drink a quarter of a cup, three to four times daily. Rhodiola is considered safe and nontoxic, and is synergistic with other herbal adaptogens.

Velvet Deer Horn: Preparations made from antlers of the red deer (*Cervus elpahus*) and also of deer, elk, caribou, and other horned animals, are equally as revered as ginseng in traditional Chinese medicine. They are used for the restoration of kidney yang energy, the most robust form of qi in the body. Antlers are secondary characteristics of male deer and the fastest growing tissue produced by any mammal. Horns are harvested (without killing the animals) from young, healthy male deer when the antlers are covered with a velvety outer layer before they calcify and become hardened horn.

Since antler regeneration requires growth

factors such as IGF-I and testosterone (Sadighi 2001), traditional longevity practices and modern science may merge in the discovery of adaptogenic medications for aging. Velvet deer horn preparations are used to increase sexual energy in men, reduce fatigue, treat rheumatoid arthritis and osteoarthritis, speed healing of bone fractures, enhance recovery time after exercise, reduce tumor activity, and promote longevity. Though not all of these claims are supported by scientific evidence, the empirical basis for its use is sound and clinically well documented in the Chinese medical literature.

You can obtain sliced and traditionally prepared deer antler in Chinese herb stores. It can be made into a tea using ten slices per quart of water. Bring to a boil and simmer for one hour. Drink one cup daily in the morning away from food. Pantocrine, a commercial preparation, is available as a liquid extract or in tablets. Take 25–40 drops, or one to two tablets in the morning a half-hour before eating for three weeks, which constitutes one course. An intermission of ten days is recommended; then repeat one or two more courses.

Prolonging Health Recommendation 47— Supplement Declining Neuroendocrine Function with Natural Hormones

Once you have applied the principles and used the medications discussed in the previous sections of this chapter, evaluate your improvement. If you feel better, have more energy and greater muscle strength, and experience an uplifted mood, your neuroendocrine system is most likely beginning to function normally again. However, your hormone levels may still be low or imbalanced, and now is the time to retest your hormone levels.

If any of your key hormones still test low, consider natural hormone supplementation, hormone secretagogues, and precursor agents before you ask your doctor for hormone replacement. Of course, if your symptoms have not lessened, and the levels of key hormones are still very low, you may benefit from going directly to hormone replacement therapy.

Let's begin this section with a clarification of the difference between hormone supplementation and replacement. You supplement when hormone levels are below optimal by providing either very small amounts of all-natural hormones or substances that promote hormone production. You enhance or add to what is already there. Replacement, on the other hand, is the process of replacing insufficient hormones, which, as judged by laboratory levels, are below reference values or below optimal ranges and are not responding to enhancement. In essence, you fill up your empty hormone tank.

Most of the time, you can add very small amounts of naturally occurring hormones to improve glandular function or lift hormone levels. But when hormone levels are too low and glandular function has deteriorated beyond what supplemental assistance can enhance, you need to replace the deficient hormone with sufficient dosages.

You enhance your hormonal activity using natural medications, glandular products called protomorphogens, and low dosages of natural hormones. We begin with insulin and cortisol; then consider DHEA because of its role as a central biomarker for aging; then thyroid hormones; and last the sex hormones and human growth hormone.

Insulin: In Type I diabetes, also called insulin-dependent diabetes, the islet cells of the pancreas cease producing insulin, and as a consequence, glucose levels in the blood rise. The cause for this is still unknown, but it is thought to be due to autoimmune activity that destroys the islet cells, or to genetic patterns, which may express the diabetic gene in very young people.

> ✳ **CAUTION:** Treating abnormally low insulin levels with natural medicines, especially if you are diabetic, requires the assistance of a licensed physician. If you use insulin, never stop using this hormone without the consent of your doctor.

However, in healthy people insulin levels are rarely low. On the contrary, the main problem we face is the opposite: excessive production of insulin and the eventual insensitivity of insulin receptors. But some people can have abnormally low insulin levels and not be diabetic; that is, their glucose levels are not elevated, and in these cases promoting insulin activity in the body is helpful to restore glucose uptake by the cells.

Researchers are investigating oral insulin-like compounds called insulin mimetics (as in mimic) in a hopeful search for a replacement to the daily insulin injections required by Type I diabetics. One such promising medication is L-783,281, derived from an African fungus (Zhang 1999). Though numerous other plants are being studied for their potential as insulin mimetics, none have been developed into safe drugs; however, while we wait for research to progress, there are safe natural remedies we can use.

Several natural remedies mimic insulin in the body, including common cinnamon (*Cinnamomum verum*). Use one-quarter to one teaspoon daily on your foods, or take 200 mg of MHCP (methylhydroxychalcone polymer), a concentrated form of cinnamon. Another plant remedy with insulin activity in the body is goat's rue (*Galega officinalis*), a common flowering plant native to Europe but now extensively naturalized in America. Galega and MHCP are combined in InsuLife, a formula developed by Jonathan Wright, M.D., one of the world's leading authorities on nutritional medicine, and distributed by Life Enhancement.[46]

Also, several trace minerals have insulin-like activity in the body including selenium (Stapleton 2000), chromium, and vanadium. Lapid Pharmaceuticals, a company based in Israel, has developed the proprietary drug LP-100, an organically chelated form of vanadium, considered more bioavailable than the mineral salts of vanadium usually taken (Balasubramanyam 2001).

Cortisol and DHEA: The seriousness of excess cortisol and its ability to shorten our life span have focused my previous discussions on how to lower cortisol levels. Now, I discuss the opposite condition: low adrenal function in which both cortisol and DHEA levels are low. Since both cortisol and DHEA are produced in the adrenal cortex, you supplement cortisol and DHEA by taking adrenal cortisol extracts made from the adrenal glands of livestock such as cows or pigs. Though glandular extracts are the treatment of choice for supplementing borderline low adrenal activity, there are advantages and disadvantages to their use.

The advantages of using glandular extracts are that they are completely natural and provide low dosages of adrenal hormones as a corrective medication rather than as a drug. This assures you that you are not overdosing on steroid hormones, as often only very small amounts are needed to reestablish normal adrenal function rather than excess amounts that can suppress adrenal function and cause other harmful effects.

However, there are several disadvantages. First, glandular substances may not contain any hormones at all, or the amounts may be too low to do any good. Second, most adrenal glandular products are made from whole tissue, containing both adrenaline and cortisol. Since adrenaline can cause hyperactivity and insomnia, I do not recommend whole adrenal extracts. Use only a product that is made from the adrenal cortex, the part that contains cortisol and DHEA. Third, the amount of cortisol in extracts is not always the same.

In short, most adrenal extracts typically available at health food stores are not adequate for supplementation; however, your doctor can provide concentrated extracts of adrenal cortex containing standardized amounts of naturally occurring cortisol. The typical dosage is between 1.25 and 2.5 mg of cortisol equivalent taken in divided dosages daily, usually taken in the morning, at noon, and in the later afternoon. Do not take them before bed as your sleep could be affected.

Nutritional supplements and herbs are also helpful in restoring adrenal reserve. In most cases of borderline low adrenal function, stress reduction, rest, and improving dietary habits will correct the problem. Panthothenic acid (vitamin B$_5$), vitamin C, and ginseng are most commonly used. For adequate adrenal nutrition, if your adrenal glands are functioning insufficiently as judged by your symptoms and salivary test results for free cortisol and DHEA, take 500 mg of pantothenic acid two to three times daily with 1,000 mg of vitamin C.

Since the Chinese think highly of the kidney and adrenal function, doctors of Chinese medicine and knowledgeable acupuncturists are experts in improving adrenal function by natural methods. They use acupuncture as well as herbs such as ginseng. Licorice root (*Glycyrrhiza glabra*) extract is helpful in improving adrenal activity; however, you should not take it if you have high blood pressure. For this reason, Chinese medical experts use only small amounts of steamed licorice root at a time. Since licorice root influences both cortisol and aldosterone, an adrenal hormone that helps regulate fluid status in the body, if your blood pressure is low or if your blood pressure goes down when you stand up

(a condition that causes dizziness upon standing up too quickly), then licorice root may help your adrenal function. Take 10–20 drops of licorice root tincture twice daily, morning and afternoon.

If your DHEA levels are below optimal, but not significantly low, take 5-10 mg of DHEA in capsules or tablets, once a day either in the morning or evening. Do not take more without tracking your current DHEA-S levels in your blood or free DHEA levels in your saliva.

A newer form of DHEA, 7-Keto DHEA, is reported to have many of DHEA's benefits but

Nutritional supplements and herbs are also helpful in restoring adrenal reserve. In most cases of borderline low adrenal function, stress reduction, rest, and improving dietary habits will correct the problem. Panthothenic acid (vitamin B$_5$), vitamin C, and ginseng are most commonly used.

none of the side effects. This is mainly because it does not have the steroid hormone effect of DHEA. Though many doctors recommend 7-Keto DHEA, it is much more expensive than regular DHEA, and in my experience it does not have the same benefits. However, it is worth trying if you are unable to take regular DHEA due to excessive conversion into DHT, which causes increased oily skin and acne.

Thyroid: Begin improving thyroid function by managing your diet. Avoid foods that inhibit thyroid function, which include large amounts of soy, cabbage family vegetables (cabbage, broccoli, cauliflower, and mustard greens), rutabaga, turnips, and walnuts, almonds,

> ☀ **CAUTION:** Adding extra iodine or overdoing it with your intake of iodine-containing kelp and other seaweeds can cause an increase of dietary or supplemental iodine. Artificially increasing iodine levels can trigger autoimmune reactions, worsening a thyroid condition. Do not take iodine supplements except under the advice of a qualified health professional and then only for short periods of time lasting no longer than two to four weeks.

peanuts, pine nuts, millet, sorghum, and cassava (tapioca). A low-carbohydrate diet and low-calorie diets used for weight loss also inhibit thyroid function and result in the opposite effect: more difficulty in losing weight due to poor thyroid performance. If you have low thyroid function, eat equal-proportioned meals four to five times daily, include carbohydrates such as rice or fruits in each meal, and avoid eating too much of the thyroid-inhibiting foods.

Normal thyroid hormone synthesis depends on adequate amounts of dietary iodine.[47] Several other nutritional supplements are useful in promoting thyroid function, including selenium, copper, zinc, vitamin D, vitamin A, and tyrosine.

Tyrosine is an amino acid and the basic building block for thyroid hormone. If your thyroid function is low, take 500–1,000 mg, two to three times daily. It is a safe supplement without side effects. Adequate amounts of iodine, selenium, copper, and zinc, as well as vitamins A and D, are required for proper thyroid function. You will be taking more than enough of these trace minerals and vitamins by following the recommended dosages of nutritional supplements in this book.

After trying the nutritional approach for six to eight weeks, if your thyroid function still remains low, use a whole thyroid glandular supplement. Natural thyroid glandulars provide a range of bioavailable thyroid hormone and intermediary substances that work close to how your thyroid hormones work on their own. They can be very effective in normalizing your thyroid function. Most glandular products sold in health food stores do not contain active thyroxin, although some might contain trace amounts; preparations with active amounts of T-4 and T-3 can be obtained through a health professional or on the Internet.

If you are taking an active form, start with a quarter of a grain (usually equivalent to one 250-mg capsule) and gradually increase up to one grain of thyroxine equivalent (two capsules, two times daily). Be sure to ask your doctor if the glandular you are taking has active thyroid hormone or if it is thyroxine-free; if it is an active form, have your doctor supervise your program and check your thyroid function by a blood test.

Acupuncture is also extremely useful in correcting thyroid weakness. I generally recommend 12 acupuncture sessions at the rate of two for six weeks. At the end of the course of treatment, I recheck the blood studies. Generally, cases improve with one or two courses of treatment (12–24 sessions, and many in as few as six sessions). Practicing specific yoga postures also helps improve thyroid function; I suggest you start with a qualified yoga instructor before going off on your own.

Pregnenolone: The prohormone pregnenolone is essential for the synthesis of all steroid hormones, and I generally recommend beginning supplementation with this important substance for both men and women over 50 years old. Take 10 mg daily with the evening meal.

Androstenedione and Testosterone: Since androstenedione is involved in the syn-

Selected Phytoestrogenic Foods

Listed alphabetically:

Alfalfa	Corn	Potatoes
Anise seed	Cucumbers	Pumpkin
Apples	Fennel	Rhubarb
Baker's yeast	Garlic	Rice
Beer	Green beans	Rye
Beets	Oats	Sage
Cabbage	Olives	Sesame seeds
Carrots	Papaya	Split peas
Cherries	Parsley	Squash
Chickpeas	Peas	Wheat
Clover	Plums	Yams

thesis of testosterone and therefore also with estrogen metabolism, if your sex hormones are below optimal levels, consider supplementing with 10–25 mg of oral or sublingual androstenedione once daily. Androstenedione can be a very active prohormone in some people because it interconverts with testosterone, and has direct conversion pathways with both dihydrotestosterone and estrone. The dosage should be lowered or supplementation stopped entirely with the onset of acne or increased facial hair growth. To stimulate your own testosterone production, ask your doctor to prescribe the homeopathic preparation Testis Compositum from Heel;[48] or try glandular products made from orchic tissue (derived from bovine testicular substance).

Progesterone: Though the most common plant source of progesterone is found in wild yam root (*Dioscorea spp.*), it is not biologically available and is poorly absorbed in the intestine. This is the reason why only a synthetic version of progesterone, progestin (Provera), was available and only by prescription for many years. Newer processing techniques that allow greater bioavailabity of the progesterone molecules in wild yam now have made natural progesterone creams widely accessible.

Since progesterone levels tend to decline in women before estrogen levels, symptoms of irregular menstruation, increased symptoms of premenstrual syndrome, and the discomfort associated with uterine fibroids can appear starting as early as age 35. If you have symptoms associated with low progesterone, consider supplementing your levels by applying a quarter of a teaspoon of a two-percent progesterone cream once daily to the inner arms or thighs, or on the neck or upper chest, and alternate the areas you use. To match your natural progesterone cycle, for women with periods coming every 28–30 days, apply the cream between days 12–26 of your cycle. For those women with menstrual cycles less than 28 days, apply the cream from day 12 to the first day of your period and then stop.

Estrogen: Phytoestrogens are your best choice for supplementing estrogen levels, including soy isoflavones, lignans, and coumestans found in alfalfa and soybean sprouts. A

large number of other foods contain phytoestrogens, including apples, corn, and sunflower
seeds. I suggest that my female patients over
the age of 45 regularly include these foods in
their daily diet. Many herbs contain phytoestrogens or have estrogenic activity in the body,
including black cohosh (*Cimicifuga racemosa*),
vitex (*Vitex agnus-castus*), and the Chinese
herbal medicine dong quai (*Angelica sinensis*).
All of the herbs discussed in this section are
safe and nontoxic, and without side effects or
interactions with drugs.

Originally used by Native Americans,
black cohosh has a long history of application
for women's complaints. It contains the triter-
pene glycosides acetin and cimicifugoside, and
isoflavones, as well as a variety of other substances. German research suggests that black
cohosh decreases rising luteinizing hormone
levels in perimenopausal women, therefore
helping to stabilize estrogen activity in the
body (Duker 1991). Remifemin, a patented
extract of black cohosh made in Germany, is
my clinical choice for your hormone-balancing
regimen; for women, take one tablet, once or
twice a day.

Vitex, or chaste berry, is another herb that
appears to regulate luteinizing hormone and is
useful for symptoms arising from estrogen
imbalance during perimenopause. It may also
have an effect on lowering prolactin levels,
which are often elevated in polycystic ovarian
syndrome. I prefer the liquid extract or tincture
form of this herb, taken as 20–40 drops in
water once daily in the morning.

Dong quai, a traditional Chinese medicine
known to nearly every Asian woman, is a highly
respected herbal remedy for all gynecological
complaints. Sometimes referred to as the
"woman's ginseng," dong quai is a member of
the same family as edible celery and is a prized
adaptogenic herb for the female hormonal system. Though it does not contain active phytoestrogens, it has other effects that make it useful
for women during their reproductive years,
through menopause, and, combined with other
herbs including ginseng and licorice, in the
older years. The recommended dosage is 3–4 g
daily made into a tea; steep the sliced dried
herb in boiled water for at least one hour; drink
one cup two times daily.

Human Growth Hormone: A main hormonal biomarker for aging, human growth hormone (HGH) tends to decline steeply starting
after age 25 with suboptimal levels appearing as
early as one's forties. HGH production depends
on many factors, including a healthy liver, normal insulin function, a well-functioning hypothalamus and pituitary gland, and adequate
levels of other hormones. Optimizing HGH levels improves overall hormonal activity in your
body, provides an improved sense of well-being,
and enhances all aspects of physical performance. If you have symptoms of HGH insufficiency and your levels of IGF-I are below
optimal, consider enhancing HGH with precursor substances and releasing agents called secretagogues.

Human growth hormone secretagogues
(HGHS) are a curious form of anti-aging therapy, as they are not, strictly speaking, precursor
molecules, prohormones, or building-block
substances. Rather, they are compounds that
cause the release of growth hormone by the
pituitary gland. Specifically, these compounds
are synthetic molecules that activate receptors
in the hypothalamus and pituitary, where they
stimulate the actions of growth-hormone-
releasing substances, thereby increasing HGH
secretion (Fuh 1998).

That these compounds exist, both naturally within our body and artificially outside of
it, informs us that the pituitary, unlike other
endocrine glands, has the ability to respond to

a wide variety of stimuli that cause an increased release of HGH. For example, it is well known that heavy exercise stimulates the release of HGH, as does fasting and normal deep sleep—all major lifestyle conditions that support our goal of prolonging health.

Roy G. Smith, Ph.D., is the dean of growth hormone receptor and secretagogue research at Baylor University's Aging Research Center in Houston, Texas. Based on his work with the puffer fish (*Spheroides nephelus*), he suggests that this remarkable ability of HGH receptors to respond so readily is a highly conserved evolutionary trait approximately 400 million years old (Smith 1999). What this means is still debated among gerontologists, but what it might mean is that the secret of aging may be locked in an evolutionary puzzle hundreds of millions of years old. If we find the key, we may solve a major part of the aging dilemma—why we grow old. That, of course, is what researchers hope to find by investigating potential HGHS compounds.

As therapeutic medications for the treatment of sarcopenia and other age-related conditions, HGHS compounds offer considerable promise and have several advantages over HGH injections. First, they are taken as an oral medication, making them more convenient than injecting yourself regularly; second, they are safer and mimic the normal pulsatile release of HGH in the body (Micic 1999). The main disadvantage is that they are not as potent as synthetic HGH given by injection, and therefore are not that useful for people over age 70 with severe sarcopenia and very low IGF-I levels. However, this disadvantage makes them perfect for people in their forties, fifties, and sixties who have mild to moderate HGH decline.

HGHS compounds affect the release of HGH—as synthetic compounds they are not that specific—and they also release prolactin

and adrenocorticotropic hormone (ACTH), which might cause increased cortisol levels (Ghigo 1999). In this case, if you are taking cortisol in any form, it is wise to cut back the dose by half while on either HGHS compounds or HGH injections until you can have your hormone levels retested. HGHS compounds also have central nervous system effects, and receptors with HGHS affinity have been found in the heart, adrenal glands, ovaries, testes, lungs, and muscles. Thus, HGHS activity may be cardioprotective against damage to the myocardium (heart muscle) in older people, making it a possible treatment for early stage congestive heart failure (Muccioli 2000).

Research on HGHS compounds was first undertaken in the early 1960s, with greater emphasis on development of medications with possible therapeutic potential appearing in the mid-1980s (Bowers 2000). In the 1990s, a number of promising synthetic HGHS compounds were under investigation, including HGH-releasing peptides such as Ipamorelin, gherlin (a substance secreted in the stomach with HGH activity), nonpeptide HGHS compounds such as NN703 (tabimorelin), and HGH mimetics such as MK-677.

Unfortunately, all research on the most promising of the HGHS compounds, MK-677, a nonpeptide potent oral HGH-releasing substance developed by Merck Research Laboratories, was halted in the late 1990s. At that time FDA approval for a drug to treat aging as a condition rather than a distinct disease was questionable, and MK-677 did not show major improvement in HGH-deficient people of advanced age, making it seem a poor business risk. Merck's decision did not mean that MK-677 was ineffective, and that it did not have considerable potential as a lifestyle medication for HGH insufficiency in adults between 40 and 65 years of age. In fact, researchers have shown it to be effective in improving bone metabolism (Murphy 1999), sleep, and other age-related parameters. In at least one study, the recommended daily dosage of 25 mg raised IGF-I levels to those of young adults (Patchett 2000).

Research continues on other HGH-enhancing substances such as gherlin, a hormone-like peptide secreted by the stomach. It was discovered in 1999 by Japanese scientists and is thought to have appetite-stimulating properties with a potential to help reduce obesity (Ghigo 2001). Ipamorelin is shown to counteract the damaging effects of cortisol and improve body composition (Andersen 2001), and tabimorelin, in the nonpeptide family, has a promising future as an HGHS compound (Zdrackovic, Christiansen, et al. 2001).

Though these pharmaceutical HGHS compounds remain unavailable as clinical medications, there is little question that it is simply a matter of time before potent oral HGH-releasing drugs become available. After all, bovine growth hormone has long been in use to increase milk production in dairy cows, as well as for more rapid growth in pigs and other animals used for meat production. Unfortunately, this suggests that commercial interests may be more important to the large pharmaceutical companies that have the capability to develop such compounds than the provision of a safe, beneficial medication for the prevention of age-related conditions.

In the meanwhile, there are a number of natural HGH-releasing substances. Some are as close as your local health food store, such as amino acids and certain foods that improve HGH-I secretion and raise IGF-I levels. The most useful of these amino acids is arginine, which is combined with lysine, ornithine, and glycine for synergistic effects (Chromiak 2002). Tryptophan is a key amino acid involved in

HGH-releasing peptide formation; it is important in maintaining neurotransmitter balance and in restoring the relationship between growth hormone and insulin-like growth factor (the HGH/IGF-I axis).

Since amino acids build peptides, substances formed by the combination of two amino acids held together by an amine bond, it is not surprising that sufficient dietary protein is necessary to maintain adequate amino acid levels in the body and for building peptides, many of which stimulate HGH secretion. L-arginine is the most effective of the HGH-enhancing amino acids, and is best taken on an empty stomach in dosages between 10 and 30 g daily. When combined with L-lysine, 1,500 mg of each amino acid is equal to the higher single dosing of arginine alone (Isidori 1981).

Taking amino acids is safe; however, since arginine may stimulate human herpes simplex virus growth, if you have any form of herpes virus, do not take arginine. Also, arginine can enhance insulin activity, and should not be taken by diabetics using insulin.

Garlic can improve HGH release and is best when taken in a concentrated form containing aged garlic (Kyolic). Research indicates that high-allicin garlic (this is the kind you want to use if you have an infection because of allicin's potent antimicrobial properties) is not as effective as the aged type containing S-allyl cysteine. The recommended dosage is 4 ml twice daily (Buz'Zard 2002). Aged garlic is safe, has less odor than raw or other garlic preparations, and has the added benefits of improving cardiovascular function.

Taking advantage of the fact that amino acids, foods, and even herbs enhance HGH secretion, and the large demand for easy and inexpensive substitutes for HGH injections, many companies emerged in the late 1990s offering HGHS products. Of the hundreds that

I've reviewed and tested, few have any clinical merit. Among those that actually increase IGF-I levels is a commercial combination of amino acids, peptides, growth-hormone-releasing cofactors, and the patented HGHS compound Symbiotropin (Meditropin).[49]

This was developed by the second-generation-growth-hormone researcher James Jamieson, Ph.D.; it is available only through a physician or pharmacy. IGF-I levels increase an average of 30 percent over a course of 12 weeks of using this, which is as good as any of the pharmaceutical forms in development (Jamieson 1998). Some of my patients experience a 65 percent increase. The dosage is two effervescent tablets dissolved in water taken nightly two hours after the evening meal. It is a safe medication without known interactions.

Prolonging Health Recommendation 48— Replace Deficient Hormones with Bio-Identical Hormones

If after you have tried all of the recommendations in *Prolonging Health* Recommendation 47 and done the neuroendocrine balancing and other therapies discussed in the previous sections of this chapter, and if after three to six months on hormone supplementation your hormone levels are still not rising into the optimal range, then consider medical replacement therapies with bio-identical hormones. Bio-identical hormones are synthetic analogues having the same molecular structure as the human hormone they replace. For example, the bio-identical testosterone molecule is the same testosterone your own body produces.

However, using bio-identical hormones is only the first aspect of natural hormone replacement, and in my clinical experience,

Growth-Hormone-Releasing Substances	
Compound	**Dosage**
L-arginine	10–30 g daily
50/50 L-arginine and L-lysine	3,000 mg daily
Kyolic aged garlic	4 ml twice daily
Meditropin	2 tablets daily

there are four others. The second aspect is to use very low physiologic dosages, in contrast to pharmacological or high doses, of the hormone in order to bring your hormone levels out of extreme deficiency. Remember our discussion on genetic expression and signaling molecules. Hormones are signaling substances and can enhance positive genetic expression; they can also, if used incorrectly and especially in high dosages, trigger negative gene expression, including the initiation of cancer. A physiologic dose means one at the level your body is used to working with on its own.

The third aspect of natural hormone replacement is to only replace those that are necessary, based upon both physiological and laboratory evaluations. Do not ask your doctor to indiscriminately prescribe hormones simply because you think they might help you reverse age-related conditions or live longer. Such practices do little if anything to reverse aging; but if you work with those hormones that are deficient, you can greatly improve your function and abilities.

Synergism is the fourth aspect, and refers to the methodology of combining more than one hormone, and often four to six or more, in small amounts to mimic the body's normal hormone levels.

The fifth aspect is to follow your progress regularly with routine laboratory testing to monitor your body composition and assess possible side effects of hormone therapy as well as your general symptoms.

The Five Aspects of Natural Hormone Replacement

When considering taking prescription hormones, keep these five aspects in mind:

1. Use only bio-identical hormones.

2. Use very low to minute physiologic dosages.

3. Replace only those hormones that are below optimal ranges or close to, or below, the reference range.

4. Never use a single hormone in high dosages, but supplement and replace several hormones for their synergistic effects.

5. Follow your laboratory results regularly, making adjustment in your hormone program as needed based upon the test results, your symptoms, biomarker profile, and your doctor's advice.

How to Replace Cortisol Correctly: If your cortisol levels are too high, or if you take any form of cortisone, you may damage important organs and tissues in your body, such as your bones and heart. In this case, it is necessary to bring your cortisol levels down and into a normal range. On the other hand, your adrenal glands may be performing suboptimally, and your cortisol levels may actually be too low. In this scenario, you may be constantly tired or have hypoglycemia since cortisol helps to raise blood sugar levels. Low cortisol also contributes to chronic inflammation, arthritic joint pain, lowered immune function, allergies, and asthma.

If your fasting cortisol levels in your blood and free cortisol and 17-ketosteroids in your urine are below the reference ranges, the function of your adrenal glands may be weak. If you are not improving over a period of four to six months with the all-natural approach, you may need a prescription of hydrocortisone (Cortef), a synthetic drug whose molecular structure is identical to human cortisol. The recommended dosage is 5–20 mg daily in divided dosages, with the maximum dosage being 5 mg, four times daily.

Since cortisol is not only a major and therefore necessary hormone, but also a dangerous hormone, I recommend that you start with a low dose and gradually increase until you feel an increase in energy. Begin with 2.5 mg daily taken in the morning, and increase weekly to 2.5 mg twice daily, up to 10 mg if necessary (2.5 mg four times a day). Then review your symptoms. Are you less tired? Do you have less frequent allergic symptoms or fewer colds?

Test your free cortisol levels in your saliva, or have a blood test for fasting cortisol and a 24-hour urine test for 17-ketosteroids and free cortisol. If your adrenal function is very low, your doctor may want to put you on an even higher dosage, up to 20 mg or more daily. However, keep in mind that taking more than 30–40 mg of cortisol daily will suppress your own adrenal hormone production, cause thinning of your skin and easy bruising, and weaken your immune system.

For replacement therapy, 20 mg of cortisol daily should be the maximum dosage, and even that may be too high when taken for longer than one year and if you are concurrently taking HGH. In your *Prolonging Health* program, take the lowest dosage that gives you symptom improvement and never go higher than the reference range on your laboratory tests. In the case of cortisol, don't prescribe for yourself; follow your doctor's advice.

How to Replace DHEA: Though DHEA is available over the counter, better forms are obtained as a prescription or from your doctor in a micronized form, which is the form I recommend. Since the particle size is small, this form is easily absorbed and is more efficient for the body to utilize. Though most anti-aging doctors recommend DHEA in dosages ranging from 25–50 mg for women and 50–100 mg for men, or higher, I have found these dosages to be too high for people with chronic disease, those that are very weak, and the very elderly. Instead, I usually recommend 5–10 mg for both men and women; increase the dosage if your symptoms are not improving, up to 20–30 mg for women and 35–50 mg for men. At times much higher dosages are necessary to improve overall neuroendocrine function and steroid hormone levels.

DHEA is taken with food and is best taken in the morning. Paradoxically, when taken in the evening, DHEA improves sleep in some people, while in others it causes insomnia. Start by taking it in the morning, but consider taking it immediately after dinner to improve your sleep. Go back to the morning dose if you experience trouble sleeping.

DHEA is considered safe in the recommended dosages and is not associated with increased risk for any disease. On the contrary, research indicates that it may be protective for both cancer and cardiovascular disease. However, DHEA can cause acne, increase facial hair growth, aggravate rosacea, make your skin oilier, and sometimes cause high blood pressure.

As with all ingested steroid hormones, there is concern that extended use may cause liver damage. Patients with liver disease should take a sublingual form of DHEA or a transdermal cream applied to the skin. This method of use prevents them from going directly to the liver, as when oral preparations are ingested. When absorbed from the intestines, orally ingested steroid hormones are passed directly along to the liver through the portal vein. Avoiding this direct route places less stress on the liver.

If You Need Thyroid Hormone Replacement: The current standard for the treat-

> ※ **CAUTION:** Both DHEA and cortisol are steroid hormones and have considerable physiological activity in the body. In general, low dosages of cortisol are safe and without side effects. However, when you first start taking them, do not use them for more than six months without retesting your hormone levels. Since DHEA is an androgenic hormone, it can convert in the body to testosterone. In some cases this may be beneficial; however, it can also cause facial hair growth in women and acne in both men and women.
>
> It has also been associated with high blood pressure. Men should have their PSA (prostate-specific antigen) tested regularly if they are using DHEA. Do not use DHEA, except under medical supervision, if you have an enlarged prostate gland. Do not use DHEA if you have hypertension or are concerned about acne, and discontinue immediately if these occur. Take these hormones only under a doctor's supervision.

ment of hypothyroidism in the United States is replacement with synthetic levothyroxine (Synthroid, Levothroid, Levoxyl), synthetic liothyronne (Cytomel), or a synthetic combination of both (Thyrolar). For most medical doctors there is no other option; however, natural prescription thyroid is available and should be the starting medication of choice for people beginning thyroid replacement.

Like whole glandulars, prescription natural thyroid is prepared from desiccated porcine or bovine thyroid glands. Prescription natural thyroid contains standardized amounts of levothyroxine and liothyronne (38 mcg of levothyroxine and 9 mcg of liothyronne per 1 grain or 60 mg of UPS thyroid) and is highly purified and safe to use.

The most commonly used brand is Armour Thyroid (thyroid, USP) manufactured by Forest Pharmaceuticals.[50] Another brand, Bio-Throid from Bio-Tech Pharmacal[51] is equally effective and often preferred by anti-aging practitioners because it contains fewer chemical additives. Both use glands from hormone-free animals, a healthy choice in this age of feed contaminants. Your pharmacy may have to special order these, or you can order them yourself through an Internet pharmacy with a prescription from your doctor. A better choice is to use a compounding pharmacy that specializes in bio-identical hormones, individualized prescriptions, and specialized delivery systems such as transdermal creams.

For hormone balancing, the milder version of hormone replacement, in those whose thyroid tests are outside the optimal ranges but still within the laboratory reference ranges and those for whom supplemental approaches did not work, I recommend you start with 15 mg (a quarter of a grain) of prescription thyroid. Take it in the morning before 10 A.M. and gradually increase every week until you are taking 60 mg (one grain) daily in the morning on an empty stomach. You may find that you get more benefit by dividing the dosage between morning and afternoon (between noon and 3 P.M). If the afternoon dosage keeps you awake at night, discontinue it and take your thyroid only in the morning.

Generally you will not need more than one grain to feel improvement in energy and to see many of the symptoms disappear. If you do not find that you are improving, your problem may not be thyroid related or you may require a higher dosage. For cases of true hypothyroidism, dosages as high as 180 mg (three grains) are often required. Consult your doctor if you are not improving.

As people age, even if their general thyroid activity approximates normal, there is typically a progressive decline in the amount or activity of T3. This is due to inadequate thyroid hormone metabolism and faulty conversion of T4 to T3, the more biologically active thyroid hormone of the two and approximately four times as potent as T4. If your T3 levels are even borderline low over a sustained period of time, many of the classic age-related changes such as thinning and falling hair, dry skin, and fatigue may appear. Therefore, if you are over 50, routinely test total T3 *and* free T3 levels in your blood. If your free T3 is below optimal, and in some cases it can be low even when taking Armour thyroid or Bio-Throid, which contains some T3, you may need to replace just T3 or increase the dosage of T3 in addition.

The diagnosis of hypothyroidism is based upon an elevated level of thyroid-stimulating hormone (TSH) and low circulating T4, and should be treated with Armour or Bio-Throid. However, there are several gradations of thyroid dysfunction, especially during aging, which are often missed upon routine examination and evaluation based on TSH values only. Consistent low readings for under-the-arm or oral temperature frequently accompany low thyroid function.

The assessment of functionally low thyroid includes a normal TSH level within the reference range of 0.35–5.5 mIU/mL, but above 3.5 mIU/mL; a free T3 level below or at the low end of the normal range of 2.3–4.2 pg/mL; and an oral temperature of less than 98.2° F (Milner 1999), or an underarm temperature of 97.8° F or lower.

The underarm temperature test for assessing thyroid function was proposed by Broda O. Barnes, M.D., and is performed by taking your temperature with a basal thermometer under your arm before you get out of bed in the morning (Barnes and Galton 1976).

How to Take Your Basal Temperature

Buy a basal thermometer from a drug store. Basal thermometers differ from regular (mercury) fever thermometers. A chart for recording your temperature usually comes with the basal thermometer; keep both by your bed.

- Before getting out of bed in the morning, place the thermometer under your arm for several minutes (up to ten minutes and no less than five).

- It is very important to take your temperature at approximately the same time every morning and before you get out of bed.

- Record the readings directly after taking your temperature.

- Continue daily for at least one month.

- If you are menstruating, start on Day 1 (the first day of show of blood) and continue until the start of your next period.

Remember, our goal is to enhance hormone activity and restore neuroendocrine function for the purpose of prolonging health and achieving our maximum life span. Our purpose here is not the treatment of hypothyroidism or any other endocrine disease, which we'll leave to your doctor or endocrinologist. We also do not want to increase levels of blood hormones at the expense of causing additional neuroendocrine imbalances.

If you suspect that you are not suffering from hypothyroidism, but may have symptoms of low thyroid and fit the profiles discussed above, consider replacing T3 using a compounded slow-release form. Start at a low dose of 7.5 mcg, increasing by 7.5 mcg every two days until your oral temperature reaches 98.6° F and your basal temperature reaches at least 98.0° F, which usually happens between 25 and 50 mcg. However, some people require considerably higher dosages and need close monitoring by their doctor. Once normal body temperature is attained, retest your thyroid hormones by a

> **CAUTION:** Consult your doctor if feel you need more than one grain of natural thyroid daily or more than 25 mcg of T3 alone. Discontinue immediately if you experience agitation, insomnia, headaches, high blood pressure, or rapid heartbeat.

blood test and have your doctor evaluate the results.

Essentially, you want to correct the lab test results and bring your thyroid hormone levels into optimal ranges, restore normal body temperature, and not experience any side effects of excess thyroid hormone. Symptoms of excess thyroid include headaches, nervousness, agitation, sweating, irregular and rapid heart rate, and insomnia. If unchecked, excess thyroid medication abuse can lead to hyperthyroidism, high blood pressure, and osteoporosis.

Thyroid hormone function is synergistic with other hormones, including HGH, cortisol, and melatonin. To benefit and balance hormone activity in the entire body, all of my patients with low thyroid take 0.5–1.0 mg of melatonin directly before bed nightly even if they do not have sleep problems. Women with menstrual abnormalities, such as PMS, irregular cycles, or infertility, and those experiencing the symptoms of perimenopause may need balancing of their estrogens and progesterone before their thyroid functions normally. However, that subject is beyond the scope of this book. If you suspect other hormonal imbalances, consult with a doctor qualified to evaluate your condition.

How to Use Progesterone Correctly: In the previous section, we discussed supplementing progesterone in women who had normally functioning ovaries and progesterone production but who needed a little extra progesterone to balance their body's estrogen. In this section we consider the use of progesterone to oppose estrogen replacement; restore bone density; control uterine fibroids; provide neuroprotection; protect against cancer during aging, and produce anti-senescence benefits.

Progesterone is generally safe even in high dosages and is routinely used by more and more women. Its use for premenstrual syndrome is supported by a number of medical doctors, notably John R. Lee, M.D. author of *Natural Progesterone: The Multiple Roles of a Remarkable Hormone* (Lee 1993), and Katharina

Research has shown that as an anti-senescence hormone, progesterone improves bone density, protects the brain and heart, prevents cancer, has antistress properties, and improves immunity by protecting the thymus gland, as well as other functions in addition to its reproductive role in younger women.

Dalton, M.D., author of *Once A Month: Understanding and Treating PMS* (Dalton 1999) and other books on progesterone. The big question is this: What dosage is necessary for prolonging health in the later years once menstruation has stopped and pregnancies are over? What role does progesterone play during aging?

To answer that, we need to review briefly progesterone's action in the body. It is primarily for the preparation and maintenance of pregnancy. The ovaries produce progesterone cyclically during the monthly cycle with the highest levels reached just after mid-cycle (ovulation). If pregnancy occurs, progesterone pro-

duction is taken over by the placenta and increases, with levels peaking at the third trimester. However, once menopause occurs, ovarian production declines to nearly zero.

Besides maintaining pregnancy, progesterone plays other roles in the body. It acts as an antiestrogen and antitestosterone compound in the brain and other tissues, and may also play a role in stabilizing the damaging effects of cortisol. It increases the flow of calcium ions into nerve cells in the brain, and dampens the release of neurotransmitters that influence mood. In some people, this is exactly the effect they want, as progesterone calms the nervous system and acts like an antianxiety agent (Vliet 1995).

Thierry Hertoghe, M.D., refers to progesterone as the "serenity hormone" (Hertoghe 2002). Interestingly, this effect can make some women feel tired or even lazy and lethargic, and some even complain that progesterone makes them depressed rather than serene. If progesterone makes you feel too relaxed or significantly depresses your mood, it may not be for you, your dose may be too high, or you are not balancing it with enough estrogen and testosterone.

Research has shown that as an anti-senescence hormone, progesterone improves bone density, protects the brain and heart, prevents cancer, has antistress properties, and improves immunity by protecting the thymus gland, as well as other functions in addition to its reproductive role in younger women.

Ray Peat, Ph.D., was among the first researchers to recognize the anti-aging benefits of progesterone. He describes it as the "most protective" hormone that the body produces (Peat 2001). So, if progesterone protects the fetus during pregnancy, can it protect us during aging? This question remains to be answered, but because of its safety and possible benefits, progesterone is an important hormone for women in the *Prolonging Health* plan.

For perimenopausal and younger women, progesterone dosages typically range from 100 to 400 mg daily, which may be too high for post-menopausal women. Replacement dosages during aging are much less, ranging from 10 to 100 mg daily, though occasionally your individual requirement may be higher. The dosage depends on your individual needs, based upon how well you respond, if you experience any side effects, and what progesterone levels you attain on a lab test after you have been using progesterone for at least three months. If you use progesterone creams, you can easily monitor your progress using salivary testing with a goal to attain the middle of the reference range. Still, serum progesterone is the standard most anti-aging doctors use and the target range on a blood test is 1.5–4.5 ng/mL. But what preparation and form are best?

Not too long ago, there were no natural oral progesterone medications. I remember in the early years of my practice that women who required progesterone received monthly injections. Since modern micronized progesterone was developed by Joel Hargrove, M.D., of Vanderbuilt University in Tennessee, oral preparations have become available, which absorb well from the gut and are not associated with liver toxicity. Progesterone also absorbs readily through the skin, so you can choose between a compounded capsule, a transdermal cream, or even a vaginal suppository.

Natural bio-identical progesterone, as is natural estrogen, is derived from Mexican wild yam or soybean oil. Creams are supplied in a 2-ounce tube or 30-gram jar, with percentages of progesterone ranging from three to ten percent. For example, a ten-percent cream con-tains 100 mg of progesterone per gram (1 gram = 1/4 teaspoon). If your doctor prescribes 100 mg of progesterone daily, apply 1/4 teaspoon to the thin skin on your neck, upper chest, or inner arms. Always apply a transdermal cream to clean, dry skin and rub it in briskly to facilitate absorption. Also, alternate locations every few days so as not to build up hormone residues in your skin. If you want 50 mg daily, use 1/8 teaspoon of a ten-percent cream, or have a five-percent cream compounded and apply 1/4 teaspoon.

For a low-dose use during aging, ten-percent natural progesterone combined in vitamin E oil (Progest-E Complex)[52] is the treatment of choice. Each one-ounce bottle contains 2,800 mg of natural progesterone. One drop of the oil contains 3 mg of progesterone, with an average dosage of three to four drops per day equaling about 10 mg of progesterone. This form absorbs very well and has the added advantage of the antioxidant properties of vitamin E. Take one to four drops daily, as recommended by your doctor, by mouth, rubbed into the gums, or applied to the skin as you would a transdermal cream. Women under 45 years old and perimenopausal women follow a cyclical method using progesterone from day 12 to 26 as described previously. Postmenopausal women require continuous use in the lower ranges. Progesterone is safe in the recommended dosages.

Though men produce very little progesterone, during aging their levels become even lower. As we discussed, testosterone levels drop in older men and estrogen levels can rise, and along with exposure to xenoestrogenic substances in the environment, estrogen levels may rise, so taking progesterone may benefit some men. Progesterone receptors occur in the lining of the blood vessels, and adequate levels of progesterone provide cardiovascular protection

> ✳ **CAUTION:** Though even large do-
> sages of natural micronized proges-
> terone are considered safe, do not take oral
> progesterone if you have any form of liver
> disorder or suffer from yeast infections.

and may give men with a risk for heart disease
a preventative edge.

If you are a man over 50, and your lab studies indicate rising estradiol or estrone levels,
high testosterone levels from using a transdermal cream or other form of testosterone, or you
have excess conversion of testosterone to DHT,
consider adding progesterone to your regimen.
Take 2.5–5 mg of natural progesterone in vitamin E oil or as a transdermal cream applied to
the same areas described above. Monitor your
progesterone levels with saliva testing. After
three to six months of use, reduce the dosage if
your salivary levels increase to above the reference range.

For the purposes of prolonging your
health, never use synthetic progestins like
Provera, the injectable contraceptive Depo-
Provera, or those found in birth control pills.
These preparations are not bio-identical, and
according to medical studies they are associated with numerous side effects and risks,
including acne, increased blood clotting and
stroke, liver disease, and cancer—the opposite
effect we want in prolonging our health.
Prometrium (progesterone USP), a pharmaceutical micronized form of progesterone derived
from plant sources, is available, but its draw-
back is that it comes in only two strengths, 100
mg and 200 mg tablets, and contains dyes
(D&C yellow #10 and FD&C red # 40), which
may be objectionable for those wanting all-
natural sources.

Though natural progesterone is considered
non-toxic and generally safe, a few side effects

are possible with long-term use or in those
women sensitive to progesterone. These
include a feeling mild euphoria—though some
women say they experience depression or
lethargy—and alterations in the menstrual
cycle, including spotting and irregular menstruation, in pre-menopausal women. It may also
cause acne, and when progesterone cream is
applied to the same area day after day, it can
cause fatty deposits to form under the skin
where the cream was applied.

**What's Safe? How to Individualize
Estrogen Replacement Therapy:** Nothing is
more controversial in the realm of hormone
replacement than estrogen, and for good reason. David Zava, Ph.D., is a biochemist with
expertise in breast cancer treatment, and director of ZRT Laboratory, a salivary hormone reference lab in Portland, Oregon. He calls
estrogen the "angel of life and the angel of
death," because of its important but paradoxical roles in health and disease.

For decades, naturopathic physicians have
adamantly held to the opinion that excess and
improper use of estrogen causes cancer and
abnormal gene expression. Confirmation of
our position came in 2001 when the American
Heart Association halted the largest study on
estrogen replacement before its completion
because of side effects from the therapy
(Grady, Herrington, Bittner, et al. 2002). The
combination in question was one that 15 million women were taking: Premarin (an estrogen
medication prepared from the urine of pregnant mares) and progestin (synthetic progesterone) (Nelson 2002).

What is difficult to fathom is that oral
estrogens—already known to cause cancer, gall-
stones, and liver disease—and progestins that
have a long list of known side effects including
blood clots, were so widely used. If this wasn't
cause for alarm, the side effects from the com-

bination of the two were even more extensive and included nausea, vomiting, breast swelling and pain, irregular vaginal bleeding, headaches, yeast infections, fluid retention, weight gain, and changes in blood sugar metabolism. Where does that leave women who want the benefits of estrogen replacement but not the risks?

Estrogen is the feminizing hormone that gives shape to the female form, smoothes the skin, prevents wrinkles, and keeps the eyes, mouth, and vagina moist. It prevents depression, enhances sexual interest and pleasure, promotes sound sleep, protects the bones, and supports the immune system. Research shows that it improves blood supply to the brain and may have a role in preventing Alzheimer's disease. In my clinical experience, women like the positive effects of estrogen, and for good reason, but they are very scared of its cancer risks. It is because of these benefits that estrogen replacement will not likely go away. But what is the best way to approach estrogen replacement for the purpose of prolonging health?

As with all the hormones discussed in this chapter, make sure how you use estrogen is consistent with the five aspects of hormone replacement: (1) use natural bio-identical estrogens; (2) use the lowest, physiologic dose possible to achieve results; (3) after practicing the hormone balance and supplementing methods discussed in this chapter, use estrogen only if your laboratory values are below optimal ranges, and never exceed those ranges; (4) never use any form of estrogen alone, but combine it with progesterone and other hormones for their protective and balancing effects; and (5) have your estradiol and estrone levels checked at least once a year.

There are three forms of bio-identical estrogen available: estrone (E1), estradiol (E2), and estriol (E3). Jonathan Wright M.D., was among the first to recommend a combination of all three estrogens (called "tri-est," for triple estrogen), in a ratio of 80 percent E3, ten percent E2, and ten percent E1 (Wright 1997). This was supposed to approximate the normal proportion of estrogens in the body and work in a synergistic manner to obtain clinical effectiveness. In my clinical experience, this approach works well for most women; however, for some women there is not enough estradiol in a tri-est formula to reduce hot flashes and other annoying symptoms of perimenopause, nor to slow bone loss. Also, though the largest amount in the formula is estriol, considered the safe estrogen, it does not readily convert into estradiol and does not absorb well in the gut.

To remedy this, compounding pharmacists mix estrogen, combining progesterone along with them in the formula, as a transdermal cream in 1.25 mg, 2.50 mg, and 5.00 mg strengths. Since estrone is linked to many of the side effects from estrogen replacement, many naturopaths prefer bi-est, composed of estradiol and estriol. Both of these are compounded by a pharmacist based upon the physician's prescription. The average starting dosage is 2.5 mg of bi- or tri-est with 50–100 mg of progesterone. Apply 1/4 teaspoon once daily on a cyclical or continual basis according to your doctor's directions. In general, postmenopausal women should apply the cream every day. Observe changes in your symptoms and body composition, and retest your blood levels in three months. If your estradiol levels are improving, tri-est or bi-est may be for you. If not, consider changing to estradiol alone, combined with progesterone.

The generally recommended starting dose is 0.5 mg of estradiol (equivalent to 2.50 mg of bi- or tri-est) with 50–100 mg of progesterone. A compounding pharmacist can make a combination of estrogens with progesterone, and even add in testosterone or other hormones,

> ✳ CAUTION: Since estrogen is potentially dangerous, identifying risks before you begin is wise. These include a previous incidence of breast or other form of cancer, and liver disease. Oral estrogen, even bio-identical forms, may reduce liver function. To prevent this always use transdermal creams. Some women have hypersensitive estrogen receptors, and any amount of estrogen in any form causes side effects. These include breast tenderness, nipple soreness, and vaginal bleeding. In these cases, if your doctor cannot find a balanced solution when combining progesterone and testosterone, it is best to avoid the use of estrogen entirely.

based on your doctor's prescription and what is individually right for you. Apply estrogen cream in the same manner as progesterone cream.

Replacing Lagging Testosterone: Testosterone is an anabolic hormone that effectively builds muscle size, increases strength, and improves overall body composition. If you want to optimize your physical performance, reduce the depression associated with aging, sleep better, have more sexual desire and energy, increase bone and muscle mass, and reduce fat, consider using testosterone. It is nearly impossible to increase your testosterone levels with natural supplements, so if your testosterone levels are below the reference range, you may benefit from prescription strength testosterone replacement. But how much testosterone do you need?

In evaluating your testosterone levels, keep in mind that men also need to measure free testosterone. Sometimes, total testosterone levels are in acceptable ranges but free testosterone is low. In this case, you may ask your doctor to prescribe testosterone for enhancement purposes, using small amounts to raise the levels of total testosterone along with free testosterone. Also, if you're over age 55 when evaluating testosterone function, always measure sex hormone binding globulin (SHBG) at the same time. SHBG is produced in the liver, and levels of both testosterone and estrogen, as well as other hormones, influence SHBG production. Though SHBG production tends to decline with age, higher levels of testosterone tend to suppress SHBG, and estrogen tends to increase the liver's production of SHBG. HGH supplementation also suppresses its production.

SHBG exerts a great influence on the bioavailability of testosterone in the body, as it binds tightly to DHT. Total testosterone levels change in tandem with SHBG in order to maintain constant levels of free testosterone. Therefore, if SHBG levels are low, and total testosterone levels are normal, more peripheral conversion of testosterone to DHT could take place, causing acne and increased facial hair growth, but loss of hair on the scalp. If SHBG levels are too high, more estrogenic activity may be taking place, and consequently more testosterone is bound and unavailable for use, or too much testosterone is being converted to estrogen, resulting in the same thing—not enough testosterone available for the tissues.

Oral estrogens, which I do not recommend, do the same thing. They tend to block the liver's production of IGF-I, resulting in lower levels of IGF-I and HGH, while increasing SHBG and growth hormone binding protein (GHBP), but are moderated to some degree by progesterone and testosterone (Ho 1998).

Though there are numerous testosterone preparations such as injectables, gels, pills, and patches, for the purposes of the *Prolonging Health* program the preferred form is bio-identical natural testosterone in a transdermal

Changes in Plasma Levels in Selected Hormones in Women

Hormone	Levels in Women 20–30 years	Levels in Women over 60 years	Level to Consider Supplementing	Level to Consider Replacing
Estradiol, 17-Beta (pg/mL)	19–528	0–31	Below 45	Below 35
Estrone (pg/dL)	19–140	14–103	As a rule, declines in estrone, estriol, and total estrogen levels are not used to guide timing for supplementation or replacement, but are useful for monitoring replacement therapy.	
Total estrogens (pg/mL)	61–437	Less than 40		
Progesterone (ng/mL)	0.2–28.0	0.0–0.7	Below 1.5	Below 0.5
Follicle-stimulating hormone, FSH (mIU/mL)	1.5–9.1	23.0–116.3	Above 35[1]	Above 65
Luteinizing hormone, LH (mIU/mL)	0.0–76.3	5.0–52.3	LH levels are not directly used to guide estrogen supplementation or replacement, but may serve as a guide when monitoring replacement therapy	
Testosterone (ng/mL)	14–76	15–70	Below 30	Below 20
DHEA-S (ng/dL)	65–380	17–90	Below 250	Below 150
Androstenedione (ng/dL)	47–268	30–150	Below 150	Below 50
Pregnenolone (ng/dL)	10–230	10–230	Below 150	Below 100
Insulin-like growth factor, IGF-I (ng/mL)	90–360	71–290	Below 200	Below 150
Sex hormone binding globulin, SHBG (nmol/L)	18–114	18–114	SHBG levels reflect availability of testosterone and estrogen, and tend to fall during aging, though they can also rise when estrogen levels decline. Optimal levels are around 25–60.	
Leptin (non-obese, ng/mL)	1.1–27.5	1.1–27.5	Reduced levels in the lower end of the reference range may contribute to weight gain. Weight loss is necessary, or leptin injections may be helpful.	

Women over 35 years old should test progesterone and DHEA-S levels; those over 45 should consider adding estradiol and FSH to the test; and those over 50 should consider having the remaining studies done. Supplemental and replacement recommendations apply to symptomatic women over 35 and nonsymptomatic women over 50 years.[2]

1. Rising FSH levels signal the approach of menopause and are very elevated in postmenopausal women. Estradiol replacement tends to lower FSH levels, and is useful in guiding therapy in the early stages of estrogen replacement.

2. Reference ranges based on lab values used by Laboratory Corporation of America. LabCorp: 358 South Main Street, Burlington, NC 27215; http://www.labcorp.com/

> **CAUTION:** Though natural testosterone tends to improve prostate tissue structure and function, in some cases testosterone replacement may complicate underlying cancerous changes. Always have your doctor perform a prostate exam and a PSA test before you start taking testosterone in any form.

cream or lotion. The starting dose for men is generally 100 mg daily (ten-percent testosterone cream) applied by rubbing 1/4 teaspoon into the upper chest, inner arms, or sides of the abdomen once daily. Have your testosterone levels checked three months after you begin your regimen and adjust the dosage accordingly.

The goal for testosterone replacement is to increase the levels of total testosterone so that they are in the upper range of the reference values, and to enhance the levels of free testosterone so that they fall within the reference values. A testosterone range that is safe and provides muscle, mood, and energy enhancement in men is usually between 650 and 850 ng/mL. In addition, it is necessary to prevent too much conversion of testosterone into excess amounts of DHT or estrogen.

Though testosterone is considered a male hormone, women require sufficient amounts to synthesize estradiol and to balance other female hormones. The starting dosage for women is 5–10 mg (0.5–1.0 percent testosterone cream) applied daily, but even this dosage can be too high in many women who develop facial hair growth and acne. If this happens, discontinue and discuss your options with your doctor. Often, the reason is that estrogen and progesterone levels are not high enough to offset the masculine characteristics caused by the testosterone. However, in some cases, receptors for DHT in the hair follicles and skin are simply too sensitive and you will not be able to take testosterone.

Natural testosterone replacement is generally safe, but it can lower sperm production, cause infertility in both men and women, lower total cholesterol and HDL, and it can increase the number of red blood cells. So far, none of these have been linked to an increased risk for disease; however, as with all hormone replacement therapies, it is important to proceed cautiously.

How to Supplement Human Growth Hormone Safely: There are three ways to increase IGF-1 levels and enhance HGH: (1) lifestyle and diet; (2) oral secretagogues; and (3) injections of synthetic HGH. A healthy diet, sunlight exposure, strenuous exercise, and plenty of deep sleep support natural release of growth hormone. Detoxification and fasting also improve HGH levels; the amino acid arginine assists growth hormone production. Do not jump into taking advertised substances that claim to raise IGF-1 levels. Use only recognized products and take them only if you have a clearly demonstrated need based on symptoms, age, clinical profile, disease condition, and blood tests.

However, if the methods cited above have not raised your IGF-I levels into the optimal range, consider injections of recombinant growth hormone (rHGH), also called somatotropin. This is a prescription substance, though it may be obtained in Mexico and other countries without a prescription, or from off-shore pharmacies over the Internet. It is produced by a special strain of *E. coli* bacteria containing the identical 119 amino acids that constitute naturally occurring pituitary human growth hormone.

For replacement purposes in adults, the most commonly recommended compound is Humatrope, manufactured by the French pharmaceutical company Eli Lilly. Other excellent

Changes in Plasma Levels in Selected Hormones in Men

Hormone	Levels in Men 20–30 years	Levels in Men over 60 years	Level to Consider Supplementing	Level to Consider Replacing
Testosterone (ng/mL)	241–827	Tends to fall below 400	Below 600	Below 400
Free testosterone (pg/mL)	9.3–26.5	6.6–18.1	Below 10	Below 6.6
Dihydrotestosterone, 5-alpha, DHT (ng/dL)	25.0–99.0	Tends to fall	Levels tend to fall with age, but can rise when using transdermal creams. DHT levels should remain constant.	
DHEA-S (ng/dL)	280–640	28–175	Below 350	Below 250
Androstenedione (ng/dL)	57–265	57–265	Below 150	Below 50
Pregnenolone (ng/dL)	10–200	10–200	Below 100	Below 50
Insulin-like growth factor, IGF-I (ng/mL)	114–492	71–290	Below 250	Below 150
Sex hormone binding globulin, SHBG (nmol/L)	13–71	13–71	SHBG levels reflect availability of testosterone and estrogen, and tend to fall during aging, though they can also rise. Optimal levels are around 25.	
Luteinizing hormone, LH (mIU/mL)	1.5–9.3	3.1–34.6	LH levels may increase temporarily as testosterone falls, then may eventually decline to levels below the range if gonadal function is absent.	
Estradiol, 17-Beta (pg/mL)	3–70	3–70	Estrogen levels can decrease in men as they age, but also have a tendency to rise. Elevated levels are considered unacceptable.	
Estrone (pg/dL)	12–72	12–72	No supplementation or replacement required for men.	
Total estrogens (pg/mL)	40–115	40–115		
Leptin (non-obese, ng/mL)	0.5–13.8	0.5–13.8	Reduced levels in the lower end of the reference range may contribute to weight gain. Weight loss is necessary, or leptin injections may be helpful.	

Men over 45 years old should consider testing for total testosterone and DHEA-S levels; those over 50 should consider adding the remaining studies. Supplemental and replacement recommendations apply to symptomatic men over 45 and nonsymptomatic men over 55.[1]

1. Reference ranges based on lab values used by Laboratory Corporation of America. LabCorp: 358 South Main Street, Burlington, NC 27215; http://www.labcorp.com/

brands are also available, such as Norditropin, made by Novo Nordisk in Denmark. The typical dosage for adults is by body weight, with an average replacement range from 0.5 to 1.0 IU per day.

However, when applying all of the dietary, lifestyle, nutritional, and herbal recommendations in this book, you can achieve effective results with considerably lower dosages. In this case, daily

> **CAUTION:** A prescription is required for rHGH and you will also need instructions from your doctor on how to do the injections yourself. However, like all of the stronger medications listed in this book, if you notice any unusual symptoms, discontinue immediately and discuss it with your doctor. Although low dose rGH injections or oral secretagogues are without significant risk, long-term use can cause receptor resistance, making them less effective. Your doctor should monitor long-term use (more than one year) of HGH-enhancing substances, even in low dosages. Do not take rHGH without a doctor's supervision.

dosages of 0.25 to 0.5 IU, or even less in some people, taken for three months, are sufficient to achieve symptom improvement and improve body composition without causing side effects (Gillberg, Bramnert, et al. 2001). At that time, and if your IGF-I levels have improved, you can reduce the times you inject HGH to three times a week. Often, a combination of daily use of an oral secretagogue with a bi-weekly injection provides significant benefits at less cost and with less risk.

In the dosage I typically recommend, HGH enhancement is usually safe and without significant side effects. However, minor side effects may occur, such as swelling caused by fluid retention. It this occurs, reduce your dosage and discuss your symptoms with your doctor. Never use HGH if you have cancer, have a history of cancer, or are at high risk for any form of cancer.

Common Side Effects of HGH Replacement

- Fluid retention
- Carpal tunnel symptoms (tingling and numbness of the wrist, palm, and first three fingers)

- Muscle and joint pains
- Tinnitus (ear ringing)

Symptoms of HGH Deficiency

- Reduced lean body mass and increased abdominal obesity
- Reduced strength and less exercise capacity
- Depressed mood and easily upset, with less self-control
- Increased social isolation
- Feeling of incompetence
- Fatigue
- Thin, dry skin
- Poor venous circulation
- Cold hands and feet
- Reduced bone density
- Falling eyelids, cheeks, buttock, and triceps muscles under the arms

Replacing Other Hormones: A comprehensive discussion of anti-aging hormones would not be complete without mentioning several other important hormones. Though not "super-hormone" stars like DHEA and HGH, these lesser known molecules play just as important a role in regulating and balancing the neuroendocrine system, one of our main goals in *Prolonging Health*. These other hormones include serotonin, newly discovered thalamine, erythropoietin, relaxin, leptin, aldosterone, calcitonin, androstenedione and androstenediol, vitamin D_3, eicosanoids, and thymus extracts. We have already reviewed several of these, so let's finish our discussion with the most important of these.

INJECTABLE THYMIC EXTRACTS: Thymic hormones from the thymus gland are considered by some anti-aging experts to be the missing

Safety and Additional Information on Thymus and Other Glandular Extracts Derived from Cows

Oral thymic extracts are considered safe and nontoxic and may be used for chronic viral conditions. However, there are several conditions in which their use is contraindicated: during pregnancy; if you have thymus tumors, myasthenia gravis, multiple sclerosis, or untreated hypothyroidism; or are on immune suppressive therapy to prevent organ transplant rejection. With the exception of synthetic thymosin, thymic extracts are made from calf's thymus glands, and derived mainly from European countries.

There is currently no evidence of contagion of BSE (bovine spongiform encephalopathy), or mad cow disease, through the use of bovine extracts for medicinal purposes. However, the German government issued a warning in 1994 stating the possibility of transmission of this disease through glandular tissue products. Before you use any glandular product, consult with your doctor, or contact the manufacturer or a governmental agency that reports on current safety issues related to BSE.

link in preventing age-related diseases. I agree. Numerous research studies have been conducted on these as immune modulators for the treatment of chronic viral conditions and there is growing interest in their use as anti-aging medications.

Several high-quality prescription-strength thymic extracts are produced in Germany. Two of these are Thymomodulin, made by Ellen Pharmceuticals, and Thym-Uvocal by Mulli, which are safe medicines. Another is Thymoject made by Biosyn; each 2 ml ampoule contains 100 mg of biotechnologically produced polypeptides made from bovine thymus glands.[53] Both injectable ampoules and oral tablets are available from many of these German companies.

Thymus Mucos, also from Germany, comes only in an oral form; but injectables are the preferred form because that way the medication gets directly into the bloodstream. The Italian-made thymic extract Leucotrofina A is also an excellent medication. Since these substances are not licensed drugs in the United States, injectable medications are available only through alternative avenues such as buyers' clubs or International Anti-aging Systems over the Internet.

The synthetic immunomodulating drug Thymosin alpha-1 is used for these same purposes. Zaduxin, a proprietary form of it, is licensed in 20 countries worldwide (excepting the United States, where it is classified as an orphan drug for the treatment of hepatitis B) for the treatment and prevention of influenza. Several studies have shown that thymosin improves the outcome of HCV patients when it is given with interferon. HIV/AIDS patients have also reported benefits from taking thymosin. It increases interleukin-2 receptors on T cells, increases maturation of T cells, and increases the production of gamma and alpha interferon. Although it is an injectable drug and requires a prescription, some AIDS health groups import it from Italy or other countries and it may be possible to obtain it over the Internet.

The dosage for injectable thymic extracts is one ampoule injected intramuscularly every day or every other day. A course typically consists of three weeks of injections, with an intermission of two weeks. Resume thymic therapy as needed to prevent infections and cancer, treat chronic viral infections, improve energy, and reduce age-related weakened immunity. Do not inject thymic extracts without a doctor's supervision.

ALDOSTERONE: The hormone aldosterone is secreted by the adrenal glands and increases the absorption of sodium to help the body retain water and control blood pressure. A deficiency manifests as urgency to urinate immediately after drinking water, low blood pressure, dizziness when standing up quickly due to a condition caused by a rapid drop in blood pressure, constant fatigue but feeling much better when lying down, and craving for salty foods. Aldosterone is measured in serum or a 24-hour urine sample. Licorice root tends to increase aldosterone activity in the body, but should not be used if you have high blood pressure. Fluronef, a steroid drug, is the medical treatment for low aldosterone and must be prescribed by a medical or osteopathic doctor.

CALCITONIN: This hormone produced in the thyroid gland is involved in calcium metabolism and bone breakdown, and low levels have been associated with migraine headaches and stomach ulcers. The main use for calcitonin is in the treatment of advanced osteoporosis; it is used as a nasal spray prepared as a synthetic hormone, and it requires a prescription.

THALAMINE: A newly discovered pineal hormone, injectable thalamine is an anti-senescence medication under investigation in Russia. It is not available in the United States at this time, but oral preparations may hold promise as complementary treatment with melatonin for restoring neuroendocrine balance and synchronicity in the body.

ERYTHROPOIETIN: One of a growing number of hormone-like growth factors, erythropoietin promotes the production and differentiation of red blood cells and is used in medical treatment of serious cases of chronic anemia as seen in kidney disease. For its energy and physical performance-enhancing properties, endurance athletes have used it in excessive dosages to provide them a competitive edge. Deficiency of erythropoietin causes anemia, fatigue, and pallor—all conditions often seen in the elderly.

Though some anti-aging doctors are experimenting with low doses of this substance, erythropoietin hasn't yet made it into the standard circle of anti-senescence drugs. Too much can make your blood too thick, causing clotting and stroke, and it should be used only in low dosages of 500 IU two to three times a week while under a medical or osteopathic doctor's supervision.

RELAXIN: Though the precise role of this hormone's physiological function in the body remains unknown, relaxin levels rise considerably during pregnancy. It is known that it participates in maintaining pregnancy and preparing the uterus for delivery. In addition, research suggests that relaxin has a wider range of activities than once thought, including increasing heart rate and the regulation of fluid balance in the brain. It has been used effectively for the treatment of fibromyalgia, and is thought to increase energy and stamina, as well as improve collagen, making ligaments stronger and skin softer. It is available without a prescription from pure porcine sources. Take 20–40 mcg twice daily.

LEPTIN: Derived from the Greek word *leptos*, this newly discovered hormone is associated with regulation of body weight, metabolism, and reproductive function. Most leptin in the body is produced in fat cells, though small amounts are also made in the stomach and in the placenta. Leptin receptors are found in large numbers in the hypothalamus and perhaps in other parts of the neuroendocrine system as well. It may play a significant role in neuroendocrine adaptation during fasting and calorie restriction (Shimokawa 1999, 2001).

Leptin levels are higher in women, obese people, and people with insulin resistance independent of body fat (Fisher 2002), and these levels change with age, exercise, and steroid hormone function. Though recombinant leptin is commercially available and is used in research, it has not yet found a place in anti-aging therapies. This may change within the decade, however, as new functions for leptin are discovered, including influence on growth hormone secretion, immune function, cancer, and aging.

ANDROSTENEDIONE, ANDROSTENETRIOL, AND ANDROSTENEDIOL: Metabolites of the prohormone DHEA have been shown to act as immune protective substances during infections from a wide variety of microorganisms including human herpes viruses, bacteria, and parasites (Loria 1996). Androstenedione, the precursor hormone for testosterone, is useful in raising testosterone levels in women and also in aging men; it is not as immunologically active as its metabolites androstenetriol and androstenediol.

Researched extensively in animal models by Roger M. Loria, Ph.D., of the department of microbiology and immunology at the Medical College of Virginia Commonwealth University in Richmond, Virginia, both of these hormones restore immunity after radiation damage (Loria 2000), improve endocrine regulation during infections (Padgett 1997), modulate immune cell activity and function, protect against lethal viral and bacterial infections (Ben-Nathan 1999; Loria 1988), protect against cancer (Huynh 2000), and may also have anti-cortisol properties.

Androstenedione is available over the counter and is taken in dosages ranging from 5 to 25 mg. Since it can raise testosterone levels, particularly in women, discontinue if you experience signs of androgen excess such as increased facial hair or acne. Androstenetriol and androstenediol are available for research purposes; however, several pharmaceutical versions are in the pipeline for use in elderly people for immune enhancement.

The mechanisms that run the neuroendocrine system are complex and interrelated. Think of them in layers, building in complexity. They compose a lacework of biological functions between cells and your body as a whole organism. Hormones do not exist in a vacuum, but are part of the extraordinary biological milieu that is your body. They circulate to every part of your body; communicate with each cell; interface biochemically with every molecule; and with the genetic material that provides your physiological blueprint.

Hormones are chemical messengers that play a significant role in health and aging by regulating neuroendocrine function. In doing so they moderate the effects of stress, improve energy, promote sleep, stimulate appetite and sexual behavior, and influence the features of aging. Hormones are thus *modifiable* aging factors that we can change to prolong our health and retain youthful vigor as we age.

The ten most important hormones for prolonging health are these: insulin, cortisol, DHEA, pregnenolone, progesterone, melatonin, thyroid, estrogen, testosterone, and HGH.

- Insulin is the most critical; without proper regulation it can signal the initiation of accelerated aging.

- Cortisol is a double-edged sword: if it is too low, you feel tired; if too high, it can cause the hypothalamus to atrophy and imbalance other hormones.

• DHEA is the most common anabolic steroid hormone in your body and is frequently low in chronic disease, autoimmune disease, aging, and when you are under long-term stress.

• Pregnenolone is the precursor hormone behind all steroid hormones. It protects the brain and nerve cells, improves memory, and helps regulate sex steroid hormone production.

• Progesterone provides protection from a wide array of age-related factors and balances estrogen's negative effects.

• Melatonin is a neuroendocrine regulator and can help reset your biological clock. Along with DHEA, it buffers the negative effects of stress hormones and enhances the activity of HGH, thyroid, and the thymus.

• Thyroid improves your metabolism, lifts energy, and benefits the entire neuroendocrine system.

• Estrogen maintains a woman's feminine form, improves memory, promotes restful sleep, brightens mood, enhances sexual pleasure, removes wrinkles, and improves brain function during aging.

• Testosterone improves mood, sleep, skin texture, body composition, and energy. It drives the libido and restores youthful sexual vigor.

• HGH supplementation is very controversial, but it is the hormone that provides the most anti-aging benefits. It improves body composition, increases strength and endurance, improves sexual performance, firms and lifts up sagging muscles, fills out thinning lips, and promotes hair growth.

Remember: hormones work synergistically with each other. Do not supplement one without another. Only increase levels of those that show need based upon your age, laboratory testing, and symptoms. To work best, hormone therapy should be tailored to your individual metabolism, age, genetics, and health condition.

Summary of *Prolonging Health* Recommendations for Neuroendocrine Balancing

• *Prolonging Health* Recommendation 41— Get Your Hormones Tested

• *Prolonging Health* Recommendation 42— Improve Insulin Signaling with Nutritional Medications

• *Prolonging Health* Recommendation 43— Achieve Neuroendocrine Balance by Neutralizing Excess Cortisol
  • DHEA, 5–15 mg daily in the morning with food
  • Phosphatidylserine, 100–300 mg daily with food
  • Gerivitol, oral or injectable

• *Prolonging Health* Recommendation 44— Achieve Neuroendocrine Balance by Restoring Synchronicity with Melatonin
  • Take melatonin directly before bed but after the lights are out, in ranges of 0.5 to 3.0 mg. Combine it with 5 mg of zinc and 10 mg of vitamin B_6. To enhance melatonin's effect, take 50–150 mg of 5-HTP and 400 mg of SAMe after dinner.

• *Prolonging Health* Recommendation 45— Achieve Neuroendocrine Balance by Regulating Your Hormonal Pathways
  • Soy isoflavones, 50–100 mg twice daily with food
  • Lignans, 1–2 tablespoons of fresh ground flaxseed meal daily
  • Indole 3-carbinol (I3C), 200–800 mg daily with food
  • Saw palmetto, 320 mg of the lipophilic extract containing 85 percent fatty acids and sterols daily with food

• *Prolonging Health* Recommendation 46— Use Herbal Adaptogens to Reset the Hormonal Axis
  • Ginseng, 100–250 mg of the standardized extract one to two times daily, away from food

- Siberian Ginseng, 250–500 mg daily, away from food
- Ashwagandha, 150–300 mg daily (2 to 5 mg of withanolides), away from food
- Rhodiola, 360–600 mg (1% rosavin) or 100–170 mg (3.6% rosavin) daily, away from food
- Velvet deer horn, 25–40 drops or 1–2 tablets of Pantocrine daily, in the morning away from food

- *Prolonging Health* **Recommendation 47—Supplement Declining Neuroendocrine Function with Natural Hormones**
  - Low insulin, 200 mg of MHCP (methylhydroxychalcone polymer) daily, with food
  - Low cortisol, 1.25 and 2.5 mg (cortisol equivalent) of adrenocortical extract in 3–4 divided dosages daily, away from food
  - Low thyroid, tryrosine 500–1,000 mg, 2–3 times daily; whole natural thyroid glandular 1/4–1 grain (one 250-mg capsule per day to two capsules twice a day)
  - Pregnenolone, 10 mg daily, with dinner
  - Androstenedione, 10–25 mg of oral or sublingual androstenedione daily
  - Progesterone, 1/4 teaspoon of a 2 percent progesterone cream daily
  - Estrogen: use dietary phytoestrogens (soy isoflavones, lignans, coumestans) and herb estrogen balancers (black cohosh, vitex, dong quai)
  - Human growth hormone: use amino acids (arginine, lysine, ornithine, glycine, tryptophan) and take Meditropin, two effervescent tablets dissolved in water taken nightly two hours after dinner

- *Prolonging Health* **Recommendation 48—Replace Deficient Hormones with Bio-Identical Hormones**
  - Cortisol, 5–20 mg or hydrocortisone 4 times daily, away from food
  - DHEA, 5–30 mg for women; 5–50 mg for men of micronized DHEA morning or evening, with food
  - Thyroid, 1/4–3 grains of desiccated thyroid (38 mcg of levothyroxine and 9 mcg of liothyronne per 1 grain or 60 mg of UPS thyroid) first thing in the morning, away from food
  - Progesterone, 10–100 mg cream or 50–100 mg oral daily
  - Estrogen, 1/4 teaspoon of 1.25–5.00 mg transdermal tri-est cream daily
  - Testosterone, 1/4 teaspoon of 10% natural testosterone cream for men; 0.5–1.0% cream for women
  - Human Growth Hormone, 0.25–1.0 IU of recombinant HGH injected daily or 3 times weekly

15 *Prolonging Health* Modifiable Aging Factor 9: Immune System Decline—How to Prevent Immunosenescence and Promote Immune Competence

As we age, our immune function can decline significantly, leaving us as older people more vulnerable to infections, more susceptible to autoimmune diseases, and more prone to cancer. In fact, unhealthy older people can have combinations of chronic degenerative illness and at the same time suffer from autoimmune illness, infections, and multiple types of cancer.

Age-related weakening of the immune system allows latent viruses to surface, reactivating infections such as common herpes zoster virus, which causes the painful condition of shingles. It predisposes us to more severe and even life-threatening infections from common bacteria and viruses, such as pneumonia and influenza; it contributes to cancer by allowing the cell proliferation that causes tumor formation to occur; and it contributes to autoimmune diseases such as rheumatoid arthritis.

However common this scenario is among the general population of elderly people, scientists are unclear about the connections. Are immune cells irreversibly programmed for immunosenescence, the term used to describe an aging immune function (Pawelec 1997)? Is the immune system, like other parts of the body, a "victim" of cumulative environmental factors? These include oxidative damage from ultraviolet radiation, toxic chemicals, toxicity from long-term use of multiple pharmaceutical drugs, along with changes in neuroendocrine status such as increased levels of the stress hormones cortisol and adrenaline. Or is immunosenescence a *combination* of cellular, genetic, and environmental factors (Hodges 1997)?

In this chapter, I discuss the nature of the immune system, what is known about age-related changes and immunosenescence, and the causes of immune dysfunction and decline. Then I introduce the methods that can help reverse it.

The Immune System Is an Intercommunication Network

The simple view of the immune system's role in health is that it protects us from invading pathogens such as viruses, bacteria, protozoa, molds, and parasites, as well as allergens, natural and man-made toxic substances, and also helps prevent cancer. It does this by recognizing self from non-self, or what belongs in our body for growth and survival, and what is foreign and therefore dangerous. Substances that instigate an immune response are collectively referred to as antigens; those that trigger allergies are allergens; those that cause cancer are carcinogens.

According to the conventional model of immunology, the immune system operates as a watchdog or policeman, guarding and defending us from everything that doesn't belong to our biology. However, in recent years, this model has undergone profound changes largely due to the discovery of hundreds of new immune substances previously unknown to science. The simple view is not sufficient to explain complex immune processes, or to determine the immunological changes that occur during aging.

According to Rita B. Effros, Ph.D., a gerontologist at the School of Medicine at the University of California at Los Angeles, contemporary scientific terminology that describes what were previously thought of as random occurrences that happened during aging might be exchanged for terms like "cross wiring" or "remodeling." These terms better fit the complex adaptive changes that the immune system goes through during aging (Effros 2001).

In the new immunology model, the immune system is still seen as a defense system, but also as a communication system interpreting signals between the environment and immune system and having interactions with other parts of the body such as the neuroendocrine system—a communication system that affects every aspect of the body, including the aging process. Therefore, the immune system is better thought of as a sensory organ that monitors the body on a cellular and molecular level through a network of chemical intercommunications to maintain homeostasis, rather than as a linear system of biological insults and reactions.

Another way scientists are beginning to look at the immune system is through the lens of evolutionary biology. The evolutionary model proposes that if the internal environment is disturbed by an infectious microorganism, threatened by physical injury or by biochemical disruption from within, the immune system works rapidly to neutralize the offending agent and restore balance and homeostasis. It also learns from its experience and remembers; it evolves novel strategies to cope with *future* insults. This model better serves our purposes because prolonging health requires a comprehensive understanding of how the body works in order to develop antisenescence methods that are effective and safe.

The immune system has organ, tissue, cel-

In the new immunology model, the immune system is still seen as a defense system, but also as a communication system interpreting signals between the environment and immune system and having interactions with other parts of the body such as the neuroendocrine system—a communication system that affects every aspect of the body, including the aging process.

lular, and molecular elements. The major organs and tissues of the immune system include the thymus gland, bone marrow, tonsils, adenoids, the bronchial-associated lymphoid tissue (BALT) in the lungs, the lymph nodes, spleen, and gut-associated lymphoid tissue (GALT). GALT is composed of lymph nodes in the large intestine and the Peyer's patches in the small intestine. The immune tissue system also includes the mucosa-associated lymphoid tissue (MALT). These are composed of diffuse immune tissues and cells lining the body's cavities, including the respiratory, gastrointestinal, and urinary tracts. Molecular immunological elements include immune cells, proteins, and cytokines.

White blood cells are responsible for the immune response. They are divided into lymphocytes, basophils, neutrophils, eosinophils, and monocytes. The lymphocytes form the main immune cells and form two classes of immune cells: B cells and T cells. B cells mature in the bone marrow, T cells mature in the thymus gland. Neutrophils and monocytes are involved in initial immune response to infection; eosinophils and basophils are involved in the allergic response. Let's look more closely at the lymphocytes because of their importance in the aging immune system.

How lymphocytes develop within the thymus into T cells is poorly understood. It seems to involve a complex series of biological events that take place in different microenvironments in the thymus gland (Anderson and Jenkinson 2001). T cells differentiate further into a vast number of immune cells; the most important of these are the CD4+, CD8+,[54] and natural killer (NK) cells. T cells secrete cytokines; these are proteins that affect the behavior of other cells and are closely involved in the immune response. They help to activate other immune cells and are further differentiated into T helper 1 and 2 cells (T_H1 and T_H2). Both types assist B cells to make antibodies. CD8+ T cells have a killer cell (cytotoxic) function against viruses and other pathogenic microorganisms that invade cells. NK cells also have cytotoxic activity and directly kill cancer and virus-infected cells.

B cells make protein substances called immunoglobulins, which can be as numerous and as specific as there are different chemical structures. This enables the immune system to protect us from nearly every imaginable infectious microorganism we might encounter by making matching antibodies against pathogenic antigens. However, your immune system does not horde or stockpile all of the antibodies; it operates from memory and creates new or adapted antibodies only upon demand.

T and B cells work together to initiate an immune response, which is thought to consist of two types: innate and adaptive. In response to a pathogenic insult, the body's initial response is mediated by innate immunity. It eliminates or contains the infection, but it doesn't develop a memory system to recognize the pathogen if it occurs again. That is the function of adaptive immunity. This focuses on the specific pathogen causing the infection and sets into motion a recognition system that creates *lifelong* immunity to the same infectious organism.

For example, when you were exposed to the measles virus as a child, your immune system responded by neutralizing and eliminating it from your body. It created a *specific memory* for that virus so if you were exposed to it again, antibodies against measles would be swiftly made, preventing you from reexperiencing the infection. That is innate and adaptive immunity working together.

Innate immunity was once thought to be a "hard-wired" fixed system that operated as an aggressive first line of defense. It is now known that the innate response is a highly sophisticated system involving numerous chemical substances and that it is also fully integrated with the adaptive response. Adaptive immunity is enhanced by vaccinations, and both innate and adaptive immunity are improved with proper nutrition, stress reduction, adequate rest and sleep, and sufficient amounts of antioxidants and other vitamins and minerals. These are also benefited by adaptogenic and immunomodulating herbal medicines such as astragalus, a traditional Chinese herb with tonic and immune-regulating effects.

Besides lymphocytes and other white cells, immunity is mediated by numerous proteins in the blood collectively called complement, and by a variety of biochemical substances collectively called cytokines and chemokines. These immune substances facilitate intercommunication between immune cells and even between chemical substances of the pathogenic organisms and your cells.

There is apparently little or no conscious awareness by the brain that the immune system is vigilantly at work. Unless symptoms like fever from an infection develop, you have no perception of the immune system's constant surveillance activity, how it is removing microbes, neutralizing cancer cells, and protecting your tissues from harmful toxins and toxic environmental substances. That the immune system is usually silent makes its relationship to the aging process difficult to monitor until the symptoms of a disease appear, the worst among them being cancer. However, a faulty immune system allows for numerous other age-related diseases as well, such as cardiovascular diseases and autoimmune disease such as rheumatoid arthritis.

Your Aging Immune System

The immune theory of aging proposes that the immune system and its cellular components set the stage for aging. Scientists who support this theory have found that there are a number of universal age-related biomarkers that suggest that one or more aspects of the immune system act as pacemakers for the aging process. The most significant of these occurs in the thymus gland, which undergoes a major reduction in size and function, called thymic involution (George 1996).

T lymphocytes, one of the most important immune cell types, mature in the thymus gland through a complex molecular process involving thymic hormones. These hormones also circulate in the blood, and though little is known about how thymic hormones influence immunity, researchers consider them important for a well-functioning immune system. The biological significance of the immune system during aging has been intensively researched.

Autopsies performed on dead older people indicate that atrophy of the thymus gland is universally present. A 60-year-old person's thymus can be 95 percent smaller than its full adult size. This reduction in size is correlated with declining immune function, primarily with a steep decrease in the number of T cells in unhealthy elderly people. However, some studies show that T cell numbers remain unchanged in *healthy* older people, though the percentage of functioning T cells decreases. This suggests that the thymus is capable of T cell development throughout life and that this function is therefore not age dependent (Rodewald 1998).

Though clinical observation clearly shows an increased incidence of disease among elderly people and research suggests that numerous cellular changes occur in the general population of older people, researchers have discovered evidence that contradicts these facts. We still do not know enough about the immune system during aging to resolve these contradictions; meanwhile stress and cumulative environmental factors may play a larger role than previously thought.

Evidence from centenarian studies shows that healthy centenarians do not have more diseases or infections than younger people and their immune cells were not affected by age. In fact, healthy centenarians have well-preserved immune systems. However, when sick centenarians were compared with healthy centenarians, the sick group had significantly reduced immune function (Rabin 1999). This suggests that age-related immune decline may be more linked to environmental factors such as stress and diet rather than to genetics or the aging process alone.

Therefore, preventing disease by prolonging health influences immunity, which is intimately connected to hormone function, and directly affects the health span. Thus preventing immunosenescence and promoting immune competence are critical factors in achieving maximum longevity, as, obviously, you cannot live long if you die early from an infection or cancer.

Changes in Immune Cells During Aging: The most noticeable changes in the immune system during aging occur among T cells. These changes include a shift from a predominance of CD4+ cells to CD8+ cells, suggesting a change in the immune system's focus from mounting responses to acute infections to managing more persistent chronic disease processes and intracellular infections as seen in chronic viral diseases such as Epstein-Barr virus, repeated influenza infections, hepatitis virus, cytomegalovirus, and cancer. Other shifts in immune cell populations occur, as well as an overall reduction in T cell numbers. Interestingly, women experience fewer of these changes than men, which is perhaps another reason why women live longer.

T cells produce a number of substances, including cytokines, integral to a well-functioning immune system. One group of cytokines, the interleukins, displays significant changes with age. For example, as T cell number and function decline, interleukin-2 (IL-2) levels decrease; this causes further decline in T cells because the presence of IL-2 is necessary for T cell growth. This decline causes them to divide less frequently, and therefore they become too old to function normally in the absence of IL-2. Imbalances of IL-2 are also associated with an increase in autoimmune diseases (Kroemer 1989). This is why measuring levels of IL-2 serves as a good biomarker of the aging immune system.

Levels of another important cytokine called interleukin-6 (IL-6) increase with age. This substance is linked to osteoporosis, chronic inflammation, and other age-related disorders. Levels of tumor necrosis factor alpha (TNF-alpha), a pro-inflammatory cytokine also involved in autoimmune diseases and cancer, are increased in older people (Armstrong 2001). IL-6 and TNF-alpha are good overall biomarkers for age-related changes in immune status.

T cell regeneration may be another key in understanding the aging immune system. Studies on T cell regeneration using animal models show that the thymus is important for regenerating T cells. In humans, subjects lacking the thymic capacity to regenerate T cells have reduced numbers of CD4 helper cells, a type of T lymphocyte that is reduced in HIV infection as well as in aging (Mackall 1997).

Activity of other white blood cells is reduced during aging. These include macrophages, monocytes, neutrophils, and eosinophils. While the cell count of natural killer cells remains unchanged, their cell-killing or cytotoxic function may be reduced in older people. When NK cells are depleted or their activity reduced, tumor formation and susceptibility to viral infection increase; both are conditions that can be fatal in older people (Cerwenka 2001).

As with hormonal communication, the immune decline associated with aging may be more of an intercommunication problem between immune cells, hormones, and other components of the immune system rather than immune incompetence caused by aging. Research suggests that numerous substances are involved in "signal transduction," a process whereby immune cells communicate with one another. Without specific protein markers on the surface of T cells, such as CD28 and CD69 antigens (Pioli 1998) that apparently decline with age, the immune system is unable to respond to foreign pathogens or developing cancer cells.

Another recently discovered signal transduction factor termed *Stat3* has been shown by researchers to be vital to maintain the architecture of the thymus gland. As mentioned, this gland is important for the production of T cells and prevention of immune system decline, and ultimately it may be one key in controlling the aging process (Sano 2001).

Signaling defects also occur among older people in the ability of cytokines to cross the blood-brain barrier, thereby reducing the fever response to infection. Clinically, it is well known that older people have a reduced fever response to acute infection and often succumb to influenza or pneumonia because their immune system cannot mount an aggressive enough initial response. One such cytokine involved in eliciting a fever is interleukin-1 beta; its ability to cross the blood-brain barrier is markedly reduced in older people (McLay 2000). These findings suggest that communication between the brain and its functions in immune activity in the rest of the body is impaired during aging.

Age-Related Immune Changes

Reduced	Increased
Total number of T cells	Interleukin-6
Percentage of viable T cells	TNF-alpha
Interleukin-2	CD8
IgM response	ANA
NK cell function	
CD4	
Percentage of B cells	

A number of immunological changes related to aging have been documented, including increased autoimmune activity simultaneously with decreased function of the innate and adaptive aspects of the immune system.

The total number of B cells may be reduced in elderly people, or at least the percentage of viable B cells, the lymphocytes that produce antibodies by interacting with T cells. This causes a significant decline in antibody function. The first type of antibody produced at the onset of an infection is called IgM (one of five immunoglobins); in elderly people IgM production may be compromised. Reduced production of antibodies allows infections to occur.

Autoantibodies, immune substances that react against your own tissues (as occurs in rheumatoid arthritis or autoimmune thyroid disease), are increased during aging. Antinuclear antibody (ANA), a general marker for autoimmune disease activity found in a blood sample, also tends to be increased in older people, signifying autoimmune or self-destructive processes are at work in the body. Researchers in Japan have found that persistent ANA elevations in otherwise healthy older people may indicate immune activity against selected genetic material; this hints at a possible genetic-immune connection (Xavier 1995).

Older people do not respond as well as younger ones to vaccines and may experience more side effects, though at least one study has shown that healthy older people do not have any more side effects than others do (Allsup 2001). This suggests that healthy older people have sufficient immune function to produce antibodies from the vaccine and thereby reap the benefit.

Other Factors That Influence the Aging Immune System: Though immune-related molecular and cellular changes occur commonly in elderly people, my clinical experience suggests that many of these changes, especially in those people under stress, start gradually, beginning as early in life as the forties or fifties, or perhaps even earlier. Some gerontologists supportive of the immune theory of aging suggest that stress to the mother during pregnancy affects the immune function of her offspring even later in life, through the activity of cortisol and other stress hormones. They further contend it can also indirectly affect the offspring's predisposition to disease and aging itself.

Cumulative damage by chronic infections and the oxidative damage caused by the inflammation of infectious illnesses further reduce immune function and tax the immune system's capacity. HIV is an obvious example of an infection that compromises immunity. Other less formidable chronic infections also weaken immunity over time, including hepatitis C virus (HCV), human herpes virus 6 (HHV-6), cytomegalovirus (CMV), and the sexually transmitted bacteria chlamydia (*Chlamydia trichomatis, C. pneumoniae*). Referred to as the "silent epidemic," more than four million new cases of chlamydia infection occur in the United States each year. These and other "stealth" infections increase the risk for cardiovascular disease, neurodegenerative diseases such as Alzheimer's disease and Parkinson's, liver and kidney disease, and cancer (Ewald 2000).

Hormone decline is closely associated with immunosenescence. Hormones involved include DHEA, GH, melatonin, estrogen, and thyroid hormones. Low and even low normal levels of the thyroid hormone triiodothyronine (T3) are common in aging and contribute to low NK cell activity (Kmiec 2001).

Mucosal immunity, the part of the immune system that protects against foreign pathogens entering the body when we breathe and eat,

can be significantly reduced in elderly people. This may explain why the elderly are particularly susceptible to respiratory infections such as influenza and pneumonia (Shugars 2001). Cytotoxic T cells may also be reduced in mucosal immune deficiency.

Since immune cells are first produced in the bone marrow, age-related changes in bone health and bone marrow status, such as occur in osteoporosis, may cause a decrease in the overall numbers of stem cells. Or they may cause defects in the normal pathways of T cell development and significantly alter immune status. B cell generation within the bone marrow is strongly influenced by the activity of cytokines, and abnormal levels of substances such as IL-6 reduce the viability of T and B cells, thus predisposing us to chronic infections, autoimmune diseases, and cancer.

Factors That Cause Immunosenescence

- Low DHEA
- Elevated cortisol
- Stress
- Thymic involution
- Diabetes and insulin resistance
- Chronic infections
- Poor diet
- Low nutrient density
- Excess oxidation
- Genetic changes
- Environmental toxins
- Pharmaceutical drugs
- Low thyroid function (decreased serum T3)
- Age-related changes in the bone marrow

The Aging Immune System and Cancer

Throughout this book, I have repeatedly emphasized that the ultimate enemies of longevity are cancer and old age. My clinical opinion is that all of the late-onset degenerative diseases (cardiovascular disease, diabetes, arthritis, osteoporosis, and even neurodegenerative diseases) are preventable. If they do occur and are caught early enough, they can be effectively treated using an integrated approach that combines modern Western diagnostic techniques with natural medicines and a healthy lifestyle.

Many types of cancer are also preventable, such as lung cancer, predominantly caused by smoking cigarettes. However, the underlying processes of cancer are so ancient and appear so intimately interwoven into the fabric of our biological evolution that in order to prolong health and reach our maximum life span, we have to remain cancer free.

For evolutionary biologists investigating the reasons for aging, the fundamental questions are these: Why do we grow old? Why do we get tumors? Are the two related in such a way that we can learn about aging from studying tumor mechanisms? Evidence suggests that cancer and senescence are related, but what is that relationship (Krtolica 2002)? What role does the aging immune system play in cancer development?

There seems little question that oxidative damage, DNA damage, inflammation, and neuroendocrine imbalances can contribute to tumor formation. Tumors do not develop independent of other factors; they are not foreign parasites that invade your body. They are the result of mutations that take place in normal healthy cells that undergo alteration in order for oncogenesis to take place. How this occurs is also still unknown to scientists.

However, in healthy centenarians, nature apparently solved this dilemma of aging and cancer, leaving old age the winner. Therefore, it is our job to discover what nature's solution is in order to prevent cancer from killing us while we age. Then we will have only old age itself left—the final enigma in unraveling the mystery of longevity and perhaps even that of immortality.

In terms of evolution, when we contemplate the human body, we are looking at a biological masterpiece containing ancient genes and newly evolved structures, all put together in an astounding array of chemical and biological processes. Unfortunately, we know little about most of them, but what we do know is fascinating and provides clues to the aging-cancer dilemma.

It appears that the aging process itself may activate a number of genetic mechanisms that influence a cell's proclivity for tumor proliferation. These include an imbalance in the telomere "fail-safe" mode and other mechanisms that inhibit tumor formation by limiting cellular proliferation (Weinstein 2002). As discussed earlier, telomeres are noncoding material at the tips of chromosomes and they shorten over time with each cell division. The telomere theory of aging (refer back to chapter 1) hypothesizes that repair procedures renew telomere length up to a point, then, unable to maintain replicative integrity, telomeres shorten and aging results.

Unbelievably, though normal cells do not live forever, tumor cells are immortal, as demonstrated by recent research (Kim 1994). They divide relentlessly, apparently without regard for the laws that seem to govern every other cell in the body. What is the difference between the immortality of tumor cells and normal healthy cells that age? How does that relate to the human quest to become immortal?

The answers may lie with the telomeres again, and with telomerase, the enzyme responsible for maintaining the length of telomeres in normal cells (Campisi 2001). Apparently, cancer cells have a way of turning telomerase on and using it to replicate continuously, assuring their immortality. Scientists have found that when they block telomerase (or genetically engineer mice that have lower amounts of telomerase), cancer cells are prevented from dividing. Unfortunately, the trade-off is a shortened life span, since without telomerase, the division of normal cells is reduced.

Fortunately, nature has a solution to the telomerase dichotomy in the form of two proteins. The genes p53 and WRN encode proteins to prevent normal cells from turning into cancer cells. Described as "the guardian of the genome," p53 is activated by any number of stressors, such as damage to DNA or telomere loss. It is thought to be responsible for initiating repair, suppressing tumor formation, and possibly even arresting senescence.

However, even in the p53 gene, we see a similar phenomenon as with telomerase: when mice are engineered to have high p53 activity, they are resistant to tumors as expected, but age prematurely (Tyner 2002). The WRN protein, considered a longevity molecule, helps to rebuild telomeres and is used by about ten percent of cancer cells to maintain their immortality.

Though the aging-cancer riddle continues to frustrate gerontologists and oncologists, it appears that many of these theories are at least loosely linked. For example, the SIR2 protein, a gene thought to control the rate of aging, can suppress p53 activity, allowing cells to live longer. Also, cellular responses to telomere abnormalities involve both telomerase and p53 activity. There are alternative pathways that allow cells to express life, death, or cancer, including the WRN model as an alternative to telomerase.

Then there is apoptosis, programmed or voluntary cell death—cell suicide. Apoptosis not only helps to shut down abnormal and diseased cells, such as cancer and those cells infected with viruses, but it participates in body changes during growth and development. For example, human embryos resemble fish in the early stages of development, but in order to grow fingers instead of fins or flippers, the fish-like cells must die to be replaced by human cells. It appears that evolutionary processes have designed a system of multiple fail-safe mechanisms—alternative pathways, pleiotropic possibilities, mutations in cell phenotype, and countless other biological wonders—that if we could understand would provide us clues to preventing cancer and help us live longer. Ironically, for our body to live, cells must contain within themselves the programming on how to die.

By now, you may be more comfortable with the ironies and paradoxes of aging, including the aging-cancer dilemma. We have yet another question: What can we do now to prolong our health and prevent cancer to achieve maximum longevity? This is where the immune system comes in. A normal cell must undergo alterations to become a cancer cell, and an intact well-functioning immune system helps to prevent these initial changes and/or eliminate mutant cells, thus preventing cancer. This fact is the clue to an immune strategy.

How to Prevent Immunosenescence and Promote Immune Competence

My experience with healthy elderly patients has convinced me of several facts. Immune function does not automatically decline with age. Those who remain healthy are no more susceptible to infection, cancer, or autoimmune disease than younger people are. Immune function can be enhanced through diet, exercise, vitamin and mineral supplementation, and by using specialized immune-modulating medicines. These methods not only improve immune function, but also promote positive genetic expression, making cells immune from the changes that allow cancer to develop.

The major targets for immune enhancement and reversing immunosenescence are the thymus gland, the bone marrow, and the mechanisms responsible for intercellular communication. Reversing thymic degeneration, or at least replacing thymic hormones, is essential for maintaining a healthy T cell population. Methods that support a good blood supply and promote bone integrity contribute to viable bone marrow, which is essential for the production of immature T cells. By maintaining hormonal balance through a well-regulated neuroendocrine system and improving signal transduction, your cells can communicate better.

Nutrients play an important role in maintaining immune function. Elderly people often eat less and have poorer nutrition than younger people do, so it is important that you follow the *Prolonging Health* dietary recommendations all your life. Many individual vitamins and minerals are necessary for strong immunity. For example, calcium is necessary for signal transduction. A deficiency in calcium contributes to poor bone health, which in turn reduces the bone marrow's ability to create mature T cells.

But it also halts intercellular communication among immune cells and inhibits the production of cytokines, the proteins responsible for coordinating the immune response. Microminerals, nutritional substances other than calcium, magnesium, and phosphorus, which are macrominerals, have been shown to enhance NK cell function in older people (Ravaglia 2000).

For example, zinc supplementation helps to reverse the thymus gland degeneration (Mocchegiani 1995). Vitamin E appears to be not only a superb general antioxidant capable of preventing cardiovascular disease, but it's also a cancer preventative and enhances T cell function in older people. Researchers have demonstrated that vitamin E improves T cell responsiveness (Beharka 1997) and promotes cellular immunity in aging (Moriguchi 1998).

Prolonging Health Recommendation 49— Get Your Immune Functions Tested

If you have a chronic illness or are over 65, consider having your blood tested to evaluate your immune status. Your doctor will have to order these tests for you, though members of the Life Extension Foundation can order many of these tests without a doctor. Here are four to consider:

ANA: Antinuclear antibody (ANA), also referred to as the fluorescent antinuclear antibody test (FANA), is a sensitive screening test to evaluate the presence of autoimmune or self-induced inflammation. In a situation of persistent immune activity, immune cells may attack your own tissues, causing more inflammation and increased cellular destruction. ANA is elevated in systemic lupus erythematosus, Sjögren's syndrome, rheumatoid arthritis, polymyositis, inflammation of the kidneys and the lungs, during viral or bacterial infections, and with colitis and liver inflammation. It may be elevated in elderly people with an underlying autoimmune disorder (Xavier 1995). Healthy people do not have elevated ANA.

Lymphocyte Function: Test your total white blood cells (WBC), total T cells (CD3+), helper T cells (CD4+), cytotoxic T cells (CD8+), total B cells (CD20+), and NK cell count and activity. If your immune system is strong, your total white cells should be between 4,500 and 8,500. Since the reference ranges for the different types of lymphocytes vary depending on which laboratory you use, I cannot give you optimal values for these tests. Your results should fall within the normal reference ranges provided by your medical laboratory.

Cytokines: Test for interleukin-2 (IL-2), interleukin-6 (IL-6), and tumor necrosis factor-alpha (TNF-alpha). Low levels of IL-2, with high levels of IL-6 and TNF-alpha, signify chronic inflammation and a predisposition to degenerative disease. Optimally, keep them within your laboratory's normal reference ranges.

Microbial Antibodies: To be thorough, consider testing for common infectious microorganisms. These include bacterial antibodies (*Chlamydia, Helicobacter pylori*); fungal antibodies (*Candida albicans*); and viral antibodies (Epstein-Barr virus, cytomegalovirus, human herpes simplex viruses I and II, human herpes virus-6, hepatitis B and C viruses, human immunodeficiency virus). Healthy people do not test positive for these.

Prolonging Health Recommendation 50— Use Immunomodulators to Boost Immune Function

Specialized natural medications that enhance immune function, called immunomodulators, contribute to immune system function. These include Chinese medicinal herbs such as astragalus (*Astragalus membranaceus*), ginseng (*Panax ginseng*), and cordyceps (*Cordyceps sinensis*); yeast-derived substances such as beta-1, 3-D-glucan; Amazonian herbal extracts such as cat's claw (*Uncaria tomentosa*); and European herbal extracts such as Iscador, a Swiss preparation made from mistletoe (*Viscum alba*). Let's review these in more detail.

Astragalus: A traditional Chinese tonic, astragalus is typically used to promote the innate immune function in people who are prone to frequent colds and minor cases of influenza. The polysaccharide components in astragalus are believed responsible for its immune-enhancing activity, including stimulation of interferon production, increasing immune cell activity, and facilitating destruction of tumor cells. Use it as a tea by simmering 9–30 g of the dried sliced root, easily obtained at a Chinese herb store; or take two to three 500-mg capsules, two times daily. Astragalus is a safe herb with no known side effects or interactions.

Ginseng: Widely used for its neuroendocrine and adaptogenic uses (see chapter 17), ginseng also is useful as an immunomodulating medication for individuals who suffer from fatigue concurrently with immune deficiency (Scaglione et al. 1990). Both astragalus and ginseng help to restore the body's natural physiological balance and normal homeostasis. The recommended dosage is 100–250 mg daily of the standardized extract containing four to seven percent ginsenosides.

Cordyceps: A highly valued traditional Chinese medicine, cordyceps prepared in the traditional manner is composed of the dried body of the larvae of a moth on which it grows. However, modern preparations are available that commercially cultivate the fungus without having to infect moths to obtain its medicinal activity. Cordyceps increases levels of interferon, interleukin-2, and helper T cells, and stimulates natural killer cell activity, all of which tend to decline during aging. Take 500–1,000 mg of the extract three times daily before food. It is considered safe and can be taken over a long period of time; it has no known interactions with drugs.

Beta 1, 3-D glucans: Beta-glucans are components of fungal cell walls and are commercially derived from mushroom species and common baker's yeast (*Saccharomyces cerevisiae*). They have a number of immune-enhancing properties that help to stimulate innate immunity and are effective in the prevention of common viral illnesses such as colds and flu, as well as for adjunctive care in the treatment of fungal and parasitic infections. As a substance, beta 1, 3-D glucans is considered safe and nontoxic, with no known drug interactions.

To prolong health and improve immune function in aging, take 100–250 mg daily. For the adjunctive treatment of cancer and other conditions associated with immune decline during aging, daily dosages of 1,500–3,000 mg are required (Keller 2000).

Uncaria Extract: Cat's claw (*Uncaria tomentosa*) is a large woody vine that grows in the upper Amazon region of Peru. Research has shown that uncaria extracts have immunomodulating properties, and it has been investigated as an anticancer medication, an anti-inflammatory (Sandoval-Chacon 1998), an antiviral (Williams 2001), and a DNA repair agent (Sheng 2000). If you have an elevated ANA or an autoimmune disorder, consider taking uncaria extract. The form I recommend is the water-soluble extract C-MED 100. Take 350 mg of C-MED 100, standardized to eight percent carboxy alkyl esters, twice daily away from food.

Iscador: A Swiss preparation made from wild mistletoe growing on pine, apple, oak, and other trees, Iscador (called Iscar in the United States) is a widely used cancer medication in Germany, Switzerland, and other European countries (Murphy 2001). Besides its use in the treatment of cancer, it has value as an immunomodulating medicine. Researchers have demonstrated Iscador's effectiveness in increasing total lymphocyte count and stimulating immune cell activity (Gorter 1998), including that of natural killer cells. Having been shown to increase life expectancy in can-

Researchers have demonstrated Iscador's effectiveness in increasing total lymphocyte count and stimulating immune cell activity, including that of natural killer cells. Having been shown to increase life expectancy in cancer patients, Iscador is an extraordinary natural medication with considerable potential as an immune-enhancing substance to be used during aging.

cer patients (Grossarth-Maticek 2001), Iscador is an extraordinary natural medication with considerable potential as an immune-enhancing substance to be used during aging.

Iscador has been in clinical use for more than 80 years and has an excellent safety record. It is an injectable medication that requires a prescription from a medical or osteopathic doctor. If you choose to use Iscador, carefully review its uses with your doctor. It can be taken concurrently with hormone therapies, most herbs, and homeopathic medications; however, individual contraindications may apply. Due to possible interactions, do not use it at the same time as pharmaceutical drugs except with your doctor's approval and directions.

Prolonging Health Recommendation 51— Take a Thymus Extract

Extracts prepared from the thymus glands of animals, refined proteins such as thymic protein-A, and injectable natural and synthetic thymic preparations such as thymosin alpha-1 or beta-4 are useful in rebuilding your immunity.

Whole Thymus Extracts: Most commercial thymus extracts are derived from calf thymus glands prepared as a dried powder to the manufacturer's specifications. These forms contain only trace amounts of thymus hormones, so I do not recommend them to my patients. However, the Canadian company Atrium Biotechnologies produces concentrated, whole, live-cell bovine thymus tissue extracts.[55] Live-cell extracts and injections have been popular in Europe for decades as rejuvenation therapies. Atrium manufactures their products to European standards. NatCell Thymus is an oral liquid preparation that arrives frozen and must be kept frozen until use. Thaw one vial by rubbing it between your palms, and drink the entire contents two times weekly. Also available as a sublingual spray, NatCell Thymus can be obtained through your doctor.

Thymic Protein-A: Considered one of the leading natural thymic immune-supporting medications, BioPro thymic protein-A contains concentrated thymus hormone proteins that have been shown to stimulate helper T-4 cell function (Rosenbaum et al. 2001). It comes in individual packets containing a white powder that dissolves in your mouth for efficient sublingual absorption. Take one to two packets, but not with food or after eating. Thymic protein-A is a safe substance without interactions or side effects.

Injectable Thymic Extracts: Several high-quality prescription-strength thymic extracts are produced in Germany. Thymomodulin (Leucotrofina is an Italian version) made by Ellen Pharmaceuticals and Thym-Uvocal made by Mulli are safe injectable medicines for restoring thymic hormone levels. Injectable medications go directly into the bloodstream and have a greater therapeutic effect in the body than oral preparations do.

Synthetic thymic extracts are also effective in improving immune function. Thymosin alpha-1 and beta-4 are used for this purpose. Research has shown that thymosin increases the maturation of T cells, the production of the cytokines gamma and beta interferon, and promotes wound healing (Huff 2001; Billich 2002). Consider these if your immune function is weak, your white blood cell or lymphocyte counts are low, or if you have a chronic viral infection.[56] The dosage for injectable thymic extracts is one ampoule injected intramuscularly every other day, for a course of two to three weeks or longer.

Significant immune system decline is evident in unhealthy and sick older people, but immune decline is not universal in the aging process since healthy centenarians have normal immune function. This suggests that the immune system is a highly complex process involving multiple organ as well as molecular and cellular factors, and is influenced by and influences other systems, principally the neuroendocrine system, but is also dependent on genetic factors.

Scientists do not agree on the underlying causes of immunosenescence, but regardless of conflicting theories, by the time you reach "older" age, the integrity of your immune system will likely be compromised. This reduction in protective capacity is caused by a host of factors including environmental and cellular changes, and it influences the fact that most cancers occur in older people. A healthy immune system is essential to prolonging your health and achieving maximum longevity.

Summary of *Prolonging Health* Recommendations to Boost Your Immunity

- *Prolonging Health* Recommendation 49— Get Your Immune Functions Tested
  - Test your antinuclear antibody (ANA). Though it is often elevated in elderly people, healthy people do not have high ANA.
  - Test your total white blood cells (WBC), total T cells (CD3+), helper T cells (CD4+), cytotoxic T cells (CD8+), total B cells (CD20+), and NK cell count and activity. For optimal health, your total white cells should be between 4,500 and 8,500; your lymphocyte levels should fall within the laboratory's reference ranges.
  - Test your cytokines: interleukin-2 (IL-2), interleukin-6 (IL-6), and tumor necrosis factor-alpha (TNF-alpha); keep them within your laboratory's normal reference ranges.
  - If you suspect an infection, get your antibodies tested for infectious microorganisms.

- *Prolonging Health* Recommendation 50— Use Immunomodulators to Boost Immune Function
  - Drink astragalus tea (simmer 9–30 g of the dried sliced root for one hour), or take two to three 500-mg capsules, two times daily.
  - Consider taking 100–250 mg of ginseng (4–7 percent ginsenosides) daily.
  - Take 500–1,000 mg of cordyceps extract three times daily before food. Take 100–250 mg daily of beta 1, 3-D glucans. If you have cancer or a viral infection, take 1,500–3,000 mg daily.
  - Consider taking Iscador injections if you have had cancer.
  - Take 350 mg of uncaria extract C-MED 100, standardized to 8 percent carboxy alkyl esters, twice daily away from food, to boost your immune system and lower inflammation.

- *Prolonging Health* Recommendation 51— Take a Thymus Extract
  - Consider taking an oral thymus extract such as NatCell Thymus or thymic protein-A at least three times weekly if your immune system is weak.
  - Get thymic extract injections (Thymomodulin, Leucotrofina, Thym-Uvocal, thymosin alpha-1, or thymosin beta-4) if your white blood cell count is low or you have a chronic virus.

16 *Prolonging Health* Modifiable Aging Factor 10: Neurodegeneration—How to Revitalize Your Aging Brain

It has been said that even if we resisted frailty, avoided cancer, and lived long enough, we would all eventually succumb to dementia (Yankner 2000). Nothing frightens us more, aside from death itself, than the specter of an elderly person whose mental functions have declined so much that that person is classified as having Alzheimer's disease. Such a person, completely dependent on others, has lost all human dignity, living in a twilight world of childishness, mental vacancy, or sometimes in the psychotic behavior of dementia.

Is the "inevitable" deterioration of mental function another aging myth? Can neurodegeneration be prevented? If so, to what degree and by what methods? Can the aging brain be revitalized, and if so, how?

Inspiring examples of the brain's unflagging creative and mental abilities in older people include a long list of notables: Leo Tolstoy, Claude Monet, Linus Pauling, Manuel de Oliveira, and Stanley Kunitz. At the age of 95, Kunitz was still creating new poems and reading to live audiences, and was named poet laureate of the United States. Tolstoy (1828–1910) wrote until age 82, when he suffered a fatal infection, which he caught while traveling by train. The French artist Monet (1840–1926) still painted at 86, just

before he died of lung cancer. Linus Pauling (1901–1994), the only person to win two unshared Nobel prizes (one in 1954 for chemistry and the other in 1962 for peace), continued to write and publish scientific papers and serve as the director of the Linus Pauling Institute into his nineties. Oliveira, called Portugal's "ageless wonder," is considered one of the world's greatest movie directors and, at 93, directed the film *I'm Going Home*, which won recognition at the Cannes International Film Festival in 2001.

We are on the threshold of undreamed of possibilities in the neurobiology and neurophysics of the aging brain. The individuals just cited are examples of what we too might achieve, perhaps at even older ages. However remarkable these examples are as individual cases, they do not answer the fundamental questions presented above, nor do they reveal what the mind and consciousness are.

In the last decade of the twentieth century, the dualistic paradigm that separated spirit from the body, the body from the brain, and the brain from the mind, and which had already influenced scientific thinking for several hundred years, started to give way to the holistic paradigm of body/mind/spirit as a unity. However better the holistic model is, it does not convey the interrelationships of the many different biological phenomena in the body, and it does not tell *where* consciousness is, what the mind is, or explain the consciousness/mind connection.

Antonio R. Damasio, M.D., is head of the neurology department at the University of Iowa College of Medicine in Ames and adjunct professor at the Salk Institute for Biological Studies in San Diego, California. He says that by the year 2050 "sufficient knowledge of biological phenomena" will transform the landscape of neurobiology (Damasio 1999). Paralleling these advances is a similar curve in the neurobiology of aging, pharmacology, cellular and molecular gerontology, and genetics. These sciences combined may bring us for the first time closer to glimpsing "the ghost in the machine," the consciousness underlying the body-mind connection.

In this chapter we explore the remarkable human brain and the changes it endures in aging. We'll see how to revitalize its cognitive abilities, memory, and creative capacity with a wide array of natural medicines and selected pharmaceuticals. But first we need to learn how the brain and nervous system function.

The Brain and Nervous System

Our brain, a product of several hundred million years of evolution, is an extraordinary structure. Its architecture includes three divisions: cerebrum, cerebellum, and brain stem. The cerebrum is the frontal part of your brain, located just behind your forehead, composed of two halves called the right and left hemispheres, and covered by a thin layer of "gray matter" called the neocortex. The neocortex folds along the many canyons of the cerebrum, and if spread flat would cover an area approximately two and a half square feet.

Neurologists and neurobiologists, scientists and physicians who study the brain, divide the cerebrum into four areas, or lobes, and propose that each controls a different function. The frontal lobe (the front part of your brain) is responsible for abstract problem solving; the temporal lobes (located on the front sides of your brain) control memory, language, and hearing; the parietal lobes (located on the sides behind the temporal lobes) are influential in processing sensory information; and the occipital (located at the back) governs vision.

Behind the cerebrum lies the cerebellum, the part of your brain that controls movement and muscle coordination and processes kinesthetic memory. This is the function that provides skilled athletes, dancers, martial artists, and yoga masters the ability for their muscles to remember sequences of movement in order to perform complex physical acts. This function allows us, as we age, to become more coordinated, as illustrated by the saying "practice makes perfect." Traditionally, tai chi masters are generally older individuals who don't reach their peak performance until they are 60 or older, which suggests that some brain-body functions actually improve with age.

The brain stem, situated at the upper end of your spinal column and behind the cerebrum, is the first part of the brain formed during fetal development. It is often referred to as the "reptilian" or primitive brain since it was also the first part of the brain to evolve. It is responsible for relaying sensory information from the body to the brain and controls basic physiological processes such as breathing and heart rate.

The entire brain, composed of these three parts and other tissues, weighs about three pounds (1.5 kilograms) and contains an estimated 100 billion brain cells. There are two types of brain cells: neurons and glia, and there are over 50 known subtypes. Neurons, functioning as a communications network, do the majority of the brain's work, and are composed of several types of proteins that make up the different neuronal structures. Neurons are separated from each other by a microscopic gap (10–20 nanometers) called a synapse, which allows electrical and biochemical signals to pass from one neuron to the next.

This neuronal "talk" involves neurotransmitters (protein substances such as serotonin) and specialized enzymes that bathe the synaptic gap and destroy neurotransmitters as quickly as they are released in order to maintain a fresh supply of neurotransmitters. Neurotransmitters are the chemical messengers that help brain cells communicate with one another and are built from proteins. More than 500 substances that have the potential to act as neurotransmitters have been discovered in the brain. However, only a few are characterized as neurotransmitters, and these include acetylcholine, dopamine, and serotonin.

Another part of the brain important to our discussion on aging is the limbic system. This is often referred to as the "feeling brain" and is part of the cerebrum. Unlike the neocortex, or "the thinking brain," which makes up the coating of the brain tissue, the limbic system lies deep within the cerebrum and rests just on top of the brain stem. It is composed of the hippocampus, the amygdala, the hypothalamus, the thalamus, and the pituitary gland—all structures that are critical to health and aging.

In Alzheimer's disease, the hippocampus is among the first tissues to deteriorate, an event thought to be responsible for much of the memory loss associated with this condition. The hippocampus is also vulnerable to the damage caused by long-term cortisol excess, a problem common to both stress and aging. The amygdala is largely responsible for processing emotions; the hypothalamus is closely related to managing homeostasis and bodily functions such as temperature and metabolism; it also sends messages to the pituitary gland, which in turn controls hormone secretion in other glands such as the thyroid and adrenals. The thalamus, an area of the brain just above the hypothalamus, acts as a relay station for nerve impulses from the body to the brain.

What makes the brain run? Though fatty acids obtained from the diet are the building blocks of the brain's tissue, composing about two-thirds of it by weight, glucose is the main energy source of the brain, and a constant supply of it is necessary for the brain to function properly. The pancreas, liver, neuroendocrine system, and other body systems work together to provide steady levels of glucose to the brain.

The Aging Brain—The Root of Aging?

Like all other parts of our body, the brain ages. Perhaps, as some gerontologists believe, aging even begins in the brain, in which case neurodegeneration, the gradual loss of neuron activity and function (neurons are brain cells), could be the root of the aging brain.

Alzheimer's, Huntington's, and Parkinson's diseases, as well as memory loss, are associated with the neurodegeneration of aging. Like the other aspects of aging we've discussed, neurodegeneration is not a single event, but a compound and complex process involving molecular, cellular, hormonal, and metabolic factors. It is characterized by reduced cerebral blood flow, neurotransmitter deficiency, structural deterioration and reduced neuronal plasticity (adaptability), neuroendocrine imbalances, and disrupted cholinergic activity. Nerve cells that are critical for memory and learning use the neurotransmitter acetylcholine to function and are said to exhibit cholinergic activity. A decrease in this function is associated with loss of the brain's cognitive function.

As we age, many events happen. Mitochondrial defects accumulate. DNA mutations allow for the replication of less viable cells. Chronic inflammation results in damage to neural tissue. Repeated viral and bacterial infections may contribute to additional damage to nerve cells. Free radical molecules accelerate oxidative damage to cell membranes and other parts of the neuron. Declining hormonal activity in neurons dampens the immune response in the brain. Poor blood flow due to reduced heart function, sticky blood, or high blood pressure plays a significant role in neurodegeneration.

What We Know About Neural Aging: Contrary to the scientific dogma that persisted for decades, even with the lack of sound evidence, we now know that our brain continues to produce new neurons at least into our seventies and that it loses few, if any, of its neurons during life. We have all of our "marbles" after all. Unfortunately for many aging individuals, many of those marbles may be cracked and chipped; even so, those who follow the recommendations in this chapter will likely benefit, with improved brain function.

Though the number of brain cells remains relatively constant throughout life, the brain does reduce in size. Marilyn S. Albert, Ph.D., is professor of psychiatry and neurology at the Harvard Medical School and director of the Gerontology Research Unit at Massachusetts General Hospital in Boston. She says the average brain shrinks by 6 to 16 percent between the ages of 30 and 80 (Albert 1997). This decrease in overall volume of the brain is caused by a reduction in myelin, the protein substance that forms a protective coating on nerve sheaths; there is a 45-percent decrease in myelinated fibers. So even if you retain all of your nerve cells, do they work as well?

At the Sixth International Symposium on Neurobiology and Neuroendocrinology of Aging, in Bregenz, Austria, in 2001, Carol A. Barnes, Ph.D., of the University of Arizona in Tucson, presented a list of things we know about neural degeneration. She reported that the cellular function of neurons is well preserved during aging. Ironically, though there is little overall cell loss, selective *deterioration* does

Contrary to the scientific dogma that persisted for decades, even with the lack of sound evidence, we now know that our brain continues to produce new neurons at least into our seventies and that it loses few, if any, of its neurons during life. We have all of our "marbles" after all.

occur in cellular activity and intercommunication between cells is impaired. Barnes explained that even though memory and other cognitive functions tend to decline with aging, compensatory mechanisms make up for these age-related changes, which can be even more powerful than the original brain function (Barnes 1976).

Perhaps this is one reason why healthy older people tend to become wiser with age, as we know that intelligence remains stable across the entire life span and that according to yogic science, deeper levels of conscious awareness are more available to us as we age.

Two other features of neurodegeneration are also important to discuss: neural plasticity and hippocampal aging. Our nervous system has to remain flexible in order to adapt to all the environmental and psychological stressors that occur in the process of living. This adaptation is referred to as neural plasticity. The brain remodels itself throughout life, much as bones and other tissues do, requiring new nerve cells for repair and regeneration.

In 1998, a joint effort by Peter S. Eriksson, Ph.D., of Sahlgrenska University Hospital in Goteborg, Sweden, and Fred H. Gage, Ph.D., of the Salk Institute for Biological Studies in San Diego, California, discovered that even in the mature human brain, particularly the hippocampus—the gateway to memory and learning—neurogenesis occurs (Eriksson 1998). This is an incredible discovery because it informs us that the creation of new nerve cells is possible. That suggests that not only can our cognitive abilities improve as we get older, but also perhaps there is a way to reverse neurodegeneration.

However, atrophic changes in the hippocampus do occur with aging, leading to memory loss and difficulty in spatial navigation. The hippocampus is where our "cognitive maps" are stored; these are memories of how we get from one place to the other, avoiding obstacles in the process. Have you ever been to Florida? If so, you'll notice that in retirement areas for the elderly, grocery store aisles are wider and turning lanes along the highway are marked well in advance of the actual turn. No one wants older people getting lost while on their way to the grocery store or between the fruit and cereal sections once they're in the store.

Just as hormone production is decreased in aging, the level of neurotransmitters—the chemical messengers that make all neural activity possible—is less and the number of receptor sites they stimulate is also reduced. Among the most important of these neurotransmitters is dopamine, the brain chemical associated with pleasure and brain metabolism.

Dopamine is part of a family of neurotransmitters called catecholamines, which also includes epinephrine and norepinephrine; all are synthesized from the amino acid tyrosine. In fact, according to Nora Volkow, M.D., associate laboratory director in Life Sciences at Brookhaven National Laboratory in Upton, New York, approximately six percent of the total number of these receptors are lost between the ages of 20 and 80 (Volkow 2001). Other researchers have documented loss of dopamine receptors (Amenta et al. 2001), and changes in the interactions between different brain chemicals (Segovia 1999). Loss of dopamine is associated with Parkinson's and Alzheimer's disease; pharmacologically improving dopamine metabolism appears to make some improvement in these late-onset neurodegenerative conditions.

Levels of serotonin, related transporting chemicals (Kuikka 2001), and serotonin receptors (Sheline 2002) also decrease in aging. Serotonin (5-hydroxytryptamine, 5-HT) is the neurotransmitter responsible for contentment, sensitivity to pain, sleep, appetite, and sexual behavior; its levels are associated with age-related changes in mood. Like melatonin, to which it is chemically related, serotonin is found in nearly all living things. Serotonin also influences processes related to memory and learning, and it can activate the HPA-axis, thereby influencing the secretion of pituitary hormones. Along with other neurotransmitters, serotonin plays an essential role in overall neuroendocrine balance.

Although serotonin can be obtained from dietary sources, endogenous (inside the body) 5-HT is synthesized from the amino acid tryptophan in neurons of the central nervous system. Its highest concentrations are in the hip-pocampus and other areas of the brain, but large amounts are also produced in the gut. Referred to as the "second brain" (Gershon 1998) or enteric nervous system, the gut has independent sites of neural integration and processing. It does "think" like the brain; per-haps there is something in the saying, "follow your gut."

Acetylcholine, the most abundant neuro-transmitter in the body, is primarily involved in nerve and muscle activity and in controlling muscle tone. It also plays an important role in maintaining cellular homeostasis (how cells maintain their equilibrium), and is involved in memory and learning. Acetylcholine deficiency may cause light sleeping, poor concentration, and forgetfulness, and it has been associated with Alzheimer's disease.

What We Don't Know About the Brain-Aging Continuum: The aging brain and the aging process parallel each other so closely that one doesn't occur without the other. This is not surprising. As one disruption occurs in the bio-logical web, reverberations simultaneously take place in other parts. Eastern philosophy pro-poses that underlying all living phenomena is an intrinsic energy, or life force, but the inter-linking connection between these parts is still a mystery to Western-trained scientists. One of the more promising candidates for a unifying mechanism underlying the brain-aging contin-uum is how body cells and systems are affected by changes in natural rhythms.

Age-related circadian rhythmic changes were first described in 1974 by Colin S. Pittendrigh (1919–1996). He was a professor of biology at the University of Montana in Bozeman and was instrumental in founding the field of chronobiology, the search for an "internal clock" and the study of biological rhythms (Pittendrigh 1974). At the molecular

level, our biological clock is actually a system of oscillating levels of proteins, principally in the form of hormones, controlled by genetic tran-scription (Lewis 1995). The implication of the disruption of circadian rhythms and the result-ant hormonal changes might prove to be an important addition to the many theories of aging. Melatonin, for example, acts as a neu-roendocrine modulator and may be the key that regulates our internal clock.

The circadian release of pituitary and pineal hormones is altered during the aging process, but it is still not clear if declining lev-els of hormones such as growth hormone and melatonin are simply age-related phenomena, or if they happen in concert with other changes. My guess is they are orchestrated through neuroendocrine connections that, in turn, strongly influence brain function, and that the underlying mechanisms of aging are closely associated with a disruption in the *rhythms* and pulsations of life.

Many Biochemical and Environmental Factors Influence Brain Aging: Putting theo-ries aside, let's explore the many biochemical and environmental factors that influence brain aging and see what we can do to prevent and reverse neurodegenerative changes in the brain.

As discussed earlier, glucose is the primary fuel for brain activity, and we also know that glucose metabolism tends to decrease with age, while insulin resistance increases. Deficient glucose levels cause hypoglycemia, and the lack of available glucose in the brain causes mem-ory loss, confusion, and mood swings. Excess glucose, as well as too much insulin, damages brain cells and causes excessive oxidation. In addition, in some older people insulin levels drop too low, causing levels of glucose to rise, unless glucagon, cortisol, and growth hormone are also deficient. In this case, insulin, glucose, and cortisol levels may be low, which ironically may actually prolong life span, but the person with this condition is hypoglycemic, suffers from adrenal insufficiency, and tends to feel chronically weak, tired, and depressed.

The opposite is true when stress causes a rise in cortisol in the bloodstream. This happens through a complex pathway of signaling and releasing substances that starts in the amygdala and hypothalamus and ends in the adrenal glands, which release stress hormones. Excess cortisol, after circulating through the body in the blood, reaches the hippocampus, which tells the hypothalamus to send a message to the adrenal glands to stop releasing cortisol.

Under normal circumstances, this system works well, maintaining cortisol within tight ranges. However, in instances of continuous stress, or when the neuroendocrine system is imbalanced due to any number of age-related factors, cortisol levels build and damage to hippocampal and hypothalamic cells results. This further unbalances the HPA-axis and eventually the entire neuroendocrine system. Researchers have found that elevated cortisol levels in salivary samples are often found in depressed people, who also tend to have a smaller hippocampus and as a consequence suffer from memory loss—much like that seen in older people.

General slowing of mental ability and loss of short-term memory are the most commonly reported age-related changes in brain function. Much of this may be caused by lack of exercise and poor diet. Sedentary lifestyle and lack of fitness reduce the efficiency of the heart's function of pumping blood, including to the brain, and without sufficient blood flow, the brain cannot function well.

Brain function is also not well supported by a diet that does not supply adequate amounts of antioxidants, proteins, essential fatty acids, and proper carbohydrate balance. Accumulated chemical and metabolic toxic substances cause additional damage to brain tissue and nerve cells. Chronic inflammation and infections are another source of neuronal damage. Due to age-related hormonal decline, the brain does not have sufficient hormones, such as estrogen, testosterone, melatonin, and thyroid, to function properly.

How to Revitalize Your Brain

You can prevent brain aging by reducing the accumulation of toxic metals, improving detoxification pathways, reducing inflammation, taking antioxidants, using amino acids, supplementing your diet with essential fatty acids, and taking brain-enhancing medications. Herbal medications that improve cerebral blood flow (such as ginkgo) are important in a program to reduce neurodegenerative effects and reverse brain aging. Specialized "brain boosters" or nootrophics, neuroprotective compounds, neurotransmitter regulators, and synthetic cognitive-enhancing drugs all contribute to improving brain function.

Since the early 1970s, when the first generation of cognitive-enhancing drugs first appeared on the market (second generation arriving in the 1990s), research neuropharmacologists have investigated treatments for Alzheimer's disease. Unfortunately, most of these drugs have shown modest cognitive improvement at best and virtually no effect in reversing Alzheimer's. Some of these pharmaceutical compounds have use in improving memory, enhancing cognition, and reducing depression, but because these drugs are well presented in other books, such as *Smart Drugs* by Ward Dean, M.D. (Dean 1993), I will focus

Selected Cognitive and Neuroprotective Natural Compounds

Compound	Actions	Daily Dosage
5-hydroxytryptophan (5-HTP)	Serotonin precursor	50–300 mg
Phosphatidylcholine	Acetylcholine precursor	3,000–9,000 mg
L-alpha glycerylphosphorylcholine (GPC)	Acetylcholine precursor; restores muscarinic receptors	500–750 mg
Dimethylaminoethanol (DMAE)	Acetylcholine precursor; reduces lipofuscin	100–150 mg
Galantamine	Acetylcholinesterase inhibitor; restores nicotinic receptor sensitivity	16–32 mg
Huperzine-A	Acetylcholinesterase inhibitor	50–200 mcg
Phosphatidylserine	Improves neurotransmitter function; increases acetylcholine and dopamine release; improves glucose levels in the brain; reduces excess cortisol levels; stimulates nerve growth factor	100–300 mg
Vinpocetine	Antioxidant; improves oxygenation; improves red blood cell plasticity; inhibits platelet aggregation; increases glucose levels in the brain	10–30 mg
Acetyl-L-carnitine	Transports fat into mitochondria; reduces lipofuscin; cytoprotective effects; prevents apoptosis; participates in acetylcholine formation	500–2,000 mg

the majority of this discussion on natural compounds that are safe and effective in preventing age-related cognitive decline, restoring brain plasticity (adaptiveness), and normal function, and for revitalizing your brain.

There are several aspects to improving brain function, including diet, exercise, and stress reduction. Other ways include the use of antioxidants to protect neurons from oxidative damage; detoxification to remove accumulated toxic substances that damage brain tissue; hormonal balancing; improving microcirculation; reducing inflammation; and lowering the body's load of infectious microorganisms. These have all been discussed in previous modifiable aging factor chapters. So let's focus on aspects specific to brain function that we haven't previously discussed: neurotransmitters, nootrophic neutraceuticals, and neuroprotective and brain-enhancing compounds.

Prolonging Health Recommendation 52— Balance Your Neurotransmitters with Precursor Compounds

The first step in revitalizing your brain is to provide sufficient amounts of the building blocks that constitute its structure and contribute to substances that perform cognitive functions. These include amino acid precursor substances, acetylcholine precursors, and other compounds. Though we are still learning about the influences of neurotransmitters in aging, and since we know that neurotransmitters are built from proteins, it seems prudent to provide sufficient amounts of the precursor amino acids tyrosine and tryptophan in the diet, as well as in dietary supplements.

Tyrosine: A nonessential amino acid, L-tyrosine is not required from dietary sources since it is synthesized from phenylalanine, another amino acid. But it is important for the structure of most proteins in the body and serves as the precursor for several neurotransmitters including dopamine; it is also used to convert T4 to T3, as it is part of the structure of the thyroid hormone molecule. Tyrosine is found in animal and vegetable proteins, and the free form of tyrosine is also found in fermented dairy products such as yogurt. It is prepared commercially as a nutritional supplement, which is not associated with any side effects in the recommended dosage of 500–1,500 mg daily.

Possible drug interactions with tyrosine may occur with MAO inhibitors, such as phenelzine sulfate (Nardil), causing possible high blood pressure; therefore tyrosine should not be taken at the same time. It is best used with other amino acids, including phenylalanine; vitamin B_6, folic acid, and copper are required for its synthesis in the body.

Tryptophan: This is one of the eight essential amino acids. Since it cannot be readily synthesized in the body, tryptophan must be obtained in the diet or from nutritional supplements. The metabolism of tryptophan is complex, but essentially it converts to 5-hydroxytryptophan (5-HTP), which converts to serotonin (5-HT). Though tryptophan has powerful mood-enhancing and sleep-inducing properties, it was banned by the FDA in 1989 for over-the-counter use. This was after 37 people

contracted eosinophilia-myalgia syndrome (EMS) from a contaminated lot of tryptophan. However, it remains available by prescription, in Mexico, or from offshore pharmacies; it can be used in 500–1,500 mg dosages.

5-HTP: Since 5-HTP is an intermediary metabolite in the conversion of tryptophan to serotonin, it is often used as an alternative. 5-HTP is made commercially from tryptophan or processed from the seeds of griffonia (*Griffonia simpliciflora*), a medicinal tree related to carob found in West Africa. It is used in dosages of 50–300 mg daily. In some instances, dosages as high as 600 mg are required to improve serotonin levels. However, these higher dosages may metabolize into too much serotonin, possibly causing nausea, diarrhea, and vomiting in some people. Reports of overdosing are rare; 5-HTP appears to be safe within the recommended dosages. The addition of vitamins B_6 and B_5 help convert 5-HTP to serotonin.

Phosphatidylcholine: Choline is an essential nutrient widely distributed in foods. It is necessary for the structure and function of all cells and plays a number of important roles in the body such as a precursor for a variety of signaling molecules; it also serves as the precursor for phosphatidylcholine and acetylcholine. A phospholipid substance that forms a major component of cell membranes, phosphatidylcholine has liver-protective effects, is involved in cell membrane composition and repair, and is the precursor for the neurotransmitter acetylcholine, and several other chemical substances. It is useful in the treatment of depression along with omega-3 fatty acids, and may have a role in the management of Alzheimer's disease.

Phosphatidylcholine is found in soy, sunflower seeds, and eggs, and is commercially prepared as lecithin, as well as in a 90 percent concentrate available as a nutritional supplement in soft-gel capsules. The typical daily dosage of the supplement form is between 3 and 9 g. It is a safe substance with no known side effects or interactions with drugs.

L-Alpha Glycerylphosphorylcholine (GPC): A compound that plays an important role as a natural acetylcholine precursor is L-alpha glycerylphosphorylcholine (GPC). A byproduct of phosphatidylcholine, GPC is effective in slowing the structural changes in the brain that are associated with age-related cognitive decline. It helps to restore muscarinic receptors, which, along with nicotinic receptors, are necessary for acetylcholine to communicate with nerve cells. It also increases the release of dopamine; and it appears to potentiate the effects of growth hormone releasing hormone in the pituitary gland, resulting in improved levels of growth hormone in the body (Ceda 1992).

The sum of these effects improves brain plasticity and has corrective effects on cognitive decline during aging. GPC is safe and well tolerated, with occasional gastrointestinal irritation, headache, and nausea reported. The typical dosage is 500–750 mg daily.

Dimethylaminoethanol (DMAE): DMAE, another natural acetylcholine precursor, is produced in the body and is chemically similar to choline. Only small amounts are converted into acetylcholine, yet it has been shown to help remove lipofuscin, an aging pigment; it is useful in the treatment of age-related mood disorders such as depression and anxiety. Its use has been associated with restlessness and muscle tension in the back of the neck and head, but it is otherwise considered safe. Therapeutic dosages range from 100 to 1,000 mg per day; in some individuals it can inhibit choline uptake in the brain, so I usually recommend using it as a medication at 100–150 mg daily.

Prolonging Health Recommendation 53— Balance Your Neurotransmitters with Acetylcholinesterase Inhibitors

It's unfortunate that we cannot directly supplement acetylcholine, but we can take substances that block the enzyme acetylcholinesterase, which breaks down acetylcholine, thereby protecting our existing stores of this important neurotransmitter. Though there are several acetylcholinesterase drugs, such as donepezil (Aricept) and rivastigmine (Exelon), there are also natural acetylcholinesterase inhibitors: galantamine and huperzine A.

Galantamine: An alkaloid substance derived from the bulbs of several different flowering plants in the *Amaryllidaceae* family, galantamine functions as an acetylcholinesterase inhibitor. It also improves the sensitivity of an important acetylcholine receptor, the nicotinic receptor. It is readily absorbed and safe in the recommended dosage of 16–32 mg daily.

Huperzine A: Also a plant alkaloid, huperzine is derived from club moss (*Huperzia serrata*), a traditional Chinese herb. It is used to improve cognitive function and, like galantamine, huperzine has mild effectiveness in the treatment of Alzheimer's disease. It absorbs well when taken orally, and though it is considered generally safe, because of possible adverse effects including dizziness, blurred vision, sweating, and nausea, it should be used with caution by those with a history of seizures, arrhythmias, and asthma.

Though it does not have adverse reactions with most drugs, it can have additive effects and possible adverse interactions with synthetic acetylcholinesterase inhibiting agents; it should not be used concurrently with these drugs. The average dosage is 50–200 mcg daily.

Prolonging Health Recommendation 54— Take Melatonin

Melatonin regulates the body's internal clock and is used to manage sleep disturbance, improve mood, and reduce jet lag. It is necessary to provide neuroendocrine balance in the brain, and is involved in neurotransmitter metabolism. A typical dose I recommend is 0.5–3 mg of melatonin nightly.

Prolonging Health Recommendation 55— Take Enough B Vitamins

B vitamins appear important for neurogenesis and act as cofactors in neurotransmitter synthesis. It is well known that both the mother's diet before and during pregnancy and the infant's diet require vitamins B_{12} and folic acid for normal brain development. In addition to a B-complex supplement, I recommend 1,000–2,000 mcg of vitamin B_{12} and 1–5 mg of folic acid daily.

Prolonging Health Recommendation 56— Take Nootrophic Neutraceuticals and Neuroprotective Compounds

Nootrophics are substances that improve cognitive function. They include a growing list of natural substances, such as L-alpha glycerylphosphorylcholine (GPC), phosphatidylserine, vinpocetine, huperzine-A, and acetyl-L-carnitine.

Phosphatidylserine: A phospholipid found in all cells of the body, with the highest concentration in brain cells, phosphatidylserine (PS) facilitates the storage, release, and activity of several neurotransmitters, and helps cellular intercommunication in the brain. It helps release dopamine, increases acetylcholine production, improves brain glucose metabolism, lowers excess cortisol levels, and boosts nerve growth factor necessary for the generation and health of neurons. Supplementation with PS improves memory, mood, learning, and concentration.

It is derived from bovine cortex or soybeans, and though not available in the United States, the bovine source is the preferred form in Europe. PS derived from soy lecithin has been shown to be equally effective, and is considered very safe and without interactions, with the exception that PS may enhance the effects of blood-thinning drugs and should not be used if you are taking Coumadin and heparin. The typical dosage is 100–300 mg daily.

Vinpocetine: Another plant-derived medication, vinpocetine comes from an alkaloid found in the African periwinkle (*Vinca minor*). It improves cerebral blood circulation, improves oxygen utilization, exerts antioxidant activity, improves red blood cell plasticity and inhibits clumping of platelets; it also raises glucose levels in the brain. It improves concentration and memory, and reduces age-related effects in the brain. Further, it can reduce seizure activity and may have benefits in lowering blood pressure, as well as improving the outcome after a stroke. It is considered safe and without interactions, but since it affects blood circulation, it should not be used at the same time as blood thinners. It absorbs best with food, and the dosage is typically 10–30 mg daily.

Acetyl-L-Carnitine: Related to the amino acid carnitine, acetyl-L-carnitine occurs naturally in the body, where it is involved in the transportation of fats into the mitochondria. It improves learning and memory, counteracts depression in the elderly, and has neuroprotective effects. It also reduces lipofuscin formation in the brain, improves immune function and receptor sensitivity for several neurotransmitters, benefits heart function, improves sperm count, and has antioxidant activity. Acetyl-L-carnitine has cell-protective properties and prevents excessive cell death. It also helps in the formation of acetylcholine, decreases glycation, and is neuroprotective. It is safe and without side effects in dosages ranging from 500 to 2,000 mg daily.

Prolonging Health Recommendation 57— Use Neuroprotective Hormones

Several hormones protect the brain from the degenerative effects of aging, toxic chemicals, excess cortisol, and xenobiotic substances. These include pregnenolone, progesterone, and estrogen (see chapter 14). Of the three, pregnenolone is the most neuroprotective.

Pregnenolone: Concentrations of pregnenolone in the brain decline with age. It is a useful medication to restore brain function. Pregnenolone improves memory, exerts a positive influence on neurotransmitters, increases neurogenesis (in particular, neurogenesic activity in the hippocampus), and improves cognitive function. It has a buffering effect on stress and promotes better sleep. It also has mild anti-inflammatory activity and may play a role as a complementary medicine in the management of the low-grade chronic inflammation associated with aging. Men and women over 50 should consider taking 30–100 mg of pregnenolone daily after dinner.

Prolonging Health Recommendation 58— Fortify Your Brain with Cognitive-Enhancing Herbs

Several of the nootrophic compounds already discussed, such as galantamine, huperzine A, and vinpocetin, are derived from plants. However, in this section, we focus our discussion on several herbs that improve cognitive function, including ginkgo extract, the Ayurvedic herb bacopa, and the Chinese herbs polygonum and gastrodia.

Ginkgo: Though the modern form of ginkgo was discovered in extracts from the leaves of the Asian ginkgo tree (*Ginkgo biloba*) by Japanese researchers in 1966, ginkgo has a long history in traditional Chinese medicine, where the seeds are used in the treatment of asthma and to reduce excess urination. The active constituents in the leaves include flavone glycosides and terpene lactones: ginkgolides and bilobalide. Investigations into the therapeutic effects of pharmaceutical ginkgo biloba extract (GBE) were principally performed in the early 1960s by German researchers who developed the currently used standard of 24 percent glycosides and 6 percent terpenes.

The Japanese have since developed a more concentrated form of GBE, standardized to 28 percent glycosides and 7 percent terpenes. In my clinical work, I use an even stronger form standardized to 32 percent glycosides and 9 percent terpenes (referred to as the 32/9 extract). This extract can be obtained from Pure Encapsulations[57] and is presently the highest potency available for the treatment of age-related cognitive decline.

GBE improves microcirculation in the brain and to the extremities. This makes it useful for improving brain function and in the treatment of conditions of reduced blood flow in the legs such as intermittent claudication, a condition characterized by cramping and leg pain after walking. Regular usage of GBE improves memory, reduces depression, reduces tinnitis and vertigo, and treats age-related cognitive decline. It is safe to use, but because it improves blood circulation and also reduces platelet aggregate (clumping), it should not be used with blood-thinning drugs. The typical dosage is 120–240 mg of the 24/6 standardized extract, taken two to three times daily, or 160 mg of the 32/9 extract twice daily.

Bacopa: The extract of this herb is prepared from the leaves of the semitropical plant *Bacopa monniera.* Called *Brahmi* in Ayurvedic medicine, where it is traditionally used for memory enhancement and to promote sleep, in modern herbal medicine it is prepared in a standardized extract containing 20 percent bacosides and used as a cognitive-enhancing substance. It also has antioxidant activity, anti-inflammatory properties, and acts as a cardiotonic. Bacopa is safe and without side effects or interactions, and is taken in dosages of 100–300 mg of the standardized extract.

Polygonum: This is classified by traditional Chinese medicine as a "yin and blood tonic," which means a substance that restores kidney and liver function. It treats dizziness, blurred vision, graying hair, insomnia, and generalized weakness—all conditions associated with aging (Bensky 1986; Yin 1992). Polygonum (*Polygonum multiflori*) is safe to take regularly over a long period of time. It is synergistic with other Chinese herbal tonics, such as ginseng, and is often combined with them to enhance its effects. Modern herbal practitioners combine it with bacopa, ginkgo, and other natural nootrophics for the treatment of age-related cognitive decline.

Polygonum is safe and is taken as a traditional tea using 10–30 g of the prepared root, or as a 10:1 extract in capsules at a dosage of 250–500 mg daily.

Gastrodia: Like polygonum, gastrodia (*Gastrodia elata*) is a traditional Chinese herbal medicine backed by several thousand years of use. It is taken to improve symptoms that accompany reduced brain function including dizziness, insomnia, restlessness, and poor memory; it is valued for the treatment of seizures, hypertension, and to promote recov-ery after a stroke (Wang 2002). Research studies indicate that gastrodia provides neuroprotection in the hippocampus (Kim 2001), affects neurotransmission in the brain (Ha 2001), improves cerebral blood flow (Jingyi 1997), and has antioxidant properties (Liu 1992).

Gastrodia is combined in formulas with polygonum as in Tianman and Shouwu Formula (*tianma shou wu pian*) or other herbs, such as Cerebral Tonic Pills (*bu nao wan*) and Gastrodia Dispel Wind Formula Tablets (*tianma chu feng pu pien*) (Fratkin 1986). These patented formulas can be bought at Chinese herb shops or from your acupuncturist. The dosage is different for each preparation, but generally it is 5–10 pills two times daily.

Aging and declining brain function appear to parallel each other in what is called the brain-aging continuum. The brain has the capacity to remain plastic and adaptive throughout life given the right environment, diet, exercise, adequate blood flow, hormonal balance, and neurotransmitter activity. If the body itself is free of the major degenerative diseases of aging, it seems possible that brain function can be improved and age-related brain decline prevented.

However, improving brain function best takes place in the context of a comprehensive approach in which *all* aging factors are addressed. To what degree restoration of brain function and halting neurodegeneration are possible is still unknown, but it depends on many factors, principally the rebuilding of brain tissue through enhanced neurogenesis. Lowering cortisol, normalizing insulin, and supplementing deficient levels of estrogen, progesterone, testosterone, thyroid hormone, growth hormone, pregnenolone, and DHEA all promise some improvement in preventing neurodegeneration and eliciting neurogenesis.

Still, these measures may be inadequate to compensate for advanced late-onset neurodegenerative conditions, such as Alzheimer's. Though still in their infancy, "smart drugs" and other synthetic mood- and cognitive-enhancing substances will play an increasing role in the treatment of age-related neurodegenerative disorders. A number of scientifically studied natural medicines are available for the treatment of cognitive decline associated with aging, providing complementary therapy in a complete prolonging health plan.

Summary of *Prolonging Health* Recommendations for Revitalizing Your Brain

- *Prolonging Health* Recommendation 52— **Balance Your Neurotransmitters with Precursor Compounds**
  - Take 500–1,500 mg of L-tyrosine daily.
  - Take 500–1,500 mg of L-tryptophan daily.
  - Take 50–300 mg of 5-HTP daily.
  - Take 3–9 mg of phosphatidylcholine daily.
  - Take 500–750 mg of L-alpha glycerylphosphorylcholine (GPC) daily.
  - Take 100–150 mg of dimethylaminoethanol (DMAE) daily.

- *Prolonging Health* Recommendation 53— **Balance Your Neurotransmiters with Acetylcholinesterase Inhibitors**

- Take 16–32 mg of galantamine daily.
- Take 50–200 mcgs of huperzine daily.

- *Prolonging Health* Recommendation 54— **Take Melatonin**
  - Take 0.5–3 mg of melatonin nightly.

- *Prolonging Health* Recommendation 55— **Take Enough B Vitamins**
  - Take 1,000–2,000 mcg of vitamin B_{12} and 1–5 mg of folic acid daily.

- *Prolonging Health* Recommendation 56— **Take Nootrophic Neutraceuticals and Neuroprotective Compounds**
  - Take 100–300 mg phosphatidylserine (PS) daily.
  - Take 10–30 mg of vinpocetine daily.
  - Take 500–2,000 mg acetyl-L-carnitine daily.

- *Prolonging Health* Recommendation 57— **Use Neuroprotective Hormones**
  - Take 30–100 mg of pregnenolone daily.

- *Prolonging Health* Recommendation 58— **Fortify Your Brain with Cognitive-Enhancing Herbs**
  - Take ginkgo extract: 120–240 mg of the 24/6 standardized extract, two to three times daily; or 160 mg of the 32/9 extract twice daily.
  - Take 100–300 mg of bacopa extract daily.
  - Take 250–500 mg of polygonum extract daily.
  - Consider taking gastrodia.

17 The Practice of *Prolonging Health:* Five Longevity Strategies for Reaching Your Maximum Life Span

Up to this point, I have presented information supporting my hypothesis that by preventing disease and prolonging your health, you can live a healthier, productive, and longer life. I reviewed the changes that occur during aging and discussed state-of-the-art aging research. I discussed biomarkers, explained what laboratory tests are most useful in evaluating the effects of aging on your body, and outlined how to determine your age-point. I presented the science behind the modifiable aging factors, and outlined what you can do to prevent them from occurring or lessening their effects.

Now, in this chapter, I organize these concepts into practical methods and present a coherent plan of five comprehensive strategies to safely and effectively assist you in prolonging your health and maximizing your life span. By following these strategies, you can put the *Prolonging Health* model into practice.

The Five Longevity Strategies

I. Restore Homeostasis

II. Eat for Longevity

III. Practice Periodic Caloric Restriction

IV. Exercise for Maximum Longevity

V. Use Life-Extending Nutritional Supplements

Longevity Strategy I—Restore Homeostasis

In my experience, the healthiest and longest-lived people have several things in common. First, and most important, their lifestyle supports health and longevity. Second, they have an intrinsic vitality that emanates from them as a vibrancy of spirit, conveying a sense of superb physical health. It is as if they just took a hike in the mountains: that's how it seems to everyone who is fortunate enough to meet them. We learn how to protect, sustain, enliven, and regenerate our own inner source of energy by following their example.

Third, such people have an indomitable spirit manifest in their personality as gratefulness and equanimity; this prevents the stresses of life from accumulating and taking a disastrous toll on their body, mind, and emotions. Such people have achieved this without drugs or hormones, or even vitamins.

Think how effective your program can be if you combine the *Prolonging Health* lifestyle, modeled on the longest-lived among us, with the latest and best information on longevity medications, nutrients, and hormones. Of course, possessing a healthy genetic base, avoiding infections, living in an environment as free as possible from toxic chemicals and excessive amounts of electromagnetic radiation, and residing in a geographical location that supports health and longevity are equally important. Let's look at a few examples of such people.

My Taoist teacher, Share K. Lew, is an example of a modern master who has attained longevity naturally. Born in Guangzhou province (Canton), China, in the early part of the twentieth century, Master Lew entered a traditional Taoist kung fu temple on a sacred mountain at the age of 14, where he lived and practiced under the guidance of his mentor until the Japanese invasion in 1938. After leaving the temple, he traveled to Hong Kong and then San Francisco, where he continued his study in kung fu with his uncle in Chinatown. Now in his mid-eighties, Lew is free of all late-onset diseases and continues to teach the method of energy cultivation, qi gong, to students in Europe and the United States.

The Yupik Eskimos of St. Lawrence Island, among whom I lived during the winter and spring of 1967–68, are remarkable in many ways. Living on a diet consisting of 90 percent meat and fat from walrus, seal, whale, and fish, with the occasional sea bird or egg, they remain robust and vital well into their seventies and eighties, sometimes attaining ages up to 104. In fact, a male is considered still among the "young people" until at least age 45, at which time, if he hasn't yet married, he is expected to settle down to family life. During the long daylight of late spring, it was not uncommon for me to see men in their mid-eighties setting off for a day's walk of up to 20 miles across the tundra.

Okinawa, an island south of Japan, has become the modern-day Shangri-La. Made famous by the landmark book *The Okinawa Program* (Willcox, Willcox, and Suzuki 2001), Okinawans have the world's longest life expectancy and health span. Among their many characteristics, they maintain considerably higher levels of DHEA, testosterone, estrogen, and other hormones in their later years than do their American counterparts.

An American example of natural longevity achieved was Paul Bragg, the father of the American health foods movement. He was active well into his nineties, when he died during a surfing accident in Hawaii. Another is Bill Haast, founder and director of the Miami Serpentarium. Well into his nineties, Bill remains actively engaged in his work with poisonous reptiles, handling cobras and other venomous snakes daily for the purpose of extracting venom for the antivenom drug and research market. Bill Galt is founder of the Good Earth Restaurants and Peace Leaders International, the latter a group of businessmen volunteers who teach leadership and negotiating skills. At 73, Galt bicycled for a month in northern Europe, supervised the construction of a new home in a remote area along the Sea of Cortez in Baja California, Mexico, attended several intensive yoga retreats, and carried on an active consulting business.

How do they do it? Though from different parts of the world and from varying backgrounds, each of these individuals or groups has one thing in common: their vital energy remained strong throughout their life. The balance between genetics and environment works in them to maintain homeostasis and promote health and longevity. In addition, their lifestyle and diet, behavior and psycho-spiritual outlook, along with lifelong daily habits such as walking, support the state of equilibrium in which longevity is possible.

Their bodies are in balance with their environment; their lifestyle and diet support positive genetic expression and minimize negative genetic expression; and they are free of all of the late-onset degenerative diseases and cancer. In addition, they have a refined outlook on life that includes psychological and spiritual means of maintaining mental and emotional equilibrium. In effect, their homeostasis is perfectly functioning.

Homeostasis is the overall equilibrium your body maintains between its internal envi-

Due to improper diet and inadequate nutrition, lack of overall fitness, environmental stresses including xenobiotic and toxic chemical substances, and the effects of psychological stress on key neuroendocrine functions, our genetic architecture is weakened and negative gene expression occurs. This in turn triggers the effects of the ten modifiable aging factors.

ronment and the external environment in order to survive, remain disease free, and produce offspring. It may not determine our life span, but it is the central mechanism that keeps us healthy and prevents senescence as we age.

As we've discussed, health and longevity should be natural to our life. Due to improper diet and inadequate nutrition, lack of overall fitness, environmental stresses including xenobiotic and toxic chemical substances, and the effects of psychological stress on key neuroendocrine functions, our genetic architecture is weakened and negative gene expression occurs. This in turn triggers the effects of the ten modifiable aging factors. The end result of this chain of events is disruption of homeosta-

sis; we are unable to function normally and we age. Eventually, the insidious erosion of aging leads us towards what we are taught is inevitable senescence—except we now know that this is reversible.

Five functional systems or biological mechanisms in the body maintain homeostasis. Each must be in top form for you to prolong health and attain longevity. The process of prolonging health begins when you reverse the ten modifiable aging factors and restore homeostasis. You can do this through addressing the *Prolonging Health* recommendations found in this next section.

Five Biological Mechanisms That Maintain Homeostasis

1. Biological clock
2. Neuroendocrine system
3. Renal system (kidneys and electrolytes)
4. Metabolism
5. Cardiovascular system

Prolonging Health Recommendation 59— Reset Your Biological Clock

The eminent biopsychologist John Gibbon, Ph.D., calls the body's biological clock the "primordial context." This is the inescapable underlying process that influences all organisms, in all eras, of all life on Earth (Wright 2002). Our cells ebb and flow in the fluid matrix of our body, much like the changing tides of the sea; they are regulated by biological pacemakers set to a master "clock" in our brain, which, in turn, is synchronized with the celestial rhythms, the passage of time, light and dark cycles, and the changing seasons.

Researchers are finding that in different genes specific proteins influence the workings of our biological clock. These include melanopsin, a pigment found in the eye that is thought to communicate light sensations to the brain, which sets our internal clock to light and dark cycles (Berson 2002). While scientists figure out the mechanism of mitotic cell division, telomeres, and cellular senescence, we can meanwhile begin to prolong our health by following a lifestyle in accord with our biological clock.

The neuroendocrine system plays an important role in maintaining the body's internal connections between the biological "time-pieces" in our cells and brain. It is therefore integral to homeostasis. The hypothalamus in the brain plays a role in regulating our internal clock and hormone production in the body. The clinical focus of most anti-aging doctors is on hormone replacement therapy. But before we can safely and effectively replace declining hormone levels, we have to restore the integrity of the entire neuroendocrine *system*. We do this through diet, exercise, the use of adaptogenic herbs such as ginseng, and with melatonin (see chapter 14).

Take these steps to reset your biological clock:

- Take 0.5–3.0 mg of melatonin nightly before bed.

- Get regular, deep sleep.

- Replace deficient estrogen, testosterone, DHEA, pregnenolone, and growth hormone.

Your body clock is functioning well if you fall asleep easily and stay asleep through the night for at least six to seven hours without waking. Other signs of a well-functioning biological clock are getting sleepy in the evening when darkness falls; waking gently with the ris-ing sun (not having to always use an alarm clock to wake you); not having to take long naps during the day; having regular daily bowel movements; and having a normal appetite.

Prolonging Health Recommendation 60— Rehydrate to Improve Your Kidneys

The body's renal system, composed of the two kidneys and utilizing numerous hormones, is responsible for maintaining the fluid and electrolyte balance in the body, without which we couldn't remain alive. From the view of traditional Chinese medicine the kidneys are the organs most responsible for longevity. Homeostasis is dependent on healthy kidneys and a well-functioning renal system.

Water is necessary for life. The human body requires adequate hydration regularly throughout the day, every day of your life, to function properly. Images of the Fountain of Youth and miraculous waters have a universal association with longevity, and for good reason. During aging, tissue hydration is impaired because of reduced kidney function, hormonal imbalances, improper uptake of water by the cells, and other reasons. Hydration or water intake is important for maintaining protein structure and the conformation of nucleic acids such as DNA. Thus keeping your body well hydrated is an important longevity factor.

The recommendation of drinking six to eight 8-ounce glasses of pure water each day is a good start. However, when you are ill, exercising vigorously, exposed to higher temperatures, and/or aging, your need for water increases. Therefore, with six to eight glasses of pure water each day as a starting point, increase by one glass for each additional hour of exercise, and by another one or two glasses if the weather is hot, you are sweating heavily, or you are exercising in a heated room or using a sauna. This brings the total up to 12–14 glasses of water daily. Herbal teas, soups, juices, coffee, some carbonated drinks, and the fluid contained in foods help to hydrate the tissues but should not be considered a replacement for pure water or part of the intake count.

Unfortunately, older people tend to be less active and experience reduced thirst so they drink less than the recommended minimum of six to eight glasses of water daily. In addition, due to bladder weakness, when they increase their water intake, there is a tendency to urinate more, especially at night. The inconvenience of frequent urination makes them drink less water and leads to a cycle of reduced water intake and dehydration.

For my older patients who are chronically dehydrated, I recommend molecularly altered water. This is purified water with extra oxygen in a form engineered to make it more efficiently utilized by tissues. This provides hydration advantages that even pure spring water does not have. By using altered water, you can drink less and prevent dehydration. One such water is Penta, manufactured by Bio-hydration Research Lab[58] in San Diego, California, by a patented process that changes the molecular shape of water into clusters that have thinner connections between water molecules. This alteration substantially increases the water absorption of your cells.

Don't drink water from the tap. It often contains organic and inorganic contaminants and is unfit to use in your *Prolonging Health* program (Leviton 2001). Use pure spring or filtered water instead. Do not drink distilled water, except if during a detoxification regimen, as it contains no minerals.

Here's a simple feedback mechanism to help you know how your hydration is going. Look at your morning urine. During the night, your kidneys filter your blood by removing impurities and placing them in the urine for excretion. Morning urine is therefore more concentrated with substances. It should be slightly yellow, but not very dark yellow or brown, and should not have a strong smell. During the day, your urine should be clear or have a faint yellow color. If your urine is too dark, you are not drinking enough water.

Here's another way to check to see if you're dehydrated. Pinch the skin on the back of your hand, just in front of your wrist. If it springs back, you're well hydrated. But if a ridge remains where you pinched up the skin or it slowly returns to normal, you are dehydrated. In this case, drink more water until when you do the pinch test your skin springs back quickly.

Prolonging Health Recommendation 61— Replenish Electrolytes

As you age, not only is your ability to absorb water lessened, but your ability to absorb the trace minerals contained in water and food is also reduced. Electrolytes are minerals in the bloodstream that help maintain homeostasis and promote normal cell function.

The cells' utilization of macrominerals (calcium, magnesium, and phosphorus) and trace minerals (zinc, selenium, and boron) is likely reduced. Minerals are important in maintaining bone formation and structure, muscle contractility, immune function, acid-alkaline balance, and many other functions in the body. Partly because of this, bone mineral density is reduced and osteoporosis becomes common in elderly women, but it can also occur in men (Fatagyerji 1999).

Osteoarthritis, a disease characterized by inflammation and joint pain (in advanced stages it causes calcium deposits around the joints), is one of the most common complaints of the elderly; it is also influenced by mineral metabolism. Other age-related conditions affected by unbalanced minerals include heart disease and immune function.

Many trace minerals play key roles as cofactors (coenzymes) in important enzyme reactions; they serve as antioxidants and help regulate glucose and hormones. Not only is it critical to make sure your mineral levels are adequate, but it is also important to maintain a balance between them, as with calcium to magnesium, and sodium to potassium. Without a proper balance, the cells cannot function properly and degenerative diseases gradually develop.

Over time, some minerals can accumulate to toxic levels. Iron, an essential component of hemoglobin, which carries oxygen in the blood, is the best known of these. However, it readily reacts with oxygen to generate free radicals. Since humans cannot easily excrete iron, its absorption in the gut is tightly regulated and under control by three known genes. Mutations in any of these genes can lead to excessive iron absorption in which iron overload (hemochromatosis) may cause organ damage, particularly to the liver (Kaplan 2000).

Mineral metabolism can be improved through diet, supplementing macrominerals such as calcium and trace minerals; exercise, hormone balancing, and adequately hydrating your body with sufficient quantities of water. Many pharmaceutical drugs deplete minerals, so have your pharmacist review any medications you are taking to see if they cause significant mineral loss or vitamin depletion. Avoid supplementation with iron unless you have testing done by your doctor for iron deficiency anemia or other conditions caused by low iron levels.

Tea and other natural dietary substances help to control iron levels in your body. I don't advocate the regular use of electrolyte-enhanced water. It's fine for after sports events, but chronic use may skew the electrolyte profile. It's better to get minerals from the diet and supplement to necessary dosages on an individual basis.

Prolonging Health Recommendation 62— Reenergize Your Metabolism

As we age, we gradually lose the ability to produce and utilize energy. Advanced age is associated with loss of energy, which is characterized by lack of vitality, increased fatigue, muscle weakness, and frailty. However, other conditions also exhibit these traits to a greater or lesser degree, such as after long periods of inactivity, chronic infections and during certain stages of acute infections, blood loss such as after surgery or childbirth, anemia, during long periods of fasting or from chronic malnutrition, and when recovering from a severe illness. In all of these cases, the predominant characteristic is decreased energy. But what is decreased? For that matter, what is energy?

The physical energy of the body is produced through the metabolism of foods. It is manifested in the body when glucose is utilized. In the human body, energy is created as a result of glucose and oxygen metabolism; though created through metabolism, energy is generated in the mitochondria of the cells. Called the power plants of the cell, and therefore of the whole body, the mitochondria transform oxygen and nutrients, such as glucose, into energy and produce water and carbon dioxide as by-products.

A number of enzymes and coenzymes, such as CoQ10, are required to complete the process; the energy created is stored in a molecule called adenosine triphosphate (ATP). This process, called the citric acid or Krebs cycle, allows us to function, work, and carry out all physical activities related to living. Disruption of this process causes fatigue, and eventually manifests in aging.

Normal metabolism requires a healthy diet, sufficient enzymes, adequate trace minerals, a well-functioning neuroendocrine system, healthy liver function, adequate hydration, effective oxygenation, active cellular function, and positive genetic expression. Enhanced metabolic func-

As you age, your body also loses its ability to store water in the tissues. Along with reduced protein synthesis, which produces collagen and elastin, this contributes to the drying and wrinkling of your skin. Dehydration is very common in older people, so to prolong health and age well, the first step to improving your organ reserve is to get enough water.

tion requires regular strenuous physical exercise and deep breathing practices, such as pranayama or qi gong. In order to prolong your health and achieve your maximum life span, it is necessary to reenergize your metabolism so it becomes highly efficient with the right balance of nutrients and from a minimum of food.

If you tire easily, are fatigued without physical exertion, have a poor appetite, feel tired in the morning upon waking, and find it hard to gain or lose weight, your metabolism is underfunctioning. To reenergize your metabolism, follow the dietary and exercise recommendations presented later in this chapter.

Prolonging Health Recommendation 63— Rebuild Organ Reserve

One of the hallmarks of aging is a gradual decline in the ability of your vital organs, the heart, liver, and kidneys, to respond to the

demands of living, such as defending you against infections, managing inflammation, and handling stress. This age-related diminishment of organ function is referred to as a loss of organ reserve. It is caused by protein damage and therefore by reduced size and function of tissues such as muscles and organs, largely composed of proteins. The mechanisms that cause this damage are oxidation, glycation, methylation, inflammation, DNA mutations, and abnormal cellular metabolism (all modifiable aging factors and previously discussed), as well as poor hydration.

As you age, your body also loses its ability to store water in the tissues. Along with reduced protein synthesis, which produces collagen and elastin, this contributes to the drying and wrinkling of your skin. Dehydration is very common in older people, so to prolong health and age well, the first step to improving your organ reserve is to get enough water.

If you are chronically underweight, are gradually losing weight, and have lost muscle mass, most likely you have poor organ reserve. If you have an advanced case of any of the age-related conditions associated with the modifiable aging factors, such as cardiovascular disease, Type II diabetes, or hypothyroidism, you may also have low organ reserve.

As a general principle, you rebuild your organ reserve through following the *Prolonging Health* recommendations. These serve as guidelines to promote protein, fluid, electrolyte, vitamin and mineral, and neuroendocrine balance.

If your weight is normalizing, your energy is increasing, you have more muscle and greater strength, and have reversed all the disease conditions associated with aging, you are effectively rebuilding your organ reserve.

Prolonging Health Recommendation 64— Neutralize Stress

If you want to be healthy and live a long life, you have to learn to reduce the effects of stress on your body. Note I did not say "no stress," as that is impossible in life. All the examples of long-lived individuals that I've mentioned in this book are people like you and me, who have had their share of serious stress. It's just that for them stress did not overwhelm their body systems, and they were able to return to balance after the stressful events with their homeostasis intact.

Our bodies are made to cope with some stress, and function better with the right amount of stress. However, overwhelming stress or insidious stress that goes on for years disrupts our neuroendocrine system and accelerates aging. There are many different stress-reduction therapies including meditation, but our body's natural way to neutralize stress is through sleep and rest cycles. Sometimes, actively attempting to achieve stress reduction is more stressful. To neutralize stress, get enough sleep and rest.

Rest and repose are different from sleep and they are mandatory for a healthy life-style. This includes adequate rest between repetitions of weight lifting or stretching, as well as during the day or evening (after dinner) when the body is allowed to relax and unwind. When possible, an afternoon siesta will help to calm your nerves and recharge your mind and body to finish the rest of your day in a better mood and with more energy for the evening with your family. Studies have shown that a 15–20 minute siesta refreshes the mind and body but longer than that disrupts sleep.

Repose is relaxing and includes vacation time away from work schedules and routines; it includes social time with friends, walks on the beach or in the woods, gardening, visits to art museums, and listening to good music, among many possibilities. Traditional religions set aside one day each week for rest and worship–a custom to which we should perhaps consider returning. Meditation provides deep rest and is highly recommended for people suffering from any chronic disease, viral illness, or mood disorder.

Sleep is important in order to feel recharged in the morning, and it also promotes proper body functioning, helps maintain organ reserve, relaxes the mind, and restores the spirit. Importantly, it also enhances and regulates the immune system, aids in the recovery from illness, and helps in the prevention of disease. Humans, like all animals, require a restorative sleep cycle each day, and without adequate sleep you will find it difficult to recover from illness and to live longer.

Numerous scientific studies support the profound effect that sleep has on our well-being. Studies have shown that disrupted sleep, an increasingly common condition among modern urban people, decreases levels of natural killer cells. Lack of sleep causes extra-susceptibility to infections such as colds and influenza. Stress, lack of rest between periods of work or activity, and disruption of regular deep sleep make us more vulnerable to infections. Long sound sleep, even in the daytime, is one of the best remedies for the flu. J. Allan Hobson, Ph.D., a professor of sleep science at Harvard University, contends that the universal exhortation of mothers to their children to "get a good night's sleep" may be one of the best natural remedies available to ward off infections.

Scientists link deep sleep with hormone production. For example, growth hormone is mainly released at night, and deep sleep promotes more growth hormone production. Eve Van Cauter, Ph.D., researches sleep at Northwestern University in Chicago (Van Cauter 2000). She says that poor sleep adversely affects glucose metabolism and growth hormone production. People who are stressed produce too much cortisol at night, which is just the time when it's supposed to be low in the body. Too much cortisol disrupts sleep and causes abnormal glucose levels at night.

In the elderly, sleep tends to be shallow and interrupted and, because of this, they are fatigued and less alert during the daytime and so have to take a nap. This makes it so they can't sleep at night. They tend to go to bed earlier and then wake up in the middle of the night. When they wake up and turn on the lights, their melatonin secretion is suppressed and low levels of melatonin make it difficult to fall back to sleep. So, in order to prolong your health, it is essential that you promote natural sleep.

The need for sleep in a healthy person ranges from six to ten hours each night, the average being eight hours. When one is ill, or when the immune system is fighting off an infection, the sleep requirement moves towards the higher end. Get nine to ten hours of good sleep each night, and up to 12 hours if you have an active infection. However, to prolong your health and achieve maximum longevity, you need *moderate* and *regular* amounts of deep sleep. Though everyone's rhythms are different, try to go to bed before 10 P.M. and get an average of eight hours of uninterrupted sleep each night. Many people do well on six to seven hours. Find your own optimal sleep time, but no matter how many hours that is, it is important to sleep deeply.

Too much sleep can be just as bad as not enough. Daniel F. Kripke, M.D., a professor of psychiatry at the University of California at San Diego, studied the sleep habits of 1.1 million people ranging in age from 30 to 102 (Kripke 2002). The results of his study suggest that life span can be reduced by sleeping too much (Kripke 2003). According to Dr. Kripke, the risk of death increases by 34 percent in those who sleep ten hours as compared with those who sleep seven to eight hours. The risk of an early death also increases for those who sleep too little, but not as much as for those who sleep too much.

Here are some suggestions to help you sleep:

- Follow a regular schedule: Go to sleep and get up at the same time. Try not to nap for longer than 15–20 minutes during the day, and don't make a routine of napping every day.

- Get vigorous exercise at regular times each day.

- Get at least two hours of natural light in the morning and afternoon each day.

- Don't drink beverages with caffeine late in the day, or at all, if you are sensitive to caffeine.

- Keep your blood sugar levels from falling too low during the night by eating a snack before bed. Try a cup of warm chamomile or other herb tea with honey.

- Don't drink alcohol to help you sleep. You may fall asleep more easily after drinking, but it also makes you wake up after a few hours.

- Create a safe and comfortable place to sleep. Make sure there are locks on all doors and smoke alarms on each floor. Keep the temperature evenly regulated, not too hot or cold.

- The sleeping room should be dark, well ventilated, and as quiet as possible. The darker your room, the more melatonin you'll produce.

- Develop a relaxing bedtime routine. Do the same things each night to tell your body that it's time to wind down. Some people watch the evening news, read a book, or soak in a warm bath.

- Take melatonin (0.5–3 mg) regularly. Make sure you take it before sleeping but just after turning out the lights.

- Try valerian root (200–600 mg of the extract containing 0.2–0.8 percent or higher concentration of valerenic acid) or kava-kava (150–500 mg of the extract containing 30 percent kava lactones). Take these an hour before bed.

If you have chronic sleep problems that aren't helped by these natural means, see your doctor or a sleep specialist for a sleeping medication.

Longevity Strategy II—Eat for Longevity

As we age, regularity appears to make the body more efficient. When we eat is no exception to this. A good starting point is three regular meals each day, except when fasting or on a hypoglycemic diet (which recommends four equal meals), composed of a variety of fresh vegetables, meats, fish, and poultry, seasonal fresh ripe fruits, an assortment of seeds and nuts, and the inclusion of garden spices and herbs. Eat a variety of different foods; don't eat the same food more than two times per week. All food should be organically raised, whenever possible.

Eating a natural diet does not come easily. It requires a new understanding of how important foods are to your health and the need to eliminate certain unhealthy food choices or habits. It is not the purpose of this book to go into diets in detail; rather, I want to point out the importance of a healthy diet that can prolong health. Let's take a look at some dietary recommendations that will help you prevent disease, prolong your health, and foster longevity.

Prolonging Health Recipes

The following recipes are from the kitchen of Chef Everett Williams.[59] The style is a healthy fusion of Asian, French, and American cuisines. These recipes will give you an idea of how to work with the *Prolonging Health* dietary guidelines. Use organic, free-range meats and organically grown fruits and vegetables whenever possible. These are high protein, low carbohydrate, and high in nutrient-dense foods. Enjoy.

Coconut Bouillabaisse

This is a seafood soup in a light coconut broth with a hint of lemon grass; serves four.

Ingredients:
4 ounces fresh halibut
4 ounces fresh Ahi tuna or salmon
8 large shrimp
8 large sea scallops
1 cup coconut milk
3 cups chicken broth
1 stalk lemon grass
1 stalk celery
1 cup snow peas
1 medium carrot
1 tablespoon of fresh ginger
1 tablespoon of fresh garlic
1 medium onion
1/4 cup fresh cilantro
olive oil
sesame oil

Clean and dice the fish. Trim the scallops and remove the shell from the shrimp, but leave the tail on.

Wash and cut the vegetables, cutting the celery and carrots diagonally. Chop the garlic and ginger finely.

Heat a wok or large saucepan on high heat. Add 4 tablespoons of olive oil and bring just to the smoking point. Add the fish, searing on all four sides. Add the vegetables. When they are 3/4 cooked, add the ginger and garlic.

Sauté one minute more; add the chicken broth, then the coconut milk.

Bring to a boil, and add the shrimp and scallops. Add the lemon grass.

Simmer until fully cooked. Serve and top with fresh cilantro and drizzle sesame oil on top of each bowl.

Salt and pepper to individual taste; or add a small amount of soy sauce or lemon or lime juice.

Total protein per person = 25 g

Grilled Chicken Breast Caesar Salad

This is a healthy salad that makes a complete meal; serves 4.

Ingredients:
Four 4-ounce organic free-range chicken breasts
1 head romaine lettuce
6 cloves of fresh garlic
1 whole organic egg
1 small can of anchovies
1 organic lemon
1/4 cup cold-pressed virgin olive oil
fresh thyme and rosemary
salt and pepper
Parmesan cheese

Clean the chicken breasts; remove the skin and fat; wash in cold water.

Peel and dice 2 garlic cloves. Finely chop the thyme, rosemary, and garlic, then place in a mixing bowl.

Roll the chicken breasts in the herbs; add 1 tablespoon of olive oil and a pinch of salt and pepper; set them aside.

Clean and wash the romaine lettuce; let it drain in a colander.

Put the remaining 4 cloves of garlic, 1/4 cup of olive oil, 1 whole egg, and 1/2 can of anchovies in a blender. Blend at high speed until creamy. This is your Caesar dressing.

Grill the chicken breasts and set aside to cool.

Arrange whole leaves of lettuce on plates.

Cut the chicken breasts on the diagonal into 4–6 slices each, and place alongside the lettuce.

Drizzle the Caesar dressing over the top. Squeeze fresh lemon juice over the lettuce and chicken. Garnish with parmesan cheese and the remaining whole anchovies.

Total protein per person = 28 g

Healthy Vegetarian Stir Fry

This traditional stir fry uses organic vegetables and tofu over brown rice; serves 4.

Ingredients:
1 pound of organic firm tofu
1 large organic carrot
2 stalks of organic celery
1 organic red bell pepper
1/2 pound of snow peas
1/4 pound of bean sprouts
1 large red onion
4 garlic cloves
1 tablespoon of chopped ginger
olive oil, soy sauce, sesame oil
2 cups of brown rice
regular or black sesame seeds

Wash the tofu and cut into small squares; let drain for several minutes.

Mix the tofu in 1/4 cup of soy sauce and 2 tablespoons of sesame oil in a bowl; marinate for 30 minutes.

Cook the brown rice.

Preheat oven to 450° F

Wash and slice the carrots and celery diagonally. Wash and dice the red pepper. Wash and clean the snow peas, bean sprouts, and cilantro. Peel the onion; slice it into small slivers.

Drain the tofu and place it on an oiled baking sheet. Bake until lightly brown on all four sides.

Turn the tofu every 10 minutes to achieve even browning. When cooked, set the tofu aside.

Heat a wok or large sauté pan on high heat; add 1 tablespoon of olive oil.

Add all the vegetables except the bean sprouts.

Sauté until the onion is translucent. Add the garlic and ginger. Sauté two more minutes; then add the bean sprouts. Add soy sauce and finish cooking for a few more minutes; then remove from the stove and set aside.

Place 1/4 cup of brown rice on each plate and cover with the sautéed vegetables. Put the tofu squares on top of the vegetables. Garnish with a few sprigs of cilantro, and finish by drizzling 1 teaspoon of sesame oil over the top of each dish. Sprinkle with sesame seeds.

Total protein per person = 20 g

New York Steak Entrée

This all-American dish is made with organic, free-range beef and fresh, organically raised vegetables. It's high in protein and low in carbohydrates; serves 4.

Ingredients:

Two 6–8 ounce organically raised "New York" steaks
1 large spaghetti squash
1 pound of baby carrots
1 pound of oyster or other available fresh mushrooms
fresh thyme, rosemary, and parsley
nutmeg
olive oil
salt and pepper

Preheat oven to 450° F

Cut the spaghetti squash in half. Remove the seeds. Rub the inside of the squash with olive oil, and salt and pepper.

Place the prepared squash on a baking sheet and bake for 45 minutes or until tender.

When the squash is tender, remove the flesh with a fork and season with olive oil, a pinch of salt, and a dash of nutmeg.

Lower the oven temperature to 425° F.

Wash and finely chop the herbs.

Heat a large sauté pan on high heat; brown the steaks on all sides.

Place the browned steaks in a pan with the herbs and lightly cover with olive oil; marinate for 30 minutes.

Place the marinated steaks on a baking sheet and cook in the oven at 425° F until rare, medium, or well done (as desired); let them stand for about 10 minutes.

Peel, wash, and then steam the carrots.

While the steaks are cooking, sauté the mushrooms in olive oil until slightly brown.

Slice the cooked steaks on the diagonal, allowing 3–4 ounces per person. Place 1/2 cup of the cooked squash in the center of the plate. Arrange the sliced meat on one side of the plate. Place the baby carrots on the other side. Garnish the meat with mushrooms. Finish with a few sprigs of fresh parsley in the center.

Total protein per person = 28 g

Prolonging Health Recommendation 65— Eliminate Sugar

You will have to eliminate foods that promote disease. The most destructive among these is refined sugar. It stimulates insulin release from the pancreas and is a contributing factor in hypoglycemia, insulin resistance, obesity, and diabetes. Refined sugar consumption is linked to osteoporosis, dental cavities, high blood pressure, and atherosclerosis, and increases triglyceride levels. If you want to prolong your health, stop using refined sugar. Instead, use a minimal amount of natural sugars from honey, fruit juices, and maple syrup. Eat whole fruits and a small amount of dried fruits such as dates or figs.

Prolonging Health Recommendation 66— Eat Foods with Vitality

Foods should be alive and full of energy. Years ago, I learned much about the natural diet from my mentors, notably Dr. Bernard Jensen, who taught that food is our best medicine. One of his most important lessons was that when food is served it should retain its vital energy, or life force—called *prana* in yogic philosophy and *qi* by the Chinese. Look at the color of a food after cooking. If it retains its natural color (vegetables are bright and vibrant), its vital energy is still present.

The maxim is: if vitality is present in the foods, health will follow in the body. The Chinese are experts at this and traditionally eat only freshly picked vegetables; even when fish is eaten, the fish is alive and still flopping before it is prepared for cooking.

In your diet, food sources are critical. Carbohydrates should be unrefined, high-fiber, with a low glycemic index; proteins should be principally from vegetable sources, such as seeds, nuts, and legumes, but organically raised lean meats and poultry as well as fish and shellfish are allowed. Fats should be unsaturated oils, rich in omega-3 oils, as from flaxseed and fish. Eat plenty of vegetables. They are a source of natural fiber; vegetables and meat are the most nutrient-dense foods. Four to six servings of fresh vegetables a day is a minimum, prepared as vegetable soups, salads, raw fresh juices, or steamed, baked, or sautéd. Frozen and canned vegetables don't count as fresh.

Growing your own vegetables or getting them direct from a farm is even better than buying them in a grocery store.

Prolonging Health Recommendation 67— Emphasize Alkaline Foods

Eat more alkaline foods than acid-forming foods. Our body works better when it is slightly alkaline, while too much acid makes us more prone to infections and promotes accelerated aging. Acid-forming foods include red meat, sugar, wheat products such as breads and pasta, coffee, and vinegar. Alkaline foods are fish and chicken, honey, rice and corn, herbal teas, and most vegetables.

Ripe fruits are alkaline forming, but citrus can be too acidic for some. Don't overconsume orange juice and citrus fruits. Apples, pears, peaches, and plums are healthy alkaline fruits. Eating low-acid and more alkaline foods gives you more energy, helps prevent disease, and can foster longevity.

Prolonging Health Recommendation 68— Get Enough Protein

Dietary protein is necessary to build muscle, maintain organ reserve, and repair tissues. On average, our body absorbs 70–90 percent of protein from plant sources and 80–100 percent from animal protein sources. These percentages suggest that animal proteins are better than plant proteins; however, both sources are good and should be combined to make up a balanced protein requirement. I recommend eating protein from animal and plant sources at each meal.

We can absorb about 25 grams of protein at a time. Therefore, divide your daily protein intake so that you are eating protein foods in the morning for breakfast and lunch. Eat fewer protein foods for dinner, as they can be too stimulating and may keep you from falling asleep. Eating a light evening meal promotes deep sleep. However, your body needs proteins while you're asleep to carry out repair processes. To facilitate protein repair, you could take a protein supplement between seven and nine P.M. (see chapter 11).

On average, I recommend 65–85 grams of protein daily for men and women. These should be derived from a variety of animal and plant sources. However, to build muscle and repair damaged tissue, your body requires more protein, as much as 125 grams or more per day. The *Prolonging Health* program advises you to build and maintain muscle and to repair degraded proteins; therefore, for optimal success you need 85–125 grams of protein each day. In order to utilize this much protein, you have to exercise regularly.

To get this much protein each day, eating 25 grams of protein per meal (three to four ounces of fish, meat, or poultry contains about 24 grams), you have to have at least two high-protein snacks (a protein supplement or a handful of seeds or nuts). Try to get at least 80 percent of your protein needs from dietary sources; then supplement the remaining 20 percent with whey protein. Many Westerners are allergic to soy, so I do not recommend commercial soy protein products. Also, soy protein does not absorb well in the gastrointestinal tract; as you get older, it becomes important to consume protein that has 100 percent absorption. Traditional soy products such as tofu or miso, however, are well absorbed and make healthy additions to meals.

Consume enough protein, but don't overeat protein foods or take too much protein supplement at a time. To improve protein digestion, take a digestive enzyme that contains hydrochloric acid at the same time as your protein meal or snack.

Protein-Rich Foods
Animal Sources:

- Lean meat and poultry, 3 oz = 24–28 g
- Fish and shellfish, 3 oz = 18–22 g
- Milk, 1 cup = 8 g
- Yogurt, 1 cup = 9–10 g
- Cheese, 1 oz = 7 g
- Cottage cheese, 3/4 cup = 24 g
- Eggs, 1 whole or 2 egg whites = 7 g

Vegetarian Sources:

- Almonds, 1 cup = 26 g
- Lentils and dry beans, 1 cup = 15 g
- Vegetables, 1 cup = 3–4 g
- Grains:
  - Bread, 1 slice = 3 g
  - Rice, 1 cup = 5 g
  - Bagel, 1 medium = 8 g
- Soy foods:
  - Firm tofu, 4 oz (1/2 cup) = 10 g
  - Regular tofu, 4 oz = 5 g
  - Tempeh, 4 oz = 24 g

Prolonging Health Recommendation 69— Eat Nutrient-Dense Plant Foods

Your body utilizes the nutrients contained in whole fresh foods better than those found in nutritional supplements. Therefore, don't rely exclusively on nutritional supplements. They are meant to supplement your diet, not to replace food. Make sure you include an abundance of nutrient-dense plant foods (phytonutrients) in your diet. Many of these can be juiced, making them more concentrated and better for you. I recommend one to two glasses of fresh juice a week, or more if you have the time to juice. However, don't overuse juices to the exclusion of consuming whole foods.

Nutrient-dense plant foods include the cabbage family (cruciferous vegetables including green and purple cabbage, broccoli, Brussels sprouts, cauliflower, collards, and kale); soybeans (tofu, tamari, soy sauce, tempeh, green soybeans in the pod, and soybean sprouts); carotene-containing foods (carrots, yellow and orange squash, and cantaloupe); quercetin-containing foods (apples, onions); lycopene-containing tomatoes; and chlorophyll-containing foods (alfalfa, chlorella, spirulina, wheat grass, and all green leafy vegetables). Nutrient-dense plant foods tend to be alkaline. Include more of these foods in your daily diet.

Prolonging Health Recommendation 70— Include Longevity Dietary Nutrients from Foods and Herbs

Certain foods have more longevity benefits than others. Henry Mallek, Ph.D., author of *The New Longevity Diet,* calls these foods "long-lost factors in the anti-aging equation." Though eating a well-balanced, healthy diet promotes wellness and prevents disease, and nutrient-dense foods prolong health, longevity foods have the potential to extend your life span. These foods contain nutritional factors beyond vitamins and minerals. They include conjugated linoleic acid, flavonoids, isothiocyanates, lignans, monoterpenes, nucleotides, phytates, phytosterols, protease inhibitors, saponins, organosulfur compounds, and tannins. Many of these substances are found in foods and herbal teas. Be sure to include several of them in your weekly diet.

Conjugated linoleic acid: An essential fatty acid, conjugated linoleic acid is found in milk, beef, and lamb. It helps to regulate cell division and growth, promotes normal body

composition, enhances immunity, and prevents cancer. If you are not allergic to milk products, eat some organic yogurt several times a week; if you are not vegetarian, eat organically raised beef and lamb once or twice a week.

Flavonoids: There are more than 4,000 known flavonoids. These substances are concentrated in the seeds, flowers, bark, peel, or skin of plants. The flavonoid family includes citrus bioflavonoids, rutin, quercetin, and polyphenols. They fight infections from bacteria and viruses, reduce inflammation, have antioxidant activity, prevent blood clots, and promote the body's natural detoxification processes. Flavonoids are found in green tea, citrus, apples, onions, grapes, and red wine.

Isothiocyanates: These substances are mainly found in cruciferous vegetables, but also occur in turnips, kohlrabi, rutabaga, Chinese cabbage, bok choy, horseradish, radish, and watercress. Isothiocyanates have been shown to be especially effective in fighting lung and esophageal cancers, and they can lower the risk of gastrointestinal and respiratory tract cancers. Consuming isothiocyanate-rich vegetables can reduce cancer by preventing cancer cells from being activated, counteracting the toxic effects of carcinogens that have been activated, and speeding up the removal of cancerous cells and their toxic by-products from the body.

Lignans: These are female hormone–like substances that include enterolactone and enterodiol and which balance estrogen in the body. Including lignans in the diet of men and women helps prevent cancer. They are found in large amounts in flaxseed and oil, but are also present in whole grains, nuts, berries, and other oil seeds such as sesame. Lignans are found in herbs such as the traditional Chinese medicine *Schisandra chinensis.* High-fiber diets provide more lignan than low-fiber ones. Take one to four tablespoons of ground flaxseed a day. Use one to two tablespoons of organic flax oil with your food three to four times a week. Eat a palmful of different raw seeds and nuts several times a week. Try seasoning your food with a teaspoon of sesame oil.

Monoterpenes: The two best known monoterpenes are D-limonene and perillyl alcohol. D-limonene is used as a cleaning agent, a pesticide, and a nutritional supplement. Monoterpenes control the spread of cancer, protect DNA, and promote positive genetic expression. They are found in the essential oils of many plants including caraway, dill, bergamot, peppermint, spearmint, lavender, cherries, and tomatoes; they are found in the rinds of lemons, oranges, and grapefruit.

To obtain monoterpenes, drink mint or spearmint tea, or add a few sprigs of fresh mint to a pitcher of pure water. Let it stand for 30 minutes or longer, chill in the refrigerator, and drink with your meals. Here's another way to get monoterpenes. Add a slice of lemon, lime, or orange to a glass of pure water; or grate organic lemon or orange rind to garnish side dishes.

Nucleotides: These are necessary for making and repairing DNA and RNA, and improve immune function (Yamauchi 2002). The importance of sufficient nucleotides in infant formulas in order to support growth and development, a process that requires 480 mg daily of nucleotides, is recognized. Nucleotides are equally important in adults, and to prevent aging we need upwards of 700 mg a day. They are found in nutritional yeast, meat, fish, poultry, plant shoots, sprouts, and baby corn. Many of these foods can be purchased in Asian markets and nutritional yeast is available in health food stores.

Phytates: These longevity nutrients protect the body from the harmful oxidative effects of iron, copper, and other minerals. They chemically bind them so they are unavailable for the body to absorb. Phytates boost natural killer cell activity to fight against viruses and cancer, and they have antioxidant properties. Associated with plant fiber, which reduces the risk of colon cancer, they reduce cholesterol and triglycerides.

Inositol hexaphosphate (IP6)[60] is a by-product of the metabolism of dietary phytates and is commercially prepared from rice bran. It helps to regulate cell function, is involved in intercellular communication, and has anti-cancer properties (Vucenik 1998). Dr. Shamsuddin, M.D., Ph.D., of the University of Maryland, discovered that IP6 taken together with inositol, a B vitamin, exerted anticancer properties (Grases 2002; Shamsuddin 1999).

The typical daily dose is 800–1,200 mg of IP6 with 200–300 mg of inositol. For cancer patients or those at high risk of cancer, Dr. Shamsuddin recommends doses in the range of 4,800–7,200 mg of IP6 along with 1,200–1,800 mg of inositol. For best results, take this nutraceutical on an empty stomach and away from other vitamins. As a cancer preventative, I recommend taking a two-week course of IP6 and inositol once or twice a year.

Phytates are found in corn, sesame and sunflower seeds, peanuts, wild rice, soybeans, split peas, and whole grains. Phytates have been called "anti-food" because in high dosages they can be toxic to the body. In small amounts they are beneficial to the body, but do not consume excessive amounts of these foods.

Phytosterols: These are a group of fat compounds closely related to cholesterol found in plants. They have anti-inflammatory properties, help to lower cholesterol in humans, and may have anticancer properties. The most active phytosterols, beta-sitosterol and beta-sitosterolin, are useful in the treatment of

Longevity Foods

Yogurt

Green tea

Apples

Grapes

Almonds

Figs

Dates

Red wine

Cruciferous vegetables

Watercress

Flaxseed and flaxseed oil

Nutritional yeast

Baby corn

Sprouts

Bamboo shoots

Rice bran syrup

Peaches

Plums

Soybeans

Garlic

Chocolate

autoimmune disorders such as rheumatoid arthritis. Dietary sources of phytosterols include spices, seeds and nuts, okra, whole grains, and cruciferous vegetables.

Moducare[61] is a nutraceutical formulation of phytosterols (20 mg of total plant sterols and 200 mg of sterolins); the typical dosage is two capsules, three times daily for one week, and then one capsule, three times per day thereafter. In severe cases of chronic inflammation, higher dosages (three to four capsules, three times daily) are required.

Protease Inhibitors: These protect DNA from damage and have anticancer properties. They are found in green leafy vegetables, fruits (principally peaches and plums), corn, soybeans, potatoes, and sweet potatoes. Eat more of these foods to prevent cancer and prolong your health.

Saponins: These substances are a natural plant detergent. Plants containing saponins form a creamy, soapy texture when mixed with water. The name comes from the Latin *sapo*

(soap) because of the detergent action that they exhibit. They are found in soybeans and other dried legumes such as pinto, kidney, black, and lima beans, and lentils. Ginseng, sarsaparilla, licorice, aloe, and other herbs contain high amounts of saponins. They have immune-enhancing properties, lower cholesterol, and have anticancer activity. Eat small amounts of the above foods and take saponin-containing herbs.

Organosulfur Compounds: Organosulfur compounds are found in plants belonging to the allium family, such as garlic, chives, leeks, shallots, scallions, and onions. They are distinguished by their strong odor and are reported to protect against stomach, colorectal, esophageal, colon, mammary gland, and lung cancers, though the exact mechanisms of their cancer-preventive effects are not clear. Organosulfur compounds appear to exert a modulating effect on several enzymes in the body that are involved in detoxifying carcinogens. Use these in cooking and salads, and add small amounts when you make fresh vegetable juice.

Tannins: Plant tannins are yellowish-white to brown-colored substances found in common foods and beverages. These include grapes, legumes, red wine, tea, coffee, and chocolate. Tannins have powerful antioxidant properties, are toxic to a wide range of microorganisms, and have anticancer activity. Include tannin-containing foods and beverages in small but regular amounts in your diet.

Longevity Strategy III—Practice Periodic Calorie Restriction

Animals that hibernate have a longer life span. Vegetables last longer when kept refrigerated and a frozen fish does not spoil. However, I prefer not to be frozen, kept on ice, submerged in cold water, or sleep all of the time in order to live longer. A balance between the absence of disease, vigorous quality of life, and maximum life span potential is what we strive for. One way to achieve that is by practicing calorie restriction.

To maintain homeostasis and to live long, it is not enough only to eat well and avoid foods with chemical residues. You must also know how to *not* eat. Calorie restriction, the only way to increase life span that has been proven by both scientists and yogis, is the voluntary restriction of food intake sufficient to lower total calorie consumption so that metabolism slows down. This is followed by a number of other physiological changes and stabilizes homeostasis. Calorie restriction has been shown to lengthen maximum life span in laboratory test subjects including yeast, fish, fruit flies, worms, mice, and monkeys.

Consider the research of Stephen R. Spindler, Ph.D., a professor of biochemistry at the University of California at Riverside and founder of Life Span Genetics, a company researching possible pharmaceutical interventions to reverse negative gene expression. Dr. Spindler strongly supports the theory that the rate of aging is influenced by diet. He contends that when you are well fed, you age faster and have a higher incidence of cardiovascular disease, cancer, and diabetes.

Tests with laboratory animals have proven, and Indian yogis and Chinese Taoists have demonstrated, that a diet with fewer calories lowers the incidence of all of the degenerative diseases associated with aging and extends life span. Dr. Spindler's studies, which used microanalysis of 11,000 genes in mice livers, suggest that calorie restriction for as short as four weeks reverses liver damage and reverses the negative genetic expression associated with the

aging phenotype (Spindler 1991, 2001). His studies suggest that calorie reversals can lower biological age and renew cells.

Roy Walford, M.D., a professor of pathology at the University of California at Los Angeles, is one of the pioneers of the life extension movement and considered the father of the caloric restriction. In his *Beyond the 120*

Tests with laboratory animals have proven, and Indian yogis and Chinese Taoists have demonstrated, that a diet with fewer calories lowers the incidence of all of the degenerative diseases associated with aging and extends life span. Studies suggest that calorie reversals can lower biological age and renew cells.

Year Diet, Dr. Walford systematically presents his case for lowering the amount of food you eat. He emphasizes that to be effective calorie restriction requires achieving maximum metabolic balance. This means that the energy you expend in work and activity has to be *less* than the energy generated by your cells. To generate energy, you must eat high nutrient density foods such as fruits and vegetables and get enough protein (Walford 2000).

Though Dr. Walford's experiments brought calorie restriction to the forefront of aging research during the 1970s, he was not the first to discover the diet and aging connection. As early as 1935, Clive McCay, M.D., of Cornell University in Ithaca, New York, experimented with calorie restriction. He raised rats from birth on a restricted feeding plan supplemented with vitamins and minerals. Dr.

McCay's experiment showed that the calorie-restricted animals had less disease, were more active, and lived twice as long as the laboratory rats fed on a standard diet. In human terms, that's equivalent to being more than 150 years old.

George S. Roth, Ph.D., and his colleagues at the National Institute on Aging are coming closer to unraveling the reason why calorie restriction works. In a number of studies using rodents and rhesus monkeys, Roth has shown that a 30–50 percent calorie restricted diet, supplemented with nutrients, significantly extends life span. He also postulates that there is no increase in life span without calorie restriction (Roth 2001, 2002). This is an extraordinary finding. It informs us that calorie restriction is the only known way of extending our life span. Antioxidants help reduce the shortening of life span due to disease, but they do not extend life span. But is reducing what we eat, and eliminating much of the tastier foods such as desserts, worth a few extra years?

It seems that calorie restriction not only extends life span, but has beneficial effects on many systems in the body. In one study performed by Julie A. Mattison, Ph.D., a colleague of Dr. Roth and a researcher at the University of Arizona in Tucson, calorie restriction improved 90 percent of 300 measured biomarkers in the tested animals. It also significantly reduced the number of tumors and other diseases associated with aging (Mattison 2002).

Additionally, a number of the biomarkers improved. Results demonstrated that the calorie-restricted animals were healthier; they also had normal glucose levels, improved insulin sensitivity, and improved secretion of important hormones such as melatonin (Mattison 2001).

Many researchers contend that results from studies in worms and insects, or even short-lived rodents, do not translate to humans, but Dr. Roth's work demonstrates that calorie restriction prolongs health and extends life in both rodent and primate models. Further substantiation of the calorie-restriction theory is offered by research that has demonstrated that it universally extends life span in a wide range of species from spiders to fish (Gerhard 2001). But people are not monkeys, spiders, or fish, so does calorie restriction benefit humans?

The work that has been done suggests lifelong calorie restriction also extends human life span. Studies show that Okinawans, whose diets have 40 percent fewer calories than the average American diet, live considerably longer. Are there any other examples or historical precedents to prove the claims of calorie restriction?

The answer is found in Eastern longevity practices with its history of several thousand years. Longevity practitioners in the East emphasized fasting and low-calorie vegetarian diets. People in India, China, Tibet, Nepal, and other Eastern countries continue such practices to this day. Such practices not only validate the modern premise of calorie restriction, but offer us insights into the experience of long-term food restriction and provide us invaluable practical advice on how to carry out a safe and effective calorie restriction program.

Proponents of calorie restriction would like us to believe that calorie-restricted animals jump around the cages with boundless energy and joy. This is not always the case. So before we discuss my recommendations, it is important to know a few facts about calorie restriction. First, calorie-restricted laboratory animals may live up to 40 percent longer, but when food is severely restricted in mice experiments, the animals become overly hungry and display agitated behavior, sometimes even trying to jump out of their cages.

Second, though calorie restriction extends

life span and reduces metabolism, the experimental animals produce less energy and are less active. They experience reduced fitness and their muscle mass declines. When they are required to be more active, as when researchers make them run on a treadmill, many of the benefits gained from calorie restriction are lost.

So, to prolong health effectively, we have to find an optimal *individualized balance* between getting enough food, the right quality of food, and the longevity benefits from eating less. In addition, we must retain muscle mass without overexercising and losing the benefits obtained from a calorie-restriction regimen.

Researchers have shown that though calorie-restricted laboratory animals live longer, levels of nearly all of the hormones involved in their metabolism go down, including thyroid, IGF-I, and growth hormone. Additionally, steroid hormone levels tend to decline in the calorie-restricted animals, though melatonin levels increase (Mattison 2001).

Paradoxically, with the exception of increased melatonin levels, these findings don't quite fit the current neuroendocrine theory of aging. The neuroendocrine theory contends that aging is related to declining levels of anabolic hormones (GH, IGF-I, estrogen, DHEA, testosterone) and increased levels of catabolic hormones (insulin, cortisol). In contrast, proponents of the calorie-restriction model contend that an extended life span is associated with decreased levels of anabolic hormones.

So how do we solve these problems and use the beneficial effects of calorie restriction to increase our life span? I suggest a sensible and effective solution is *periodic* calorie restriction alternated with *moderate* caloric intake of nutrient-dense and longevity foods, high protein, low carbohydrates, and moderate fat, along with careful use of hormones and nutritional supplements.

Effects of Calorie Restriction

- Lower incidence of diabetes, cancer, and cardiovascular disease
- Improved insulin sensitivity
- Improved liver function
- Improved neuroendocrine balance
- Improved pancreatic function
- Increased life span
- Lower blood sugar levels
- Reversal of aging gene expression

Prolonging Health Recommendation 71— Practice Periodic Caloric Restriction

The principle of caloric restriction advocated in this book is derived from Eastern longevity practices, Oriental and naturopathic medicine, my own clinical experience, and the research of scientists such as Drs. Wolford and Roth. For optimal results, the practice of caloric restriction should be consistent with the four goals of the *Prolonging Health* program. To enable us to achieve our maximum life span, a program must reduce our biological age, help us maintain the age-point, reverse premature aging, and improve our body composition and quality of life. Therefore, I advocate periodic caloric restriction and not a permanently restricted diet.

Periodic caloric restriction means eating a low-calorie diet for one to four weeks, and alternating this with a normal- to moderate-calorie diet. A moderate-calorie diet is in the range of 1,500 calories daily. This is approximately 30–50 percent of that of the average American diet, and about the number of calories consumed by Okinawans. For periodic caloric restriction, reduce your total calorie intake further. Consume about 1,200–1,400 calories each day. You can go as low as 800 calories for three to nine days if you are a small person in good health or a person of average weight.

Eat the same types of nutrient-dense and longevity foods I've recommended, only in smaller amounts. You can practice calorie restriction as part of a detoxification program, or on its own. I suggest that you do this for at least one to four weeks every three to four months.

On the alternate months, eat a diet moderate in calories. However, if you are exercising heavily, you need more calories. During periods of weight training for muscle gain or increased strength, increase your protein intake as well as overall calories. For these purposes, you may need to increase your total daily calories to 2,400–3,000. However, for maintenance return to the moderate calorie diet of 1,500–2,000 calories.

Some people feel very good on a calorie-restricted diet and choose to stay on this regimen for longer than the recommended time. However, remember to be careful not to lose muscle when practicing caloric restriction. It is best not to go longer than four weeks at a time. Additionally, since one of the mechanisms by which caloric restriction slows aging is reducing metabolism, those who practice it over a long period of time may have less energy. This makes it hard to exercise, and muscle mass and strength decline. When practicing caloric restriction, rest and do not overexercise. Light stretching, yoga, tai chi, and walking are beneficial. If you are weight training, you can continue, but reduce the weights you lift and perform your repetitions more slowly.

Longevity Strategy IV—Exercise for Maximum Longevity

By age 40, most people rarely exercise, and if they do, they do not exercise as vigorously as they did when they were younger. However, it is never too late to benefit from exercise. Studies have shown that men and women 50 years and older who exercise regularly can improve their cardiovascular fitness, lower levels of blood fats such as cholesterol, strengthen their bones, achieve normal body composition, and improve their overall quality of life (Yataco 1997). Numerous studies by exercise physiologists and sports medicine physicians have proven the positive effects of exercise for elderly people. Here are a few:

- Exercising increases appetite and helps your metabolism work better. After three months of regular exercise, expect to eat 15 percent more calories while losing four to five pounds of body fat (Hakkinen 1998).

- Weight training counteracts the catabolic (tearing down) effects of aging and age-related conditions such as insufficiency of kidney function (Castaneda 2001).

- Retired professional athletes who continue to train regularly, even if not competitively, retain their aerobic capacity.

- Endurance training in men can reduce age-related loss of aerobic capacity by 50 percent (Vincent 2003).

- There is little difference between men and women in terms of exercise; both benefit from it (Fitzgerald 1997).

- Weight training may improve insulin tolerance (Duncan et al. 2003) and help restore IGF-I, GH, and DHEA levels (Borst 2002).

- Weight training improves bone density (Teixeira 2003); and even moderate exercise helps strengthen bones (Hagberg 2001).

- Regular exercise improves balance and reduces the risk of falling accidents (Taggart 2002).

- Exercise improves body composition (Evan 1995).

There is no question that exercise improves health. What many people do not know is that overdoing it, or doing intense repetitive exercise, can increase oxidative damage to cells, which causes tissue damage and accelerates aging, and produce a higher risk of respiratory infections; it can also trigger latent viruses. A Danish study showed that intense exercise decreases levels of natural killer cells and lymphokine-activated killer cells. Make sure that you get sufficient rest after exercise. Take a day off between intensive exercising.

The goals of exercise are to achieve balance, flexibility, core strength, muscle strength, and aerobic fitness. But what is the best exercise?

Excellent exercises, such as hatha yoga and tai chi, originated in Asia and are now available in the West. These are not just exercises but complete systems of physical and mental health, which train mind, body, and spirit. Hatha yoga is the master exercise for the body and mind. Tai chi is a good exercise for the nervous system and mental-emotional state, and has profound positive effects on the body. Research studies have been done on both hatha yoga and tai chi practitioners and have confirmed their benefits. My own Chinese tai chi and Indian yoga masters are living proof of this. Rarely ill and very active even into their eighties and nineties, these extraordinary individuals taught me much of what I know and practice in my own life.

More available for Americans are gym exercises such as weight training with equipment and using cardiovascular machines. We are also more inclined to walk, bicycle, jog, or swim than to practice yoga or tai chi, which many Americans find boring. The best way to make use of the gym is by combining a variety of exercises, often referred to as cross-training, so that all parts of your body are worked out,

not only one system or area. A combination of light weight training, swimming, bicycling, or walking, isometrics, and stretching seems to produce the best results and the least injury.

My recommendations are to vary your program to include two to three days of weight training alternated with two to three days of aerobic activity each week. These should be your main exercises, allowing an hour and a half for each workout. Include stretching and some isometric exercises with these as warmups. On off days perform a minimum of 20 minutes of isometrics and stretching at home. Take one to two rest days each week.

Think about how much time each week you can devote to physical exercise and schedule it into your calendar. Start gradually and work towards higher levels of training. Find a fitness instructor and work together to design an exercise program that fits your individual needs. If you have access to good quality yoga or tai qi instruction, begin classes and attend regularly. If you are not able to do any of these, start walking at least three times per week for a minimum of 30 minutes each time. Whatever exercise regimen you begin, be patient. Don't push yourself, and avoid injury.

Prolonging Health Recommendation 72— Improve Your Balance

As we age, there is a tendency to lose physical balance. Some of this is due to age-related changes in the vestibular system of the inner ear. The human inner ear contains two divisions. These are the hearing portion, or cochlea, and the balance portion, or vestibular system. The vestibular system in each inner ear consists of a network of tubes (the semicircular canals) and sacs (the vestibule). These tubes are filled with fluid, and as the position of your head changes, the fluid moves within the inner ear and bends tiny hairs found in the sensory cells inside the ear canal.

Bending these hairs initiates nerve impulses that pass along the vestibular nerve to the brain. The impulses provide information to the brain about changes in head position in relation to your body and surroundings. The brain sends commands to the muscles of your body; these commands allow you to maintain your balance as you sit, stand, or move about.

Balance is a complex function requiring healthy vestibular function, neuromuscular coordination, and muscle strength. You can improve your balance by strengthening your muscles as in weight training, yoga, or tai chi, and by dancing. In my clinical experience, balancing exercises alone are not sufficient to help improve balance. Strength and coordination are required as well. Muscle tension and misalignment of the vertebrae in the neck, and the effects of degenerative discs in the cervical spine can also cause problems with balance. Chiropractic or osteopathic adjustments, acupuncture, massage, and physical therapy may also help to improve balance. Since the progressive loss of balance is one of the biomarkers of aging, it's important that you improve and maintain your balance to lower biological age.

Prolonging Health Recommendation 73— Become More Flexible

As we age, we become stiffer and our tendons and ligaments grow less elastic. You may become more flexible by stretching regularly, practicing yoga, and doing other forms of stretching exercises. A complete flexibility program should begin with the spine and encompass every joint and ligament in the body. I recommend that for every hour of weight lifting, resistance training, or cardiovascular exer-

cise you perform, you stretch for at least 30 minutes. Many people find that alternating yoga classes with weight training provides a balance between strength and flexibility.

Prolonging Health Recommendation 74— Work on Your Core Strength

Core strength is what holds your spine erect, keeps your stomach from sagging, and gives martial artists like Jackie Chan the ability to perform physical feats that seem impossible to us. In Asian philosophy, core strength is called internal energy. This is achieved by holding different postures for several minutes, as done in yoga positions or martial arts poses. Take a yoga class or if you're up to it, practice qi gong. This is a style of exercise that involves holding standing postures for long periods of time while practicing deep breathing. Another system, called Pilates, improves flexibility and helps you become stronger.

Prolonging Health Recommendation 75— Gain More Muscle

The best way to gain muscle is by weight training, but other forms of resistance exercise also work. These include isometrics and Pilates.[62] These involve the use of specialized equipment that develops core strength, flexibility, and overall muscle strength without overworking any one muscle group or tiring the body. Pilates is an excellent exercise system, and I often recommend it for elderly people.

Weight training builds muscle, helps gain strength, improves balance, improves walking ability, boosts performance in other exercises, and promotes blood flow to hard-to-reach parts of the body. It also stimulates hormone production (Hakkinen 2002). Exercise in general is a potent releaser of growth hormone (Nindl 2001; Kraemer 2001). The more intense the exercise and the more frequently you perform it, the more growth hormone is released. Research suggests that when older people use a combination of oral GH secretagogues with exercise, they lose weight and increase muscle mass, and their body composition improves (Wideman 2002). Research also shows that testosterone levels increase with heavy resistance training (Hakkinen 2002).

Muscle mass declines with aging, so practice some form of resistance training at least three days each week. This will help prevent sarcopenia or the muscle wasting commonly seen in the elderly; it will help improve your neuroendocrine balance, prevent insulin resistance, and maintain a healthy body composition.

Prolonging Health Recommendation 76— Improve Your Cardiovascular Fitness

Walking, swimming, and aerobic styles of yoga such as Ashtanga improve your cardiovascular fitness. I agree that we should improve our cardiovascular fitness, but first we need to improve our balance, increase our muscles, become stronger, develop core strength, and become more flexible; then we can add aerobic exercises. Your health will greatly improve when you follow the exercise recommendations in this section, leaving cardiovascular exercises for last.

It is commonly thought that cardio-workouts are the best way to exercise. On the contrary, they often are the worst. If you begin exercising by pushing your heart rate, as is typically recommended, you can stress your body. This uses up glucose and raises your levels of adrenaline and cortisol; it causes the release of glycogen from the muscles and liver, raising glucose levels and causing the release of

insulin. Though the burst of adrenaline and cortisol temporarily makes you feel good, forcing the secretion of even more can exhaust your adrenal glands.

This is the opposite effect of what we want. These are catabolic hormones after all, and in the long term they accelerate aging. Also, if your pancreas produces too much insulin during exercise, you can become hypoglycemic and feel exhausted.

Our exercise goals are to increase the levels of anabolic hormones such as testosterone and growth hormone, decrease the catabolic ones such as insulin and cortisol, and restore neuroendocrine balance and prolong our health. Avoid the hormonal imbalances caused by intense aerobic forms of exercise and instead practice moderate, regular exercise. Diana Schwarzbein, M.D., author of *The Schwarzbein Principle II*, advises resistance, flexibility, and cardiovascular training in a 2-1-1 ratio. The *Prolonging Health* exercise recommendations advise that you improve your balance and develop core strength as well.

Longevity Strategy V—Use Life-Extending Nutritional Supplements

Nutritional supplementation is essential to enhance the nutrient density of your diet. This increases the micronutrient saturation of your tissues, which is especially important as one ages. Supplements are required to provide sufficient antioxidant protection against accumulated oxidative damage; cofactors and enzymes are necessary for metabolism; precursor molecules are needed for proteins, hormones, and neurotransmitters; and neuroprotective substances must be obtained to promote the brain's cognitive function.

Under optimal circumstances, we should be able to obtain enough of these nutrients directly from our food. But we don't have optimal circumstances with regard to food. Most Americans have access to plenty of food—in fact, too much food of all kinds—but the standard American diet, appropriately abbreviated as SAD, is deficient in many essential nutrients. It is particularly low in micronutrients, such as trace minerals and important antioxidants such as vitamin E, but it's high in calories in the form of refined carbohydrates and the wrong kinds of fats. The typical American way

Our stressful modern lifestyle and repeated exposure to toxic environmental pollutants, even in micro amounts, as well as to an increasing variety of microbial agents, dictate that optimal nutrition can be obtained only by supplementing our diet with commercially prepared nutrients. These problems are compounded as we age, complicated by the fact that older people generally have less appetite so they eat less.

of eating does not promote health, and it is the main contributing factor to all of the late-onset diseases associated with aging.

Our stressful modern lifestyle and repeated exposure to toxic environmental pollutants, even in micro amounts, as well as to an increasing variety of microbial agents, dictate that optimal nutrition can be obtained only by supplementing our diet with commercially prepared nutrients. These problems are compounded as we age, complicated by the fact

that older people generally have less appetite so they eat less (Mowe 2002). They typically do not have enough energy to prepare foods properly, preferring to eat easily prepared prepackaged foods or in restaurants; this contributes to a lower nutritional status among the elderly (Bates 2002) and predisposes them to degenerative diseases (Mowe 1994).

Researchers investigating the relationship of nutrients and aging have found that the lower overall nutritional status caused by poor diet contributes to reduced amounts of important vitamins and minerals such as carotenoids (Olmedilla 2002), tocopherols, magnesium (Vaquero 2002), chromium, folate, and vitamins B_6 and B_{12} (Selhub 2002). Lack of these nutrients is associated with heart disease, cataract formation, diabetes, and a variety of diseases associated with aging.

Keep in mind that taking vitamins and minerals is not a replacement for eating healthy food. Rather, it *complements* a healthy, nutrient-dense diet. An increasing volume of research shows that micronutrients provided in the diet and through supplementation can prevent disease, enhance health, and promote genetic stability (Fenech 2002). Also, many common prescription and over-the-counter drugs and other substances deplete important nutrients, and should be avoided when possible.

To prolong your health, supplement your diet in an organized way. Begin with a high quality multivitamin-mineral formula, then get optimal amounts of individual antioxidants. Ensure adequate calcium balance; get enough omega-3 and omega-6 essential fatty acids; take a digestive enzyme; and include specialized nutrients for your individualized health needs. To round off your nutritional supple-

Selected Nutrient-Depleting Drugs

Drug	Depleted Nutrients
Alcohol (including in cough syrups and herbal tinctures)	Vitamins A, B_1, B_3, B_{12}, biotin, choline, folate
Antihistamines	Vitamin C
Nonsteroidal anti-inflammatory drugs (Motrin, Celebrex)	Folic acid
Metformin (Glucophage)	Vitamin B_{12}
Phenytoin (Dilantin)	Vitamins B_{12}, D, K; calcium, folic acid
Salicylates (aspirin)	Vitamin C, folic acid, potassium, sodium
Steroid drugs (prednisone)	Vitamins B_6, C, D
Tetracycline antibiotics	Vitamins B_1, B_2, B_3, B_6, B_{12}, K, biotin, calcium, magnesium, iron, inositol, *Lactobacillus acidophilus* and *Bifidobacteria bifidus*
Valproic acid (Depakote)	Folic acid, carnitine

Source: Pelton 2000.

ment program, use specialized nutraceutical substances that influence the modifiable aging factors.

Prolonging Health Recommendation 77— Take a Multivitamin-Mineral Formula

The best general nutritional supplement is a multiple vitamin and mineral formula that includes a variety of nutrients in low to moderate, but adequate dosages. Products that have nutrients in too high dosages, usually B vitamins, or that require you to take more than six capsules or tablets daily, are often difficult to swallow and hard on the digestive system. Taking one or two capsules with meals is much more manageable.

A multivitamin-mineral supplement serves to *supplement* the diet, and is not meant to raise the blood levels of any specific nutrient. In order to boost the antioxidant defenses, we'll increase the dosage of individual antioxidants to optimal levels, and beyond if necessary, in order to maintain adequate blood levels of vita-

mins C and E, selenium, and coenzyme Q10 for wellness and to retard aging.

A dietary supplement that promotes health and prevents senescence should include a mixture of different nutrients including vitamins, macro and trace minerals, enzymes, lipids, amino acids, phospholipids, and other nutritional factors that approximate the nutrients contained in foods. Of course, no commercially prepared formula will ever duplicate nature's complexity, but some are better than others.

For my patients, I often recommend products such as those from Thorne Research[63] or Life Factor Research,[64] though there are several other good products available, such as those designed by the Life Extension Foundation.[65] Another, Optigene Professional,[66] is a specialized nutraceutical anti-aging dietary supplement with C-Med 100, a DNA repair substance derived from the Peruvian herb *Uncaria tomentosa*. This citation of specific brand products is not an endorsement, but merely a report from my clinical practice.

Recommended Amounts of Individual Nutrients Contained in a Multivitamin-Mineral Formula

Nutrient Range	Form	Recommended Dosage
Folic Acid	Calcium folinate	800 mcg
Biotin		200–400 mcg
Trimethylglycine		100 mg
Vitamin B_1	Thiamine	10–50 mg
Vitamin B_2	Riboflavin, riboflavin-5-phosphate	10–25 mg
Vitamin B_3	Niacin, niacinamide	50 mg
Vitamin B_5	Calcium pantothenate	250–500 mg
Pantothene		50 mg
Vitamin B_6	Pyridoxine HCL, pyridoxal 5-phosphate	10 mg
Vitamin B_{12}	Cyanocobalamin, methylcobalamin, adenosylcobalamin	1,000 mcg
Paraaminobenzoic acid (PABA)		200 mcg
Choline	Bitartrate, citrate	100–250 mg
Phosphatidylcholine		150 mg
Inositol		250 mg
Vitamin A	Palmitate, acetate	5,000 IU
Beta-carotene		5,000 IU
Mixed carotenes		12,500–25,000 IU
Lutein		500–750 mcg
Lycopene		3 mg
Citrus bioflavonoids		500–1,000 mg
Vitamin C	Ascorbic acid, ascorbyl palmitate	250 mg
Vitamin E	d-alphatocopherol, mixed tocopherols	400–500 IU
Vitamin D_3	Cholecalciferol	400 IU
Vitamin K		80–100 mcg
Calcium	Amino acid chelate, citrate	250–500 mg
Magnesium	Citrate, aspartate	250–500 mg
Potassium	Aspartate, citrate, chloride	90–150 mg
Selenium	Selenomethionine, picolinate	200 mcg
Zinc	Methionate, picolinate, succinate	15–30 mg
Copper	Amino acid chelate	1–1.5 mg
Chromium	Picolinate, polynicotinate	200 mcg
Molybdenum	Sodium molybdenum, picolinate	125 mcg
Iodine	Potassium iodide	75–225 mcg
Manganese	Gluconate, picolinate	5–15 mg
Silicon		10 mg
Boron		3–5 mg
Vanadium	Sulfate, picolinate	100 mcg

Spread the amount you take throughout the day, during or immediately after your meals, so the body absorbs the supplemental nutrients along with those in your food. Clinical evidence suggests that nutrients work *synergistically,* as in nature, and that they also tend to work better in the body and cause fewer imbalances, such as those sometimes associated with high-dose single nutrients, when combined with a multivitamin and mineral product.

Typical Nutritional Supplement Mistakes

Correct nutritional supplementation is a science all its own, which includes not only providing effective nutrients, but ensuring their absorption and making adjustments due to individual variability. Here are some typical mistakes people make when taking supplements:

- Taking too many supplements, and often skipping meals in the process, can unbalance dietary nutrition with the wrong calorie mixture of proteins, carbohydrates, and fats, and by providing inadequate fiber.

- Taking supplements of poor quality or of low nutrient value.

- Not taking sufficient dosages of the right supplements.

- Taking too high a dosage of an individual supplement, causing imbalances in other nutrients.

Prolonging Health Recommendation 78—Get Optimal Amounts of Antioxidants

The second most important aspect of your supplemental nutrient plan is to ensure that you are getting enough antioxidants in dosages beyond the optimal recommended range. Granted, antioxidants occur in foods and many are included in your multivitamin-mineral formula, but to obtain optimal results in your *Prolonging Health* program, several critical antioxidants are necessary in higher dosages than obtained in food or in your multivitamin-mineral formula.

In a German study, researchers found that even in people eating a good diet and taking nutritional supplements, blood levels for key nutrients, particularly folate (Mattson 2002) and vitamin E, were still below reference values (Beitz 2002). Therefore, it is essential to ensure that your daily intake of antioxidants not only is sufficient, but provides high enough dosages of key antioxidants, especially vitamins C and E, and coenzyme Q10, to bring your blood levels into the upper end of the reference ranges for these nutrients as measured by a lab test.

Oxygen is a double-edged biological sword: we need it to survive, but it causes tissue degradation. The observation of this scientific paradox led to the oxidative damage or free radical theory of aging (discussed earlier in this book), which theorizes that gradual cumulative oxidation occurs throughout our body, especially to our genetic material and mitochondrial DNA, and that it is inevitable and responsible for aging. To compensate for oxidative stress and the formation of free radical molecules, our bodies evolved very effective antioxidant mechanisms, which operate perfectly during youth, but falter later in life. In addition, naturally occurring antioxidant substances in foods support the antioxidant defenses within our body.

As an extension of the oxidative theory of aging and concepts of antioxidant defenses, scientists hypothesized that by supplying additional antioxidants (zinc, vitamins C and E), we should be able to improve our antioxidant status, and thereby reduce the effects of free radicals on our body, and even reverse aging. They

Optimal Longevity Ranges for Antioxidants

Antioxidant	Recommended Form	RDA	Typical Therapeutic Dosage	Optimal Longevity Range
Vitamin C	Ascorbic acid; calcium-magnesium-potassium ascorbate; ascorbyl palmitate	35–95 mg	200–2,000 mg	up to 10,000 mg
Vitamin E	d-alpha tocopherol; mixed tocopherols	15–30 mg	200–500 IU	up to 1,600 IU
CoQ10	Ubiquinone; Idebenone	none	30–60 mg	up to 1,200 mg
Vitamin B$_2$	Riboflavin hydrochloride; riboflavin-5-phosphate	1.7 mg	10–100 mg	up to 400 mg
Vitamin B$_6$	Pyridoxine hydrochloride; pyridoxal hydrochloride; pyridoxal-5-phosphate	2 mg	50–100 mg	up to 500 mg
Vitamin B$_{12}$	Cyanocobalamin; methylocabalamin; adenosylcobalamin (coenzyme B$_{12}$)	0.3–2.6 mcg	1,000 mcg	up to 4,000 mcg
Selenium	Selenium picolinate	10–75 mg	200–400 mcg	up to 1,200 mcg
Zinc	Zinc picolinate; zinc methionine	5–19 mg	15–25 mg	up to 250 mg
Lipoic Acid	Alpha-lipoic acid	none	25–100 mg	up to 600 mg
Carotenes	Beta-carotene as natural mixture of *all-trans* and *cis* forms; mixed carotenoids	none	25,000–100,000 IU	up to 300,000 IU
Astaxanthin	Astaxanthin	none	2.5–5.0 mg	up to 20 mg
Arginine	L-arginine	none	500–1,000 mg	up to 30 grams
Lysine	L-lysine	none	500–1,000 mg	up to 6 grams
Cysteine	N-acetylcysteine (NAC)	none	200–500 mg	up to 5,000 mg
Glutamine	L-glutamine	none	500–2,000 mg	up to 40 grams
Glutathione	reduced L-glutathione	none	50–100 mg	up to 300 mg

To calculate your antioxidant needs, refer to the list of antioxidants and then look at the label on your multivitamin-mineral formula. Subtract the dosages in your multivitamin-mineral product from those on the list and make up the difference by adding individual antioxidants. For example, if your multivitamin-mineral formula contains 15 mg of zinc, and the chart's optimal range is 25 mg, then you need to add another 10 mg of zinc daily.

References: The Linus Pauling Institute, *The New Recommendations for Dietary Antioxidants*; Pelton, R., et al. *Drug-Induced Nutrient Depletion Handbook*; Crayhon, R., Designs for Health, *Supplement Monograph Manual*; Roberts, A. J., et al. *Nutraceuticals: The Complete Encyclopedia*; Gaby, A. R. and Wright, J. V., *Nutritional Therapy in Medical Practice.*

found that supplementing the diet with antioxidants, while not reversing aging, had wide-ranging beneficial influences in the body, including prevention of cancer, cardiovascular disease, and neurodegenerative disease, perhaps even influencing the outcome of Alzheimer's dementia. Today, scientists continue to investigate the effects of antioxidants on cellular and molecular aging, and with very promising results.

Taking the antioxidant hypothesis a step further, doctors, pharmaceutical and nutritional supplement companies, and individual life extensionists experimented with other naturally occurring antioxidant substances that have anti-aging potential. They found that *com-*

bining antioxidants with nutritional supplements improved results.

The basic antioxidants necessary for health, and in higher dosages to enhance antioxidant defense and retard aging, are vitamins C and E, selenium, zinc, and the carotene family. Several other common nutrients, including the amino acid arginine, and members of the B vitamin family, especially folate and vitamins B_6 and B_{12}, have antioxidant properties, as well as the ability to lower toxic oxidizing molecules such as homocysteine. Researchers have found that newly discovered antioxidant substances such as coenzyme Q10 exert powerful antioxidant activity in the cell (Linnane, Zhang, et al. 2002). Several antioxidants, such as lipoic acid and acetyl-L-carnitine, exert their activity at the level of the mitochondria (Hagen 1998). Others, notably N-acetylcysteine and thioproline, a substance found in shiitake mushrooms that binds cancer-causing nitrates, enhance glutathione activity (Miquel 2002). As discussed, glutathione is a naturally occurring antioxidant in the body.

The longevity range is much higher even than the typical recommended therapeutic dosages, and considerably higher than the recommended daily allowances (RDA). There are several reasons for this: (1) due to biochemical individuality, some people require unusually high dosages to achieve physiological effects; (2) to treat the effects of aging, cumulative oxidative stresses, and active or occult disease processes, more of each is needed; and (3) continual exposure to toxic environmental chemicals requires increased antioxidant protection, so dosages higher than normal are required to maintain health.

To assess your nutrient status and gauge your daily intake of antioxidants, periodically test the levels of at least five key antioxidants

> ☀ **CAUTION:** Never take mega dosages of any nutrient without knowing whether you are allergic or sensitive in any other way to that substance, or whether it has any interactions with medications you may be taking. Do not increase any nutrient towards the extreme end of the antisenescence range without the support of a nutritionist or other health care professional knowledgeable in the use of nutritional substances for anti-aging.

in your blood: vitamin C, vitamin E, coenzyme Q10, selenium, and the carotenes. Your doctor can order these tests from any standard reference lab. AAL Reference Laboratories[67] offer a panel that includes all of these plus a few other tests. If money is not a hindrance, I recommend the comprehensive oxidative panel performed by Genox Laboratories,[68] which involves both urine and blood tests as described in part 3.

Prolonging Health Recommendation 79— Ensure Adequate Calcium and Mineral Balance

Minerals play a number of key roles in your body, serving as coenzymes in numerous metabolic reactions, providing the composition of bones and teeth, and helping to maintain a wide variety of biochemical processes. If you follow the *Prolonging Health* dietary principles and take a multivitamin-mineral formula and added antioxidants, your daily intake of all microminerals, such as zinc and boron, and of most macrominerals (with the possible exception of calcium) should be sufficient.

Calcium needs vary according to eating habits, race, gender, and age, but in general adequate levels of calcium are necessary to maintain the structural integrity of the skeleton, the normal function of muscle contraction, blood coagulation, cell membrane function, and hormone secretion (Griffin 1996). Calcium also functions as a second messenger within the cell, relaying messages to the cell about the arrival of proteins and growth factors at the receptor sites on the cell's surface.

Calcium metabolism is tricky, for too much or too little causes considerable dysfunction in the body. The concentration of calcium outside of the cell is 1,000 times greater than intracellular (inside the cell) calcium; this tells us that too much calcium is undesirable. Improper calcium metabolism leading to excess intracellular calcium can cause hypertension and even lead to cell death. Calcium inside the cell is controlled by a wide range of substances including hormones and neurotransmitters, as well as the correct balance of other minerals, particularly sodium. That is why excess salt in the diet causes so many problems in the body.

Cellular calcium homeostasis is tightly controlled by three hormones: parathyroid and calcitonin (both secreted by the thyroid gland) and vitamin D_3; it is regulated by the kidneys via a dynamic exchange of calcium between the blood and bone. Vitamin D_3, also called calciferol, is both a vitamin and a steroid hormone (Farach-Carson 2003). It facilitates calcium absorption and is necessary for bone formation and metabolism. Vitamin D_3 may arrest the autoimmune processes that contribute to diabetes, rheumatoid arthritis, and lupus; it may reduce cancer growth (Gruber 2002); it influences gene expression (Theodoropoulos 2003); and it prevents osteoporosis (Willis 2002).

Serum calcium levels, found on all standard chemistry panels when you have a blood test, is maintained between a narrow range of 8.5 and 10.5 mg/dL. However, since abnormal values are seen only in serious bone disease, as in metastatic cancer, knowing your serum calcium levels is not particularly useful for evaluating calcium status in the body.[69] For this, calcium levels in hair are better. Hair mineral analysis is readily performed at home or in the doctor's office by clipping small amounts of hair from the back of your head, the pubic region, and under your arms; the hair is then sent to a lab for analysis (Bralley 2001). Optimally, total serum and hair calcium results should fall directly in the middle of the reference ranges.

Since nearly 75 percent of dietary calcium comes from dairy products in the standard American diet, those people avoiding dairy products for health reasons are at risk for calcium deficiency. Excess use of refined sugar and high-phosphorous-containing products such as sodas, as well as too much red meat, can inhibit calcium metabolism.

Absorption is another issue. The average American diet supplies about 750 to 1,000 mg of calcium daily, but calcium is poorly absorbed in the gut, so only one-third of this ingested amount makes it into the body. The same, or worse, is true with calcium supplements: only a fraction (as low as 5–20 percent in the case of calcium carbonate from oyster shell and dolomite) of the elemental calcium is absorbed. Calcium citrate, a form of calcium bound to citric acid, is absorbed only slightly better, up to about 30 percent.

The form of calcium that absorbs the best is an amino acid chelate. It is produced by a process in which an organic molecule (an amino acid) is attached to a mineral. True amino acid chelates, such as calcium glycinate, histindinate, and lysinate, are absorbed up to 45 percent and are considered the most bioavailable form of calcium. But even the absorption of amino acid chelated calcium can be inhibited by dietary factors. Low-fat, high-fiber, high-carbohydrate diets prevent calcium absorption, lowering the absorption percentage to less than 20 percent. Calcium absorption also decreases with age, so it is wise to use a combination of different forms of calcium, including an amino acid chelate.

In 1994, the National Institutes for Health (NIH) set optimal calcium intake guidelines for older adults at 1,500 mg daily. In 1999, the National Academy of Science recommended 1,000 mg per day. So what is the optimal amount of dietary calcium? In general, most people do not get enough calcium, especially as they age, so they need to take additional calcium to supplement dietary sources.

Calcium requirements are highest during the growth years between 10 and 20, and for those over 50. Total dietary calcium for older people should range from 1,000 to 1,500 mg daily from a wide variety of natural sources, including cultured dairy products such as yogurt and some cheese (if you are not allergic to the proteins in milk), green leafy vegetables, legumes, soy (as in tofu), fish, seaweeds, and seeds and nuts.

The many factors that inhibit calcium absorption mean you should supplement your dietary intake of calcium with at least 500 mg of calcium citrate, or better, with an amino acid chelated form. If you do not drink milk or consume other dairy products, increase your supplemental intake to 750–1,000 mg daily; if you have osteoporosis, increase your supplemental intake to 1,200–1,500 mg.

Here are a couple of tips to know if you are getting enough:

Calcium Levels in Selected Foods

Food	Portion	Amount of Calcium
Sardines	3.5 oz	443 mg
Yogurt	1 cup	400 mg
Milk	1 cup	300 mg
Figs	10 dried	269 mg
Bok choy	1 cup	158 mg
Wakame	3.5 oz	150 mg
Tofu	1/2 cup	130 mg
Almonds	24 dried	75 mg
Halibut	3.5 oz	60 mg
Spinach	1/2 cup	28 mg
Carrots	1 medium raw	19 mg

- If your muscles cramp easily, especially at night, you are not getting enough calcium into your tissues; increase your dosage by 250 mg daily until the cramping stops.

- If your hair analysis reveals low calcium, or your serum calcium levels are below the middle of the range, increase your calcium supplementation by 250 mg daily.

Take calcium throughout the day along with your multivitamin-mineral formula with meals. However, do not take more than 500 mg at a time, as much of it will not absorb. The balance of your calcium supplement is best taken in the evening, after dinner. You improve calcium regulation in the body by maintaining healthy kidney function, through weight-bearing exercise, and restoring hormonal balance.

Prolonging Health Recommendation 80— Boost Your Omega-3 and Omega-6 Essential Fatty Acid Intake

Essential fatty acids (EFAs) are fats and oils essential for health that must be supplied in the diet. EFAs provide the structural material that composes all cell membranes, and they are necessary to many other functions in the body including the production of eicosanoids. Eicosanoids are a family of compounds derived from polyunsaturated acids that act as paracrine and autocrine hormones to regulate many cell functions.

Eicosanoids play crucial roles in a variety of physiological and pathophysiological processes, including regulation of smooth muscle contractility and various immune and inflammatory functions. They are involved in nearly every metabolic process in the body, from the control of insulin to serving as autocrine hormones and signaling molecules, and all are critical functions for prolonging health.

Among the three main groups of eicosanoids are prostaglandins. These are hormone-like substances that influence inflammation, blood clotting, heart rate, and the integrity of blood vessel walls. The pain and swelling associated with an injury are medicated by prostaglandins, as are the lower abdominal cramping that some women experience before their period, some forms of headaches, and a variety of chronic conditions such as cardiovascular disease. Aspirin and other nonsteroidal anti-inflammatories inhibit prostaglandin synthesis, which is one of the mechanisms that make these drugs effective in pain control.

Since eicosanoids are synthesized in the body from EFAs, it is necessary to supply adequate amounts of both omega-3 and omega-6 EFAs in the diet by eating fish, seeds, nuts, avocados, and natural plant oils such as olive oil. However, unless you are eating large amounts of coldwater fish such as salmon and halibut, EFA supplementation is necessary.

Excellent sources include flax oil, evening primrose oil, black currant oil, borage seed oil, cod liver oil, and oil from other coldwater fish such as sardines. The ideal ratio of omega 3 to 6 is 1:4, and as EFA balance promotes health, it is wise to obtain the bulk of your EFAs from foods. However, it is difficult to eat enough fish and olive oil to maintain sufficient levels of fatty acids in the body, so some supplementation is usually necessary.

There is no consensus on adequate daily amounts of EFAs, nor on the ideal supplemental dosage. In addition, the variety of sources and the percentages of the different types of EFAs make it difficult for one to know what is best. From my clinical experience, most people do not get enough EFAs in their diet or from supplements, so to prolong health I recommend a variety of different forms, primarily from diet sources.

Supplement with one teaspoon of flax oil daily with food; one tablespoon of cod liver oil one or two times weekly; and 1,000 to 2,000 mg of EPA/DHA fish oil daily with food. Each 1,000-mg capsule should contain 300 mg of EPA and 200 mg of DHA, the balance being made up of other oils. You may also wish to add small amounts of oil of evening primrose, borage seed, or black currant seed. The upper limit for daily fish oil supplementation is 9–10 g. In *The Omega RxZone*, Barry Sears recommends at least 2.5 g of fish oil daily as a beginning dosage, gradually increasing the dose until you feel better, experience more mental clarity, have less muscle aches and joint pain, and experience enhanced physical performance (Sears 2002). Jonathan Goodman, N.D., author of *The Omega Solution*, proposes that the total combined amount of dietary and supplemental EFAs be about 10 g daily (Goodman 2001).

Recommended Essential Fatty Acid Supplements

- 10 g total from combined dietary and supplemental sources

- 1 tablespoon of cod liver oil, 1–2 times weekly

- 1 teaspoon of flax oil, daily

- 1,000–2,000 mg of EPF/DHA fish oil daily

Fish oil supplements are considered safe. However, if you take too much, you may experience excessive or easy bleeding, increased LDL cholesterol, and excess oxidative activity in the body. Take all oil supplements with food for better absorption.

Prolonging Health Recommendation 81— Take Digestive Enzymes

As people age, their pancreatic function declines and fewer digestive enzymes are available to break down food than when they were young. Foods also contain enzymes, but that may not be adequate to compensate for your own lack of enzymes. Taking a broad-spectrum plant-based or pancreatic enzyme during your meals can greatly improve the digestion and absorption of foods and nutrients (Chambon-Savanovitch 2001).

I recommend pancreatic enzymes for people over age 50, for those with chronically poor digestion, and when eating a high-protein diet. Symptoms of poor digestion include abdominal distention, constipation, diarrhea, and stomach pain after eating or lower belly pain more than 20 minutes after meals.

Digestive enzymes are rated by strength as established by the United States Pharmacopoeia (USP). Each standard "X" contains not less than 25 USP units of amylase, 2 USP units of lipase, and 25 USP units of protease. Most digestive enzymes are supplied as 4X pancreatin per 500-mg tablet or capsule. The typical dosage is one to three capsules with or immediately after meals. Some nutritionists recommend higher dosages or more concentrated enzymes; up to 10X pancreatin. Pancreatic enzymes are generally well tolerated and have no side effects or interactions in the recommended dosages.

As people age, they tend to have difficulty digesting proteins. This causes them to eat less meat and other foods high in protein. Yet to prolong our health, it is necessary to keep consuming optimal amounts of protein. Therefore, take hydrochloric acid with your pancreatic digestive enzymes. Hydrochloric acid assists protein digestion, renders the stomach sterile against orally ingested pathogenic microorganisms, prevents bacterial or fungal overgrowth of the small intestine, encourages the flow of bile and pancreatic enzymes during eating, and facilitates the absorption of a variety of nutrients including folic acid, vitamin C, beta-carotene, iron, calcium, magnesium, and zinc. Numerous studies have shown acid secretion declines with age and that impaired hydrochloric acid production is associated with a variety of clinical conditions.

Hydrochloric acid is available as betaine hydrochloride and glutamic acid hydrochloride. The potency of a capsule or tablet preparation may vary from 5 to 10 grains (1 grain = 64.75 mg). A typical dosage of hydrochloric acid is 5–80 grains taken with meals three times a day. The recommended method when starting to take hydrochloric acid is to begin with 5–10 grains with each meal and increase by capsule or tablet until gas, bloating, and belly pain are gone. Be sure to take a hydrochloric acid supplement with your protein powder drink. Hydrochloric acid supplements are safe, but if you take too much, your stomach will burn. If this happens, reduce the dosage or discontinue.

Prolonging Health Recommendation 82— Use Longevity Nutraceuticals

To live to over 120, you need other substances, specifically seven specialized nutritional substances that are so potent they fall into a category of their own. They're called *longevity nutraceuticals*, that is, natural medications that can help modulate the ten aging factors and boost the effectiveness of your *Prolonging Health* program.

The Seven Longevity Nutraceuticals

1. Acetyl-L-carnitine

2. Carnosine

3. Creatine

4. L-alpha glycerylophosphorylcholine (GPC)

5. L-carnitine

6. Nicotinamide adenine dinucleotide (NADH)

7. S-adenosyl-methionine (SAMe)

The nutraceutical agents discussed below have all been shown to be safe and effective medications, and they have a long history of use by life-extensionists and body builders. Most of the research on these compounds has been performed in Europe, Japan, and Russia, though all these substances are available over the counter in the United States. Make sure that you add one or all of these medications to your supplement regimen in the recommended dosages; start on the low end of the recommended range, and gradually increase the daily dose towards the upper end. These substances are safe and generally without side effects, but discontinue if you experience any gastrointestinal discomfort or other reactions.

Acetyl-L-carnitine: A form of L-carnitine, acetyl-L-carnitine has been extensively researched for its neuroprotective properties (Tolu 2002; Bigini 2002). It enhances metabolism in the mitochondria and therefore increases energy and endurance; it has antioxidant properties (Liu 2002) and is a precursor for acetylcholine, a neurotransmitter that helps cognitive function and treats depression (Pettegrew 2002). It also decreases glycation (the negative combination of glucose and proteins). There are no known contraindications,

and it is considered a safe substance, without interactions with drugs. It is synergistic with lipoic acid and other antioxidants. The typical dosage is 500–2,000 mg daily.

Carnosine: This nutraceutical is composed of the amino acids beta-alanine and L-histadine. It is found in highest concentrations in the heart, neurons, and muscle cells, and appears to address nearly all cellular and metabolic aging factors (Hipkiss 2001). It is an antioxidant (Kang 2002) and prevents glycation (Seidler and Yeargans 2002). It protects against DNA damage, has neuroprotective properties (Tabakman, Lazarovici, and Kohen 2002), and enhances immunity and protects against cancer. Carnosine has been shown to improve aging skin and eyes, promote wound healing, and enhance exercise performance (Suzuki 2002). It is safe, without known drug interactions. Carnosine is synergistic with vitamin E and coenzyme Q10. Use it in dosages ranging from 50 to 500 mg daily.

Creatine: After being synthesized from the amino acids L-arginine, glycine, and L-methionine, creatine is transported to the skeletal muscles, heart, and brain, where it is metabolized into creatine phosphate and released into the blood. Though sufficient amounts of creatine can be obtained from meat, these amounts may not be adequate to maintain and build muscle during aging. Since sarcopenia is the characteristic body type of advanced age, maintaining muscle mass and strength is necessary as people age. Creatine has energy-promoting activity during nonaerobic exercise such as weight training, and supplementing creatine appears useful in building muscle (Haub et al. 2002).

There are several forms of creatine on the market, but the better one is creatine monohydrate; it can be taken in dosages ranging from 5 to 20 g daily, divided into two to three portions throughout the day. It is a safe substance and there are no reported drug interactions, though coffee may interfere with creatine's beneficial effects. Since it can potentially elevate serum creatine levels, a lab marker for kidney function, it should not be taken by anyone with any type of kidney condition. In high dosages it can cause diarrhea, and muscle cramping has been reported as well.

L-alpha glycerylophosphorylcholine (alpha GPC): Alpha GPC is a by-product of phosphatidylcholine synthesis, and serves as a precursor molecule for acetylcholine. It increases several phospholipids in the brain, restores neurotransmitter receptors, enhances cognitive function and improves memory, and has been used to treat the effects of stroke. It is also considered a growth hormone releasing agent, and is extensively used by body builders (Ceda 1992). It is a safe substance, without side effects or interactions, and is synergistic with phosphatidylcholine and related substances. The typical daily dosage is 100–500 mg.

L-carnitine: L-carnitine plays a role in cellular metabolism in the mitochondria and the synthesis of acetylcholine in the brain. It is naturally synthesized in the body from the amino acids lysine and methionine; since deficiency can occur, supplementing with L-carnitine is used in the prevention and treatment of cardiovascular disease, kidney and liver disease, diabetes, and low sperm count. It is an active free-radical scavenger, prevents lipofuscin accumulation, and may improve immune function in patients with chronic viral diseases. L-carnitine can enhance physical performance and increase exercise tolerance.

It is considered very safe in dosages typically ranging from 1 to 99 g spread out in two or three installments per day. L-carnitine is synergistic with many of the nutritional supplements we've discussed, including vitamin C, coenzyme Q10, lipoic acid, chromium, and the B-vitamin family.

Nicotinamide adenine dinucleotide (NADH): NADH is the activated form of niacin (vitamin B_3). It plays a central role as a coenzyme in energy production in the cell, for which it has been called the "energy of life" coenzyme. It was discovered in 1934 by the American medical researcher Nathan Kaplan, and developed as a nutraceutical medication by Jorg Birkmayer, M.D., Ph.D., in Austria, where it has been studied in the treatment of Parkinson's disease. It can be used in Alzheimer's disease, in the treatment of depression, and with chronic fatigue patients, for whom it appears to improve energy as well as alertness and concentration.

It is safe and without side effects, and is taken typically in dosages of 5–20 mg daily. It is controversial which form is best, but most doctors prefer the ENADA form from Austria. NADH is synergistic with L-tyrosine, 5-HTP, coenzyme Q10, L-carnitine, phosphatidyl serine, and vitamins C, B, and E.

S-adenosyl-methionine (SAMe): A synthetic form of a natural metabolite of the amino acid methionine, SAMe is a multipurpose longevity compound. It is able to help maintain mitochondrial function, prevent DNA mutation, and restore cell membrane and receptor function; it is also neuroprotective, has antidepressant activity, and protects the liver from damage from inflammatory cytokines, alcohol, and drugs. SAMe has been used in the treatment of osteoarthritis and rheumatoid arthritis.

SAMe has been called the "daytime melatonin," because its synthesis during the day helps melatonin synthesis at night. Like melatonin and other substances in the body, the production of SAMe is pulsatile, with highest levels occurring just before sunset, after which levels drop as melatonin levels begin to rise.

It's considered safe, though some people have reported dry mouth and nausea after using it. The typical dosage of SAMe is 800–1,600 mg daily, taken in two divided dosages starting at 400 mg, two times daily. It can affect brain neurotransmitters, so do not take SAMe with antidepressant drugs. The benzodiazepine antianxiety drugs Valium and Xanax suppress melatonin and disrupt the natural circadian rhythm, and may also adversely influence SAMe cyclicity.

Summary of Dosages for the Seven Longevity Nutraceuticals

Substance	Anti-Senescent Dosage
Acetyl-L-carnatine	up to 2,000 mg
Carnosine	up to 500 mg
Creatine	up to 20 grams (20,000 mg)
Alpha GPC	up to 500 mg
L-carnitine	up to 9 grams (9,000 mg)
NADH	up to 20 mg
SAMe	up to 1,600 mg

damage to your cells and accelerate aging. Natural therapies, though slower working, are the only manner in which to correct age-related diseases and reverse cellular and metabolic aging factors.

If any one of the ten modifiable aging factors is particularly challenging for you, specific nutrients may be necessary. In these cases, the dosage is generally considerably higher than the norm. If you have any of the late-onset diseases associated with aging, have a tendency towards a particular disease by genetic predisposition or lifestyle, or have strong risk factors for any of these diseases, you have to work actively at reversing the specific aging factors involved in your disease risk or condition. To accomplish this, work with your doctor on a drugless healing plan using natural medicines, diet, and lifestyle changes to correct the underlying causes of these diseases.

Prolonging Health Recommendation 83— Add Specific Nutrients to Address Individual Modifiable Aging Factors

Making improvements in your diet and taking general nutritional supplements may help prevent disease and improve your health. However, if you have a chronic, degenerative, age-related, or genetic disease, specialized attention may be required to treat your condition effectively.

The occurrence of age-related diseases increases after the age of 50, so actively preventing them becomes a bit like having a second job. The end stage of these aging factors is degenerative disease, and if you already have one or more, then you have to work specifically on reversing them one by one. Treating age-related diseases by only controlling the symptoms with pharmaceutical drugs does not cure the condition or reverse the underlying causative factors. This type of treatment creates drug-induced imbalances that cause additional

Your body requires many nutrients to function properly, most of which can be supplied in a healthy diet. However, for optimal function, sufficient amounts of these nutrients can be obtained only by taking additional amounts in supplemental form. In order to prolong your health and achieve maximum longevity, supplementing these nutrients is essential.

To build an effective and safe nutritional supplement plan, start first with lifestyle and diet, then include a broad-spectrum multivitamin-mineral formula, ensuring that you are getting adequate nutrition and preventing the marginal deficiencies that are common as people age.

Next, in order to optimize your antioxidant defenses, build upon this foundation by adding individual antioxidants. Ensure that you have sufficient amounts of calcium, as well as omega-3 and omega-6 essential fatty acids.

Take pancreatic digestive enzymes and hydrochloric acid to help improve your nutritional status. Include advanced nutraceutical medications that have proven effective in preventing age-related conditions, reversing the main aging factors, and prolonging health. Take specific nutrients to treat age-related disease and prevent any of the ten modifiable aging factors to which you are susceptible.

Summary of *Prolonging Health* Recommendations and Five Strategies for Achieving Your Maximum Life Span

- **Longevity Strategy I—Restore Homeostasis:** *Prolonging Health* begins when you reverse the ten modifiable aging factors and restore homeostasis. You do this by addressing the following *Prolonging Health* recommendations:

- *Prolonging Health* Recommendation 59—
  Reset Your Biological Clock

- *Prolonging Health* Recommendation 60—
  Rehydrate to Improve Your Kidneys

- *Prolonging Health* Recommendation 61—
  Replenish Electrolytes

- *Prolonging Health* Recommendation 62—
  Reenergize Your Metabolism

- *Prolonging Health* Recommendation 63—
  Rebuild Organ Reserve

- *Prolonging Health* Recommendation 64—
  Neutralize Stress

- **Longevity Strategy II—Eat for Longevity:** Eat a healthy diet composed of a variety of fresh vegetables, meats, fish, and poultry, seasonal fresh ripe fruits, an assortment of seeds and nuts, and the inclusion of garden spices and herbs. Follow the following recommendations:

- *Prolonging Health* Recommendation 65—
  Eliminate Sugar

- *Prolonging Health* Recommendation 66—
  Eat Foods with Vitality

- *Prolonging Health* Recommendation 67—
  Emphasize Alkaline Foods

- *Prolonging Health* Recommendation 68—
  Get Enough Protein

- *Prolonging Health* Recommendation 69—
  Eat Nutrient-Dense Plant Foods

- *Prolonging Health* Recommendation 70—
  Include Longevity Dietary Nutrients from Foods and Herbs
  - CONJUGATED LINOLEIC ACID: Consume organic yogurt several times a week; if you are not vegetarian, eat organically raised beef and lamb once or twice a week.
  - FLAVONOIDS: Consume green tea, citrus, apples, onions, grapes, and red wine.
  - ISOTHIOCYANATES: Consume cabbage, broccoli, turnips, kohlrabi, rutabaga, Chinese cabbage, bok choy, horseradish, radish, and watercress.
  - LIGNANS: Consume flaxseeds and flaxseed oil, whole grains, nuts, berries, sesame oil, and herbs such as Schisandra chinensis.
  - MONOTERPENES: Consume caraway, dill, bergamot, peppermint, spearmint, lavender, cherries, and tomatoes; incorporate rinds of lemons, oranges, and grapefruit in your cooking.
  - NUCLEOTIDES: Consume nutritional yeast, organically raised meat, fish, poultry, plant shoots, sprouts, and baby corn.
  - PHYTATES: Consume corn, sesame and sunflower seeds, peanuts, wild rice, soybeans, split peas, and whole grains.
  - PHYTOSTEROLS: Consume spices, seeds and nuts, okra, whole grains, and cruciferous vegetables.

- PROTEASE INHIBITORS: Consume peaches, plums, corn, soybeans, potatoes, and sweet potatoes.
- SAPONINS: Consume pinto, kidney, black, and lima beans, and lentils. Drink ginseng, sarsaparilla, and licorice teas; use aloe.
- ORGANOSULFUR COMPOUNDS: Consume garlic, chives, leeks, shallots, scallions, and onions.
- TANNINS: Consume grapes, legumes, red wine, tea, coffee, and chocolate.

- **Longevity Strategy III—Practice Periodic Calorie Restriction:** To maintain homeostasis and live long, practice calorie restriction by following this recommendation:

- *Prolonging Health* **Recommendation 71— Practice Periodic Caloric Restriction:** Reduce your total calorie intake to about 1,200; go as low as 800 calories for three to nine days if you are a small person in good health or a person of average weight. Eat nutrient-dense and longevity foods in smaller amounts.

- **Longevity Strategy IV—Exercise for Maximum Longevity:** Exercise to prevent disease and maintain muscle mass by following these recommendations:

- *Prolonging Health* **Recommendation 72— Improve Your Balance**

- *Prolonging Health* **Recommendation 73— Become More Flexible**

- *Prolonging Health* **Recommendation 74— Work On Your Core Strength**

- *Prolonging Health* **Recommendation 75— Gain More Muscle**

- *Prolonging Health* **Recommendation 76— Improve Your Cardiovascular Fitness**

- **Longevity Strategy V—Use Life-Extending Nutritional Supplements:** Nutritional supplementation is essential for enhancing the nutrient density of your diet.

- *Prolonging Health* **Recommendation 77— Take a Multivitamin-Mineral Formula**
  - ACETYL-L-CARNITINE: Take 500–2,000 mg daily.
  - CARNOSINE: Take 50–500 mg daily.
  - CREATINE: Take up to 20 g daily, divided into two to three portions throughout the day.
  - L-ALPHA GLYCERYLOPHOSPHORYLCHOLINE (ALPHA GPC): Take 100–500 mg daily.
  - L-CARNITINE: Take up to 9 g daily.
  - NICOTINAMIDE ADENINE DINUCLEOTIDE (NADH): Take 5–20 mg daily.
  - S-ADENOSYL-METHIONINE (SAMe): Take 600–1,600 mg daily, taken in two divided dosages starting at 400 mg, two times daily.

- *Prolonging Health* **Recommendation 83— Add Specific Nutrients to Address Individual Modifiable Aging Factors**

18 Mastering the Ten Modifiable Factors of Longevity

If you have been following the advice presented throughout this book, you have altered, if not transformed, your lifestyle to one that promotes health and prolongs life; changed your diet to prevent disease and foster longevity; started taking a multivitamin-mineral to ensure nutrient protection; added extra antioxidants in order to enhance antioxidant defenses and protect against genetic damage; ensured that you have enough calcium; and included essential fatty acids.

In themselves, these steps can effectively prevent all of the late-onset diseases associated with aging, but to live to over 120, other medications become necessary. To achieve this, you've taken at least one of the seven longevity nutraceuticals and have begun to restore your neuroendocrine balance with bio-identical hormones and supportive adaptogenic herbs. What's left to do?

It's time to integrate the practice of the *Prolonging Health* program into your lifestyle and to master it. You can do this by implementing the recommendations I've discussed; by working with your doctor as you find necessary to help you achieve your *Prolonging Health* goals; and by individualizing your program so that it is fine-tuned to your body and genetics. In this manner, prolonging your health becomes a way of life. When you put the *Prolonging Health* program to work, you benefit because your lifestyle prevents disease and promotes positive genetic expression. In this way you can extend your life span.

The rule for prolonging your health is to take it seriously. In the beginning of your program, you can make gradual changes, but as you age, more effort becomes necessary. At that time, partial effort will yield partial results. You have to transform each of the modifiable aging factors into longevity factors. If you take prolonging your health seriously, you will achieve better results.

Before we proceed further, let's reestablish our goals based upon what we learned. The goals of *Prolonging Health* are to:

- Prevent degenerative and genetically caused diseases associated with aging.

- Improve your quality of life by reducing depression, improving strength, increasing independence, enhancing arousal and sexuality, and restoring energy.

- Reverse premature aging and lower your biological age.

- Achieve maximum life span of 90, 100, 110, 150 years, or more.

To meet these goals, several criteria must be met. The criteria for *Prolonging Health* and achieving your maximum life span are:

- Shift the age-point and lower biological age.

- Keep out of, or just within, the aging zone.

- Prevent metabolic imbalance by managing glucose and insulin, and never reach the metabolic critical point.

- Prevent and reverse all of the ten modifiable aging factors.

- Practice a lifestyle that fosters longevity by following the five longevity strategies.

By keeping the *Prolonging Health* goals and criteria in mind, you can *transform* each of the ten modifiable aging factors into *longevity factors*. Rather than accelerating aging, these become positive influences that promote health and longevity. Remember, each of the aging factors is *modifiable*, and largely under your control. Here's what can happen as you successfully modify each aging factor:

- **Modifiable Aging Factor 1—Oxidative Damage** is caused by the negative effects of excessive oxidation and inadequate antioxidant protection. You transform this aging factor into a longevity factor by taking antioxidants, eating a healthy diet, and avoiding environmental conditions like over-exposure to radiation that cause oxidative damage. When oxidative processes are re-tooled in the body, healthy oxygen utilization prevents the late-onset diseases associated with aging and promotes longevity.

- **Modifiable Aging Factor 2—Genetic Damage** is associated with oxidative damage and caused by toxic environmental chemicals foreign to the body. You transform this aging factor into a longevity factor by taking antioxidants, getting enough folic acid, and taking DNA repair medications. When genetic damage is minimized and DNA repair mechanisms are working optimally, your genes express positive attributes, cancer is prevented, and you age more slowly.

- **Modifiable Aging Factor 3—Impaired Detoxification** is caused by excessive exposure to environmental toxic chemicals, overuse of prescription drugs, faulty diet, and poor liver function. You transform this aging factor into a longevity factor by eating a healthy diet, avoiding exposure to toxic substances including pharmaceutical drugs, improving liver function, and following a regime for detoxification and cleansing of the tissues and cells. When your detoxification pathways are fine-tuned and you have eliminated most of the toxic buildup in your body, you renew your tissues and cells, prevent cancer, restore energy, and the clean cellular environment keeps you young and healthy.

- **Modifiable Aging Factor 4—Insulin Resistance** is caused by consuming processed sugar, overeating refined carbohydrates, and a sedentary lifestyle. You transform this critical aging factor into a longevity factor by avoiding sugar, eliminating refined carbohydrates from your diet, exercising regularly, and taking nutrients and natural medicines that reverse insulin resistance. This results in insulin sensitivity and healthy glucose metabolism, which prevents high insulin levels from turning on the molecular switch that controls accelerated aging.

- **Modifiable Aging Factor 5—Impaired Protein Synthesis and Glycation** is caused by the same conditions that cause insulin resistance, oxidative damage, and impaired detoxification, and is a natural consequence of aging. You transform this pivotal aging factor into a longevity factor by completing all the recommendations for modifiable aging factors 1–4 and taking natural medicines that prevent and reverse glycation. This helps you maintain muscle, repair tissues, and restore organ reserve, and promotes positive genetic expression.

- **Modifiable Aging Factor 6—Chronic Inflammation** is caused by wear and tear to your body from the normal activities of daily life, overexercising, infections, poor diet, and immune system malfunction. You transform this aging factor into a longevity factor with natural anti-inflammatory medicines and modulating inflammation with essential fatty acids. This keeps you free from arthritis, cardiovascular disease, and Alzheimer's disease, and protects against autoimmune conditions like rheumatoid arthritis. Normalizing chronic inflammation stops accelerated aging.

- **Modifiable Aging Factor 7—Impaired Cardiovascular Function and Sticky Blood** is caused by all of the conditions in aging factors 1–6: oxidative stress, genetic damage, accumulation of toxic chemicals and waste products, insulin resistance, abnormal protein synthesis, and chronic inflammation. Nearly all cardiovascular disease is due to faulty diet and lack of exercise. When this aging factor is transformed it becomes your key to longevity. With a strong, healthy heart, and clean, smooth-flowing blood, your entire body and brain will have an abundant supply of healthy blood. A strong heart and healthy circulation keep you alive and thinking clearly.

- **Modifiable Aging Factor 8—Declining Hormone Function** is a natural change that occurs with aging, but is influenced by stress, diet, exercise, and genetics. Once transformed through balancing the neuroendocrine system and replacing lagging hormones, this aging factor becomes a powerful longevity factor. It can even reverse some of the effects of aging.

- **Modifiable Aging Factor 9—Immune System Decline** contributes to many of the diseases associated with aging, particularly autoimmune diseases and cancer. It is caused by the repeated challenges our immune systems face over a lifetime of infections, allergic responses, and exposure to toxic substances, and is linked to declining thymic hormone production. When transformed by replacing deficient thymic hormone and taking immunity-boosting natural medicines, a well-functioning immune system keeps us from dying of these diseases.

- **Modifiable Aging Factor 10—Neurodegeneration** is caused by declining neurotransmitter levels, reduced regeneration of nerve cells in the brain, lower hormone levels, and oxidative damage. We transform this aging factor into a longevity factor by taking nootrophics, exercising regularly, reducing inflammation, and keeping our heart strong. A revitalized brain improves our thinking, memory, and mood, and prevents Alzheimer's. Neuro-regeneration allows you to enjoy the physical benefits of the *Prolonging Health* program during an extended life span.

In this chapter, I present eight more recommendations to help you master the ten modifiable aging factors and achieve maximum longevity. Before we discuss these final recommendations, by way of an inspiring example, let me introduce you to another of my patients.

Trisha was referred to me by her medical doctor for natural hormone balancing. At the time of her first visit she was 64 and had few physical complaints other than occasional low back pain. She was taking Premarin and Provera, and a prescription-strength pain reliever and an anti-inflammatory for her back pain. She told me that her goal was to be drug free and that she wanted to take only natural hormones.

After her physical examination, I ordered blood and saliva tests. These included a complete chemistry panel, blood counts, homocysteine, insulin, DHEA-S, estradiol, progesterone, testosterone, IGF-I, and sex hormone binding globulin. Her chemistry and blood counts were within the normal reference ranges, but her homocysteine was slightly elevated at 11.6 μmol/L. Even on Premarin and Provera, her estradiol and progesterone levels were below optimal. This made it relatively easy for me to switch her to natural hormones without having to gradually taper her off her prescription-strength hormones.

Her DHEA-S level was 128 µg/dL and her testosterone was 55 ng/dL. These were not too bad for her age, but the DHEA-S left room for improvement. Her insulin levels were low at 3.5 µIU/mL, but this was in her favor, as I didn't have to treat her for insulin resistance. Her morning salivary cortisol level was 7.5 ng/mL, which was just over the reference range (1–6 ng/dL). This suggested that her adrenal glands might be slightly overactive in response to stress. Her IGF-I levels were below the optimal range and her sex hormone binding globulin was within the reference range.

My initial program included natural tri-est and progesterone creams, melatonin, oral DHEA, a multivitamin formula, extra calcium, folic acid, licorice root extract, and ginkgo extract. Six months later, her cortisol levels had improved and were in the middle of the reference range. Her insulin levels had improved and her steroid sex hormones were beginning to balance, with increases in estradiol, progesterone, and DHEA-S, along with a slight decrease in her testosterone. She reported feeling considerably better, had more energy, and was not taking any pain medications.

The next year, I repeated the same tests and added thyroid tests (TSH, T3, free T3, T4, and free T4). I also increased the dosage of pregnenolone, which was well below the optimal range. Her thyroid test results were within acceptable ranges, but her free T3 was just below the optimal range. Her homocysteine has dropped to 7.3 µmol/L. Her cholesterol was 170 mg/dL, triglycerides 47 mg/dL, HDL at 94 mg/dL, and LDL at 68 mg/dL. Her cholesterol/HDL ratio was 1.8 and her triglyc-

eride/HDL ratio was 0.5. Her fasting glucose was 79 mg/dL. Her estradiol, progesterone, and testosterone levels were continuing to improve.

These improved, balanced values along with a continued increase in energy are what I look for in my patients. Trisha's biological age was dropping, she was not near the metabolic critical point, and she was moving out of the aging zone. I increased the dosage of pregnenolone to her regimen, and soon she reported that she was feeling better than she had in years, that her sex life was like that of a younger woman, and that she had started taking Pilates classes.

The third year, I repeated all of her tests. Her pregnenolone levels were climbing, her DHEA-S levels were in the upper end of the optimal range, sex hormone binding globulin was within range, testosterone remained strong, her IGF-I level had doubled from the initial testing, free T3 had improved, and her progesterone level was within the optimal ranges. I was disappointed in her estradiol levels, which had fallen somewhat, so I recommended that she increase her tri-est dosage. Her cholesterol and other blood lipids continued to be in the optimal ranges. I also ordered C-reactive protein and a sedimentation rate. These were well within the normal reference ranges.

Now at age 66, Trisha's health continues to improve. She exercises regularly and is gaining muscle mass and tone. She is energetic, has an active sex life, and is not at risk for any disease. My prognosis is that she'll continue to improve and remain healthy well into her seventies. It's possible that at that time to maintain her level of health she may require growth hormone and an increasing amount of nutritional supplements. But for now, she's an example of the principles and practices of *Prolonging Health* in action.

Prolonging Health Recommendation 84— Work with Your Doctor

One of your greatest resources in your *Prolonging Health* program is your doctor. When you approach your health seriously, so will your doctor. You may prefer to use the services of a specialized anti-aging clinic (see the appendix). However, anti-aging medicine can be expensive, so I suggest that you enlist your family doctor or internist as a partner in your health program.

Share your goals and plans with your doctor. Demonstrate your willingness to take responsibility for your own health. This may mean that you will have some out-of-pocket expenses not covered by your medical insurance. Don't overwhelm your doctor with questions and demands. Be respectful of his or her time and be patient. Emphasize to your doctor your commitment to the philosophy of natural medicine, but also your willingness to cooperate in the spirit of integrative medicine. However, don't be misled by the promises made about possible new drugs for age-related conditions. Medical solutions to aging are not as simple as some would have us believe.

Jeffrey Bland, Ph.D. says (Bland 2002), "The solution to overcoming age-related chronic disease is not in finding the single cause of each one; it lies instead in better describing the system of antecedents and triggers that result in changes in mediator molecules producing specific symptoms in each patient." Bland's statement informs us that there is no "magic bullet" that will turn back the clock of aging or eradicate chronic degenerative disease in a single pharmaceutical action. Instead, by creating and living a lifestyle that promotes health and prevents disease and then working at the molecular and cellular level with natural medications, you are most likely to prolong your health and promote longevity.

Regardless of what anti-aging claims a natural medicine or drug makes, it is necessary that it be effective. Here are my criteria for anti-aging medicines. To qualify as anti-aging medicine, substances must meet #5, and at least three of the other four parameters (#1–4):

1. The medicine must have preventative effects for age-related or late-onset diseases (diabetes, arthritis, cancer, and cardiovascular, Alzheimer's, Parkinson's, and autoimmune diseases).

2. The medicine must have disease modification effects (reducing symptoms, altering trajectory, halting progression, and minimizing complications including risk cofactors and co-pathology of age-related conditions).

3. The medicine must have regenerative effects and reverse age-related diseases.

4. The medicine must improve the biomarker profile and lower biological age.

5. The medicine must be safe (not trigger negative genetic expression or cause cancer).

If you are proactive, informed, and successful in preventing disease and prolonging health, your blood tests will show this and the physical examinations performed by your doctor will support it. However, it is up to you to demonstrate this to your doctor. When you do this, your doctor is more likely to cooperate with you when you request specialized blood tests and prescriptions for hormones.

In the event that your family doctor will not work with you, find one who will. Medical licensing and scope of practices for the different medical specialties vary by state. In some (Arizona, Oregon, Washington), naturopathic physicians (N.D.s) can prescribe hormones and all natural substances. In other states, only licensed M.D.s can practice medicine, while some license osteopathic physicians (D.O.s). In a few states (Florida, New Mexico), acupuncturists and doctors of Oriental Medicine (O.M.D.s) can order lab tests, prescribe natural medications, and perform injection therapies. Ask your family doctor for a referral or request a referral from a medical association whose members practice anti-aging medicine (see the appendix for a list of medical organizations).

Prolonging Health Recommendation 85— Individualize Your Program

The hallmark of integrative longevity medicine is individualized therapy. Effective dosages of nutrients, hormones, and longevity medicines vary according to individual needs and metabolism. Blood and other laboratory testing provides valuable clinical information that helps individualize

> *The hallmark of integrative longevity medicine is individualized therapy. Effective dosages of nutrients, hormones, and longevity medicines vary according to individual needs and metabolism. Blood and other laboratory testing provides valuable clinical information that helps individualize therapies that are best for you.*

therapies that are best for you. Genetic testing is also helpful, and though not perfected for this purpose yet, several genetic markers are available to help individualize your program. It takes experience and intuition to individualize your program, so discuss your needs and requirements with your doctor and, if possible, work with a naturopathic physician or other doctor knowledgeable in individualizing health plans.

Adverse reactions can occur, especially when using hormones. When your doctor prescribes hormones, be sure to monitor your levels with regular blood testing. Evaluate changes in your energy, mood, and body composition. Know what the common side effects are for each hormone. Remember, many paradoxical effects are associated with hormones, such as when using growth hormone, estrogen, cortisol, and insulin. Avoid raising your hormone levels above the optimal physiological ranges. The goal of hormone replacement is not simply to reach higher levels of a specific hormone but to achieve overall neuroendocrine balance.

You may accomplish this by reducing levels of the catabolic hormones insulin and cortisol; improving levels of the growth-promoting anabolic hormones, especially growth hormone, IGF-I, DHEA, and testosterone; and providing sufficient amounts of the protective hormones pregnenolone and progesterone (in women). If you are successful, levels of your hormone-binding proteins (SHBC and albumin) and free hormones (free testosterone, free T3) will normalize.

Individualize your nutritional supplements. Take only as much as you need to achieve results. Check your levels of vitamin E, vitamin C, coenzyme Q10, and selenium to see if you are getting enough of these important antioxidants. Check your vitamin B_{12} and folate levels. Folic acid is among the most important nutrients for the prevention of aging. Based on your body weight, take lower dosages if you are smaller; take large dosages if you are a big person.

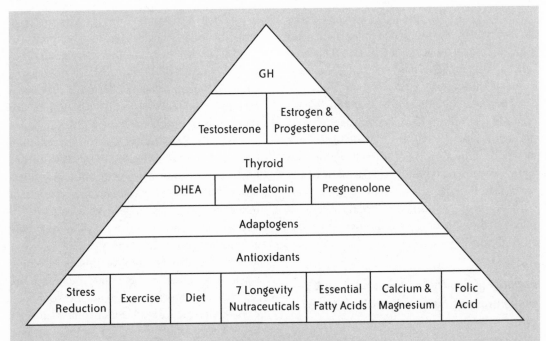

Prolonging Health Pyramid

Your *Prolonging Health* program works best when individually designed and applied comprehensively. Start with a foundation in a healthy lifestyle and include the seven longevity nutraceuticals; add antioxidants, adaptogens; then melatonin, DHEA, and pregnenolone. Add other hormones if you test low: thyroid and balance the male and female sex hormones. Growth hormone (GH) is the capstone. Use it last and only if you test low.

Prolonging Health Recommendation 86— Lower Your Biological Age and Maintain Your Age-Point

In order to resist aging, you have to remain biologically young. This is referred to as your biological age, as compared to your chronological age based on your birth date. Lowering your biological age is accomplished by improving your cardiovascular health, maintaining a high muscle-mass to body-fat ratio, and bringing levels of key hormones into the youthful range. When you accomplish this, you lower your biological age. This facilitates homeostasis and helps you maintain your age-point. To determine your progress, complete the age-point questionnaire at least once every three

months. Remember, there is no prolonging of your health without lowering your biological age, and reaching and maintaining your age-point.

Prolonging Health Recommendation 87— Avoid Your Metabolic Critical Point and Stay Out of the Aging Zone

The balance between normal and dysfunctional insulin utilization and glucose regulation is crucial in your *Prolonging Health* program. It affects your metabolic function, and without a healthy and balanced metabolism, you will most likely age more rapidly. Don't underestimate its importance. Keep your insulin levels under 10 µIU/mL and your fasting glucose less than 90 mg/dL and optimally between 78 and 85. By preventing metabolic imbalance, you avoid your metabolic critical point. This prevents a wide range of diseases and allows you to stay within the aging zone.

However, it is imperative that you remain out of or just within the aging zone, and not on the aging side. If you are already past your metabolic critical point and well within the aging zone, then you must reverse many of the aging factors. Keep your insulin, glucose, and cortisol levels within the optimal ranges. Improve the function of your pancreas and adrenal glands.

Prolonging Health Recommendation 88— Make Prolonging Your Health a Way of Life

It is necessary to practice the *Prolonging Health* recommendations and follow the longevity strategies all your life. Otherwise, your progress will be undermined and you will likely lose the gains you've made. Exercise regularly, take your nutrients, and use hormones wisely. Have annual checkups with your doctor, and get your blood tested. If you're very healthy, get checked at least once every two to four years. Make the *Prolonging Health* program a way of life.

Prolonging Health Recommendation 89— Emphasize Four Key Factors for Longevity

Not every factor, strategy, or therapy discussed in this book is of equal importance. Some are more important than others, and some are necessary for certain individuals and not for others. However, there are general principles and several key factors that apply to everyone. I've covered the principles in detail

in the ten modifiable aging factors and five longevity strategies. For those who prefer to keep it simple, here are four key factors that you cannot overlook. Longevity is associated with low insulin, healthy liver function, and high folic acid and melatonin levels. Emphasize these in your program. Here's a quick review:

Insulin Sensitivity: You cannot maintain optimal body composition, be healthy, or live long without normal insulin function (see chapter 10). It encompasses so many areas that influence aging and longevity, such that if you were to make improving your insulin sensitivity a priority you would greatly prolong your health. You can accomplish this by avoiding sugar and refined carbohydrates, eating more low glycemic index foods, reducing your total calories derived from all carbohydrates, increasing protein, and practicing periodic caloric restriction. Regular exercise helps improve insulin sensitivity, but avoid excessive exercise and exclusively performing aerobic forms of exercise such as running, aerobic dance, and spin classes. Take enough vitamin C, chromium, lipoic acid, and coenzyme Q10.

Liver Function: The liver is a key organ in your *Prolonging Health* program. It helps metabolize glucose and hormones and is the main organ of detoxification in your body. Without a healthy liver, you won't live long and your quality of life will be reduced. Practice detoxification (see chapter 9) and take liver protective substances such as milk thistle and chelidonium. Don't overeat and practice periodic caloric restriction. Get regular exercise. Avoid prescription and over-the-counter drugs that are toxic to the liver.

Folic Acid: Don't underestimate the power of this member of the B-vitamin family. You can obtain enough folic acid from your diet from eating green leafy vegetables, but optimal dosages require supplementation. If you were to take only one vitamin supplement, it should be folic acid. Take 400 mcg daily of L-5-methyl-tetrahydrofolate (the active form of folate in the body and a safe nutritional substance) and 400 mcg of folic acid daily. You can take as much as 5–10 mg of folic acid daily if you also take vitamin B_{12}.

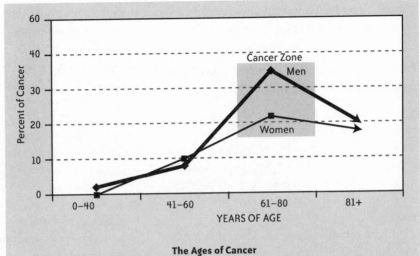

The Ages of Cancer

The incidence of cancer increases in both men and women as they age. But, beyond age 80, the incidence plateaus and may even fall.

Melatonin:

Research has shown that the only hormone that goes up during calorie restriction is melatonin. The test animals that lived longer had lower hormone values of nearly every major and minor hormone with the exception of melatonin. For a still unknown reason, longevity is associated with an increase in melatonin synthesis. You can improve melatonin production naturally by getting at least four hours of daylight exposure each day and sleeping in a darkened and quiet room for seven to nine hours each night. If you were to take only one hormone, I recommend melatonin. Take 0.5–3 mg each night, after the lights go out and just before going to sleep.

Prolonging Health Recommendation 90—Prevent Cancer

If you are successful in mastering the ten modifiable aging factors, you may be able to prevent the main causes of accelerated aging and early death. You may also prevent cancer by following these same recommendations.

However, you must remain vigilant against cancer. As you age and your immune system declines, your chances of developing cancer increase greatly. If you use hormone replacement therapy improperly or take too much of it, you may increase your risk of cancer. Exposure to toxic chemical substances at any time in your life may trigger cancer activity in your body.

Early detection is valuable but is not a replacement for prevention. If you are age 50 or older, consider these diagnostic tools to detect early signs of cancer. Have a mammogram (for women) and prostate sonogram (for men); have a whole body CT scan with contrast dye; take the cancer marker blood tests. Discuss with your doctor other tests such as a colonoscopy for intestinal polyps.

Boost your immune system (see chapter 15); regulate your neuroendocrine system and don't abuse anti-aging hormone therapies (see chapter 14); take antioxidants (see chapter 7) and guard your DNA against damage (see chapter 8); practice regular detoxification (see chapter 9); and eat a healthy diet and practice periodic caloric restriction (see chapter 17).

Prolonging Health Recommendation 91— Achieve Maximum Longevity

Science focuses on the biological mechanisms that cause aging in hopes of answering the question of what aging is and what causes it. However, those who are aging want to know what to do. Their question is: can *my* aging be controlled even if science doesn't know what causes it?

There is considerable evidence that it can, and that has been the topic of this book. As I've described in the previous chapters, though scientists have found what they think are longevity genes, most likely there is no one particular longevity or death gene that turns on or off at a set time in our lives. If there were, we would stay youthful considerably longer than we do, and probably age more quickly.

Starting at a young age, we age slowly over time and, as I've explained, aging is influenced by numerous biological, environmental, genetic, and other factors. Therefore, to effectively resist aging, we have to exert a positive influence on as many of the ten modifiable factors associated with aging as we can. Once we've done that, we have to prevent cancer. If we can do that, barring accidents, we will likely live out our natural life span. What if we want to live longer? What is the upper limit of the human life span?

By following the advice presented in this book, and with favorable genes, I am confident that some people can live to 95 or 100. We know that it is possible for a human to live about 120 years. Some researchers, such as Steven Austad, Ph.D., believe the upper limit is 150, or greater. Therefore, theoretically speaking, if the rate by which we age is malleable, and

if we can positively influence how we age by modifying those factors that accelerate aging and contribute to the degenerative diseases associated with aging, we should be able to become supercentenarians. However, do these practices guarantee that we will live longer?

Though there is no guarantee about anything in life, it is reasonable to assume that by positively influencing the trajectory of aging, it is possible that we can live to 150 or longer. It follows that if we improve and maintain physiological function, we should age more slowly. However, even if we master the ten modifiable aging factors and transform them into longevity benefits, and defeat cancer, if we continue to age we would probably shrivel down to nothing. Is there a point at which aging stops? Can we be immortal?

Though the desire to extend life beyond nature's limits is as strong as ever, the elixir of immortality continues to elude us. The desire to discover the Fountain of Youth and to search for immortality is universal among humans. This quest is lodged in our subconscious and we are reminded of it by those who took up the search: Eastern yogis and Taoists, medieval alchemists, the Spanish conquistador Ponce de Leon, and in our own times scientists, anti-aging doctors, and life extensionists. All have contributed to our knowledge of the practice of resisting aging.

Michael R. Rose, Ph.D., a professor of evolutionary biology at the University of California at Irvine, is a leading researcher in aging and a proponent of immortality. Dr. Rose proposes that in our early to mid-nineties, our chances of getting cancer or dying from the diseases associated with aging diminish greatly and eventually disappear (Rauser 2003; Rose 2000). That leaves us with only old age. However, it is biologically feasible that a biologic and metabolic equilibrium could be achieved. In this scenario, further aging is postponed and our life span extends towards yet unknown limits.

The desire to live long is universal and timeless. Effective ways to prolong health and resist aging exist. Since aging is a complex process, the method of resisting aging must be comprehensive and integrated. Start with well-defined goals, then establish specific criteria for reaching those goals. Find a cooperative doctor, or a team of alternative and conventional doctors, and work with them to order your blood tests and to prescribe bio-identical hormones.

As a rule, you should retest your hormones at least once a year. Use more frequently the self-evaluation tools discussed in part 1. Restoring and prolonging your health is a gradual process, but to achieve maximum longevity you must first head in the right direction.

Summary of *Prolonging Health* Recommendations for Mastering the Ten Modifiable Factors of Longevity

- *Prolonging Health* Recommendation 84— **Work with Your Doctor:** Your doctor is one of the greatest resources in your *Prolonging Health* program. When you approach your health seriously, so will your doctor.

- *Prolonging Health* Recommendation 85— **Individualize Your Program:** A hallmark of integrative longevity medicine is individualized therapy. Effective dosages of nutrients, hormones, and longevity medicines vary according to individual needs and metabolism. Work with a naturopathic physician or other doctor knowledgeable in individualizing health plans.

- *Prolonging Health* Recommendation 86— **Lower Your Biological Age and Maintain Your Age-Point:** To resist aging, you have to remain biologically young. There is no prolonging of your health without lowering your biological age, and reaching and maintaining your age-point.

- *Prolonging Health* Recommendation 87— **Avoid Your Metabolic Critical Point and Stay Out of the Aging Zone:** Without a healthy and balanced metabolism, you will age more rapidly. By preventing metabolic imbalance, you do not unfavorably tip your metabolic critical point. Keep your insulin, glucose, and cortisol levels within the optimal ranges.

- *Prolonging Health* Recommendation 88— **Make Prolonging Your Health a Way of Life:** Continue practicing the *Prolonging Health* recommendations and following the longevity strategies on a lifelong basis.

- *Prolonging Health* Recommendation 89— **Emphasize Four Key Factors for Longevity:** Not every factor, strategy, or therapy discussed in this book is of equal importance. Each requires an individualized approach for optimal effectiveness. However, there are several key factors that apply to everyone. Make sure that you emphasize these in your program:

  Insulin Sensitivity: You cannot maintain optimal body composition, be healthy, or live long without normal insulin function. Make improving your insulin sensitivity a priority.

  Liver Function: The liver is a key organ in your *Prolonging Health* program. Without a healthy liver, you won't live long and your quality of life will be reduced.

  Folic Acid: Don't underestimate the power of folic acid. If you were to take only one vitamin supplement, it should be folic acid.

  Melatonin: Longevity is associated with an increase in melatonin synthesis. If you take only one hormone, take melatonin.

- *Prolonging Health* Recommendation 90— **Prevent Cancer:** Remain vigilant against cancer.

- *Prolonging Health* Recommendation 91— **Achieve Maximum Longevity:** By positively influencing the trajectory of aging, it is possible that we can live to 150 or longer.

The 91 *Prolonging*

1 Complete the Biomarker Questionnaire

2 Determine Your Body Measurements

3 Use Common Laboratory Tests As Biomarkers

4 Get Your Second Level Anti-Aging Diagnostics Done

5 Evaluate Your Hormone Levels

6 Determine Your Antioxidant, Vitamin, and Mineral Status

7 Know the Condition of Your Immune System

8 Take Five More Tests to Evaluate Your Health: Chronic Inflammation, Mitochondrial Function, Genomic Status, Neurotransmitter Profiles, and Toxicology Studies

9 Complete the Age-Point Questionnaire

10 Eat Foods Rich in Antioxidants

11 Get an ORAC Blood Test

12 Take Antioxidant Supplements

13 Restore Your Glutathione

14 Get an 8-Hydroxydeoxyguanosine (8-OHdG) Test

15 Repair Your DNA with Natural Medicines

16 Follow the Five Rules of Therapeutic Detoxification

17 Follow the Five Prescriptions for Effective Detoxification

18 Get Your Insulin and Glucose Levels Tested

19 Improve Your Insulin Sensitivity with Smart Dietary Changes

20 Restore Your Insulin Sensitivity with Nutritional Supplements

21 Improve Your Liver Function to Restore Normal Glucose Metabolism

22 Consume a Regenerative Protein Supplement

23 Take Vitamin B_6 and Other Synergistic Nutrients with Your Protein Supplement

24 Take Carnosine

25 Get Tested for Chronic Inflammation

26 Avoid Foods That Promote Inflammation

27 Consume Foods That Reduce Inflammation

28 Take Probiotics

29 Take Fish Oil

30 Get Enough Folic Acid, Vitamin B_6, and Vitamin B_{12}

31 Take TMG

32 Take Niacinamide

33 Use Red Yeast Rice Extract

34 Take Anti-Inflammatory Herbs

35 Eat a Better Diet

36 Get Some Exercise

37 Reduce Your Stress

38 Lose Some Weight

39 Take Nutrients That Improve Cardiovascular Homeostasis

40 Take Herbs That Improve Cardiovascular Health

41 Get Your Hormones Tested

42 Improve Insulin Signaling with Nutritional Medications

43 Achieve Neuroendocrine Balance by Neutralizing Excess Cortisol

44 Achieve Neuroendocrine Balance by Restoring Synchronicity with Melatonin

Health Recommendations

19 Final Thoughts on Prolonging Your Health

Ultimately, to truly understand aging, we must, biologically speaking, understand life. But that is no easy task. The "big" question in science, says Mae-Wan Ho, Ph.D., a distinguished researcher in the physics of organisms at the Open University in Milton Keynes, England, is this: "What is life?" Ho proposes that "life must reside in the patterns of dynamic flow of matter and energy that somehow makes the organisms alive, enabling them to grow, develop and evolve" (Ho 1998).

It is these underlying patterns that we work with in *Prolonging Health* by improving neuroendocrine balance, resetting the biological clock, reducing inflammation, improving blood circulation and heart function, and all of the other aspects of health and aging we've discussed—mastering these help us live longer.

But just living longer is not enough. We must be healthy enough to continue to pursue our dreams; everyone, older people especially, need productive roles in society. In traditional cultures, elders are revered as repositories of wisdom; in some indigenous cultures, whose histories extend tens of thousands of years into the past, this wisdom is substantial.

Modern Western culture, on the other hand, has no model to compare with such lineages that reach into antiquity. What will large numbers of long-lived older people in the future do? Where will they go?

In a letter to the journal *Nature* in 2001, Jared Diamond, M.D., says our survival through 99.9 percent of human history has depended on information passed on through memory and verbal knowledge (Diamond 2001). Animals are largely instinctual, and are governed by genetic traits and conditioning. Humans, on the other hand, rely largely on information transmitted by the spoken word, by writing, and now by electronic transmission through the television and Internet.

Modern people will rely more on electronic and published information rather than turning to the traditional repositories of wisdom—our elders. But, does the current form of information provide us with the wisdom necessary for continued survival? Is more information, divorced from the natural element of human wisdom, the next step in human evolution? Where will it lead us?

Ken Dychtwald, Ph.D., says in *Age Power* that we need more "elder heroes," in whom advanced age is empowering rather than debilitating (Dychtwald 1999). Dr. Dychtwald paints a similar picture in his earlier book, *Age Wave*. In it age is associated with ascending evolution instead of the descending spiral of degeneration that typically accompanies aging (Dychtwald 1990).

What Dr. Dychtwald and others have realized is that only with age do special human qualities and abilities develop. Will such qualities as wisdom, so cherished by traditional cultures, blossom among the bio-enhanced and narcissistic life extensionists?

Wisdom is not simply a by-product of the biological aging process. Such abilities occur gradually, subtly, and over decades, as the fruit of experiences lived and endured by a body that is capable of withstanding the events of time and aging, and in one who has prolonged his physical and mental health into advanced age.

Eastern sages suggest that this combination of prolonged health and longevity is possible. In the modern West, we have seen examples of this in Mother Theresa, former U.S. president Jimmy Carter, and the naturopathic physician Hazel Parcells, who lived to be 103 (Dispenza 1997). From that vantage point, individuals who have aged well can serve society by bestowing their insight and wisdom if such wisdom is cherished by future generations. In such an individual, an extended adulthood becomes one of continual self-renewal.

Frederic M. Hudson, Ph.D., in *Mastering the Art of Self-Renewal*, suggests that a self-renewing adult is a reflection of a resilient society (Hudson 1999). If that is true, then perhaps a large number of healthy older people with full mental and emotional faculties will promote a new social order and reconstruct the ecological mistakes of past generations. Dr. Hudson organizes the qualities of such an elder into ten characteristics: they commit to values and purposes, connect to the world around them, require solitude and quiet, know how to pace themselves, value contact with nature, are cre-

ative, are playful, adapt to change, are always in training, and are future oriented.

This is very different, perhaps even suggestive of a transcendent difference, from the search for panaceas and the imaginary benefits of anti-aging techniques so prevalent today. It is a deepening of the values that make us human. It is the distillation of human character passed on generationally, not merely information, that may restore our culture.

In light of this, I suggest that a new theory of gerotranscendence is developing, one that offers a perspective very different from the one found in the West for the last several hundred years. It is similar to the ageless wisdom of the East, but it is not Eastern philosophy that will eventually ignite such a movement. The experiential nature of living beyond cultural expectations and living beyond biological limitations is what will change our way of aging.

Lars Tornstam, Ph.D., of Uppsala University in Sweden, suggests that there is a contemplative dimension to older age, characterized by alterations in how we perceive time and space, the disappearance of the fear of death, the seeing of immortality as in the genetic chain and not in our individual body, and an acceptance of the mystery of life and death (Tornstam 1997). The importance of self, so overwhelmingly demanding in early and mid-adult life, falls away like the wearing out of old but comfortable shoes. In its place is the realization that all of the events in one's life are patterned as a whole rather than being individual fragmented events, a mosaic of events and memories.

But more than that, gerotranscendence is not the monk's cloistered life of contemplation on fixed forms of belief, or the yogi's physical gymnastics and breath control, but more like a wandering Taoist. Nature becomes more important, as do simple things like children's laughter, or living another day of life. Perhaps it is this ability to live more in the present moment that brings happiness and a sense of wonder.

Wrinkles and creases, suggests James Hillman, Ph.D., the distinguished Jungian psychologist and professor, in *The Force of Character and the Lasting Life,* are not merely signs of aging, but lines that define character (Hillman 1999).

Perhaps the gerotranscendental elders of the next 40 to 60 years will not only introduce the unknown back into the scientifically narrow definition of the known, but will also pick up where Henry David Thoreau left off and guide us away from the brink of ecological disaster into a brave and good new world.

Though a unified theory of aging remains elusive, I propose that prolonging health is possible by following an effective, safe, and comprehensive integrated longevity program. In doing so, you can most likely remain free of disease and live a long and productive life. The recommendations in this book will help you prolong your health and may help you attain the age of 90 or more. From there, you are pioneering the way towards the upper limits of human life span.

Appendix A
Finding the Right Doctor to Oversee
Your *Prolonging Health* Program

It is difficult to say exactly what makes the "right" doctor, but the right doctor is the one who helps you get better. The second best doctor is one who does not make you worse, and refers you to the right doctor. The third best is one who makes you feel better by managing your symptoms, but is not able to actually resolve your condition.

If you are reasonably healthy and are going for an annual physical exam, need an acupuncturist to treat a knee strain, or a chiropractor to work on a stiff neck, you need only to find the doctor who provides you with the best service for the most reasonable fee. It is largely a matter of shopping the phone book, your insurance company's physician directory, or calling a referral service. This, however, is the wrong approach when looking for a doctor who specializes in anti-aging and longevity medicine.

Prolonging your health and treating diseases that arise during aging are serious matters. For this you need the best doctor available, one who is knowledgeable about *your* specific condition and individual needs, has the time and willingness to work with *you*—a person you can trust and develop a professional rapport with over several years.

Patients are often the worst judge of who is the right doctor. Though there is no guarantee that you will chose the right doctor on the first try, here are a few rules you can apply when looking for the right doctor.

Interview Carefully: Since aging is an ongoing process, you may be seeing the same doctor every few months in the beginning and then once or twice a year. At the time of your first visit or interview, consider asking a few questions as a way of interviewing a doctor. Ask if she has had a similar condition. What made her choose this area to specialize in? Doctors see many patients day after day and an astute physician knows who gets better and what medications and therapies tend to work better than others. Ask what her success rate is. Is she comfortable working as part of a team with alternative medicine practitioners?

Remember you want to know what *her* clinical success rate is and not the statistics because the research studies were not performed on *you*.

Show Respect: Keep in mind that the healing profession is very stressful. Do not be overly demanding or confrontational with your doctor. If she turns out to be the right doctor, you want her to think of you as an intelligent, informed, and concerned patient who will cooperate with care, rather than a difficult and stubborn patient who asks endless questions that waste time. Be on time for your visits. Be patient and understanding if your doctor is late, but inform her that your time is as valuable as hers and you expect to be treated with consideration.

Don't Assume Your Doctor Knows Everything: Many people make the mistake, based upon another medical myth that doctors are akin to deity, of thinking that their doctor knows everything. After all, the doctor is just another person like you, who may also have experienced an illness, who will age, who pays bills and taxes. If you get nervous with the doctor and later remember questions you wanted to ask, prepare a short list before you go in for your next visit. Do not bring in a packed page of questions or make it a habit of calling after your visit to ask questions that would have been much better answered while you were there. Both of these annoy and frustrate doctors.

Listen Carefully: When you ask questions, listen to your doctor's answers carefully. Ask him to write instructions down for you if you have a hard time remembering details. In my practice, being used to the memory loss and concentration difficulties many patients have with chronic illness and during aging, I explain the reasons for my treatments, summarize them, and write them down for the patient. Sometimes in a complex case, I also type out a summary and mail it to the patient.

Reveal Information: It is important to have a relationship with your doctor that is open and frank, with respect on your end and empathy on hers. Do not withhold information about other treatments, self-prescribed medications, or other therapies you are doing. If your medical doctor is opposed to alternative therapies, inquire on what grounds she bases this opinion. If her answer does not satisfy you, look for another doctor.

The same holds true for alternative medicine practitioners. If she is against allopathic medicine, you will find it difficult to communicate effectively on issues that involve medical intervention and drug therapy, and if you need a referral or are faced with a medical emergency, you will be unsupported.

If stress plays a key role in your illness, make sure you reveal this to your doctor, but don't expect her to listen to your personal problems for the whole of your visit. Save that for your therapist or psychologist.

Keep Your Doctor Informed: Tell her what you're doing to prolong your health, but don't overwhelm her with every detail about every acupuncture session or what the clerk in the health food store told you last week. It is a good idea to write out all the supplements you are taking so there is a copy in your file; update it periodically. Likewise, keep your alternative practitioner advised on what drugs you are taking but don't expect him to answer questions on prescription medications that your medical doctor has ordered. Ask the nurse, the prescribing medical doctor, or the dispensing pharmacist questions concerning pharmaceutical drugs, but don't expect your medical doctor to know everything about vitamins. Save those questions for your naturopath or nutritionist.

It is acceptable to provide your doctor with literature and information that you are reading. However, do not overwhelm him with books, and especially do not confront him with marketing pieces from nutritional companies advertising the latest cure for whatever ails you. Select sources that are related to your condition and make copies of parts of articles or highlight a paragraph or two that you think he might find interesting or that you would like him to comment on. Remember, you are there to access the doctor's expertise and not to confuse the issues of your case with extraneous information.

On Self-Care and Second Opinions: In this book, you have been introduced to several methods of treatment, different conventional and alternative medicine styles, and some Chinese medicine. There is competition among these different methods, all competing for the same health care dollar. Unless you have a referral from a trusted source, approach your medical care as you would any other business arrangement, adequately prepared and with care.

This book provides information for self-care, which is very different from care provided by a medical practitioner. You are responsible for reading the material carefully, reading the additional recommended literature, asking questions of your health care providers, making decisions on what natural medications might best suit your condition, obtaining these medications, and then adding them into your treatment schedule.

You may want to consider the option of "guided self-care" where you work with a natural medicine-oriented physician to order lab tests and monitor your progress. This objective second opinion can be invaluable in a long-term program. Do not hesitate to seek a third opinion if you or your doctor are feeling confused or you do not think you are making sufficient progress.

A Note to Your Doctor: Your patient has read my book on how to prolong their health and prevent the major diseases associated with aging. In it, I discuss the science behind the many theories of aging and present self-directed recommendations and strategies using natural medicines and bio-identical hormones.

The information contained in this book is garnered from 20 years of clinical practice, tens of thousands of patient visits, and thousands of hours of research. Knowing that my audience would include not only lay readers, but professionals like yourself, I extensively investigated and documented the material in this book with research from authoritative books, interviews with the principal scientists in the field, and prestigious medical and scientific journals. Indeed, I left out hundreds of other articles solely for the sake of space and time.

Though this book is meant to help patients navigate the complex issue of anti-aging medicine and to treat many of the conditions of aging on their own, it is not meant to replace the advice, guidance, and medical abilities of a physician. The material contained in this book is not meant to be used by your patient to challenge your practice of medicine. It is solely intended to help your patient improve their chances of preventing degenerative diseases and prolonging their health.

Appendix B
Physician-Administered and -Prescribed Therapies

Though this book provides self-directed treatments using natural medicine for conditions that may occur during aging, it is not a manual on how to specifically treat age-related diseases. Most of the medications and nutrients recommended are available without a doctor's prescription. However, for some you will need the assistance of a medical doctor (M.D.), doctor of osteopathy (D.O.), or in some states a doctor of naturopathic medicine (N.D.), all of whom have prescribing privileges. The following list includes some of the medications that require a physician's prescription:

- Antibiotics
- Antiviral drugs
- Armour and other thyroid hormones
- Estrogens
- Human growth hormone
- Hydrocortisone
- Injectable echinacea, homotoxicology medications, and Iscador
- Injectable thymus extract
- Intravenous vitamins, minerals, and amino acids
- Testosterone

Appendix C
Resources

To the best of my knowledge, all the resources listed here have extensive experience in anti-aging medicine, hormone replacement therapy, and the conditions discussed in this book. I neither endorse them nor have financial connections with them, and am not responsible for the results of any treatments or medications they may provide for you.

Doctors and Clinics:

Ageless Forever
Julio L. Garcia, MD
3017 West Charleston Blvd., Suite 70
Las Vegas, NV 89102
(702) 838-1994
http://www.agelessforever.net/aboutus.htm

The Anti-Aging Institute of San Diego
1875 Third Avenue
San Diego, CA 92102
(619) 398-2929

California Healthspan Institute
Ron Rothenberg, MD
320 Santa Fe Drive, Suite 301
Encinitas, CA 92024
(800) 943-3331
http://www.californiaantiaging.com/contact/

Cenegenics Medical Institute
851 South Rampart Blvd.
Las Vegas, NV 89145
(702) 240-4200
http://www.888younger.com

Giampapa Institute for Anti-Aging Medical Therapy
89 Valley Road
Montclair, NJ 07042
(973) 783-6868
http://www.giampapainstitute.com/index.html

Kronos Optimal Health Centre
15211 North Kierland Blvd., Suite 200
Scottsdale, AZ 85254
(866) 576-6679
http://www.kronoscompany.com

Medical Associations:

American Academy of Anti-Aging Medicine
1510 West Montana Street
Chicago, IL 60614
(773) 528-1000
http://www.worldhealth.net

American Association of Integrative Medicine
2750 East Sunshine
Springfield, MO 65804
(417) 881-9995
www.aaimedicine.com

American Association of Naturopathic Physicians
601 Valley Street, Suite 105
Seattle, WA 98109
(206) 298-0126
www.naturopathic.org

American Association of Oriental Medicine
433 Front Street
Catasauqua, PA 18032
(610) 266-1433
www.aaom.org

American Holistic Medical Association
6728 McLean Village Drive
McLean, VA 22101-8729
(703) 556-8729
www.holisticmedicine.org

American Osteopathic Association
142 East Ontario Street
Chicago, IL 60611
(800) 6211-1773
www.am-osteo-assn.org

British Association of Oriental Medicine
206-208 Latimer Road, Suite D
London, England, W10 6RE
0181-968-3469
www.demon.co.uk/acupuncture

The European Academy of Quality of Life and
Longevity Medicine
127 Avenue de l'Armée, 1040
Brussels, Belgium
(888) 878-2638
http://www.eaquall.net

National Center for Homeopathy
801 North Fairfax Street, Suite 306
Alexandria, VA 22314
www.healthy.net

Organizations:

Life Extension Foundation
P.O. Box 229120
Hollywood, FL 33022
(800) 678-8989
http://www.lef.org

Research Centers:

American Society on Aging
833 Market Street, Suite 511
San Francisco, CA 94103-182
(415) 974-9600
http://www.asaging.org

Buck Institute
8001 Redwood Blvd.
Novato, CA 94945
(415) 209-2000
http://www.buckinstitute.org

Center for Research and Education in Aging
University of California Berkeley
401 Barker Hall, UC Berkeley
Berkeley, CA 94720-3202
http://crea.berkeley.edu

Huffington Center on Aging
Baylor College of Medicine
One Baylor Plaza, M320
Houston, TX 77030
(713) 798-5804
http://www.healthandage.net

National Institute for Longevity Sciences
36-3 Gengo, Morioka
Obu, 474-8522 Aichi, Japan
http://www.nils.go.jp

National Institute on Aging
31 Center Drive, MSC 2292
Building 31, Room 5C27
Bethesda, MD 20892
(301) 496-1752
http://www.nia.nih.gov

Laboratories:

AAL Reference Laboratories
1715 East Wilshire, #715
Santa Ana, CA 92705
(800) 522-2621
www.aalrl.com

Aeron Clinical Laboratory
1933 Davis Street, Suite 310
San Leandro, CA 94577
(800) 631-7900
http://www.aeron.com

Genox Corporation
1414 Key Highway
Baltimore, MD 21230
(410) 347-7616
www.genox.com

Great Smokies Diagnostic Laboratory
63 Zillicoa Street
Asheville, NC 28801
(828) 253-0621
http://www.gsdl.com

Laboratory Corporation of American
358 South Main Street

Burlington, NC 27215
(336) 584-5171
http://www.labcorp.com

LifeScore and CancerSafe
8899 University Center Lane, Suite 100
San Diego, CA 92122
(877) 543-3726
http://www.lifescore.com
http://www.cancersafe.com

Meridian Valley Laboratory
515 West Harrison Street, Suite 9
Kent, Washington 98032
(253) 859-8700

Pantox Laboratories
4622 Santa Fe Street
San Diego, CA 92109
(888) 726-8698
www.pantox.com

Quest Diagnostics
One Malcolm Avenue
Teterboro, NJ 07608
(800) 222-0446
http://www.questdiagnostics.com

Vitamin and Natural Supplement Supplies:

Arcana Pharmacy
10820 North Torrey Pines Road
La Jolla, CA 92037
(858) 755-0288
http://www.arcanapharmacy.com

Life Factor Research
315 South Coast Hwy. 101, Suite U-6
Encinitas, CA 92024
(877) 668-5983
www.lifefactorresearch.com

Willner Chemists
100 Park Avenue
New York, NY 10017
(800) 633-1106
www.willner.com

Compounding Pharmacies:

College Pharmacy
3505 Austin Bluffs Parkway, Suite 101

Colorado Springs, CO 80918
(800) 888-9358
http://www.collegepharmacy.com

University Compounding Pharmacy
1875 Third Avenue
San Diego, CA 92101
(800) 985-8065
http://www.ucprx.com/

Physician-Dispensed Medications:

These companies distribute nutraceutical medications that your doctor will have to order for you. You cannot buy direct unless you are a health care professional.

Allergy Research carries organic germanium and other immune products: (800) 545-9960

Bezwecken manufacturers and suppliers of natural hormones to doctors: (800) 743-2256

Heel homotoxicology medications are imported from Germany by Heel/BHI: (800) 621-7644

HVS Laboratories manufactures homeopathic detoxification products: (800) 521-7722

Nutraceutics carries the growth hormone secretagogue Meditropin: (877) 664-6684

Pascoe homotoxicology medications are imported from Germany by SISU Natural Products: (877) 747-8872

Pure Encapsulations: (800)753-2277

Thorne Research produces some of the purest natural medicines available: (800) 228-1966

UltraClear Plus and other detoxification products designed by Dr. Jeffrey Bland are distributed by *Metagenics:* (800) 692-9400

Chinese Herbs:

Brion Herbs Corporation
9200 Jeronimo Road
Irvine, CA 92618
(800) 333-4372
www.sunten.com

Hepapro International
P.O. Box 7442
Laguana Niguel, CA 92677-7442
(888) 788-4372
www.hepapro.com

Mayway Corporation
1338 Mandela Parkway
Oakland, CA 94607
(800) 262-9929
www.mayway.com

Offshore Suppliers of Life-Extension Drugs:

Biogenesis Laboratories
http://www.biogenesis.co.za/index.asp

International Anti-Aging Systems
http://www.antiaging-systems.com/home1.htm

Websites:

Acupuncture.com: www.acupunture.com
The Aging Research Center (ARC):
    http://www.arclab.org/
Alternative Medicine.Com:
    www.alternativemedicine.com
American Federation for Aging Research:
    http://www.infoaging.org/bio-h.html
Anti-Aging Center, Europe:
    http://www.antiaging-europe.com/index.html
British Longevity Society:
    http://www.antiageing.freeserve.co.uk/drugs.htm

Gerontology Research Group: http://www.grg.org/
Health/Prolongevity/Anti-Aging Resources:
    http://www.aeiveos.com/resource/
LamMD:
http://www.drlam.com/opinion/ascobyl_palmitate.cfm
Maximum Life Foundation:
    http://www.maxlife.org/index.htm
National Center for Complementary and
    Alternative Medicine: www.nccam.org
Senescence Info: http://www.senescence.info/
WHO Center for Aging Studies:
    http://www.cas.flinders.edu.au/

Growth Hormone Sites:

Humatrope: http://www.humatrope.com/index.jsp
Norditropin:
    http://www.norditropinsimplexx.com/login/default.asp
Saizen: http://www.anti-aging-therapy.net/
Somatropinonline:
    http://www.somatropinonline.com/

Brain Product Sites:

Smart Nutrition: http://www.smart-drugs.com/
smart/info-ALC.htm

Appendix D
Additional Reading

Fiction:

Braver, Gary. 2000. *Elixir.* New York: Tom Doherty Associates.

Halperin, James L. 1998. *The First Immortal.* New York: Ballantine.

Hamill, Pete. 2003. *Forever.* Boston: Little, Brown and Company.

Jones, Gwyneth. 1998. *Phoenix Cafe.* New York: Tom Doherty Associates.

Wilde, Oscar. 1998. *The Picture of Dorian Gray.* New York: The Modern Library.

Hormone Balancing:

Hertoghe, Thierry. 2002. *The Hormone Solution.* New York: Harmony Books.

Schwarzbein, Diana. 2002. *The Schwarzbein Principle II.* Deerfield Beach, Florida: Health Communications.

Ullis, Karlis. 1999. *Age Right.* New York: Simon & Schuster.

Science:

Masoro, Edward J, and Steven J Austad, eds. 2001. *Handbook of the Biology of Aging.* 5th ed. San Diego: Academic Press.

Rose, Michael R. 1991. *Evolutionary Biology of Aging.* London: Oxford University Press.

Schulz-Aellen, Marie-Françoise. 1997. *Aging and Human Longevity.* Boston: Birkhauser.

Shostak, Stanley. 2002. *Becoming Immortal: Combining Cloning and Stem Cell Therapy.* Albany, New York: State University of New York Press.

Stock, Gregory. 2002. *Redesigning Humans: Our Inevitable Genetic Future.* Boston: Houghton Mifflin Company.

Endnotes

1. Consilience is a term used by the Harvard entomologist Edward O. Wilson to describe a merging of ideas between the social sciences and the mathematical sciences.

2. http://www.orentreich.org/

3. http://www.senescence.info/

4. The Life Extension Foundation: 1100 West Commercial Blvd., Fort Lauderdale, FL, 33309; http://www.lef.org/

5. http://www.cdc.gov/nccdphp/dnpa/bmi/bmi-adult-formula.htm

6. Reference values are from Great Smokies Diagnostic Laboratory: 63 Zillicoa Street, Asheville, NC, 28801; http://www.gsdl.com/index.html

7. Genox Corporation: 1414 Key Highway, Baltimore, MD 21230; http://www.genox.com/

8. AAL Reference Laboratories: 1715 East Wilshire, #715, Santa Ana, CA 92705; http://www.aal.xohost.com/index.htm

9. Great Smokies Diagnostic Laboratory: 63 Zillicoa Street, Asheville, NC, 28801; http://www.gsdl.com/index.html

10. Metamatrix Clinical Laboratory: 4855 Peachtree Ind. Blvd., Norcross, GA 30092; http://www.metametrix.com/

11. Pantox Laboratories: 4622 Sante Fe Street, San Diego, CA 92109; http://www.pantox.com/welcome.html

12. SpectraCell Laboratories: 7051 Portwest Drive, #100, Houston, TX; http://www.spectracell.com/carbs.html

13. Home Health Testing: 399 Pepper Street NE, Melbourne, FL 32907-1344; http://www.home-healthtesting.com/antioxidanttests.htm

14. Lymphocyte Evaluation, Activated Complete: test code number 2810, AAL Reference Laboratories: 1715 East Wilshire, #715, Santa Ana, CA 92705; http://www.aal.xohost.com/index.htm

15. Cellular Energy Profile: Great Smokies Diagnostic Laboratory: 63 Zillicoa Street, Asheville, NC, 28801; http://www.gsdl.com/index.html

16. ARUP Laboratories: 500 Chipeta Way, Salt Lake City, UT 84108; http://www.aruplab.com/testbltn/hemochrom.htm

17. Genovations, Great Smokies Diagnostic Laboratory: 63 Zillicoa Street, Asheville, NC, 28801; http://www.gsdl.com/index.html

18. Neuroregulatory Profile: test code number 7501, Pharmasan Labs: 375 280th Street, Osceola, WI 54020; http://www.pharmasan.com/

19. MyoSpan (with Peptide N): Neutraceutics: 3229 Morganford Road, St. Louis, MO 63116; http://www.nutraceutics.com/products.html

20. Environmental Protection Agency: Toxic Release Inventory Program; http://www.epa.gov/tri/tridata/tri00/index.htm

21. Though Rachel Carson's book *Silent Spring* was written in 1962 (Carson 1962), her environmental wake-up call has been largely ignored by politicians, physicians, and most scientists, as they prefer to focus on more glamorous callings. Despite the fact that levels of air pollution in many major North American and European cities have dropped since Carson's plea for environmental attention, the fact remains that every second of every day toxins still ravage our environment.

22. Metagenics: http://www.metagenics.com/

23. Thorne Research: 25820 Highway 2 West, Dover, ID 83825; http://www.thorne.com/about-us.html

24. Heel/BHI: 11600 Cohiti SE, Albuquerque, NM 87123-3376; http://www.heelbhi.com/

25. Among the three main groups of eicosanoids are prostaglandins; these are hormone-like substances that influence inflammation, blood clotting, heart rate, and the integrity of blood vessel walls. The other two main groups of eicosanoids are epoxyeicosatrienoic acids and lipoxygenase products. The pain and swelling associated with an injury are mediated by prostaglandins, as are the lower abdominal cramping that some women experience before their period, some forms of headaches, and a variety of chronic conditions such as cardiovascular disease. Aspirin and other nonsteroidal anti-inflammatories inhibit prostaglandin synthesis, which is one of the mechanisms that make these drugs effective in pain control.

26. MyoSpan (with Peptide N): Neutraceutics: 3229 Morganford Road, St. Louis, MO 63116; http://www.myospan.com/

27. The chemical nature of endocrine hormones varies and falls into three general categories based on what

substance they are derived from. Those in the first group are derived from a single amino acid and are called amines. Several common amino acids, such as tyrosine, are used to build hormones from which thyroid hormones and epinephrine are derived, as well as tryptophan (the precursor of serotonin), melatonin, and glutamic acid, which is converted into histamine, a substance involved in allergic immunity. The second group is composed of peptides and proteins. Growth hormone and follicle-stimulating hormone (FSH) are examples of hormones in this category. The third group comprises the steroid hormones such as testosterone and cortisol, which are derived from cholesterol.

28. Hormones range in size from 10^{-11} to 10^{-9} moles.

29. Though on the cutting edge of neuroendocrine research, the theory that hormones are produced in cells other than in the organs of the endocrine system is not new. It was first proposed in 1855 by Claude Bernard, the French physician credited with discovering the concept of homeostasis (Kvetnoy, Reiter, et al. 2000). A. G. Everson Pearse, a London professor and member of the Royal Microscopic Society, further developed this concept in the 1960s. He suggested that a specialized and highly organized system of cells was capable of producing hormone-like substances. Igor Kvetnoy, M.D., Ph.D., a Russian researcher with the Laboratory of Cell Organization at the Institute of Cytological Investigations in Valencia, Spain, goes further. He suggests that "DNES cells are regulators of homeostasis acting via neuroendocrine, endocrine, and paracrine mechanisms" (Kevtnoy, Sandvik, et al. 1997).

30. Not all hormones communicate with target cells through this receptor mechanism. Some can enter a cell by other chemical transport mechanisms, and some hormones such as the steroid family, which includes testosterone, estrogen, thyroid hormones, and vitamin D (1,25-dihydroxyvitamin D3), diffuse freely across the cell's plasma membrane. Once inside the cell, they can interact directly with receptors within the nucleus.

31. The half-life for DHEA is about 15–30 minutes, whereas that of DHEA-S is between seven and ten hours.

32. Conventional medical doctors use DHEA-S primarily to evaluate cases of hirsutism, a condition where women display excessive facial hair growth; for polycystic ovarian syndrome, which also includes hirsutism; and for Cushing's syndrome, a condition of excessive production of adrenal hormones.

33. Other substances secreted by the pineal may also play a role as anti-aging molecules, including serotonin; N-acetylserotonin, a melatonin precursor (Oxenkrug, Requintina, et al. 2001); and thalamine, a substance recently discovered in Russia that exerts a balancing effect on melatonin.

34. Thyroxin-binding protein carries about 70 percent of all circulating thyroid hormones and albumin binds to 15–20 percent; the remainder is bound to a substance called transthyretin, which delivers most of the thyroid hormone directly to cells.

35. Endocrinologists call this functional relationship the hypothalamic-pituitary-thyroid axis (HPT axis).

36. Values: LabCorp, direct analog-radioimmunoassay (RIA) for free testosterone; Laboratory Corporation of American: 358 South Main Street, Burlington, NC 27215; http://www.labcorp.com/

37. Values from LabCorp, EIA method: Laboratory Corporation of American: 358 South Main Street, Burlington, NC 27215; http://www.labcorp.com/

38. A second insulin-like growth factor, IGF-II, is also known but is considered less biologically important than IGF-I.

39. IGF-I references values from LabCorp: Laboratory Corporation of American: 358 South Main Street, Burlington, NC 27215; http://www.labcorp.com/

40. It is important to keep in mind that the research community is also in disagreement on many of these issues, and at times even appears confused by the complexity of the aging process. For the purposes of the discussion on neuroendocrine balancing as put forth in this book, the author strongly suggests, in agreement with a growing number of scientists, that it is largely the increase in the catabolic activity of insulin and cortisol that causes much of the brain and neural damage that results in decreased production of anabolic hormones. Therefore, in maintaining normal carbohydrate metabolism with normal levels of insulin and cortisol, one doesn't get the dramatic drops in the anabolic hormones and life span is increased.

41. Buck Institute for Aging Research: 8001 Redwood Boulevard, Novato, CA 94945; (415) 209-2000; http://www.buckinstitute.org/index.html

42. Thorne Research: 25820 Highway 2 West, Dover, ID 83825; http://www.thorne.com/about-us.html

43. Gerivitol: http://www.biogenesis.co.za/pi-gh3.asp

44. Neutraceutics: 3229 Morganford Road, St. Louis, MO 63116; http://www.nutraceutics.com/products.html

45. Sibergin: http://www.healthaidamerica.com/health/sibergin.html

46. Life Enhancement: http://www.life-enhancement.com/product.asp?ID=83

47. We need at least 75 micrograms (mcg) of iodine per day to prevent goiter, the enlargement of the thyroid associated with abnormal thyroid function. The thyroid gland contains the largest pool of iodine in the body, about 8,000 mcg.

48. Heel/BHI: 11600 Cohiti SE, Albuquerque, NM 87123-3376; http://www.heelbhi.com/

49. Meditrophin is manufactured by Nutraceutics: 3229 Morganford Road, St. Louis, MO 63116; http://www.nutraceutics.com/products.html

50. Forest Pharmaceuticals: http://www.forestpharm.com/

51. Bio-Tech Pharmacal: http://www.bio-tech-pharm.com/

52. Progest-E Complex: Kenogen: P.O. Box 50423, Eugene, OR 97405

53. Thymoject is manufactured by Biosyn GmbH: Schorndorfer StraBe 32, D-70734, Fellbach, Germany; http://www.biosyn.de/bs_deutsch/bs_seiten/bs_homepage.php

54. The CD (cluster of differentiation) designations refer to markers on the surface of lymphocytes that make them distinguishable from other cells.

55. NatCell Thymus: Atrium Biotechnologies, U.S. distributor: 9 Commerce Road, Fairfield, NJ 07004; http://www.atrium-bio.com/

56. Injectable thymus extracts can be obtained with a prescription from a medical doctor or you can order them over the Internet from an offshore pharmacy.

57. Ginkgo 32/9: Pure Encapsulations: 490 Boston Post Road, Sudbury, MA 01776; http://www.purecaps.com/about.html?section=about

58. Penta Water: Bio-Hydration Research Lab: 6370 Nancy Ridge Drive, Suite 104, San Diego, CA 92121 (800) 531-5088; http://www.pentawater.com/index.php

59. Published with permission from Everett Williams: Life Time Health & Nutrition, 4411 Morena Blvd., Suite 101, San Diego, CA 92117; (858) 490-9070

60. Inositol hexaphosphate (IP6): http://www.ip6-inositol.com/

61. Moducare is from Thorne Research: 25820 Highway 2 West, Dover, ID 83825; http://www.thorne.com/about-us.html

62. Pilates International: http://www.pilates.com/

63. Thorne Research: 25820 Highway 2 West, Dover, ID 83825; http://www.thorne.com/about-us.html

64. Life Factor Research: http://www.lifefactorresearch.com/

65. Life Extension Foundation: http://www.lef.org/

66. Optigene Professional: http://www.optigene-x.com/science/science.cfm

67. AAL Reference Laboratories: 1715 East Wilshire, #715, Santa Ana, CA 92705; http://www.aal.xohost.com/index.htm

68. Genox Corporation: 1414 Key Highway, Baltimore, MD 21230; http://www.genox.com/

69. Since 50 percent of calcium in the bloodstream is ionized, a form that makes it more bioavailable particularly for muscle contraction, measuring serum ionized calcium may be more useful than standard serum levels in assessing calcium status. The remaining calcium is mostly bound to albumin, and 10 percent is combined with other substance-forming compounds such as calcium citrate. The reference range for ionized calcium is 4.5 to 5.6 mg/dL.

Glossary

ADVANCED GLYCOSYLATION END PRODUCTS (AGEs): Abnormal molecules that result from pathological modifications between glucose and proteins altering their structure and function.

AGE-POINT: A time of life that occurs before declining sex hormones cause andropause and menopause. It is characterized by generalized stiffness and loss of flexibility, loss of balance, lack of muscle tone and strength, fatigue, low exercise tolerance, glucose imbalances, and declining levels of DHEA.

AGING: The irreversible, time-dependent, functional decline that converts healthy adults into frail ones, characterized by a reduced capacity to adjust to everyday stresses and increasing vulnerability to most diseases, leading to death.

AGING ZONE: This is the period of life when all the factors of aging are operative and when the physical signs of aging appear.

ANDROPAUSE: The male equivalent of menopause.

ANTI-AGING: A term that implies methods that reverse or prevent aging.

ANTI-AGING MEDICINE: The medical practice of preventing the degenerative diseases of aging and the promotion of longevity.

ANTIOXIDANT: Substances naturally manufactured in our bodies, found in foods, or supplied as nutritional supplements that help neutralize free radical damage.

ANTIOXIDANT CAPACITY: The chemical ability of an antioxidant to neutralize free radicals.

BIOLOGICAL AGE: A determination of aging based on physiological and biological function.

BIOMARKERS: The biological markers that indicate changes in critical physiological functions that occur in aging.

BRANCHED-CHAIN AMINO ACIDS (BCAAs): These are so named because of their unique branching structure and are three essential amino acids (valine, leucine, and isoleucine); they make up approximately 70 percent of amino acids in the body. They are readily absorbed and can be metabolized directly by muscle tissue. During prolonged workouts, BCAAs are burned as fuel to provide as much as 15 percent of your total energy requirement.

CENTENARIANS: Those who have lived to age 100.

CHRONOLOGICAL AGE: Your age determined by your birth date.

COMPLEMENTARY MEDICINE: A system of medical practice that uses alternative therapies to complement conventional medicine.

DYSGLYCEMIA: Abnormal metabolism and utilization of glucose in the body; associated with hypoglycemia and the early stages of diabetes.

ENDOTOXINS: Toxins produced and released inside the body.

FASTING GLUCOSE: A test that measures the amount of glucose in a sample of blood after not eating or drinking anything but water for eight hours prior to the test.

FREE RADICALS: Also called reactive oxygen species (ROS), these are unstable molecules with a missing electron formed during all metabolic activity in the body. This results in a chain reaction of unstable molecules, leading to genetic, mitochondrial, and cellular damage, and is one of the leading causes of disease and aging.

FRUCTOSAMINE: A blood test that measures the amount of proteins in the serum that are chemically combined (glycosylated) with glucose and reflects an average blood glucose level over a two- to three-week period.

GENOME: An organism's total DNA content found in the nucleus of a cell and that contains all the genetic information for the cell or organism as transmitted from generation to generation.

GENOTYPE: The internally coded inherited information carried in the genetic material that controls the formation of proteins, regulation of metabolism, and all biological processes in an organism.

GLYCOSYLATED HEMOGLOBIN: A blood test that measures the amount of molecules in a red blood cell that become chemically linked with glucose; older red blood cells and those of diabetics have a greater percentage of glycosylated hemoglobin.

GLYCOSYLATION: The process that causes glucose to combine with proteins and that damages their structure and causes abnormal function.

HOMOCYSTEINE: An intermediary metabolite in the biosynthesis of the amino acid cysteine from methionine, and an amino acid involved in cellular metabolism.

HORMONE METABOLITES: The biochemical by-products of hormone metabolism.

IMMUNOSENESCENCE: The progressive age-related weakening of your immune system.

INSULIN RESISTANCE: A condition that occurs when your body cannot respond properly to the insulin it produces and compensates for this by making more insulin.

INTEGRATIVE MEDICINE: A system of medical practice that combines the best of alternative and conventional medical therapies.

INTERMEDIARY METABOLITES: Chemicals produced during the metabolism of substances, but that are not the final product.

LIFE EXPECTANCY: Also called the mean life span, this is the average maximum age a person might expect to reach.

LIFE EXTENSION: The practice of taking nutritional supplements and hormones for the purpose of extending the maximum life span.

LONGEVITY: The attainment of a long life.

MAXIMUM LIFE SPAN: The age reached by the oldest member of a species.

MENOPAUSE: The ending of the female's reproductive capacity characterized by the cessation of menstruation and typically occurring between the ages of 48 and 52.

METABOLIC CRITICAL POINT: The shift from anabolism (upbuilding) to catabolism (taking apart) that occurs during aging. It can also be caused by overexercising or chronic dietary imbalances.

METABOLITES: The chemical by-products of metabolism.

METHYLATION: A biochemical process important in DNA repair, growth of new cells, and gene expression. When cells are unable to undergo normal DNA methylation, they are more prone to turn cancerous and age more rapidly.

MITOCHONDRIAL DNA: The genetic material contained in the mitochondria of a cell, unique and different from the DNA of the cell's nucleus.

MODIFIABLE AGING FACTORS: The environmental influences that exert a positive or negative impact on health, that influence genetic expression and affect aging, and that can be influenced by health practices.

NEURODEGENERATION: The progressive degeneration of nerve activity and cognitive function of the brain.

ORGAN RESERVE: The ability of an organ to restore and maintain its function.

OXIDATION: The chemical reaction that occurs when oxygen is combined with another substance, producing free radicals.

OXIDATIVE STRESS: The destructive load placed upon a cell by free radicals.

PERIMENOPAUSE: The time of life just before and after menopause, generally between ages 48 and 52.

PHENOTYPE: The outward physical appearance of an organism expressed through information carried in its genes and as affected by environmental influences.

PLEIOTROPY: The state in which a cell can have more than one function.

PROHORMONES: The precursors or biochemical building blocks for hormones.

PROLONGEVITY: The proactive involvement of an individual in promoting their own longevity.

PROTEIN GLYCATION: The result of a chemical reaction between proteins and glucose that forms abnormal proteins.

SARCOPENIA: A condition characterized by declining muscle mass and fat increase that causes an apple-shaped body to appear, with more fat around the waist, hips, and thighs, and with less muscle in the arms and legs.

SENESCENCE: The measurable decline in cellular function and observable changes in bodily processes that accompany aging; referred to as the aging phenotype.

SOMATOPAUSE: The age-related decline that occurs about a decade after menopause and andropause, characterized by low levels of growth hormone, sex hormones, and insulin-like growth factor I (IGF-I).

SOMATOTROPHIC AXIS: The major hormonal system controlling growth in the body. In aging, it is marked by an irreversible decline in levels of human growth hormone (HGH) and insulin-like growth factor I (IGF-I). This is thought to cause the decreased muscle mass and strength, decreased bone density, and increased body fat generally associated with the aging body.

SYNDROME X: A metabolic condition characterized by insulin resistance, elevated triglyceride levels, abdominal obesity, and hypertension.

SUPERCENTENARIANS: Those over 110 years of age.

TELOMERASE: An enzyme that protects telomeres by helping to reconstruct the broken tips, thereby preserving the integrity of the chromosomes.

TELOMERES: Specialized proteins at the tips of the chromosomes thought to be essential in their maintenance and to prevent abnormal cell division.

TOTAL ANTIOXIDANT ACTIVITY: Antioxidant capacity of individual antioxidants found in a food or other substance and a synergistic effect that is greater than the sum of its parts.

Bibliography

Ahsan, H, A Ali, and R Ali. 2003. Oxygen free radicals and systemic autoimmunity. *Journal of Clinical and Experimental Immunology* 131 (3):398–404.

Albert, MS. 1997. The ageing brain: normal and abnormal memory. *Philosophical Transaction of the Royal Society of London* 352 (1362):1703–09.

Aldridge, Susan. 2001. *Ageing successfully with complementary medicine.* Novartis Foundation for Gerontology [from www.healthandage.com.]

Allsup, SJ, M Gosney, M Regan, et al. 2001. Side effects of influenza vaccination in healthy older people: a randomized single-blind placebo-controlled trial. *Gerontology* 47 (6):311–14.

Amenta, F, F Mignini, A Ricci, et al. 2001. Age-related changes of dopamine receptors in the rat hippocampus: a light microscope autoradiology study. *Mechanisms of Ageing and Development* 122 (16):2071–83.

American Cancer Society. 2002. Cancer Facts and Figures 2002. New York: American Cancer Society.

American Heart Association. 2002. 2002 Heart and Stroke Statistical Update. Dallas, Texas: American Heart Association.

Ames, BN. 1998. Micronutrients prevent cancer and delay aging. *Toxicology Letters* 102–103:5–18.

———. 1999. Micronutrient deficiencies. A major cause of DNA damage. *Ann N Y Acad Sci* 889:87–106.

———. 2001. DNA damage from micronutrient deficiencies is likely to be a major cause of cancer. *Mutatation Research* 475 (1–2):7–20.

Andersen, NB, K Malmlof, et al. 2001. The growth hormone secretagogue ipamorelin counteracts glucocorticoid-induced decrease in bone formation of adult rats. *Growth Hormone & IGF Research* 11:266–72.

Anderson, Graham, and Eric J Jenkinson. 2001. Lymphostomal interactions in thymic development and function. *Nature Reviews Immunology* 1 (October):31–40.

Andreotti, F, F Burzotta, et al. 1999. Homocysteine and arterial occlusive disease: a concise review. *Cardologia* 44 (4):341–45.

Arivazhagan, P, K Ramanathan, and C Panneerselvam. 2001. Effect of DL-alpha-lipoic acid on glutathione metabolic enzymes in aged rats. *Experimental Gerontology* 37 (1):81–87.

Arking, Robert, and Craig Giroux. 2001. Antioxidant genes, hormesis, and demographic longevity. *Journal of Anti-Aging Medicine* 4 (2):125–36.

Armstrong, ME, HD Alexander, JL Ritchie, et al. 2001. Age-related alterations in basal expression and in vitro, Tumor Necrosis Factor Alpha mediated, upregulation of CD11b. *Gerontology* 47 (4):180–85.

Austad, Steven N. 1997. *Why We Age.* New York: John Wiley & Sons.

———. 2002. Where have we come from? Where do we stand? Where are we going? Paper read at Buck Institute Symposium: Neuroendocrine Systems and Life span Determination, September, in Novato, CA.

Azcoitia, I, LL DonCarlos, and LM Garcia-Segura. 2003. Are gonadal steroid hormones involved in disorders of brain aging? *Aging Cell* 2 (1):31–37.

Balasubramanyam, M, and V Mohan. 2001. Orally active insulin mimics: where do we stand? *Journal of Bioscience* 26 (3):383–90.

Ballou, SP, FB Lozanski, S Hodder, et al. 1996. Quantitative and qualitative alterations of acute-phase proteins in healthy elderly persons. *Age Aging* 25 (3):224–30.

Barbagallo, M, J Ligia, et al. 1999. Effects of aging on serum ionized and cytosolic free calcium, relation to hypertension and diabetes. *Hypertension* (October):902–06.

Barja, Gustavo, and Asuncion Herrero. 2000. Oxidative damage to mitochondrial DNA is inversely related to maximum life span in the heart and brain of mammals. *Journal of American Societies for Experimental Biology* 14:312–18.

Barnes, Broda O, and L Galton. 1976. *Hypothyroidism: The Unsuspected Illness.* New York: Harper & Row.

Bartke, A. 2001. A word of caution: can growth hormone accelerate aging? *Journal of Anti-Aging Medicine* 4 (4):301–09.

Bartke, Andrzej, and Mark Lane. 2001. Endocrine and neuroendocrine regulatory functions. In *Handbook of the Biology of Aging,* edited by E Masoro and S Austad. San Diego: Academic Press.

Bates, CJ, D Benton, HK Biesalski, HB Staehelin, W van Staveren, P Stehle, PM Suter, and G Wolfram. 2002. Nutrition and aging: a consensus statement. *Journal of Nutrition Health and Aging* 6 (2):103–16.

Bathum, L, L Christiansen, et al. 2001. Association of mutations in the hemochromatosis gene with shorter life expectancy. *Archives of Internal Medicine* 161:2441–44.

Bauman, Alisa. 2002. Is yoga enough to keep you fit? *Yoga Journal* September/October:85–158.

Beckman, KB, and BN Ames. 1998. Mitochondrial aging: open questions. *Annals of the New York Academy of Sciences* 854:118–27.

——. 1998. The free radical theory of aging matures. *Physicological Reviews* 78 (2):547–81.

Beharka, AA, D Wu, et al. 1997. Macrophage prostaglandin production contributes to the age-associated decrease in T cell function which is reversed by the dietary antioxidant vitamin E. *Mechanisms of Ageing and Development* 93 (1-3):59–77.

Beitz, R, GBM Mensink, et al. 2002. Vitamins–dietary intake and intake from dietary supplements in Germany. *European Journal of Clinical Nutrition* 56 (6):539–45.

Ben-Nathan, D, DA Padgett, and RM Loria. 1999. Androstenediol and dehydroepiandrosterone protect mice against lethal bacterial infections and lipopolysaccharide toxicity. *Journal of Medical Microbiology* 48 (5):425–31.

Ben-Shlomo, A, and S Melmed. 2001. Growth hormone excess and cancer. *Journal of Anti-Aging Medicine* 4 (4):373–81.

Bensky, Dan, and Andrew Gamble. 1986. *Chinese Herbal Medicine Materia Medica.* Seattle: Eastland Press.

Bensky, Dan, and Randall Barolet. 1990. *Chinese Herbal Medicine: Formulas & Strategies.* Seattle: Eastland Press.

Benson, Herbert. 1975. *The Relaxation Response.* New York: Avon Books.

Berson, DM, FA Dunn, and M Takao. 2002. Phototransduction by retinal ganglion cells that set the circadian clock. *Science* 295 (5557):1070–73.

Beshyah, SA, A Henderson, et al. 1994. Metabolic abnormalities in growth hormone deficient adults: II, Carbohydrate tolerance and lipid metabolism. *Endocrinology and Metabolism* 1:173–80.

Bessesen, Daniel H. 2001. The role of carbohydrates in insulin resistance. *Journal of Nutrition* 131:2782S–86S.

Bevan, P. 2001. Insulin signaling. *Journal of Cell Science* 114 (8):1429–30.

Bielsalski, HK. 2002. Free radical theory of aging. *Current Opinion in Clinical Nutrition and Metabolic Care* 5 (1):5–10.

Bigini, P, S Larini, C Pasquali, V Muzio, and T Mennini. 2002. Acetyl-L-carnitine shows neuroprotective and neurotrophic activity in primary culture of rat embryo motoneurons. *Neuroscience Letters* 329 (3):334.

Billich, A. 2002. Thymosin alpha 1. *Current Opinion in Investigational Drugs* 3 (5):698–707.

Birkmayer, JG. 1996. Coenzyme nicotinamide adenine dinucleotide: new therapeutic approach for improving dementia of the Alzheimer type. *Annals of Clinical Laboratory Science* 26 (1):1–9.

Birkmayer, JG, C Vrecko, D Volc, and W Birkmayer. 1993. Nicotinamide adenine dinucleotide (NADH)–a new therapeutic approach to Parkinson's disease. Comparison of oral and parenteral application. *Acta Neurologica Scandinavica* 146:32–35.

Birnbaum, MJ. 2001. Dialogue between muscle and fat. *Nature* 409 (February 8):672–73.

Biswas, SJ, and AR Khud-Bukhsh. 2002. Effect of a homeopathic drug, Chelidonium, in amelioration of p-DAB induced hepatocarcinogenesis in mice. *BMC Complementary and Alternative Medicine* 2 (1):4–12.

Blackburn, Elizabeth H. 2000. Telomere states and cell fates. *Nature* 408:53–56.

Blain, H, A Vuillemin, A Teissier, et al. 2001. Influence of muscle strength and body weight and composition on regional bone mineral density in healthy women aged 60 and over. *Gerontology* 47 (4):207–12.

Bland, Jeffrey S. 1998. *Improving Genetic Expression in the Prevention of the Diseases of Aging.* Gig Harbor, Washington: HealthComm International.

——. 2001. The neuroendocrine system and healthy aging. Paper read at New Approaches to Anti-Aging: Nutritional Neuroendocrinology, in Los Angeles.

———. 2002. Stress: Its relationship to chronic diseases of aging. Paper read at Breakthrough Approaches for Improving Adrenal and Thyroid Function, in Los Angeles.

———. 2003. Improving Health Outcomes Through Nutritional Support for Metabolic Transformation. Paper read at Improving Health Outcomes Through Nutritional Support for Metabolic Transformation, in Los Angeles.

Bland, Jeffrey S, and Sara H Benum. 1999. *Genetic Nutritioneering.* Lincolnwood, Illinois: Keats.

Blount, BC, MM Mack, et al. 1997. Folate deficiency causes uracil misincorporation into human DNA and chromosome breakage: implications for cancer and neuronal damage. *Proceedings of the National Academy of Sciences* 94:3290–95.

Boerner, Paula. 2001. Functional intracellular analysis of nutritional and antioxidant status. *Journal of the American Nutraceutical Association* 4 (1):27–40.

Borek, Carmia. 2001. Age breakers. *Life Extension* (August):39–43.

Borst, SE, KR. Vincent, DT Lowenthal, and RW Braith. 2002. Effects of resistance training on insulin-like growth factor and its binding proteins in men and women aged 60 to 85. *Journal of the American Geriatric Society* 50 (5):884–88.

Bortolotto, Luiz A, H Olivier, F Giovanna, et al. 1999. The aging process modifies the distensibility of elastic but not muscular arteries. *Hypertension* 34:889–92.

Bowers, CY. 2000. GHRP historical perspective. In *Human Growth Hormone Research and Clinical Practice,* edited by RG Smith and MO Thorner. Totowa, New Jersey: Humana Press.

Bralley, JA, and RS Lord. 2001. *Laboratory Evaluations in Molecular Medicine.* Norcross, Georgia: Institute for Advances in Molecular Medicine.

Brand-Miller, J, TM Wolever, K Foster-Powell, et al. 1996. *The New Glucose Revolution.* New York: Marlow & Company.

Branda, R, J O'Neill, E Brooks, et al. The effect of folate deficiency on the cytotoxic and mutagenic responses to ethyl methanesulfonatein human lyphoblastoid cell lines that differ in p53 status. *Mutation Research* 2001; 47351–71.

Brod, SA. 2000. Unregulated inflammation shortens human functional longevity. *Inflammation Research* 49 (11):561–70.

Broughton, Alan. 1999. *Estrogen and the Postmenopausal Woman.* Santa Ana, California: AAL Reference Laboratories.

Brown-Borg, HM, KE Borg, et al. 1996. Dwarf mice and the ageing process. *Nature* 384:33.

Brownlee, M, A Cerami, et al. 1988. Advanced glycosylation end products in tissue and the biochemical basis of diabetic complications. *New England Journal of Medicine* 318:1315–21.

Brusco, LI, M Marquez, et al. 2000. Melatonin treatment stabilizes chronobiologic and cognitive symptoms in Alzheimer's disease. *Neuroendocrinology Letters* 21:39–42.

Bryant, NJ, R Govers, and DE James. 2002. Regulated transport of the glucose transporter GLUT4. *Nature Reviews Molecular and Cellular Biology* 3 (4):267–77.

Brynin, R. 2002. Soy and its isoflavones: a review of their effects on bone density. *Alternative Medicine Review* 7 (4):317–27.

Buz'Zard, AR, QL Peng, et al. 2002. Kyolic and pycnogenol increase human growth hormone secretion in genetically engineered keratinocytes. *Growth Hormone & IGF Research* 12:34–40.

Cabot, Sandra. 1996. *The Liver Cleansing Diet.* Scottsdale, Arizona: S.C.B. International.

Cadbury, Deborah. 1997. *Altering Eden: The Feminization of Nature.* New York: St. Martin's Press.

Campany, Robert Ford. 2002. *To Live as Long as Heaven and Earth.* Berkeley: University of California Press.

Campisi, J, SH Kim, CS Lim, and M Rubio. 2001. Cellular senescence, cancer and aging: the telomere connection. *Experimental Gerontology* 36 (10):1619–37.

Capra, Fritjof. 2002. *The Hidden Connections.* New York: Doubleday.

Cardinali, DP, LI Brusco, et al. 1998. Melatonin: a synchronizing signal for the immune system. *Neuroendocrinology Letters* 18:73–84.

Carmel, R. 1997. Cobalamin, the stomach, and aging. *American Journal of Clinical Nutrition* 66 (4):750–59.

Carroll, PV, and G Van den Berghe. 2001. Safety aspects of pharmacological GH therapy in adults. *Growth Hormone & IGF Research* 11:166–72.

Carson, R L. 1962. *Silent Spring.* Greenwich, Connecticut: Fawcett Publications.

Casolini, P, A Catalani, et al. 2002. Inhibition of COX-2 reduces the age-dependent increase of hippocampal inflammatory markers, corticosterone secretion, and behavioral impairments in the rat. *Journal of Neuroscience Research* 68 (3):337–43.

Castaneda, C, PL Gordon, KL Uhlin, et al. 2001. Resistance training to counteract the catabolism of a low-protein diet in patients with chronic renal insufficiency. *Annals of Internal Medicine* 135:965–76.

Castracane, VD, and MC Henson. 2002. Leptin and reproduction. *Seminars in Reproductive Medicine* 20 (2):87–88.

Cathcart, R. 1981. Vitamin C, titrating to bowel tolerance, anascorbemia, and acute induced scurvy. *Medical Hypothesis* 7:1359–76.

Ceda, GP, G Ceresini, L. Denti, G Marzani, E Piovani, A Banchini, E Tarditi, and G Valenti. 1992. Alpha-glycerylphosphorylcholine administration increases the GH responses to GHRH of young and elderly subjects. *Hormone Metabolism Research* 24 (3):119–21.

Ceriello, A. 2000. Oxidative stress and glycemic regulation. *Metabolism* 49 (2):27–29.

Cerwenka, Adelheid, and Lewis L Lanier. 2001. Natural killer cells, viruses and cancer. *Nature Reviews Immunology* 1 (October):41–49.

Cesquini, M, AC Tenor, MA Torsoni, et al. 2001. Quercetin diminishes the binding of hemoglobin to the red blood cell membrane. *Journal of Anti-Aging Medicine* 4 (1):55–63.

Chaisson, Eric J. 2001. *Cosmic Evolution: The Rise of Complexity in Nature.* Cambridge, Massachusetts: Harvard University Press.

Chambon-Savanovitch, C, C Felgines, et al. 2001. A pancreatic extract-enriched diet improves the nutritional status of aged rats. *Journal of Nutrition* 131:813–19.

Cho, H, J Mu, JK Kim, JL Thorvaldsen, Q Chu, EB Crenshaw III, KH Kaestner, MS Bartolomei, GI Shulman, and MJ Birnbaum. 2001. Insulin resistance and a diabetes mellitus-like syndrome in mice lacking the protein kinase Akt2 (PKB beta). *Science* 292 (5522):1728–31.

Christen, Y, and JM Maixent. 2002. What is Ginkgo biloba extract EGb 761? An overview—from molecular biology to clinical medicine. *Cellular and Molecular Biology* 48 (6):601–11.

Christou, H, S Serdy, and CS Mantzoros. 2002. Leptin in relation to growth and developmental processes in the fetus. *Seminars in Reproductive Medicine* 20 (2):123–30.

Chromiak, JA, and J Antonio. 2002. Use of amino acids as growth hormone-releasing agents by athletes. *Nutrition* 18 (7-8):657–61.

Cirtser, Greg. 2003. *Fat Land.* New York: Houghton Mifflin Company.

Clark, AR, CA Purdie, DJ Harrison, et al. 1993. Thymocyte apoptosis induced by p53-dependent and independent pathways. *Nature* 362:849–52.

Clasey, JL, JA Kanaley, et al. 2000. Validity of methods of body composition assessment in young and older men and women. *Journal of Applied Physiology* 89 (6):2518–20.

Coles, L Stephen. 2001. Ten unsolved problems in longevity medicine today. Paper read at 9th International Conference of the American Academy of Anti-Aging Medicine, in Las Vegas, Nevada.

———. 2001. Table of worldwide living supercentenarian. *Journal of Anti-Aging Medicine* 4 (3):267–69.

———. 2002. Table of worldwide living supercentenarians. *Journal of Anti-Aging Medicine* 5 (1):141.

Couteur, DG Le, and AJ McLean. 1998. The aging liver, drug clearance and an oxygen diffusion barrier hypothesis. *Clinical Pharmacokinetics* 34:359–72.

Cusi, K, S Cukier, et al. 2001. Vanadyl sulfate improves hepatic and muscle insulin sensitivity in type 2 diabetes. *Journal of Clinical Endocrinology and Metabolism* 86 (3):1410–17.

Cutler, RG. 1984. Urate and ascorbate: their possible roles as antioxidants in determining longevity of mammalian species. *Archives of Gerontology and Geriatrics* 3 (4):321–48.

D'Agostini, F, RM Balansky, and A Camoirano. 2000. Interactions between N-acetylcysteine and ascorbic acid in modulating mutagenesis and carcinogenesis. *International Journal of Cancer* 88 (5):702–07.

Dalton, Katharina, and Wendy Holton. 1999. *Once A Month: Understanding and Treating PMS.* Alameda, California: Hunter House.

Damasio, AR. 1999. How the brain creates the mind. *Scientific American* August:4–9.

Dawson-Hughes, B, and SS Harris. 2002. Calcium intake influences the association of protein intake with rates of bone loss in elderly men and women. *American Journal of Clinical Nutrition* 75 (4):773–79.

Dean, Ward, John Morgenthaler, and Steven Williams Fowkes. 1993. *Smart Drugs II.* Petaluma, California: Smart Publications.

Dement, William. 1999. *The Promise of Sleep.* New York: Delacorte Press.

Dey, Lucy, AS Attele, et al. 2002. Alternative therapies for type 2 diabetes. *Alternative Medicine Review* 7 (1):45–58.

Diamond, Jared. 2001. Unwritten knowledge. *Nature* 410 (March 29):521.

Dispenza, Joseph. 1997. *Live Better Longer: The Parcells Center 7-Step Plan for Health and Longevity.* San Jose, California: Author's Choice Press.

Duker, EM, L Kopanski, et al. 1991. Effects of extracts from Cimicifuga racemosa on gonadotropin release in menopausal women and ovariectomized rats. *Planta Medica* 57:420–24.

Dukic-Stefanovic, S, and R Schinzel. 2001. AGES in brain aging: AGE-inhibitors as neuroprotective and anti-dementia drugs? *Biogerontology* 2 (1):19–34.

Duncan, GE, MG Perri, DW Theriaque, AD Hutson, RH Eckel, and PW Stacpoole. 2003. Exercise training, without weight loss, increases insulin sensitivity and postheparin plasma lipase activity in previously sedentary adults. *Diabetes Care* 26 (3):557–62.

Dychtwald, Ken. 1990. *Age Wave*. New York: Bantam.

———. 1999. *Age Power*. New York: Jeremy P. Tarcher.

Ebadi, M, P Govitrapong, et al. 2001. Ubiquinone (coenzyme Q10) and mitochondria in oxidative stress of Parkinson's disease. *Biological Signals and Receptors* 10 (3–4):224–53.

Effros, Rita B. 2001. Immune System Activity. In *Handbook of the Biology of Aging*, edited by E Masoro and S Austad. San Diego: Academic Press.

Emmert, DH, and JT Kerchner. 1999. The role of vitamin E in the prevention of heart disease. *Archives of Family Medicine* 8 (6):537–42.

Erickson, KL, and NE Hubbard. 2000. Probiotic immunomodulation in health and disease. *Journal of Nutrition* 130:403S–09S.

Eriksson, PS, FH Gage, et al. 1998. Neurogenesis in the adult human hippocampus. *Nature Medicine* 4 (11):1313–17.

Evan, WJ. 1995. Effects of exercise on body composition and functional capacity of the elderly. *Journal of Gerontology and Biological Sciences* 50:147–50.

Evans, BA, K Griffiths, and MS Morton. 1995. Inhibition of 5-alpha reductase in genital skin fibroblasts and prostate tissue by dietary lignans and isoflavonoids. *Journal of Endocrinology* 147 (2):295–302.

Evans, WJ. 2002. Effects of exercise on senescent muscle. *Clinical Orthopedics* (403 Suppl):S211–20.

Evans, W, and IH Rosenbery. 1991. *Biomarkers, the 10 Keys to Prolonging Vitality*. New York: Simon & Schuster.

Ewald, Paul W. 2000. *Plague Time: How Stealth Infections Cause Cancers, Heart Disease, and Other Deadly Ailments*. New York: The Free Press.

Faloon, William. 2002. Chronic inflammation: the epidemic disease of aging. *Life Extension* (January):13–16.

Fang, Jing, and Michael H Alderman. 1992. Serum uric acid and cardiovascular mortality. *Journal of the American Medical Association* 283-2404–10.

Fang, Jing, and Michael H Alderman. 2000. Serum uric acid and cardiovascular mortality the NHANES I epidemiologic follow-up study, 1971-1992. National Health and Nutrition Examination Survey. *Journal of the American Medical Association* 283:2404–10.

Farach-Carson, MC, and I Nemere. 2003. Membrane receptors for vitamin D steroid hormones: potential new drug targets. *Current Drug Targets* 4 (1):67–76.

Fasshauer, M, J Klein, K Ueki, KM Kriauciunas, M Benito, MF White, and CR Kahn. 2000. Essential role of insulin receptor substrate-2 in insulin stimulation of Glut4 translocation and glucose uptake in brown adipocytes. *Journal of Biological Chemistry* 275 (33):25494–501.

Fatagyerji, D, AM Cooper, and R Eastell. 1999. Total body and regional bone mineral density in men: effect of age. *Osteoporosis International* 10 (1):59–65.

Fenech, M. 2002. Micronutrients and genomic stability: a new paradigm for recommended dietary allowances (RDAs). *Food Chemistry and Toxicology* 40 (8):1113–17.

Ferroli, CE, and PR Trumbo. 1994. Bioavailability of vitamin B-6 in young and older men. *American Journal of Clinical Nutrition* 60 (1):68–71.

Fife, D, and JI Barancik. 1985. Northeastern Ohio trauma study III: incidence of fractures. *Annals of Emergency Medicine* 14:244–48.

Finkel, Toren, and Nikki J Holbrook. 2000. Oxidants, oxidative stress and the biology of ageing. *Nature* 408:239–47.

Fisher, S, M Hanefeld, et al. 2002. Insulin-resistant patients with type 2 diabetes mellitus have higher serum leptin levels independently of body fat mass. *Acta Diabetologica* 39 (3):105–10.

Fitzgerald, MD, H Tanaka, ZV Tran, et al. 1997. Age-related decline in maximal aerobic capacity in regularly exercising vs. sedentary females: a meta-analysis. *Journal of Applied Physiology* 83:160–65.

Flynn, MA, D Weaver-Osterholtz, et al. 1999. Dehydroepiandrosterone replacement in aging humans. *The Journal of Clinical Endocrinology & Metabolism* 84 (5):1527–33.

Forsblad, J, A Gottsater, K Persson, L Jacobsson, and F Lindgarde. 2002. Clinical manifestations of atherosclerosis in an elderly population are related to plasma neopterin, NGAL and endothelin-1, but not to Chlamydia pneumoniae serology. *International Angiology* 21 (2):173–79.

Franklin, Stanley S, JJ Jacobs, ND Wong, et al. 2002. Predominance of isolated systolic hypertension among middle-aged and elderly US hypertensives. *Hypertension* 37:869–74.

Frati, AC, BE Gordon, et al. 1988. Hypoglycemic effect of Opuntia streptacantha Lemaire in NIDDM. *Diabetes Care* 11:63–66.

Fratkin, Jake. 1986. *Chinese Herbal Patent Formulas*. Portland, Oregon: Institute for Traditional Medicine.

Friedlander, Y, M Kidron, et al. 2000. Low density lipoprotein particle size and risk factors of insulin resistance syndrome. *Atherosclerosis* 148 (1):141–49.

Frisco, S, PF Jacques, et al. 2001. Low circulating vitamin B (6) is associated with elevation of the inflammation marker C-reactive protein independently of plasma homocysteine levels. *Circulation* 103 (23):2788–91.

Fuh, VL, and MA Bach. 1998. Growth hormone secrete-gogues: mechanism of action and use in aging. *Growth Hormone & IGF Research* 8 (1):13–20.

Fukuyama, Francis. 2002. *Our Postmodern Future*. New York: Farrar, Straus, and Giroux.

Gemma, C, MH Mesches, B Sepesi, et al. 2002. Diets enriched in foods with high antioxidant activity reverse age-induced decreases in cerebellar beta-andrenergic function and increases in proinflammatory cytokines. *Journal of Neuroscience* 15 (22):6114–20.

George, AJT, and MA Ritter. 1996. Thymic involution with aging: Obsolescence or good housekeeping? *Immunology Today* 17 (6):267–72.

Gerhard, Glenn S. 2001. Caloric restriction in nonmammalian models. *Journal of Anti-Aging Medicine* 4 (3):205–13.

Gerisch, B, C Weitzel, C Kober-Eisermann, V Rottiers, and A Antebi. 2001. A hormonal signaling pathway influencing C. elegans metabolism, reproductive development, and life span. *Developmental Cell* 1 (6):841–51.

Gershon, Michael D. 1998. *The Second Brain*. New York: Harper Perennial.

Ghigo, E, E Arvat, et al. 1999. Endocrine and non-endocrine activities of growth hormone secretagogues in humans. *Hormone Research* 51 (Supplement 3):9–15.

———. 2001. Natural and synthetic growth hormone secretagogues: endocrine and nonendocrine activities suggesting their potential usefulness as anti-aging drug interventions. *Journal of Anti-Aging Medicine* 4 (4):345–56.

Gibson, Glenn R. 1999. Dietary modulation of the human gut microflora using the prebiotics oligofructose and inulin. *Journal of Nutrition* 129:1438S–41S.

Gillberg, P, M Bramnert, et al. 2001. Commencing growth hormone replacement in adults with a fixed low dose. Effects on serum lipoproteins, glucose metabolism, body composition, and cardiovascular function. *Growth Hormone & IGF Research* 11:273–81.

Gladyshev, Georgi P. 1999. Thermodynamic theory of biological evolution and aging, experimental confirmation of theory. *Entropy* 1:55–68.

Golden, TR., and S Melov. 2001. Mitochondrial DNA mutations, oxidative stress, and aging. *Mechanisms of Ageing and Development* 122 (14):1577–89.

Golden, TR, DA Hinerfeld, and S Melov. 2002. Oxidative stress and aging: beyond correlation. *Aging Cell* 1:117–23.

Goodman, Jonathan. 2001. *The Omega Solution*. Roseville, California: Prima Publishing.

Gordon, CM, MS LeBoff, and J Glowacki. 2001. Adrenal and gonadal steroids inhibit IL-6 secretion by human marrow cells. *Cytokine* 16 (5):178–86.

Gorter, RW, M van Wely, et al. 1998. Subcutaneous infiltrates induced by injection of mistletoe extract (Iscador). *American Journal of Therapeutics* 5:181–87.

Gould, Duncan C, Richard Petty, and Howard S Jacobs. 2000. The male menopause—does it exist? *British Medical Journal* 320 (March):858–61.

Grady D, D Herrington, V Bittner, et al. 2002. Cardiovascular disease outcomes during 6.8 years of hormone therapy: Heart and Estrogen/progestin Replacement Study follow-up (HERS II). *Journal of the American Medical Association* 288 (1):49–57.

Graeber, TG, D Eisenberg, et al. 2001. Bioinformatic identification of potential autocrine signalling loops in cancer from gene expression. *Nature Genetics* 29:295–300.

Grases, F, BM Simonet, I Vucenik, J Perello, RM Prieto, and AM Shamsuddin. 2002. Effects of exogenous inositol hexakisphosphate (InsP(6)) on the levels of InsP(6) and of inositol trisphosphate (InsP(3)) in malignant cells, tissues and biological fluids. *Life Science* 71 (13):1535–46.

Griffin, James E, and Sergio R Ojeda. 1996. *Textbook of Endocrine Physiology*. London: Oxford University Press.

Grimm, JJ. 1999. Interaction of physical activity and diet: implications for insulin-glucose dynamics. *Public Health and Nutrition* 2:363–68.

Grossarth-Maticek, R, H Kiene, et al. 2001. Use of Iscador, an extract of European mistletoe (Viscum album), in cancer treatment: prospective nonrandomized and randomized matched-pair studies nested within a cohort study. *Alternative Therapies in Health and Medicine* 7 (3):57–78.

Grossman, Terry. 2000. *The Baby Boomer's Guide to Living Forever.* Golden, Colorado: The Hubristic Press.

Gruber, BM, and EL Anuszewska. 2002. Influence of vitamin D3 metabolites on cell proliferation and cytotoxicity of Adriamycin in human normal and neoplastic cells. *Toxicology In Vitro* 16 (6):663–67.

Grune, Tilman, and Kelvin Davies. 2001. Oxidative processes in aging. In *Handbook of the Biology of Aging.* San Diego: Academic Press.

Gupta, I, A Parihar, et al. 2001. Effects of gum resin of Boswellia serrata in patients with chronic colitis. *Planta Medica* 67 (5):391–95.

Gupta, K, V Gupta, et al. 1998. Effects of Boswellia serrata-gum resin in patients with bronchial asthma: results of a double-blind, placebo-controlled, 6-week clinical study. *European Journal of Medical Research* 3 (11):511–14.

Ha, JH, SM Shin, SK Lee, JS Kim, US Shin, K Huh, JA Kim, CS Yong, NJ Lee, and DU Lee. 2001. In vitro effects of hydroxybenzaldehydes from Gastrodia elata and their analogues on GABAergic neurotransmission, and a structure-activity correlation. *Planta Medica* 67 (9):877–80.

Hadley, J, N Malik, et al. 2001. Collagen as a model system to investigate the use of aspirin as an inhibitor of protein glycation and crosslinking. *Micron* 32 (3):307–15.

Haeggstrom, JZ, and A Wetterholm. 2002. Enzymes and receptors in the leukotriene cascade. *Cellular and Molecular Life Sciences* 59 (5):742–53.

Hagberg, JM, JM Zmuda, and SD McCole. 2001. Moderate physical activity is associated with higher bone mineral density in postmenopausal women. *Journal of the American Geriatric Society* 49 (11):1565–67.

Hagen, TM, R Moreau, JH Suh, et al. 2002. Mitochondrial decay in the aging rat heart: evidence for improvement by dietary supplementation with acetyl-L-carnitine and/or lipoic acid. *Annals of the New York Academy of Science* 959:491–507.

Hagen, TM, RT Ingerstoll, et al. 1998. Acetyl-L-carnitine fed to old rats partially restores mitochondrial function and ambulatory activity. *Proceedings of the National Academy of Sciences* 95 (16):9562–66.

Hagen, TM, T Russell, et al. 1999. (R)-alpha-lipoic acid supplemented old rats have improved mitochondrial function, decreased oxidative damage, and increased metabolic rate. *Journal of American Societies for Experimental Biology* 13:411–18.

Hakkinen, K, RU Newton, SE Gordon, M McCormick, JS Volek, BC Nindl, LA Gotshalk, WW Campbell, WJ Evans, A Hakkinen, BJ Humphries, and WJ Kraemer. 1998. Changes in muscle morphology, electromyographic activity, and force production characteristics during progressive strength training in young and older men. *Journal of Gerontology and Biology Science and Medicine* 53 (6):B415–23.

Hakkinen, K, WJ Kraemer, A Pakarinen, T Triplett-McBride, JM McBride, A Hakkinen, M Alen, MR McGuigan, R Bronks, and RU Newton. 2002. Effects of heavy resistance/power training on maximal strength, muscle morphology, and hormonal response patterns in 60–75-year-old men and women. *Canadian Journal of Applied Physiology* 27 (3):213–31.

Hall, DM, et al. 2000. Caloric restriction improves thermotolerance and reduces hyperthermia-induced cellular damage in old rats. *Journal of American Societies for Experimental Biology* 14:78–86.

Hall, MR, RS Briggs, et al. 1983. The effects of procaine/haematoporphyrin on age-related decline: a double-blind trial. *Age Aging* 12 (4):302–08.

Halliwell, B, and GE Mestler. 1985. *Free Radicals in Biology and Medicine.* Oxford: Clarendon Press.

Han, SS, YS Keum, et al. 2002. Curcumin suppresses activation of NF-kappaB and AP-1 induced by phorbol ester in cultured human promyelocytic leukemia cells. *Journal of Biochemistry and Molecular Biology* 35 (3):337–42.

Hanahan, D. 1997. Signaling vascular morphogenesis and maintenance. *Science* 277:48–50.

Hanley, AJ, K Williams, MP Stern, and SM Haffner. 2002. Homeostasis model assessment of insulin resistance in relation to the incidence of cardiovascular disease: the San Antonio heart study. *Diabetes Care* 25 (7):1177–84.

Harman, D. 1956. Aging: a theory based on free radical and radiation chemistry. *Journal of Gerontology* 2:298–300.

———. 1976. The clinical gerontologist. *Journal of the American Geriatric Society* 24:452–53.

Haub, MD, AM Wells, MA Tarnopolsky, and WW Campbell. 2002. Effect of protein source on resistive-training-induced changes in body composition and muscle size in older men. *American Journal of Clinical Nutrition* 76 (3):511–7.

Head, KA 1997. Isoflavones and other soy constituents in human health and disease. *Alternative Medicine Review* 2 (6):433–50.

Heber, D, I Yip, et al. 1999. Cholesterol lowering effects of a proprietary Chinese red-yeast-rice dietary supplement. *American Journal of Clinical Nutrition* 69:231–36.

Hekimi, S, and L Guarente. 2003. Genetics and the specificity of the aging process. *Science* 299 (5611):1351–54.

Hendler, Sheldon S. 1985. *The Complete Guide to Anti-Aging Nutrients.* New York: Simon & Schuster.

Hertoghe, Thierry. 2002. *The Hormone Solution*. New York: Harmony Books.

Heydari, AR, B Wu, R Takahashi, et al. 1993. Expression of heat shock protein 70 is altered by age and diet at the level of transcription. *Molecular and Cellular Biology* 13:2909–2918.

Hidaka, H, T Ishiko, et al. 2002. Curcumin inhibits interleukin 8 production and enhances interleukin 8 receptor expression on the cell surface: impact on human pancreatic carcinoma cell growth by autocrine regulation. *Cancer* 95 (6):1206–14.

Hillman, James. 1999. *The Force of Character and the Lasting Life*. New York: Ballantine Books.

Hipkiss, AR, and C Brownson. 2000. Carnosine reacts with protein carbonyl groups: another possible role for the anti-aging peptide. *Biogenontology* 1 (3):217–23.

Hipkiss, AR, C Brownson, and MJ Carrier. 2001. Carnosine, the anti-ageing, anti-oxidant dipeptide, may react with protein carbonyl groups. *Mechanisms of Ageing and Development* 122 (13):1431–45.

Ho, KKY. 1998. Progesterone modulates the effects of estrogen on IGF-I in post menopausal women. *Growth Hormone & IGF Research* 8 (4):316.

Ho, Mae-Wan. 1998. *The Rainbow and The Worm*. London: World Scientific Publishing.

Hodges, R J. 1997. Aging and the immune system. *Immunological Reviews* 160:5–8.

Hofman, LF 2001. Human saliva as a diagnostic specimen. *Journal of Nutrition* 131 (5):1621S–25S.

Holliday, R, and GA McFarland. 2000. A role for carnosine in cellular maintenance. *Biochemistry* 65 (7):843–48.

Holzenberger, M, J Dupont, B Ducos, P Leneuve, A Geloen, PC Even, P Cervera, and Y Le Bouc. 2003. IGF-I receptor regulates life span and resistance to oxidative stress in mice. *Nature* 421 (6919):182–87.

Hooper, DC, S Spitsin, RB Kean, et al. 1998. Uric acid in EAE and multiple sclerosis. *Proceedings of the National Academy of Sciences USA* 95 (2):675–80.

Hotopf, M, PJ Rosch, and C Hart. 2002. Psychological stress and cardiovascular disease. *British Medical Journal* 325 (7359):337.

Houseknecht, KL, JP Vanden Heuvel, SY Moya-Camarena, CP Portocarrero, LW Peck, KP Nickel, and MA Belury. 1998. Dietary conjugated linoleic acid normalizes impaired glucose tolerance in the Zucker diabetic fatty fa/fa rat. *Biochemical and Biophysical Research Communication* 244 (3):678–82.

Houston, Mark C. 2002. The role of vascular biology, nutrition, and nutraceuticals in the prevention and treatment of hypertension. *Journal of the American Nutraceutical Association* supplement 1:5–71.

Hsieh, CC, JH DeFord, K Flurkey, DE Harrison, and J Papaconstantinou. 2002. Implications for the insulin signaling pathway in Snell dwarf mouse longevity: a similarity with the C. elegans longevity paradigm. *Mechanisms of Ageing and Development* 123 (9):1229–44.

Huang, MT, V Badmaev, et al. 2000. Anti-tumor and anti-carcinogenic activities of triterpenoid, beta-boswellic acid. *Biofactors* 13 (1–4):225–30.

Hudson, Frederic M. 1999. *Mastering the Art of Self-Renewal*. New York: MJF Books.

Huff, T, and CS Muller. 2001. Beta-thymosins, small acidic peptides with multiple functions. *International Journal of Biochemistry and Cell Biology* 33 (3):205–20.

Huynh, PN, WH Carter Jr, and R M Loria. 2000. 17 alpha androstenediol inhibition of breast tumor cell proliferation in estrogen receptor-positive and -negative cell lines. *Cancer Detection and Prevention* 24 (5):435–44.

Hyland, P, O Duggan, and A Hipkiss. 2000. The effects of carnosine on oxidative DNA damage levels and in vitro life span in human peripheral blood derived CD4+T cell clones. *Mechanisms of Ageing and Development* 121 (1-3):203–15.

Isidori, A, and A Lo Monaco. 1981. A study of growth hormone release in man after oral administration of amino acids. *Current Medical Research and Opinion* 7:475.

Iwamoto, T, K Hosoda, R Hirano, et al. 2000. Inhibition of low-density lipoprotein oxidation by astaxantine. *Journal of Atherosclerosis and Thrombosis* 7 (4):216–22.

Izumi, K. 1980. Effects of coenzyme Q10 on serum MDA, other serum lipids, and fasting blood sugar level in diabetics. *Japanese Journal of Clinical and Experimental Medicine* 57:1–11.

Jamieson, James. 1998. What do we really know about risks and benefits of growth hormone & IGF-1? Injections, secretagogues, and testing. *Townsend Letter for Doctors and Patients* (Dec):90–92.

Jarvill-Taylor, KJ, RA Anderson, et al. 2001. A hydroxychalcone derived from cinnamon functions as a mimetic for insulin in 3T3-L1 adipocytes. *Journal of the American College of Nutrition* 20 (4):327–36.

Jenkins, DJ, AL Jenkins, TM Wolever, V Vuksan, AV Rao, LU Thompson, and RG Josse. 1994. Low glycemic index: lente carbohydrates and physiological effects of altered food frequency. *American Journal of Clinical Nutrition* 59 (3 Suppl):706S–09S.

Jensen, Aaron W. 2002. Insulin regulates not just blood sugar but fatty acids as well. *Life Enhancement* (July):9–13.

Jingyi, W, M Yasuhiro, H Naoya, RC Seok, Y Yoshiharu, T Nagara, T Fumiko, M Shigeru, and K Junji. 1997. Observation on the effects of Chinese medicine zhenxuanyin for improving cerebral blood flow in rats with cerebral ischemia. *Journal of Traditional Chinese Medicine* 17 (4):299–303.

Johannsson, G, and JO Jorgensen. 2001. Safety aspects of growth hormone replacement in adults. *Growth Hormone & IGF Research* 11:59–71.

Jones, Kenneth, Kerry Hughes, Laurie Mischley, et al. 2002. Coenzyme Q-10: efficacy, safety, and use. *Alternative Therapies in Health and Medicine* 8 (3):42–55.

Julius, M, CA Lang, L Glieberman, et al. 1994. Glutathione and morbidity in a community-based sample of elderly. *Journal of Laboratory and Clinical Medicine* 47:1021–26.

Kalen, A, EL Appelkvist, and G Dallner. 1989. Age-related changes in the lipid composition of rat and human tissues. *Lipids* 24 (7):579–84.

Kamel, Hosam K, Arshag D Mooradian, and Tanverr Mir. 2000. Biological Theories of Aging. In *Endocrinology of Aging*. Totowa, New Jersey: Humana Press.

Kanda, H, K Hamasaki, et al. 2002. Antiinflammatory effect of simvastatin in patients with rheumatoid arthritis. *Journal of Rheumatology* 29 (9):2024–26.

Kang, JH, KS Kim, SY Choi, HY Kwon, MH Won, and TC Kang. 2002. Carnosine and related dipeptides protect human ceruloplasmin against peroxyl radical-mediated modification. *Molecular Cells* 13 (3):498–502.

Kaplan, Jerry, and James P Kushner. 2000. Mining the genome for iron. *Nature* 403:711–13.

Karasek, M. 1999. Melatonin in humans—where we are 40 years after its discovery. *Neuroendocrinology Letters* 20:179–88.

Karkanis, GB, JC Morales, et al. 1997. Deficits in reproductive behavior in diabetic female rats are due to hypoinsulinemia rather than hyperglyceria. *Hormones and Behavior* 32:19–29.

Keller, T. 2000. Compounding with B-1,3-D-glucan. *International Journal of Pharmaceutical Compounding* 4 (5):342–45.

Kelly, D, and PE Wischmeyer. 2003. Role of L-glutamine in critical illness: new insights. *Current Opinion in Clinical Nutrition and Metabolic Care* 6 (2):217–22.

Kelly, D, Z Zhong, MD Wheeler, X Li, M Froh, P Schemmer, M Yin, H Bunzendaul, B Bradford, and JJ Lemasters. 2003. L-glycine: a novel antiinflammatory, immunomod-ulatory, and cytoprotective agent. *Current Opinion in Clinical Nutrition and Metabolic Care* 6 (2):229–40.

Kelly, G. 2000. Insulin resistance: lifestyle and nutritional influences. *Alternative Medicine Review* 5 (2):109–32.

Kelly, GS. 2001. Rhodiola rosea: a possible plant adaptogen. *Alternative Medicine Review* 6 (3):293–302.

Kevtnoy, I, AK Sandvik, et al. 1997. The diffuse neuroendocrine system and extrapineal melatonin. *Journal of Molecular Endocrinology* 18:1–3.

Khaw, KT, S Bingham, A Welch, et al. 2001. Relation between plasma ascorbic acid and men and women in EPIC-Norfolk prospective study: a prospective population study. *Lancet* 357:657–63.

Kidd, Paris. 1997. Glutathione: systemic protectant against oxidative and free radical damage. *Alternative Medicine Review* 2 (3):155–76.

Kidd, Paris M. 2000. Parkinson's disease as multifactorial oxidative neurodegeneration: implications for integrative management. *Alternative Medicine Review* 5 (6):502–29.

Kim, HJ, KD Moon, SY Oh, SP Kim, and SR Lee. 2001. Ether fraction of methanol extracts of Gastrodia elata, a traditional medicinal herb, protects against kainic acid-induced neuronal damage in the mouse hippocampus. *Neuroscience Letters* 314 (1-2):65–68.

Kim, NW, MA Paityszek, et al. 1994. Specific association of human telomerase activity with immortal cells and cancer. *Science* 266:2011–15.

Kim, SJ, RJ Reiter, et al. 2000. Melatonin prevents oxidative damage to protein and lipid induced by ascorbate-Fe3+-EDTA: comparison with glutathione and a-tocopherol. *Neuroendocrinology Letters* 21:269–76.

Kitaman, Dalane W. 2000. Normal age-related changes in the heart: relevance to echocardiography in the elderly. *American Journal of Geriatric Cardiology* 9 (6):311–20.

Kluger, Jeffrey. 2002. Can we learn to beat the reaper? *Time* (January 21): 102.

Klungland, Arne, Ian Rosewell, and Stephan Hollenbach. 1999. Accumulation of premutagenic DNA lesions in mice defective in removal of oxidative base damage. *Proceedings of the National Academy of Sciences* 96 (23):13300–05.

Kmiec, Z, J Mysliwska, D Ranchoz, et al. 2001. Natural killer activity and thyroid hormone levels in young and elderly persons. *Gerontology* 47 (5):282–88.

Kolata, Gina. 1999. Pushing limits of the human life span. *The New York Times* (March 9).

Kontush, A, S Schippling, et al. 1999. Plasma ubiquinol-10 as a marker for disease: is the assay worthwhile? *BioFactors* 9 (2-4):225–29.

Kraemer, WJ, GA Dudley, PA Tesch, SE Gordon, BM Hather, JS Volek, and NA Ratamess. 2001. The influence of muscle action on the acute growth hormone response to resistance exercise and short-term detraining. *Growth Hormone and IGF Res* 11 (2):75–83.

Krimsky, Sheldon. 2000. *Hormonal Chaos: The Scientific and Social Origins of the Environmental Endocrine Hypothesis.* Baltimore, Maryland: John Hopkins University Press.

Kripke, DF. 2003. Sleep and mortality. *Psychosomatic Medicine* 65 (1):74.

Kripke, DF, L Garfinkel, DL Wingard, MR Klauber, and MR Marler. 2002. Mortality associated with sleep duration and insomnia. *Archive of General Psychiatry* 59 (2):131–36.

Kroemer, G, and G Wick. 1989. The role of interleukin 2 in autoimmunity. *Immunology Today* 10 (7):246–51.

Krone, CA, GE Elmer, JTA Ely, et al. 2001. Does gastrointestinal Candida albicans prevent ubiquinone absorption? *Medical Hypotheses* 57 (5):570–72.

Krtolica, A, and J Campisi. 2002. Cancer and aging: a model for the cancer promoting effects of the aging stroma. *International Journal of Biochemistry and Cell Biology* 34 (11):1401.

Kruch, Constance A, and Victoria A Velkoff. 1999. Centenarians in the United States: U.S. Department of Health and Human Services.

Kuikka, JT, L Tammela, KA Bergstrom, et al. 2001. Effects of ageing on serotonin transporters in healthy females. *European Journal of Nuclear Medicine* 28 (7):911–13.

Kuusisto, J, K Koivisto, et al. 1997. Association between features of the insulin resistance syndrome and Alzheimer's disease independently of apolipoprotein E4 phenotype: cross sectional population based study. *British Medical Journal* 315:1045–49.

Kvetnoy, IM, RJ Reiter, et al. 2000. Claude Bernard was right: hormones may be produced by "non-endocrine" cells. *Neuroendocrinology Letters* 21:173–74.

Lang, CA. 2001. The impact of glutathione on health and longevity. *Journal of Anti-Aging Medicine* 4 (2):137–45.

Lang, CA, BJ Mills, W Mastropaolo, et al. 2000. Blood glutathione decreases in chronic disease. *Journal of Laboratory and Clinical Medicine* 135:402–05.

Lang, CA, S Naryshkin, DL Scheider, et al. 1992. Low blood glutathione levels in healthy aging adults. *Journal of Laboratory and Clinical Medicine* 120:720–25.

Lavallee, B, PR Provost, et al. 1997. Effect of insulin on serum levels of dehydroepiandrosterone metabolites in men. *Clinical Endocrinology* 46 (1):93–100.

Lee, John R. 1993. *Natural Progesterone: The Multiple Roles of a Remarkable Hormone.* Sebastopol, California: BLL Publishing.

Leviton, Richard. 2001. *The Healthy Living Space: 70 Practical Ways to Detoxify the Body and Home.* Charlottesville, Virginia: Hampton Roads Publishing Company.

Levy, JR, B Davenport, JN Clore, and W Stevens. 2002. Lipid metabolism and resistin gene expression in insulin-resistant Fischer 344 rats. *American Journal of Physiology–Endocrinology and Metabolism* 282 (3):E626–33.

Lewis, Ricki. 1995. Chronobiology reseachers say their field's time has come. *Scientist* 9 (24).

Lin, YJ, L Seroude, and S Benzer. 1998. Extended life-span and stress resistance in the Drosophila mutant methuselah. *Science* 30 (282(5390)):943–46.

Linnane, AW, C Zhang, et al. 2002. Human aging and global function of coenzyme Q10. *Annals of the New York Academy of Sciences* 959:396–411.

Liska, DJ, and LR Leupp. 2002. Estrogen metabolism: a complex web. *Journal of the American Nutraceutical Association* 5 (3):4–14.

Lissoni, P. 1999. The pineal gland as a central regulator of cytokine network. *Neuroendocrinology Letters* 20:343–49.

Lissoni, P, F Rovelli, et al. 2000. Oncostatic activity of pineal neuroendocrine treatment with the pineal indoles melatonin and 5-methoxytryptamine in untreatable metastatic cancer patients progressing on melatonin alone. *Neuroendocrinology Letters* 21:319–23.

Liu, J, and A Mori. 1992. Antioxidant and free radical scavenging activities of Gastrodia elata Bl. and Uncaria rhynchophylla (Miq.) Jacks. *Neuropharmacology* 31 (12):1287–98.

Liu, J, H Atamna, H Kuratsune, and BN Ames. 2002. Delaying brain mitochondrial decay and aging with mitochondrial antioxidants and metabolites. *Annals of the New York Academy of Sciences* 959:133–66.

Loria, RM, DA Padgett, and PN Huynh. 1996. Regulation of the immune response by dehydroepiandrosterone and its metabolites. *Journal of Endocrinology* 150 Suppl:S209–20.

Loria, RM, DH Conrad, T Huff, H Carter, and D Ben-Nathan. 2000. Androstenetriol and androstenediol. Protection against lethal radiation and restoration of immunity after radiation injury. *Annals of the New York Academy of Sciences* 917:860–67.

Loria, RM, TH Inge, SS Cook, AK Szakal, and W Regelson. 1988. Protection against acute lethal viral infections with the native steroid dehydroepiandrosterone (DHEA). *Journal of Medical Virology* 26 (3):301–14.

Lowe, Gordon. 2001. Is sticky blood a treatable determinant of cognitive decline and of dementia? *Age and Ageing* 30:101–03.

Lukaczer, Dan. 1998. *Functional Medicine Adjuntive Support for Syndrome X, Functional Medicine Clinical Practice Protocol.* Gig Harbor, Washington: HealthComm International.

Lutsenko, EA, JM Carcamo, et al. 2002. Vitamin C prevents DNA mutation induced by oxidative stress. *Journal of Biological Chemistry* 277 (19):16895–99.

Lykkesfeldt, J, TM Hagen, V Vinarsky, et al. 1998. Age-associated decline in ascorbic acid concentration, recycling, and biosynthesis in rat hepatocytes—reversal with (R)-alpha-lipoic acid supplementation. *Journal of the Federation of American Societies for Experimental Biology* 12 (12):1183–89.

Lynch, MA. 2001. Lipoic acid confers protection against oxidative injury in non-neuronal and neuronal tissue. *Nutritional Neuroscience* 4 (6):419–38.

Mackall, CL, and RE Gress. 1997. Thymic aging and T-cell regeneration. *Immunological Reviews* 160:91–102.

Magalhães, João Pedro de. 2002. Namur, Belgium, July 17. Personal conversation.

Mantovani, G, A Maccio, C Madeddu, et al. 2002. Reactive oxygen species, antioxidant mechanisms and serum cytokine levels in cancer patients: impact of an antioxidant treatment. *Journal of Molecular Medicine* 6 (4):570–82.

Maran, RR, J Arunakaran, et al. 2000. T3 directly stimulates basal and modulates LH induced testosterone and oestradiol production by rat Leydig cells in vivo. *Journal of Endocrinology* 47 (4):417–28.

Maran, RR, R Sivakumar, et al. 2000. Growth hormone directly stimulates testosterone and oestradiol secretion by rat Leydig cells in vitro and modulates the effects of LH and T3. *Journal of Endocrinology* 47 (2):111–18.

Margulis, Lynn. 1992. *Symbiosis in Cell Evolution.* New York: W. H. Freeman.

Maritim, AC, RA Sanders, and JB Watkins. 2003. Diabetes, oxidative stress, and antioxidants: a review. *Journal of Biochemistry and Molecular Toxicology* 17 (1):24–38.

Marshall, JA, DH Bessesen, et al. 1997. High saturated fat and low starch and fibre are associated with hyperinsulinemia in a non-diabetic population: the San Luis Valley Diabetes Study. *Diabetologia* 40:430–38.

Martin, F. 1999. Frailty and the somatopause. *Growth Hormone & IGF Research* 9:3–10.

Martin, George M, and Junko Oshima. 2000. Lessons from human progeroid syndromes. *Nature* 408 (November 9):263–66.

Masoro, EJ, MS Katz, and CA McMahan. 1989. Evidence for the glycation hypothesis of aging from the food-restriction rodent model. *Journal of Gerontology* 44:B20–22.

Mattison, Julie A. 2002. Calorie restriction (CR) in monkeys. Paper read at Sixth International Symposium on Neurobiology and Neurendocrinology of Aging, July 21–26, at Bregenz, Austria.

Mattison, Julie A, GS Roth, et al. 2001. Endocrine effects of dietary restriction and aging: the National Institute on Aging study. *Journal of Anti-Aging Medicine* 4 (3):215–23.

Mattison, Julie A, Mark A Lane, and George S Roth. 2003. Calorie restriction in rhesus monkeys. *Experimental Gerontology* 38 (1-2):35–46.

Mattson, MP, II Kruman, et al. 2002. Folic acid and homocysteine in age-related disease. *Ageing Research Review* 1 (1):95–111.

Mayo, W, M Le Moal, et al. 2001. Pregnenolone sulfate and aging of cognitive functions: behavioral, neurochemical, and morphological investigations. *Hormone Behavior* 40 (2):215–17.

McCann, Jean. 2002. Wanna bet? Two scientists wager on whether humans can live to 130 or 150 years. *Scientist* 15 (3):8.

McCarthy, TL, and M Centrella. 2001. Local IGF-I expression and bone formation. *Growth Hormone & IGF Research* 11:213–19.

McCarty, MF. 2000. Increased homocysteine associated with smoking, chronic inflammation, and aging may reflect acute-phase induction of pyridoxal phosphatase activity. *Medical Hypotheses* 55 (4):289–93.

McDonald, RB. 1995. Influence of dietary sucrose on biological aging. *American Journal of Clinical Nutrition* 62 (1):284S–92S.

McFadden, Johnjoe. 2000. *Quantum Evolution.* New York: W. W. Norton.

McLay, RN, AJ Kastin, and JE Zadina. 2000. Passage of interleukin-1-beta across the blood-brain barrier is reduced in aged mice: a possible mechanism for diminished fever in aging. *NeuroImmunoModulation* 8 (3):148–53.

Meilahn, EH, B De Stavola, et al. 1998. Do urinary oestrogen metabolism predict breast cancer? Guernsey III cohort follow-up. *British Journal of Cancer* 78:1250–55.

Melov, S. 2000. Mitochondrial oxidative stress. Physiologic consequences and potential for a role in aging. *Annals of the New York Academy of Sciences* 908:219–25.

Meydani, SN, and WK Hu. 2000. Immunological effects of yogurt. *American Journal of Clinical Nutrition* 71:861–72.

Micic, D, and X Casabiell. 1999. Growth hormone secretagogues: the clinical future. *Hormone Research* 51 (Supplement 3):29–33.

Milner, Martin. 1999. Wilson's syndrome and T3 therapy, a clinical guide to safe and effective patient management. *International Journal of Pharmaceutical Compounding* September/October:1–10.

Minton, Phillip. 2000. *The Immortality Enzyme.* White Bear Lake, Minnesota: Winning Publications.

Miquel, J. 2002. Can antioxidant diet supplementation protect against age-related mitochondrial damage? *Annals of the New York Academy of Sciences* 959:508–16.

Mishra, LC, BB Singh, et al. 2000. Scientific basis for therapeutic use of *Withania somnifera* (Ashwagandha). *Alternative Medicine Review* 5 (4):334–46.

Mitchell, Teri. 2001. Radiation, unsafe at any dose. *Life Extension* (November):40–47.

Moberly, J, J Logan, P Borum, et al. 1998. Elevation of whole-blood glutathione in peritoneal dialysis patients by L-2-oxothiazolidine-4-carboxylate, a cysteine prodrug (Procysteine). *Journal of the American Society of Nephrology* 9:1093–99.

Mocchegiani, E, and L Santarelli. 1995. Reversibility of the thymic involution and of age-related peripheral immune dysfunctions by zinc supplementation in old mice. *International Journal of Immunopharmacology* 17 (9):703–18.

Mogadam, Michael. 2001. *Every Heart Attack Is Preventable.* Washington, D.C.: LifeLine Press.

Moller, David E. 2001. New drug targets for type 2 diabetes and the metabolic syndrome. *Nature* 414:821–27.

Moore, Richard D. 2001. *The High Blood Pressure Solution.* Rochester, Vermont: Healing Arts Press.

Morales, Alvaro, Jeremy PW Heaton, and Culley C Carson III. 2000. Andropause: a misnomer for a true clinical entity. *The Journal of Urology* 163 (March):705–12.

Moriguchi, S. 1998. The role of vitamin E in T cell differentiation and the decrease of cellular immunity with aging. *Mechanisms of Ageing and Development* 7 (1–2):77–86.

Mowe, M, and T Bohmer. 2002. Reduced appetite: a predictor for undernutrition in aged people. *Journal of Nutrition, Health Aging* 6 (1):81–3.

Mowe, M, T Bohmer, and E Kindt. 1994. Reduced nutritional status in an elderly population (> 70 y) is probable before disease and possibly contributes to the development of disease. *American Journal of Clinical Nutrition* 59 (2):317–24.

Muccioli, G, F Broglio, et al. 2000. Growth hormone-releasing peptides and the cardiovascular system. *Annals of Endocrinology* 61 (1):27–31.

Murphy, Christine. 2001. *Iscador, Mistletoe and Cancer Therapy.* New York: Latern Books.

Murphy, MG, MA Bach, et al. 1999. Oral administration of the growth hormone secretagogue MK-677 increases markers of bone turnover in healthy and functionally impaired elderly adults. *Journal of Bone and Mineral Research* 14 (7):1182–88.

Murray, Michael. 1996. *Encyclopedia of Nutritional Supplements.* Rocklin, California: Prima Publishing.

Myers, KA. 2002. Elevated homocysteine: a new marker for dementia? *Canadian Medical Journal* 166 (8):1068.

Nagasawa, T, and T Yonekura. 2001. In vitro and in vivo inhibition of muscle lipid and protein oxidation by carnosine. *Molecular and Cellular Biochemistry* 225 (1):29–34.

Nakamura, K, Y Yasunaga, et al. 2002. Curcumin down-regulates AR gene expression and activation in prostate cancer cell lines. *International Journal of Oncology* 21 (4):825–30.

Nearing, Scott and Helen. 1970. *Living the Good Life.* New York: Schocken Books.

Nelson HD. 2002. Assessing benefits and harms of hormone replacement therapy: clinical applications. *Journal of the American Medical Association* 288 (7):882–4.

Nesse, Randolph M, and George C Williams. 1994. *Why We Get Sick: The New Science of Darwinian Medicine.* New York: Vintage.

Nestler, JE, NA Beer, et al. 1994. Efffects of a reduction in circulating insulin by metformin on serum dehydroepiandrosterone sulfate in nondiabetic men. *Journal of Clinical Endocrinology* 78 (3):549–54.

Nihal, T, HA Morris, et al. 1999. Relationship between age, dehydro-epiandrosterone sulphate and plasma glucose in healthy men. *Age and Ageing* 28:217–20.

Nindl, BC, WC Hymer, DR Deaver, and WJ Kraemer. 2001. Growth hormone pulsatility profile characteristics following acute heavy resistance exercise. *Journal of Applied Physiology* 91 (1):163–72.

Nishizawa, Y, K Toshitaka, et al. 2001. Guidelines on the use of biochemical markers of bone turnover in osteoporosis (2001). *Journal of Bone and Mineral Metabolism* 19:338–44.

Norbury, R, WJ Cutter, and J Compton. 2003. The neuro-protective effects of estrogen on the aging brain. *Experimental Gerontology* 38:109–17.

Olivieri, O, AM Stanzial, and D Girelli. 1994. Selenium status, fatty acids, vitamins A and E, and aging: the Nove Study. *American Journal of Clinical Nutrition* 60 (4):510–17.

Olmedilla, B, F Granado, I Blanco, C Herrero, M Vaquero, and I Millan. 2002. Serum status of carotenoids and tocopherols in patients with age-related cataracts: a case-control study. *Journal of Nutrition Health and Aging* 6 (1):66–68.

Olshansky, S Jay, Bruce A Carnes, and Aline Desesquelles. 2001. Prospects for human longevity. *Science* 291 (23):1491–92.

Olshansky, S. Jay, Leonard Hayflick, and Bruce A Carnes. 2002. No truth to the fountain of youth. *Scientific American* 286 (6):92–95.

Osorio, A, MA Guiterrez, et al. 2002. Dehydroepian-drosterone sulfate and growth axis hormones in patients with ischemic heart disease. *Hormone Research* 57 (5–6):165–69.

Ostfeld, A, CM Smith, et al. 1977. The systemic use of procaine in the treatment of the elderly: a review. *Journal of the American Geriatric Society* 25 (1):1–19.

Oxenkrug, G, P Requintina, et al. 2001. Antioxidant and antiaging activity of N-acetylserotonin and melatonin in the in vivo models. *Annals of the New York Academy of Sciences* 939:190–99.

Ozmeric, N, T Baydar, A Bodur, AB Engin, A Uraz, K Eren, and G Sahin. 2002. Level of neopterin, a marker of immune cell activation in gingival crevicular fluid, saliva, and urine in patients with aggressive periodontitis. *Journal of Periodontology* 73 (7):720–5.

Padgett, DA, RM Loria, and JF Sheridan. 1997. Endocrine regulation of the immune response to influenza virus infection with a metabolite of DHEA-androstenediol. *Journal of Neuroimmunology* 78 (1-2):203–11.

Pak, JW, A Herbst, Bua Entela, et al. 2003. Mitochondrial DNA mutations as a fundamental mechanism in physiological declines associated with aging. *Aging Cell* 2:1–7.

Paolisso, G, A D'Amore, et al. 1994. Plasma vitamin C affects glucose homeostasis in healthy subjects and in non-insulin-dependent diabetics. *American Journal of Physiology* 266:E261–68.

Parham, Peter. 2000. *The Immune System.* New York: Garland Publishing.

Park, SY, and DS Kim. 2002. Discovery of natural products from Curcuma longa that protect cells from beta-amyloid insult: a drug discovery effort against Alzheimer's disease. *Journal of Natural Products* 65 (9):1227–31.

Patchett, AA, and MJ Wyvratt. 2000. The design of peptidomimetic growth hormone secretagogues. In *Human Growth Hormone Research and Clinical Practice*, edited by RG Smith and MO Thorner. Totowa, New Jersey: Humana Press.

Patrick, L, and M Uzick. 2001. Cardiovascular disease: C-reactive protein and the inflammatory disease paradigm: HMG-CoA reductase inhibitors, alpha-tocopherol, red yeast rice, and olive oil polyphenols. A review of the literature. *Alternative Medicine Review* 6 (3):248–71.

Pawelec, G, and R Solana. 1997. Immunosenescence. *Immunology Today* 18 (11):514–16.

Pearson, Durk, and Sandy Shaw. 1982. *Life Extension: A Practical Scientific Approach.* New York: Warner Books.

Peat, Ray. 2000. Growth hormone: hormone of stress, aging, and death? *Ray Peat's Newsletter* (April):1–6.

———. 2001. Aging, estrogen, and progesterone. *Ray Peat's Newsletter.*

Peat, Raymond. 1997. *From PMS to Menopause: Female Hormones in Context.* Eugene, Oregon: Ray Peat.

Perls, Thomas T, and Margery Hutter Silver. 1999. *Living to 100: Lessons in Living to Maximize Potential at Any Age.* New York: Basic Books.

Pettegrew, JW, J Levine, S Gershon, JA Stanley, D Servan-Schreiber, K Panchalingam, and RJ McClure. 2002. 31P-MRS study of acetyl-L-carnitine treatment in geriatric depression: preliminary results. *Bipolar Disorders* 4 (1):61–66.

Pierpaoli, Walter. 1998. Neuroimmunomodulation of aging: a programme in the pineal gland. *Annals of the New York Academy of Sciences* 840:491–97.

Pioli, C, S Pucci, S Barile, et al. 1998. Role of mRNA stability in the different patterns of cytokine production by CD4+ cells from young and old mice. *Immunology* 94:380.

Pittenrigh, CS, and S Daan. 1974. Circadian oscillations in rodents: a systematic increase of their frequency with age. *Science* 186:548–55.

Plenge, JK, and TL Hernandez. 2002. Simvastatin lowers C-reactive protein within 14 days: an effect independent of low-density lipoprotein cholesterol reduction. *Circulation* 106 (12):1447–52.

Proteggente, AR, A Rehman, B Halliwell, et al. 2000. Potential problems of ascorbate and iron supplementation: pro-oxidant effect in vivo? *Biochemical and Biophysical Research Communications* 277 (3):535–40.

Proteggente, AR, TG England, CA Rice-Evans, and B Halliwell. 2001. Iron supplementation and oxidative damage to DNA in healthy individuals with high plasma ascorbate. *Biochemical and Biophysical Research Communications* 288 (1):245–51.

Quaini, F, K Urbanek, et al. 2002. Chimerism of the transplanted heart. *New England Journal of Medicine* 346 (1):5–15.

Quig, David W. 2000. Molecules that detoxify. Paper read at 15th Annual American Association of Naturopathic Physicians Conference, in Seattle, Washington.

Quinn, PL, and AA Boldyrev. 1992. Carnosine: its properties, functions and potential therapeutic applications. *Molecular Aspects of Medicine* 13 (5):379–444.

Rabin, Bruce S. 1999. *Stress, Immune Function, and Health.* New York: Wiley-Liss.

Racchi, M, and S Govani. 2003. The pharmacology of amyloid precursor protein processing. *Experimental Gerontology* 38:145–57.

Rattan, SI. 1991. Protein synthesis and the components of protein synthetic machinery during cellular aging. *Mutation Research* 256 (2-6):115–25.

Rauser, CL, LD Mueller, and MR Rose. 2003. Aging, fertility, and immortality. *Experimental Gerontology* 38 (1-2):27–33.

Ravaglia, G, P Forti, F Maioli, et al. 2000. Effect of micronutrient status on natural killer cell immune function in health free-living subjects aged >/= 90 years. *American Journal of Clinical Nutrition* 71 (2):590–98.

Regelson, William, and Carol Colman. 1996. *The Super-Hormone Promise.* New York: Simon & Schuster.

Reiter, RJ. 1999. Oxidative damage to nuclear DNA: amelioration by melatonin. *Neuroendocrinology Letters* 20 (3-4):145–50.

Reiter, Russel J, and Jo Robinson. 1995. *Your Body's Natural Wonder Drug: Melatonin.* New York: Bantam Books.

Requejo, AM, P Andres, MR Redondo, et al. 2002. Vitamin E status in a group of elderly people from Madrid. *Journal of Nutrition, Health, and Aging* 6 (1):72–74.

Ridker, PM, N Rifai, L Rose, JE Buring, and NR Cook. 2002. Comparison of C-reactive protein and low-density lipoprotein cholesterol levels in the prediction of first cardiovascular events. *New England Journal of Medicine* 347 (20):1557–65.

Roberts, PR, and GP Zaloga. 2000. Cardiovascular effects of carnosine. *Biochemistry* 65 (7):856–61.

Rodewald, HR. 1998. The thymus in the age of retirement. *Nature* 396 (6712):630–31.

Rose, MR, and LD Mueller. 2000. Ageing and immortality. *Philosophical Transcripts of the Royal Society of London* 355 (1403):1657–62.

Rosedale, Ron. 2001. Insulin Resistance. Paper read at Designs for Health, November 4, Palm Desert, California.

Rosenbaum, ME, A Vojdani, M Susser, et al. 2001. Improved immunological marker in chronic fatigue and immune dsyfunction syndrome (CFIDS) patients treated with thymic protein A. *Journal of Nutritional & Environmental Medicine* 11:241–247.

Roth, GS, DK Ingram, and MA. Lane. 2001. Caloric restriction in primates and relevance to humans. *Annals of the New York Academy of Sciences* 928:305–15.

Roth, GS, MA Lane, DK Ingram, JA Mattison, D Elahi, JD Tobin, D Muller, and EJ Metter. 2002. Biomarkers of caloric restriction may predict longevity in humans. *Science* 297 (5582):811.

Rowe, John W, and Robert L Kahn. 1998. *Successful Aging.* New York: Dell.

Roy, M, L Kiremidjian-Schumacher, and HI Wishe. 1995. Supplementation with selenium restores age-related decline in immune cell function. *Proceedings of the Society for Experimental Biology and Medicine* 209 (4):369–75.

Royte, Elizabeth. 2001. *The Tapir's Morning Bath.* New York: Houghton Mifflin.

Rudman, D, AG Feller, HS Nagraj, et al. 1990. Effects of human growth hormone in men over 60 years old. *New England Journal of Medicine* 323:1–6.

Rufiange, M, M Dumont, and P Lachapelle. 2002. Correlating retinal function with melatonin secretion in subjects with an early or late circadian phase. *Investigative Ophthalmology and Visual Science* 43 (7):2491–99.

Ryazanov, AG, and BS Nefsky. 2002. Protein turnover plays a key role in aging. *Mechanisms of Ageing and Development* 123 (2-3):207–13.

Sadighi, M, C Li, et al. 2001. Effects of testosterone either alone or with IGF-I on growth cells derived from the proliferation zone of regenerating antlers in vitro. *Growth Hormone & IGF Research* 11:240–46.

Saito, H, and J Papconstantinou. 2001. Age-associated differences in cardiovascular inflammatory gene induction during endotoxic stress. *Journal of Biological Chemistry* 276 (31):29307–12.

Saito, H, C Patterson, Z Hu, et al. 2000. Expression and self-regulatory function of cardiac interleukin-6 during endotoxemia. *American Journal of Physiology–Heart and Circulatory Physiology* 279 (5):H2241–48.

Salteil, AR, and CR Kahn. 2001. Insulin signalling and the regulation of glucose and lipid metabolism. *Nature* 414 (December 13):799–806.

Sandoval-Chacon, M, JH Thompson, XJ Zhang, et al. 1998. Antiinflammatory actions of cat's claw: the role of NF-kappaB. *Alimentary Pharmacology and Therapeutics* 12 (12):1279–89.

Sano, S, et al. 2001. Stat3 in thymic epithelial cells is essential for postnatal maintenance of thymic architecture and thymocyte survival. *Immunity* 15:261–73.

Sarcletti, M, W Bitterlich, D Fuchs, and R Zangerle. 2002. Is the poorer rate of survival among patients with human immunodeficiency virus infection and anemia linked to immune activation? *Journal of Infectious Disease* 186 (1):141–42; discussion 142–43.

Sardi, Bill. 1999. *The Iron Time Bomb*. San Dimas, California: Bill Sardi.

Sastre, J, C Borras, and D Garcia-Sala. 2002. Mitochondrial damage in aging and apoptosis. *Annals of the New York Academy of Sciences* April (959):448–51.

Sastre, J, FV Pallardo, et al. 2000. Mitochondria, oxidative stress and aging. *Free Radical Research* 32 (3):189–98.

Sastre, J, FV Pallardo, J Garcia de la Asuncion, et al. 2000. Mitochondria, oxygen stress and aging. *Free Radical Research* 32 (3):189–98.

Sastre, J, A Lloret, C Borras, et al. 2002. Ginkgo biloba extract EGb 761 protects against mitochondrial aging in the brain and in the liver. *Cellular and Molecular Biology* 48 (6):685–92.

Sattin, RW. 1992. Falls among older persons: a public health perspective. *Annual Review of Public Health* 13:489–508.

Scaglione, F, et al. 1990. Immunomodulating effects of two extracts of Panax ginseng. *Drugs and Experimental Clinical Research* 16:537–42.

Schacter, F, L Faure-Delanef, F Guenot, et al. 1994. Genetic associations with human longevity at the APOE and ACE loci. *Nature Genetics* 6:29–32.

Schmeissner, PJ. 2002. Bregenz, Austria, July 25. Personal communications.

Schulz-Aellen, Marie-Françoise. 1997. *Aging and Human Longevity*. Boston: Birkhauser.

Schwarzbein, Diana. 1999. *The Schwarzbein Principle: The Truth About Losing Weight, Being Healthy, and Feeling Younger*. Deerfield Beach, Florida: Health Communications.

———. 2002. Diabetes. Paper read at Cardiovascular Disease: An Integrative Medical Approach to Prevention and Treatment, in San Diego, CA.

Sears, Barry. 1999. *The Age-Free Zone*. New York: Harper Collins.

———. 2002. *The OmegaRX Zone*. New York: Harper Collins.

Segovia, G, A Del Arco, and F Mora. 1999. Effects of aging on the interaction between glutamate, dopamine, and GABA in striatum and nucleus accumbens of the awake rat. *Journal of Neurochemistry* 73 (5):2063–72.

Seidler, NW, and GS. Yeargans. 2002. Effects of thermal denaturation on protein glycation. *Life Science* 70 (15):1789–99.

Selhub, J. 2002. Folate, vitamin B12 and vitamin B6 and one carbon metabolism. *Journal of Nutrtion, Health, and Aging* 6 (1):39–42.

Sentinelli, F, S Romeo, M Arca, E Filippi, F Leonetti, M Banchieri, U Di Mario, and MG Baroni. 2002. Human resistin gene, obesity, and type 2 diabetes: mutation analysis and population study. *Diabetes* 51 (3):860–62.

Sewerynek, E, J Wiktorska, et al. 1999. Effects of melatonin on the oxidative stress induced by thryotoxicosis in rats. *Neuroendocrinology Letters* 20:157–61.

Shamsuddin, AM, and I Vucenik. 1999. Mammary tumor inhibition by IP6: a review. *Anticancer Research* 19 (5A):3671–74.

Shapiro, K, and WC Gong. 2002. Natural products used for diabetes. *Journal of the American Pharmacy Association (Wash)* 42 (2):217–26.

Shay, Jerry W, and Woodring E Wright. 2000. Hayflick, his limit, and cellular aging. *Nature* 1 (October):72–76.

Sheline, YI, MA Mintun, SM Moerlein, et al. 2002. Greater loss of 5-HT (2A) receptors in midlife than in late life. *American Journal of Psychiatry* 159 (3):430–35.

Sheng, YZ, L Li, K Holmgren, and RW Pero. 2001. DNA repair enhancement of aqueous extracts of Uncaria tomentosa in a human volunteer study. *Phytomedicine* 8 (4):275–82.

Sheng, YZ, C Bryngelsson, and RW Pero. 2000. Enhanced DNA repair, immune function and reduced toxicity of C-MED-100, a novel aqueous extract from Uncaria tomentosa. *Journal of Ethnopharmacology* 69 (2):115–26.

Shigenaga, M, and B Ames. 1991. Assays for 8-hydroxy-2'-deoxyguansosine: a biomarker of in vivo oxidative DNA damage. *Free Radical Biological Medicine* 10:211–16.

Shigenaga, Mark K, Tory M Hagen, and Bruce N Ames. 1994. Oxidative damage and mitochondrial decay in aging. *Proceedings of the National Academy of Sciences* 91:10771–78.

Shim, M, and P Cohen. 1999. IGFs and human cancer: implications regarding the risk of growth hormone therapy. *Hormone Research* 51 (S3):42–51.

Shimokawa, I, and Y Higami. 1999. A role for leptin in the antiaging action of dietary restriction: a hypothesis. *Aging (Milano)* 11 (6):380–82.

———. 2001. Leptin and anti-aging action of caloric restriction. *Journal of Nutrition, Health, and Aging* 5 (1):43–48.

———. 2001. Leptin signaling and aging: insight from caloric restriction. *Mechanisms of Ageing and Development* 122 (14):1511–19.

Shiner, JS, and DE Uehlinger. 2001. Body mass index: a measure for longevity. *Medical Hypotheses* 57 (5):780–83.

Shippen, Eugene, and William Fryer. 1998. *The Testosterone Syndrome: The Critical Factor for Energy, Health, & Sexuality– Reversing the Male Menopause.* New York: M. Evans.

Shock, NW, RC Gruelich, R Andres, et al. 1984. Normal human aging: the Baltimore Longitudinal Study on Aging. *US Department of Health and Human Services, NIH publication* 84.

Shostak, Stanley. 2002. *Becoming Immortal: Combining Cloning and Stem Cell Therapy.* Albany, New York: State University of New York Press.

Shugars, DC, CA Watkins, and HJ Cowen. 2001. Salivary concentration of secretory leukocyte protease inhibitor, an antimicrobial protein, is decreased with advanced age. *Gerontology* 47 (5):246–53.

Smith, RG, and OC Palyha. 1999. Growth hormone releasing substances: types and their receptors. *Hormone Research* 51 (Supplement 3):1–8.

Song, MK, MJ Rosenthal, et al. 1998. Effects of bovine prostate powder on zinc, glucose, and insulin metabolism in old patients with non-insulin dependent diabetes mellitus. *Metabolism* 1 (January):39–43.

Sonntag, WE. 2002. Pleiotropic effects of growth hormone and insulin-like growth factor (IGF)-I on biological aging and life span. Paper read at Buck Institute Symposium 2002, in Novato, CA.

Sonntag, WE, JK Brunso-Bechtold, et al. 2001. Age-related decreases in growth hormone and insulin-like growth factor (IGF)-I: implications for brain aging. *Journal of Anti-Aging Medicine* 4 (4):311–29.

SoRelle, R. 2002. Inflammation-sensitive proteins: another ingredient in stroke? *Circulation* 105 (22):e9111.

Sorkin, JD, DC Muller, and R Andres. 1999. Longitudinal change in height of men and women: implications for interpretation of the body mass index: the Baltimore Longitudinal Study of Aging. *American Journal of Epidemiology* 150 (9):969–77.

Speroff, Leon, Robert H Glass, and Nathan G Kase. 1999. *Clinical Gynecologic Endocrinology and Infertility.* Sixth Edition. Baltimore, Maryland: Lippincott Williams & Wilkins.

Spindler, SR. 2001. Calorie restriction enhances the expression of key metabolic enzymes associated with protein renewal during aging. *Annals of the New York Academy of Sciences* 928:296–304.

Spindler, SR., JM Grizzle, RL Walford, and PL Mote. 1991. Aging and restriction of dietary calories increases insulin receptor mRNA, and aging increases glucocorticoid receptor mRNA in the liver of female C3B10RF1 mice. *Journal of Gerontology* 46 (6):B233–37.

Stapleton, SR. 2000. Selenium: an insulin-mimetic. *Cellular and Molecular Life Sciences* 57:1874–79.

Starke-Reed, PE, and CN Oliver. 1989. Protein oxidation and proteolysis during aging and oxidative stress. *Archives of Biochemistry and Biophysics* 275:559–67.

Stoll, Andrew L. 2000. *The Omega-3 Connection.* New York: Simon & Schuster.

Straub, RH, J Scholmerich, and B Zietz. 2000. Replacement therapy with DHEA plus corticosteroids in patients with chronic inflammatory diseases: substitutes for adrenal and sex hormones. *Journal of Rheumatology* 59 (Supplement 2):108–18.

Straub, RH, K Lehle, H Herfarth, et al. 2002. Dehyrdroepiandrosterone in relation to other adrenal hormones during an acute inflammatory stressful disease state compared with chronic inflammatory diseases: role of interleukin-6 and tumour necrosis factor. *European Journal of Endocrinology* 146 (3):365–74.

Sun, TH, DB Heimark, T Nguygen, JL Nadler, and J Larner. 2002. Both myo-inositol to chiro-inositol epimerase activities and chiro-inositol to myo-inositol ratios are decreased in tissues of GK type 2 diabetic rats compared to Wistar controls. *Biochem Biophys Res Commun* 293 (3):1092–98.

Susic, D, J Varagic, and ED Fronlich. 2001. Isolated systolic hypertension in elderly WKY is reversed with L-arginine and ACE inhibition. *Hypertension* 38 (6):1422–26.

Suzuki, Y, O Ito, N Mukai, H Takahashi, and K Takamatsu. 2002. High level of skeletal muscle carnosine contributes to the latter half of exercise performance during 30-s maximal cycle ergometer sprinting. *Japanese Journal of Physiology* 52 (2):199–205.

Tabakman, R., P Lazarovici, and R Kohen. 2002. Neuroprotective effects of carnosine and homocarnosine on pheochromocytoma PC12 cells exposed to ischemia. *Journal of Neuroscience Research* 68 (4):463–69.

Taggart, HM. 2002. Effects of tai chi exercise on balance, functional mobility, and fear of falling among older women. *Applied Nursing Research* 15 (4):235–42.

Tanaka, T, Y Morishita, et al. 1994. Chemoprotection of mouse urinary bladder carcinogens by the naturally occurring carotenoid astaxanthine. *Carcinogenesis* 15:15–19.

Tatar, M, A Kopelman, D Epstein, et al. 2001. A mutant Drosophila insulin receptor homolog that extends life-span and impairs neuroendocrine function. *Science* 292:107–10.

Tatar, M, A Bartke, and A Antebi. 2003. The endocrine regulation of aging by insulin-like signals. *Science* 299 (5611):1346–51.

Teixeira, PJ, SB Going, LB Houtkooper, LL Metcalfe, RM Blew, HG Flint-Wagner, EC Cussler, LB Sardinha, and TG Lohman. 2003. Resistance training in postmenopausal women with and without hormone therapy. *Medical Science and Sports Exercise* 35 (4):555–62.

Theodoropoulos, C, C Demers, E Delvin, D Menard, and M Gascon-Barre. 2003. Calcitriol regulates the expression of the genes encoding the three key vitamin D3 hydroxylases and the drug-metabolizing enzyme CYP3A4 in the human fetal intestine. *Clinical Endocrinology* 58 (4):489–99.

Theusen, L, JOI Jorgensen, et al. 1994. Short- and long-term cardiovascular effects of growth hormone therapy in growth hormone deficient adults. *Clinical Endocrinology* 41:615–20.

Tissenbaum, HA, and G Ruvkun. 1998. An insulin-like signaling pathway affects both longevity and reproduction in Caenorhabditis elegans. *Genetics* 148 (2):703–17.

Toliver-Kinsky, T, and J Papaconstantinou. 1997. Age-associated alterations in hippocampal and basal forebrain nuclear factor kappa B activity. *Journal of Neuroscience Research* 48 (6):580–87.

Tolu, P, F Masi, B Leggio, S Scheggi, A Tagliamonte, M De Montis, and C Gambarana. 2002. Effects of long-term acetyl-L-carnitine administration in rats. I. Increased dopamine output in mesocorticolimbic areas and protection toward acute stress exposure. *Neuropsychopharmacology* 27 (3):410.

Tornstam, L. 1997. Gerotranscendence: the contemplative dimension of aging. *Journal of Aging Studies* 11 (2):143–54.

Tyner, SD, S Venkatachalam, et al. 2002. p53 mutant mice that display early ageing-associated phenotypes. *Nature* 415 (January):45–53.

Ullis, Karlis. 1999. *Age Right*. New York: Simon & Schuster.

Ulrich, P, and A Cerami. 2001. Protein glycation, diabetes, and aging. *Recent Programs in Hormone Research* 56:1–12.

Upritchard, JE, WH Sutherland, et al. 2000. Effect of supplementation with tomato juice, vitamin E, and vitamin C on LDL oxidation and products of inflammatory activity in type 2 diabetes. *Diabetes Care* 23 (6):733–38.

Van Cauter, E. 2000. Slow wave sleep and release of growth hormone. *Journal of the American Medical Association* 284 (21):2717–18.

Vaquero, MP. 2002. Magnesium and trace elements in the elderly: intake, status and recommendations. *Journal of Nutrition, Health, and Aging* 6 (2):147–53.

Verma, PS, BR Goldin, et al. 1998. The inhibition of the estrogenic effects of pesticides and environmental chemicals by curcumin and isoflavonoids. *Environmental Health Perspectives* 106 (12):807–12.

Vidal-Puig, A, and S O'Rahilly. 2001. Controlling the glucose factory. *Nature* 413:125–26.

Viig, Jan, and Martijn Dolle. 2001. Instability of the nuclear genome and the role of DNA repair. In *Handbook of the Biology of Aging*, edited by EJ Masoro and SN Austad. San Diego: Academic Press.

Vincent, KR, HK Vincent, RW Braith, V Bhatnagar, and DT Lowenthal. 2003. Strength training and hemodynamic responses to exercise. *American Journal of Geriatric Cardiology* 12 (2):97–106.

Visser, M, M Pahor, DR Taaffe, et al. 2002. Relationship of interleukin-6 and tumor necrosis factor-alpha with muscle mass and muscle strength in elderly men and women: the Health ABC Study. *Journal of Gerontology Series A: Biological Sciences and Medical Sciences* 57 (5):M326–32.

Vliet, Elizabeth Lee. 1995. *Screaming to Be Heard*. New York: M. Evans.

Volkow, ND, L Chang, and GJ Want. 2001. Low level of brain dopamine D2 receptors in methamphetamine abusers: association with metabolism in the orbitofrontal cortex. *American Journal of Psychiatry* 158 (12):2015–21.

Vucenik, I, T Kalebic, K Tantivejkul, and AM Shamsuddin. 1998. Novel anticancer function of inositol hexaphosphate: inhibition of human rhabdomyosarcoma in vitro and in vivo. *Anticancer Research* 18 (3A):1377–84.

Wadstrom, T, and LP Andersen. 1999. Treatment of H. pylori infected mice with antioxidant astaxanthine reduces gastric inflammation, bacterial load and modulates cytokine release by splenocytes. *Immunology Letters* 70:185–89.

Walford, Roy. 2000. *Beyond the 120 Year Diet: How to Double Your Vital Years*. New York: Four Walls Eight Windows.

Walia, M, CY Kwan, and AK Grover. 2003. Effects of free radicals on coronary artery. *Medical Principles and Practice* 12 (1):1–9.

Walker, RF, and BB Bercu. 2001. Issues regarding the routine and long-term use of growth hormone in anti-aging medicine. *Journal of Anti-Aging Medicine* 4 (4):279–300.

Walter, PB, MD Knutson, A Paler-Martinez, S Lee, Y Xu, FE Viteri, and BN Ames. 2002. Iron deficiency and iron excess damage mitochondria and mitochondrial DNA in rats. *Proceeds of the National Academy of Sciences USA* 99 (4):2264–69.

Wang, AM, C Ma, et al. 2000. Use of carnosine as a natural anti-senescence drug for human beings. *Biochemistry* 65 (7):869–71.

Wang, D, G Yang, B Li, Z Li, and Y Chen. 2002. Investigation of the chemico-physical characteristics of the active components in the Chinese herb Gastrodia elata Bl. by capillary zone electrophoresis. *Annals of Science* 18 (4):409–12.

Weil, Andrew. 1995. *Spontaneous Healing*. New York: Alfred A. Knopf.

Weinstein, BS, and D Ciszek. 2002. The reserve-capacity hypothesis: evolutionary origins and modern implications of the trade-off between tumor-suppression and tissue-repair. *Experimental Gerontology* 37:615–27.

Wideman, L, JY Weltman, ML Hartman, et al. 2002. Growth hormone release during acute and chronic aerobic and resistance exercise: recent findings. *Sports Medicine* 32 (15):987–1004.

Widner, B, F Leblhuber, and D Fuchs. 2002. Increased neopterin production and tryptophan degradation in advanced Parkinson's disease. *Journal of Neural Transmission* 109 (2):181–89.

Willcox, Bradley J, D Craig Willcox, and Makoto Suzuki. 2001. *The Okinawa Program: How the World's Longest-Lived People Achieve Everlasting Health, and How You Can Too*. New York: Random House.

Williams, George C. 1957. Pleiotropy, natural selection, and the evolution of senescence. *Evolution* 11:398–411.

Williams, JE. 2001. Review of antiviral and immunomodulating properties of plants of the Peruvian rainforest with a particular emphasis on una de gato and sangre de grado. *Alternative Medicine Review* 6 (6):567–79.

Willis, MS. 2002. The health economics of calcium and vitamin D3 for the prevention of osteoporotic hip fractures in Sweden. *International Journal of Technology Assessment in Health Care* 18 (4):791–807.

Willis, R, M Anthony, L Sun, et al. 1999. Clinical implications of the correlation between coenzyme Q10 and vitamin B6 status. *Biofactors* 9 (2-4):359–63.

Wilson, CJ, CE Finch, and HJ Cohen. 2002. Cytokines and cognition: the case for a head-to-toe inflammatory paradigm. *Journal of the American Geriatric Society* 50 (12):2041–56.

Wolkow, CA, KD Kimura, et al. 2000. Regulation of C. elegans life-span by insulin-like signaling in the nervous system. *Science* 290 (October 6):147–50.

Wright, Jonathan, and John Morgenthaler. 1997. *Natural Hormone Replacement*. Petaluma, California: Smart Publications.

Wright, Karen. 2002. Times of our lives. *Scientific American* (September):59–65.

Wu, Z, JV Smith, and V Paramasivam. 2002. Ginkgo biloba extract EGb 761 increases stress resistance and extends life span in caenoraibditis elegans. *Cellular and Molecular Biology* 48 (6):725–31.

Xavier, RM, Y Yamauchi, et al. 1995. Antinuclear antibodies in healthy aging people: a prospective study. *Mechanisms of Ageing and Development* 78 (2):145–54.

Xavier, RM, Y Yamuchi, M Nakamure, et al. 1995. Antinuclear antibodies in healthy aging people: a perspective study. *Mechanisms of Ageing and Development* 78 (2):145–54.

Yamauchi, K, NW Hales, SM Robinson, ML Niehoff, V Ramesh, NR Pellis, and AD Kulkarni. 2002. Dietary nucleotides prevent decrease in cellular immunity in ground-based microgravity analog. *Journal of Applied Physiology* 93 (1):161–66.

Yankner, Bruce A. 2000. A century of cognitive decline. *Nature* 404 (March 9):125.

Yataco, AR, J Busby-Whitehead, and DT Drinkwater. 1997. Relationship of body composition and cardiovascular fitness to lipoprotein lipid profiles in master athletes and sedentary men. *Aging* 9 (1–2):88–94.

Yilmaz, B, S Kutlu, et al. 2000. Melatonin inhibits testosterone secretion by acting at hypothalamo-pituitary-gonadal axis in the rat. *Neuroendocrinology Letters* 21:301–06.

Yin, JH, XY Zhou, and XQ Zhu. 1992. [Pharmacological and clinical studies on the processed products of radix Polygoni multiflori]. *Zhongguo Zhong Yao Za Zhi* 17 (12):722–4, 762–63.

Yoon, JC, P Pulgserver, G Chen, et al. 2001. Control of hepatic gluconeogenesis through the transcription coactivator PGC-1. *Nature* 413 (September 13):131–38.

Yu, BP. 1999. Approaches to anti-aging intervention: the promise and the uncertainties. *Mechanisms of Ageing and Development* 111 (2–3):73–87.

Zdrackovic, M, T Christiansen, et al. 2001. The pharmacokinetics, pharmacology, safety, and tolerability following 7 days daily oral treatment with NN703 in healthy male subjects. *Growth Hormone & IGF Research* 11:41–48.

Zeeh, J, and D Platt. 2002. The aging liver, structural and functional changes and their consequences for drug treatment in old age. *Gerontology* 48:121–27.

Zhang, B, et al. 1999. Discovery of a small-molecule insulin mimic with antidiabetic activity in mice. *Science* 284 (May 7):974.

Zhang, Z, PF Inserra, et al. 1997. Melatonin, immune modulation and aging. *Autoimmunity* 26 (1):43–53.

Zimmerman, JA, V Malloy, R Krajcik, et al. 2003. Nutritional control of aging. *Experimental Gerontology* 38:47–52.

Zimmet, Paul, KGMG Alberti, and Jonathan Shaw. 2001. Global and societal implications of the diabetes epidemic. *Nature* 414 (December 13):782–87.

Index